D1614026

A LIFE STORY AND A GUIDE TO BETTER LIVING

ROBERTO IBÁÑEZ ATKINSON

SHIT!
I've got cancer,
What should I do?

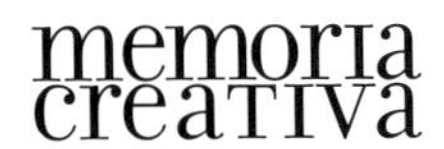

Concept, Overall Direction Roberto Ibáñez | Carolina Díaz

Texts Roberto Ibáñez | Carolina Díaz | Hernán Díaz | Lyuba Yez

Interviews Roberto Ibáñez | Carolina Díaz | Magdalena Donoso | Greta di Girolamo | Javiera Pérez | Macarena Rojas | Kristina Cordero | Sofía del Sante

Design Claudia Caviedes

Photography Jon Jacobsen | Rodrigo Basaure | Roberto Ibáñez Atkinson album

English Translation Belan Traducciones

Proof Reader Miriam Heard

Printed at Sheridan Books

Cover Photography Stuart Gibson www.stugibson.net

Back Cover Photography María Paz Calvo

Shit! I've got cancer, what should I do?

ISBN: 978-1-64007-049-3

Please review shitivegotcancer.com and share it on your social networks.

Table of contents

ACKNOWLEDGMENTS **6**

FOREWORD **8**

MY STORY: **16**

Who I am **20**

Kaboom! **34**

Forget the tie **56**

Touring hospitals through the U.S.A **68**

I'm going to live at 80% **86**

Cancer Mode ON **116**

The shadow on my lung **134**

Cancer Mode OFF **144**

The tower concept
(A new glance at life) **150**

■ What (the heck) is a melanoma **154**

■ You are what your eat **170**
(DON'T miss this chapter!)

■ Patient empowerment **192**

■ 100 Frequently Asked Questions about cancer
(with the simplest, foolproof, answers) **206**

■ 90+ people, 600+ tips **228**

■ Epilogue | Final words **470**

■ Table of contents by keyword **474**

Acknowledgements

To my mother, who has always been my strong emotional pillar and who especially embodied that role throughout this process.

To my father, who gave it his all; all his love and all his effort, and who did everything in his power to help me heal.

To my siblings, Tomás, Sebastián and Antonia, for their understanding, companionship, endless giving, generosity, and ability to understand me throughout this process.

To Pepe, my business partner, my pal, my life-long friend, just because he has ALWAYS been there. Terrific.

To the Ibáñez extended family, for their unwavering support and love throughout this process.

To María Paz Calvo –Pazita–, my wife, for loving me, understanding, for being there, and for being here in this new stage.

To Katie Schou and the Send It Foundation team, for having believed in this project since the first phone call.

To my sisters-in-law and my brother-in-law: Carolina Jara, Carolina Lavín, and Carlos Capurro, because they have been there for my family and for me throughout this process.

To Isabel Valdés, my dad´s assistant, because she was always present, helping me out in all sorts of errands and...because she is such a great listener!

To Brad Ludden and the First Descents team, for telling me on our first meeting that this could be done, that we could publish the book in the US.

To Sheridan Books, for making a special effort in the publishing of this book.

To Dawn Engle, Ivan, Elizabeth and the whole Peacejam team. None of this would be possible if it wasn't for you guys.

To Rosa Madera, who as a friend and on behalf of *Fundación Ibañez Atkinson* gave me her full support.

To Mario Valdivia, friend and a great mate during the entire first stage of my illness.

To Carolina Díaz, from *Memoria Creativa*, because she helped me write this book.

To María Teresa Sanfuentes, my psychologist, because she helped me understand my process and the growth an experience such as this brings with it.

To each of those we interviewed and their families. Without them, this book would not have seen the light.

A Stu Gibson (stugibson.net), for the cover photography of this book.

To doctors Gustavo Vial, Luis Fernando Coz, José Miguel Campero, and Benjamín Paz, because they were always ready and willing, since I was first diagnosed and up until today.

To Doctor Mercedes López, for helping me answer the questions I had when nobody was doing so.

To Francis Palisson, my friend, and dermatologist.

To Iván Mimica, chilean naturopath for being such a great guide, counsellor and good friend.

To Mark Mincolla, american naturopath resident in Boston, because he taught me to eat healthily.

To Sarah Hubbard, for seeing something nobody else saw, for her crucial help in the publishing of this book and for her kindness and generosity.

To doctor Mario Sandoval and the entire team at 110 Sport & Health Center, for helping me in the overall healing and recovery of my body over the past 3 years.

To Flavio Salazar and Diego Reyes, from *canceronline.cl,* for their help in the chapter on FAQ about Cancer.

To Trevor Zimmerman and Philip O´Connor, for being good friends, for their time spent in this project and for introducing me to the right people. Someday they will be able to say "Roberto" the way you should.

To doctor Jacoub, iris-therapist from Viña del Mar, who welcomed me into his office though he was not accepting new patients.

To the entire team of Touch, Taringa, *Celebraciones con Sentido*, Marsol, Stars, Sevilla and the team formed for this proyect who without hesitating have always given me their complete support.

To all my friends, who have followed my healing process step-by-step, LIKE the good news I post, and always have a loving gesture for me.

To all the book retailers where you can find this book, fot their help in getting it out there.

To Loreto Fuentes and Gonzalo Tagle, mother and husband of the woman who inspired me to write this book, because of their willingness, energy, and generosity in sharing with me their memories about Loreto Agurto, *Lolo*.

To all those who took the time to think about the best tips to share with others, those who, without knowing me, fully trusted this project.

To everyone who contributed to this book in one way or another. To all of you, I am truly thankful, and I have to say, without them, none of this would have been possible.

Foreword

I

I would have loved to have published this book right away after I got ill. A little over 6 years ago, I was diagnosed with a lethal form of cancer, a malignant melanoma. I immediately got lots of help. Help I am sure many others do not receive. And so, I decided to share it. A book seemed to be the best idea. I am an entrepreneur at heart and, since at the time a sense of immediacy prevailed in my every-day-life, I was just not willing to wait too long to see it published.

Luckily enough, writing a book takes time. And I say so because the first attempt was pure and utter anger. At myself. At those close to me. At the world at large. Nowadays, though, I understand it. How was I supposed not to feel angry? I was only 27 years old and, overnight, I was diagnosed with this terrifying disease.

Along with anger, which I now understand is necessary and only natural, and which, after all, helps one to survive, I felt much uncertainty. The mere fact of not knowing what would happen, and how things would sort themselves out, was at times petrifying. Now I know that it is just part of the process.

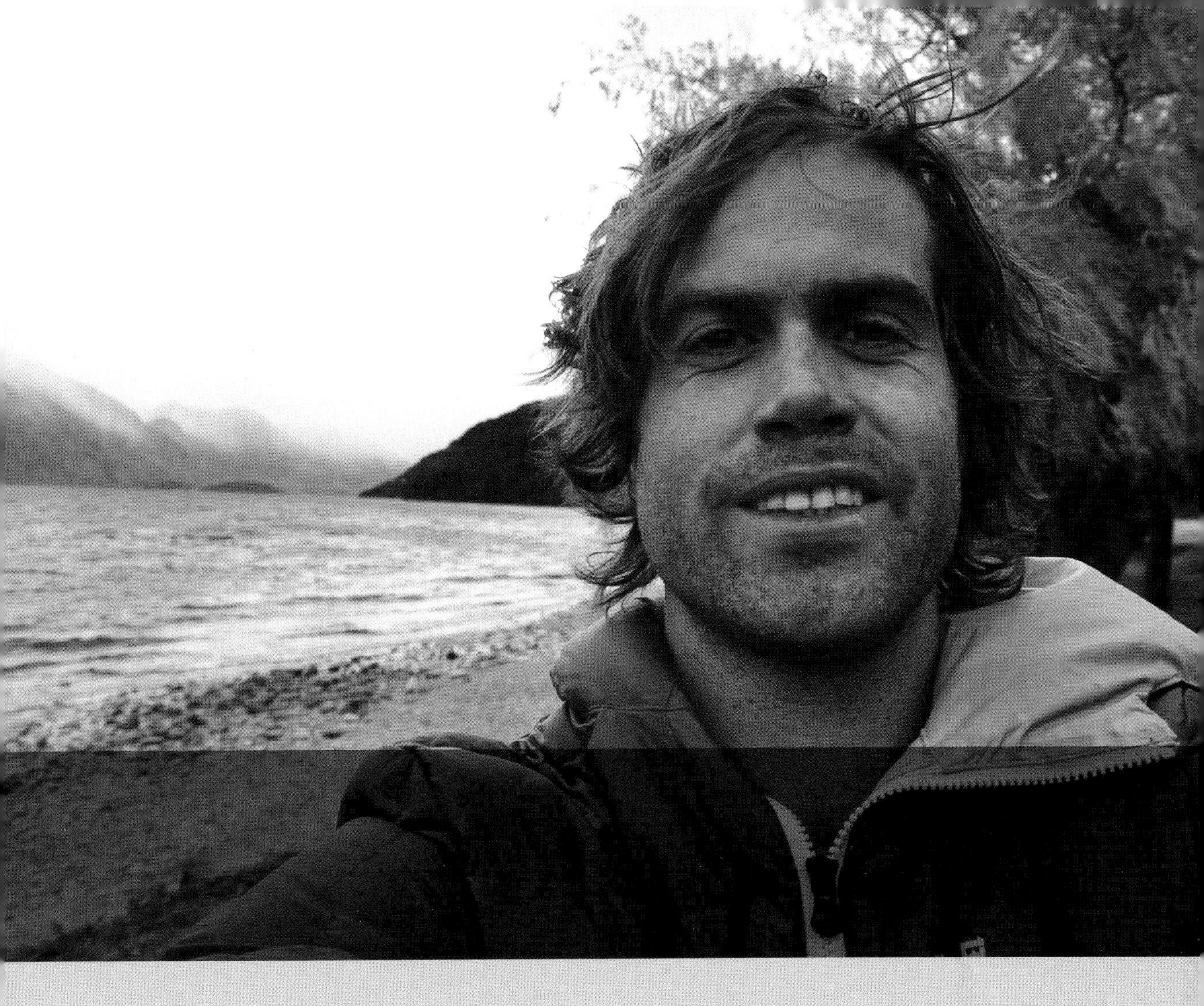

Time is wise. And, as you begin to understand what it is that you are angry about, you also understand its positives and negatives. In the end, you realize that certain things in life are simply beyond your control. And so, you continue to move forward, but this time with a lighter pace. With time comes understanding. You get it, so to speak. Anger evolves and turns into a force for good things...

About 2 years ago, I read everything I had written so far, and I knew I didn't want to leave a legacy of such angry feelings. My path had changed and I no longer identified with what seemed to be so real such a short while ago. I realized I wanted to write a book filled with hope and collaboration. So I re-wrote my story from a fresh perspective, led by the experience and knowledge the illness had brought to me, and with the peace of mind that resulted from things slowly coming back to normal. Plus, my medical exams showed that the changes I had made in my life were having positive repercussions on my health. I am now healthy –though, with this illness, you never really know–.

Of course, cancer is associated with death. Yet, when you manage to look beyond that, and you focus on the positive changes it brings about in your life, you end up cherishing this new stage. At least that is my case. I changed the way I looked at people around me, the way I acted, and also my perception of the world. I now try to look at everything through a positive prism. And even if it stemmed from cancer, I am grateful for that change.

This project has taken me 4 years, and I am happy it was so. After having announced its publication so many times, the book is finally ready and available. To all of you who were patient and generous enough to listen to my incessant chattering about this book, and who were enthusiastic in their support for this project: a BIG thank you.

I would also like to thank everyone who took part in it, those who gave the interviews, and those who contributed with their recollections, their perspective, and their experience and advice. I am certain they know this book comes to fill a gap, and that they would have liked to have had something like it at hand when their processes had just begun. That is why I organized it as a sort of travel guide: So that whoever needs it may find in it suggestions that make sense to them, that help them address some doubt, or make a decision. And that it empowers them when facing this illness, the mere mention of which inspires so much fear and uncertainty. I hope to have achieved that.

My second hope regarding this book is that, after reading it, those who have no relation whatsoever with cancer may be inspired to live the same journey of understanding that I went through. That without there being need for a diagnosis, and without the occurrence of some disaster, they may end up making a positive change in their lives. Maybe it's a lot to ask, but I truly hope to achieve that, too.

One more thing. I am not a writer, nor am I a journalist, and writing this book has been crazy. I have had help, of course. Since I had cancer I am absolutely open to receiving help from wherever it comes. Luckily, I've had the tireless participation of my family, and time has allowed for my feelings to sink in; I have thus better grounded my opinions. Yet, you will find that at times I am somewhat rash and rebellious. It's part of who I am. Having said this, I tried at all times not to hurt anybody, because nobody deserves it. But, I do give my opinion as regards the systems, phases, and *m.o.* I had to endure.

In June 2011, a month after I underwent surgery and my melanoma was removed, there was also this spark that ignited in me the need to convey knowledge and help others. My mother wanted me to meet this woman who, 3 years before, had had a metastatic melanoma similar to mine, and who was by then perfectly healthy. At the time, I did not want anything to do with other patients, let alone with their experiences or teachings. Plus, my mother had by then taken me to countless healers and shamans... even to a lady who lived with 20 cats in her house! Who would have thought back then that I would end up writing a book on precisely the experiences, testimonies, and teachings of others...

By mid-July 2011, I noticed an abnormal growth on my chest. It looked as though I was actually growing a man-breast! So, I made an appointment with my oncologist, and he explained there was a 99% chance of that abnormal breast growth being the result of lymphatic fluid in my arm seeking newer drainage paths after my lymph nodes had been removed. Even so, and just to be clear on that remaining 1%, he sent me to get a mammogram. A mammogram! Oh my! I just couldn't believe it. Where would this cancer stop? I now had to place my chest on a machine that squashes breasts to check whether or not I had a metastatic tumor in that area!

I didn't go right away. Ok, let's be honest. I just didn't fancy it. Plus, the doctor's words had calmed me down. I would get that mammogram, but only once I felt like it. Truth be told, after so many procedures, surgeries, and hospital stays, I was in no mood for another test. Still, I left the doctor's written orders in sight, in my car's cup holder, as some sort of merciless reminder. Two weeks later, my 'boob' was still the same size. Since the hospital was halfway between home and my office, one day I decided to go in there and get an appointment. To my surprise, someone had just cancelled their appointment, so they scheduled me for 20 minutes later. I felt embarrassed. I was the only man sitting in that waiting room. But I quickly got over it. Around me, each of the women waiting for that mammogram was focused solely on the news she might receive. I doubt any of them even noticed me. Just to kill time, I started reading some brochures on breast cancer and early detection.

When I walked into the examination room, a nurse requested that I undress from the waist up and then get into one of those robes that barely cover you. Then, I saw the machine that detects tumors in breasts; it looked like a huge sandwich grill. They had some trouble doing the tests on me. It is hard to place a man's breast on these machines, because there's not enough body mass to deal with. When I asked the nurse if she saw anything out of the normal, she smiled and said no, but then added I had to wait for the assessment from a radiologist.

Anyways, I went back to the waiting room, and as I was nearing the exit, a woman in her thirties approached me. She was a vibrant and beautiful brunette. She stopped me and said: 'Hey, you are Roberto Ibáñez, aren't you?' 'Yes, I am', I said, still in utter disbelief at someone recognizing me as I walked out of a mammogram, of all things. She went on: "I'm Loreto Agurto, your mother's friend whom you didn't want to meet. Sorry to stop you like this, but I saw your picture in a magazine last week, and I recognized you. I HAD to say hello'. I looked at her while in my mind I wondered what were the odds of my meeting someone in such a place and situation. I had no choice but to accept that something very magical was happening. So I gave myself that space to talk to her.

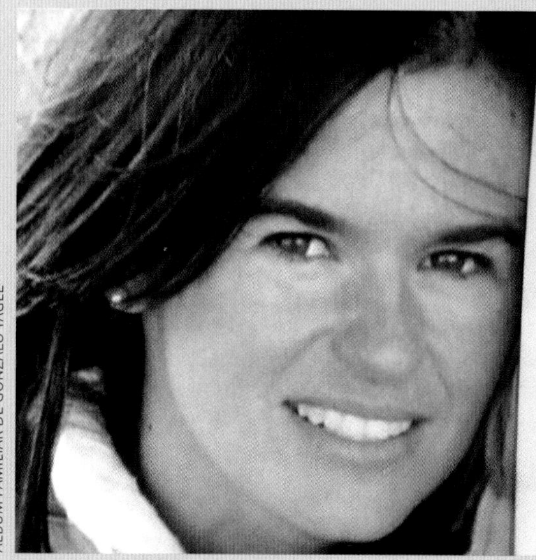

ALBUM FAMILIAR DE GONZALO TAGLE

LORETO AGURTO, THE WOMAN THAT INSPIRED ME AFTER HAVING ACCIDENTALLY MET HER

She quickly told me about her experience, and said she was aware of my case. While she talked, she smiled at me in a way that conveyed warm-heartedness and a loving nature.

I smiled back at her for the first time, while in my mind I thought: 'Man! This is someone that went through the same that I went through. And yet, she looks happy!'

Anyway, we agreed to meet that same week for lunch, and some days later, on August 5, we met at a Peruvian restaurant near my office.

Between *ceviche* and *pisco sours*, I asked her to tell me, from her point of view, what was the biggest thing cancer had taught her, what had been the most radical change she had experienced. Without a single hesitation, as though she was speaking with her heart, and not only with her voice, she said: 'Roberto, thanks to cancer, my husband and I understood how essential it is to live day-to-day and being happy with the person next to you. I realized life is a present, and that that is the way to face it. That is why I wake up every morning and try to do what I want to do, not what I have to. And, above all, I learned to set aside both ego and lies. Ego kills relationships, especially in the case of couples. *I will not yield until he does; it was his fault; I'm going to play angry; I will not let him know how I feel...* All those arguments over petty things stem from ego and lies. Once you set that aside, quarrels disappear, and you only pay attention to the things that really matter. And those, you talk and analyze together. The rest of the time, you make sure you spend it just enjoying being together".

She captivated me, I was, seduced by the charisma in her words. I could not believe it was that simple. Yet, at the same time, I knew because of my own experience that putting it in practice was not easy. How many times had I acted starting from my ego in relationships? Not only with my girlfriends. With my siblings, my parents, my friends, my workmates... I had done it a thousand times, and I kept on doing it. Ego and lies are the tools to protect ourselves, to put up a shield, so as not to be exposed and, hence, be hurt. Presenting oneself honestly, just the way one is, expressing feelings and emotions, can backfire, and even hurt if the person across from you does not think like you.

That is exactly what I told Loreto: 'Hey! But that way it's easy to end up being hurt.' She replied with that dazzling simplicity of hers: 'True, but that way you'll really find out who is next to you and whether or not it's worth it. That way you'll find your true friends, your true soul mate, and the interactions with your family will become simpler. For a while there, it won't be pleasant, but in the long run –mark my words– you will feel a better person, and you'll be much, much, happier'.

Lunch went on. We talked about other things. We laughed. She conveyed that good vibe of hers. And then, we said good-bye. But her words kept coming back to my mind, and also the way in which I had faced most relationships in my life. I kept on thinking about it. I understood that I also had to make some radical changes. If I tackled things the way Loreto was showing me, I would, for the first time in my life, be truly ME, and not the person one sometimes pretends to, or wants to, be in order to protect oneself.

A couple of days later, and as a result of all of this, I wrote a text and felt like sharing it. So I sent it to a couple of newspapers and magazines for them to publish; but the editors replied that it was far too sentimental. They were just not interested. Which is when my entrepreneurial side kicked in and said: "If they don't want to listen, I'll do it myself." And that is how this project was born, with the great advice Loreto gave me.

Today I know this book is a legacy that began with a magical encounter at a radiology center of a hospital. It is the sheer proof of the existence of the love and dedication of a survivor who shares with another one still in need. Loreto is not with us anymore, but her spirit lives on and accompanies us. I am tremendously thankful to her for having shown me life's simplicity. I hope I will be able to live that legacy to the letter.

Loreto, this book has been written in your loving memory. I promise I will do my best to live the way you taught me to, and that I will strive to convey your message of change.

Before I finish this prologue, I would like to humbly ask you –the readers– to please read the whole section entitled *My Story* and all its chapters before you decide to shape your opinion on anything or anyone. This has been quite the process, both for me and for those around me. The book includes an explanation not only of the personal changes I've gone through over the past 4 years, but also those of the people close to me. We have all changed and this book is also about making changes in our lives in the name of prevention. That is the main weapon against cancer. That is why I wrote a whole chapter on diet and nutrition, and on the direct impact the latter has on health and the body's wellbeing. That is also why one of my goals is to create awareness in all of us about the importance of wearing sunscreen and protective clothing while outside. There are very simple measures that go a long way. Teaching very young children, at the pre-school stage, to wear a hat during break-time in order to protect themselves from the sun during the hours of highest radiation, or having a sunscreen dispenser available to school children for P.E. I remember that when I began to write this book, I started to imagine that there should be huge billboards in the streets of Santiago and elsewhere in the country, with renowned athletes asserting something along the lines of "I protect myself from the sun." I'd seen this during a trip to Australia, and I guess many of them could be replicated in Chile in order to safeguard and protect the population. I imagine such matters can be regulated. My proposal is for us all to make this come true.
Another aim of this book is to collaborate. That is why there are over 90 individuals who share their stories and tips in this book. I invite all of you who would have loved to share, but couldn't, to share your story at **www.shitivegotcancer.com**

Welcome to this story!

Roberto.
Santiago, November 2015.

my story

Before we begin...

Once you begin reading, you'll realize that there are some things I really go on about, over several chapters. So I'll be upfront: this was a choice I made when I started writing.

And just to be clear: This is not a linear book, so to speak. It is a book that starts with my story and then goes on to delve into various issues that surround cancer. This perhaps unorthodox structure includes chapters that are very important to me. For instance, they deal with new and healthy eating habits, or with direct and specific answers to the most frequently asked questions when it comes to cancer.

I planned the book in this way so that each chapter could be read in independently. The aim is for the reader to be able to pick up and begin reading on any page. I wanted every chapter to have both information and data, as well as some phrase or sentence that would chime with the reader and have an impact on them. Hence the repetition. They're things I don't want readers to miss.

This book shows my life just the way it is. I didn't want to hide anything. I come from a privileged background. My family has the ability and the means to look for many, if not all, the answers. So in this book I talk about my trips to the best hospitals in the U.S., and about everything I learned, in hopes that it reaches those who do not have such privileges.

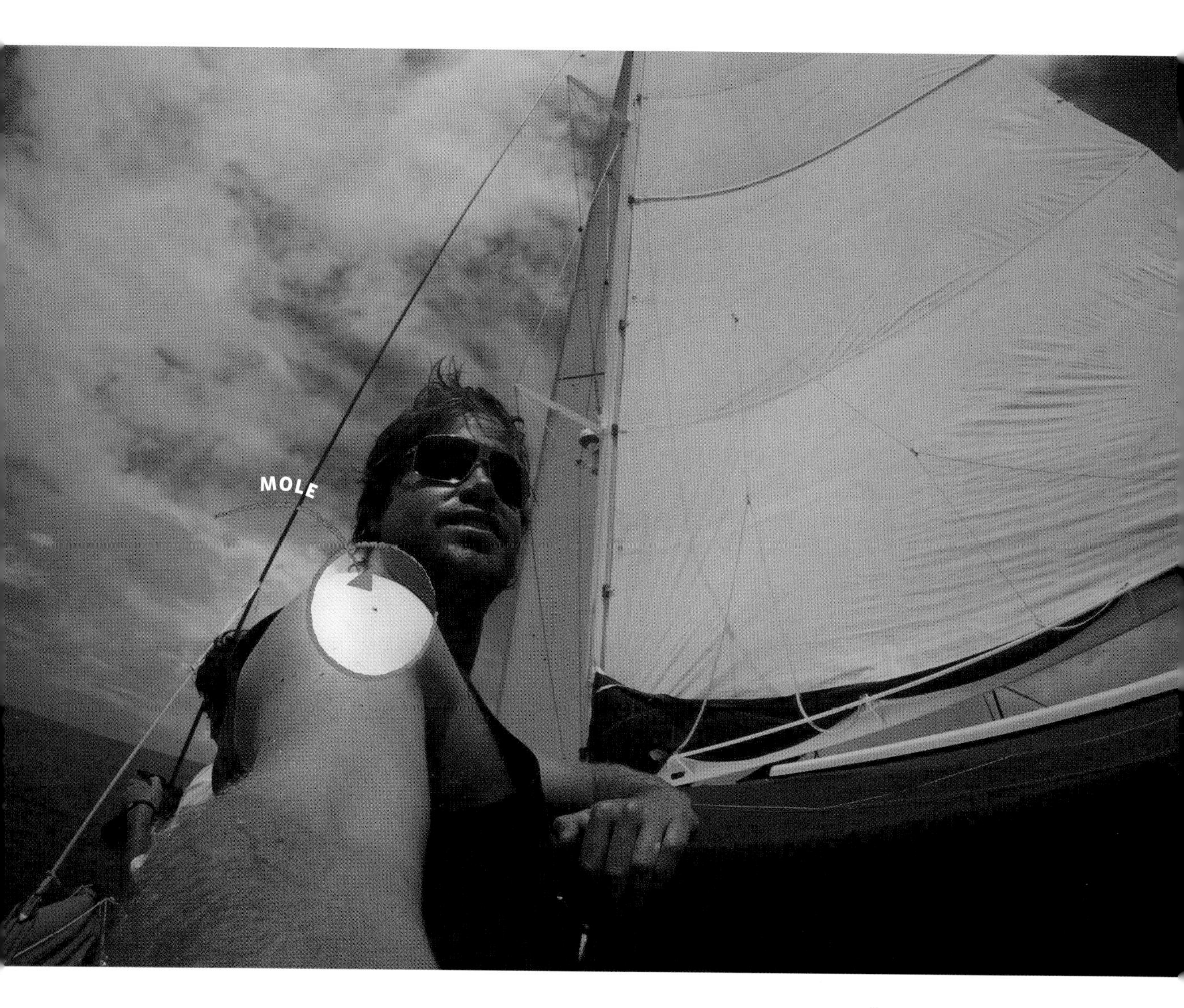

One of the few pictures I have in which the mole that triggered all of this may be seen.

Ground zero

Wednesday April 27, 2011.

Lunch; at my parents' place. 1:30 p.m.

–Hello, Roberto, how are you?

–Hey doctor! Not bad...

–Roberto, are you on your own?

–No, but hang on, 2 secs.... Ok, now I am. Tell me.

–I've got the results of your biopsy. Could you come over to the hospital so that we could talk?

–Doc, please, tell me now, over the phone. What's up?

–Roberto, the results of the biopsy show you have a malignant skin melanoma 1.5 mm thick.

– Malignant melanoma? What do you mean? What is that?

–I'd rather you came to my office so that we can talk.

–No, really, I would much rather you explained it to me right away, on the phone.

–It is a type of skin cancer.

–Ooook, aaaand? Is it dangerous?

–Please, Roberto, will you come to my office?

– Is it or isn't it dangerous?

–Yes. It is a cancer that, depending on its progress status, can be lethal.

Shit! I've got cancer... What should I do?

1. Introduction

Who I am

Unforgettable childhood memories. Unconditional family love. Experiences that have taught me to listen. To others and to myself... I have learned quite a bit over these 32 years of being Roberto Ibáñez-Atkinson.

I am the son of Heather Atkinson, a very caring and spiritual Scottish woman, and of Felipe Ibáñez, a renowned business man. My father's family created a huge company, D&S (now Walmart Chile), in which my father worked hard, over long hours, and the fruits of which have enabled us to enjoy a good life amidst an environment of hard work and responsibility. Given this background, some could be tempted to believe I am a privileged person for whom things have been easy.

In truth, my family is comprised of a big-hearted Dad who is a self-demanding businessman and who is, above all, passionate about everything he does. And of a sensitive and generous mother. I've got 3 siblings: Tomás, Sebastián, and Antonia. I am the third child. We are a family like many out there: happy, complicated, full of conflicts at times, thankful, sometimes silent, connected or disconnected depending on how things are going.

Every family has its issues, and mine is no exception. We grew up doing everything together: Sunday lunches in the dining room, supper in the kitchen every evening, spending our holidays down South fishing. I am happy to nowadays be able to say that my parents gave us a framework of simplicity and family values that we learned to cherish.

My father always taught my siblings and I that we had to earn everything through hard work. That we should strive to get things. During the summer holidays he encouraged us to work at the supermarkets. That's how I learned how to wrap a present, pack the purchased goods, stack shelves with merchandise, and knead at the bakery. It took me many summers in a row to

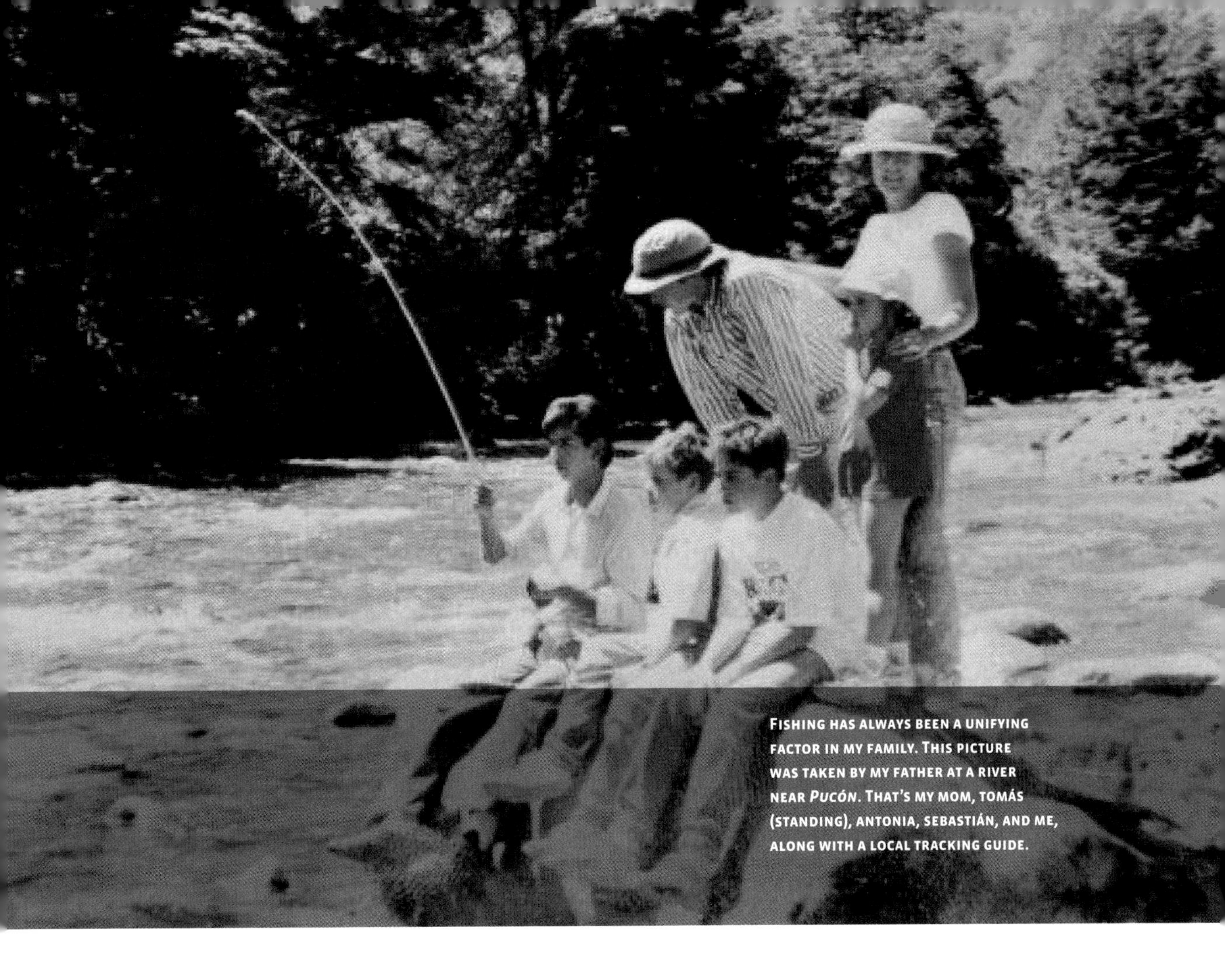

FISHING HAS ALWAYS BEEN A UNIFYING FACTOR IN MY FAMILY. THIS PICTURE WAS TAKEN BY MY FATHER AT A RIVER NEAR *PUCÓN*. THAT'S MY MOM, TOMÁS (STANDING), ANTONIA, SEBASTIÁN, AND ME, ALONG WITH A LOCAL TRACKING GUIDE.

gather a sizable experience in humility. But during that time, I discovered how exciting it is to earn your own money and, for example, use it to buy Christmas presents for your family.

That was the way it was until each of us turned 18 and entered university. Then my father would encourage us to work on one of the Boards of Directors of one of his companies. The invitation was crystal clear: "You work as the secretary, and you can earn your allowance."

I have great childhood memories of our holidays at the *Tunquelén* cabins, down South, right on the shores of Lake *Villarrica*, in *Pucón*. The 6 of us would travel there and spend a lot of time together. My Mom would make sure that things were simple and fun. Sometimes my grandfather would fly over from Scotland (to tell us his extraordinary stories of his time as a prisoner of war), and my father would fully disconnect from work. We would go out fishing, to the bakery *Pastelería Suiza,* and to buy ice-cream at *Pucono* ice-cream parlor.

We used to love being by the lake. Those are years I recall as a gift.

We later began going to our own house, cozy and family-focused. All of us siblings slept in one room, we used to talk a lot, and we would laugh and clown around. The usual. Yet, unlike the cabins, this house was far from the lake, and that sort of changed things for me. I felt as though I had lost something. The move coincided with that vulnerable stage in life which is adolescence...and so, I lived through those changes with the longing that is so typical of that transition from childhood to young adulthood.

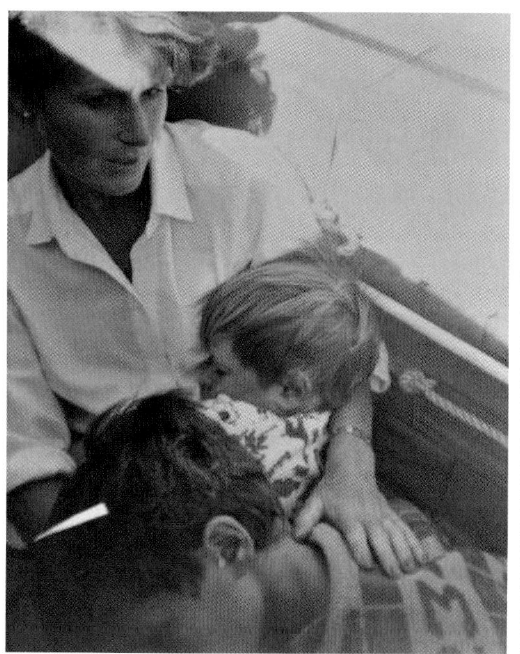

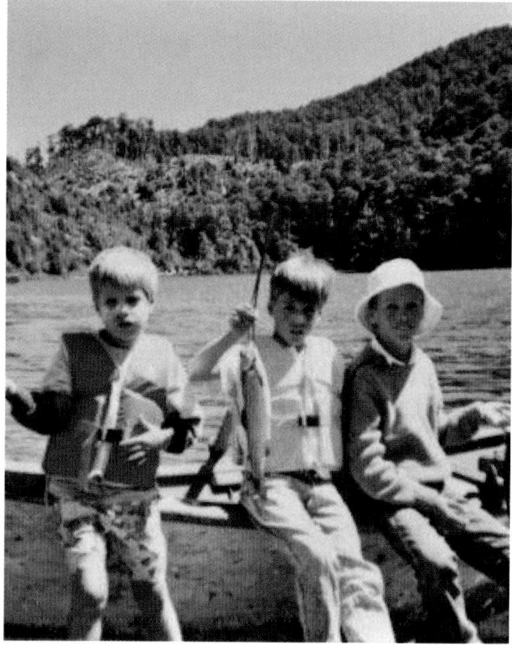

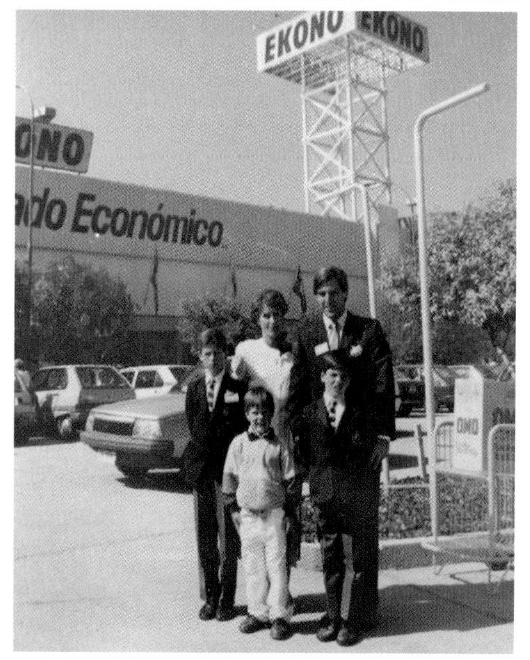

My parents gave us an environment of simplicity and family throughout our childhood. They always taught us that we had to earn things through hard work; that we had to strive to succeed

According to family and friends, I was a sensitive kind of boy, the sort that can get "stuck" in a particular emotional state and find it hard to move on. That is why I lived everything passionately. "Intense," says my sister. "With this tendency to see the glass half-empty," says my mother. They might have been right. Now that I am looking at things anew, from a sort of overview if you will, I am positive that that sensitivity has always been with me.

Maybe I just didn't know how to channel it. I say so because, since my adolescence, and for quite a while there, anger was embedded in my life. I would hear my father talking about work, I would screw up out of immaturity, I would pick fights with my siblings, and I felt an anger that, in time, turned into sadness.

I ended up seeing a therapist (who hasn't, right?) to help me sort out my very scattered feelings. During my 32 years, I have known depression, emptiness, and emotional loneliness. I now take all of this as a huge learning experience that allows me to be grateful for life's positive stages, and to feel for the suffering of others.

Since I was a little boy, my body has always expressed itself on its own. I would externalize everything and anything as some illness or other. And strange things would happen to me, such as some very odd anxiety attacks. They were like adrenalin boosts that would come out of nowhere and would make me feel as though everything was speeding up far too fast for my liking, like when you press FF in a movie.

Each episode would last about 20 minutes. Everything running Fast Forward. It seemed as though it would never stop. They still sometimes happen to me. And they are far from fun, I can tell you...

I was also one of those unfortunate children that are prone to falling ill. So much so that my siblings claim I am a hypochondriac. I came down with tonsillitis at least 4 times a year.

* My family is comprised of a big-hearted businessman of a Dad, and a very caring and spiritual Scottish mother.

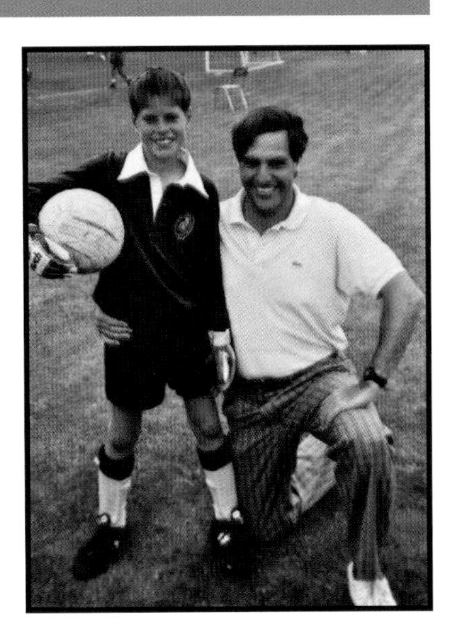

MY FATHER AND I ON A SATURDAY, FOR A SOCCER MATCH AT SCHOOL

In fact, before I found out I had cancer, I had had chronic diarrhea for 3 years. I had had endoscopies, colonoscopies, and every kind of test imaginable, but it just didn't get any better. Feeling bloated was a total nightmare, stomach aches all the time, having to run to the toilet regardless of where I was and at any given time. I suffered from acid reflux, my mouth would get sores all over. My defenses were low and, besides going to the doctor "of the month" and listening to very vague diagnoses, I didn't do much more. What else could I do? Doctors kept saying it wasn't serious, and so I kept overlooking all my ailments. But it bothered me. I hated it! Feeling like that had me tuckered out. I now know that I was prone to illnesses because I was eating incorrectly, and that I was allergic to several foods. Definitely, my body was talking to me, and had been doing so for quite a while, but I learned that later... much later.

Even so, I was always good at sports: I played rugby and tennis at school. I also skied in the winter, and used to ride my bicycle a lot. Surfing I discovered not so long ago. My real passion is kite surfing. It's a sport I came across while on exchange in Australia, back in 2005. I went there for 6 months, because I wanted to have a good time. My parents helped me fund the trip; it was the first time I ever went on my own somewhere for such a long time. I was 21 years old, and was going to the university. Once there, I stayed at a place I rented along with 5 other Chileans who became a sort of family: We were together every day, and travelled together.

That's what I was doing when I walked into a café one day and saw a poster pinned up on the wall. It read *Don't be shy, learn to fly,* and it had a picture of a guy kite surfing. I was curious, so I signed up for lessons. I gave it my all –at first it's not easy, getting the hang of it is slow and so, –I got a bit frustrated–, but I loved it. In any case, it's a sport in which you can quickly progress. You are always gaining experience; first you practice in lagoons and reservoirs, and then, when you go out to sea, it's a thousand times better, because it's not monotonous any more. I fell in love with this sport. I was fascinated by the adrenaline, by the beach, the waves, and that unique sense of being disconnected that surfaces only when it's you and your kite in the middle of the sea. It's an ever-changing relationship, because the sea is constantly changing, it's never the same.

> * My defenses had dropped and, besides going to the doctor "of the month" and listening to some vague diagnoses, I didn't do much more.

That trip back in 2005 was one of the first big experiences of my life, a break in the routine I had as a 20-something guy. At the time, I didn't spend much time thinking about what was going on, nor what was to come. I had no pre-conceived plan, I did what I felt like doing. I was doing my own thing, meeting people, and practicing kite surfing. This sport has since become central to my life, just like everything else that matters: family, friends, my job, and my pups (that I adore.) When something is as valuable to you, you make space

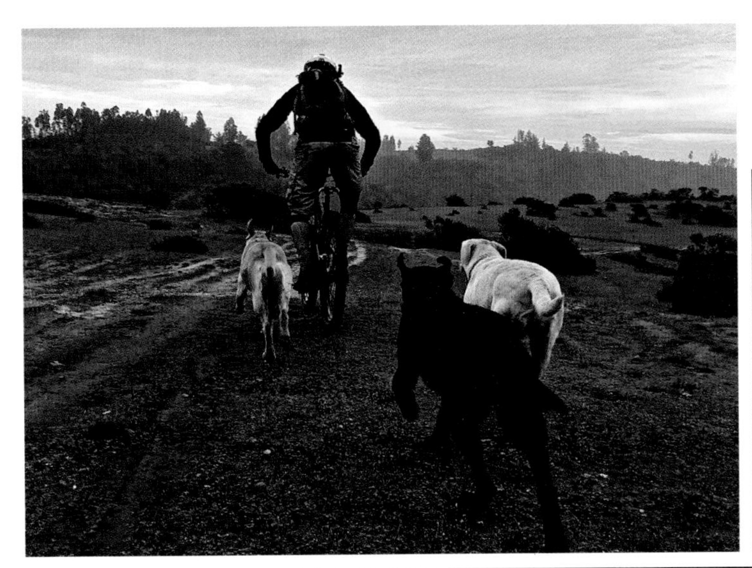

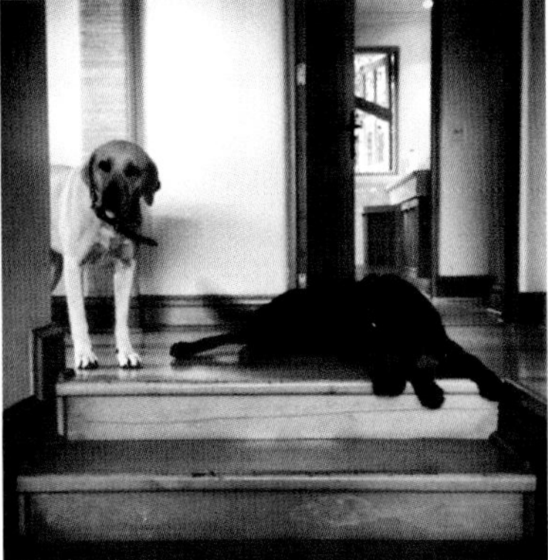

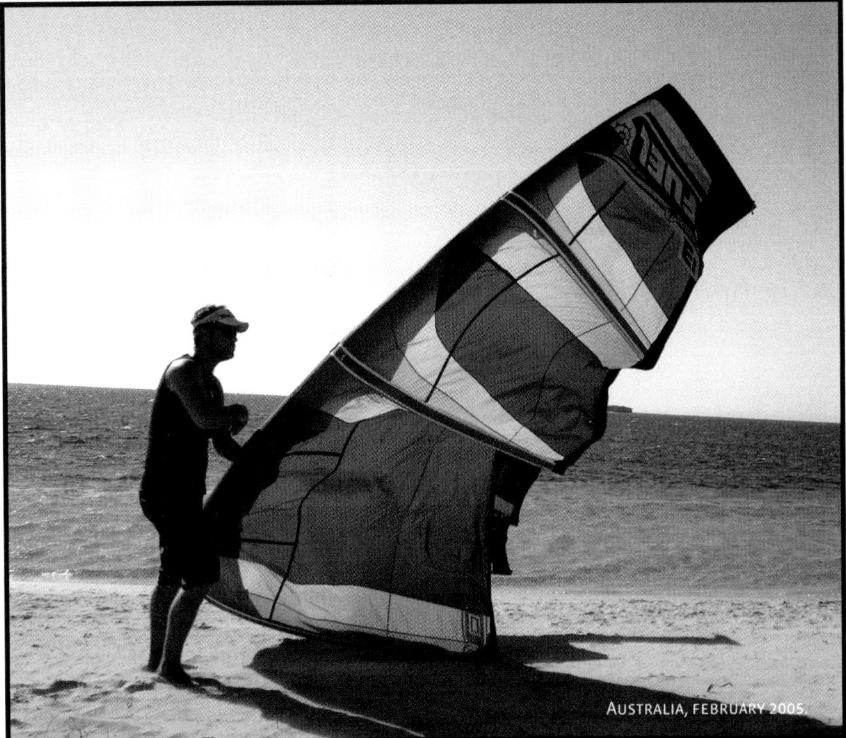

AUSTRALIA, FEBRUARY 2005.

SPORTS, NATURE, AND MY PUPS ARE KEY IN MY LIFE.

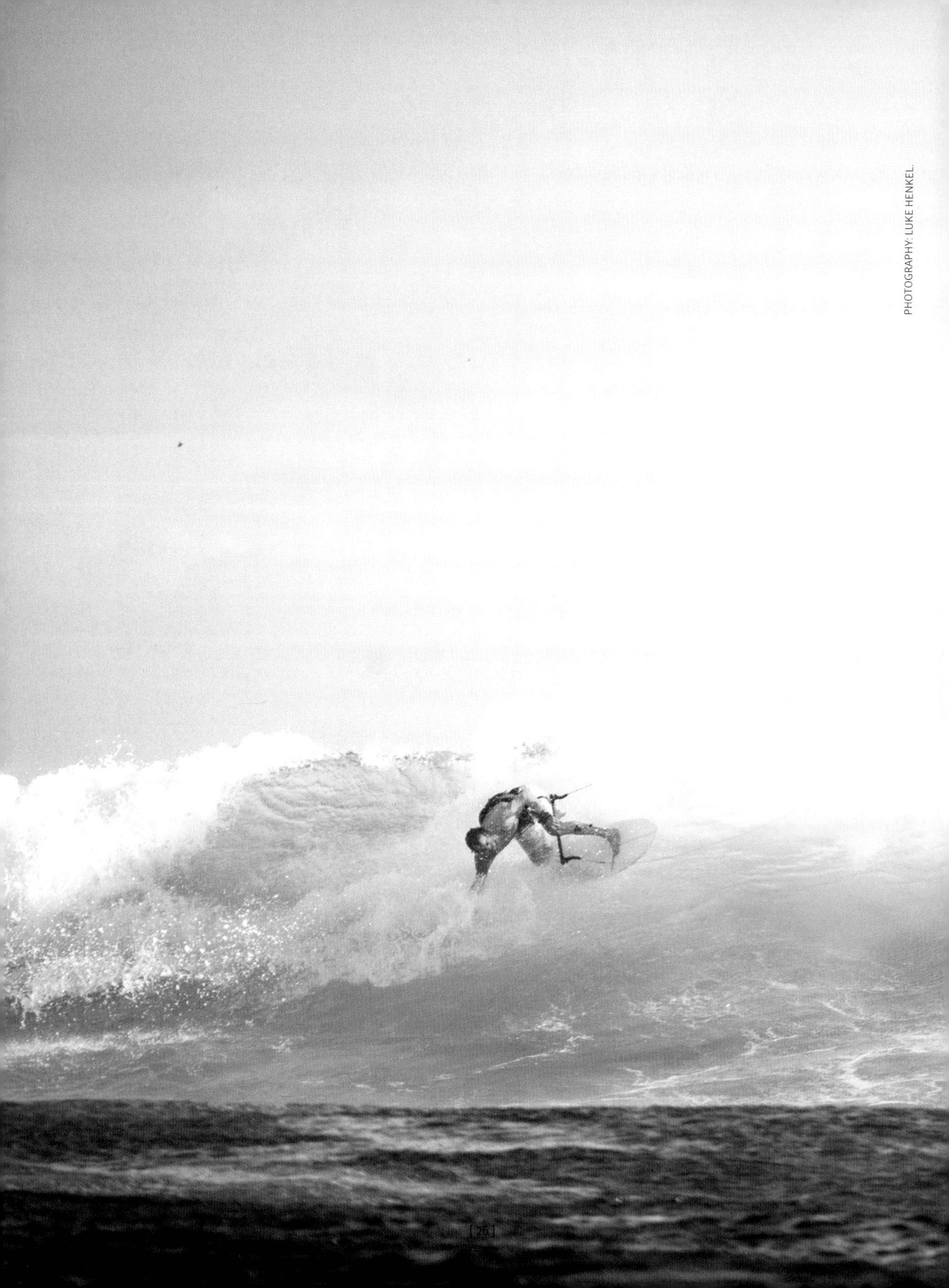

PHOTOGRAPHY: LUKE HENKEL.

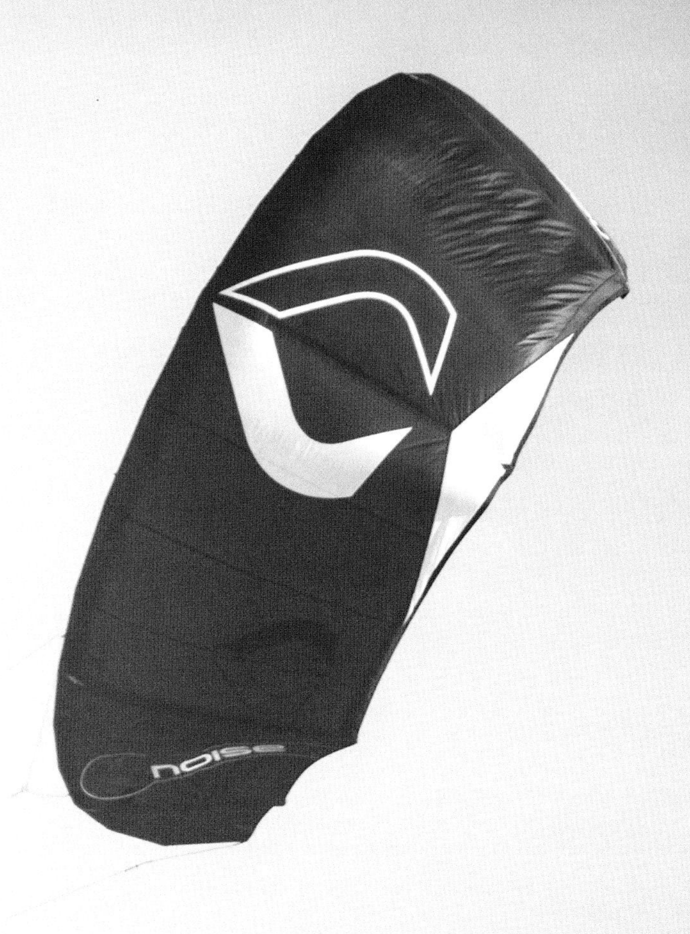

kite surf

In 2005, I fell in love with this sport. I loved its adrenaline, the beach, the waves, and that unique sense of being disconnected that embraces you while at sea. It has taken me to incredible new places. This pic was taken in Fiji, back in 2013.

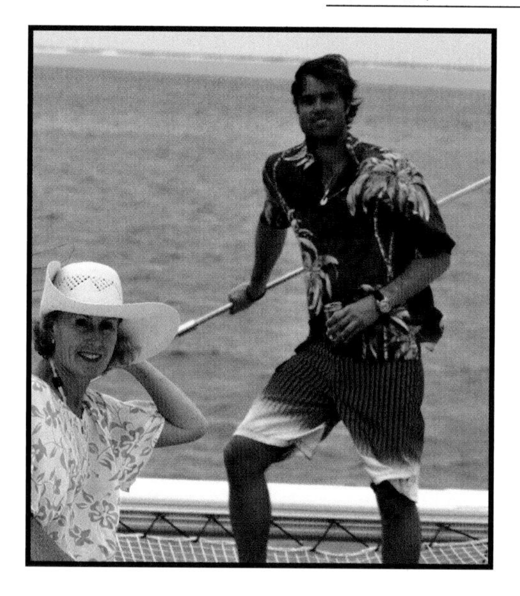

MY MOM TAUGHT ME THE MEANING OF THE WORD *BUSINESS* IN SPANISH [NEGOCIO]. IT COMES FROM THE LATIN TERMS: *NEC* AND *OCIUM*, WHICH TOGETHER MEAN "NO IDLENESS", AND ONE CANNOT COME WITHOUT THE OTHER. HERE WE ARE BOTH ENJOYING AN IDLE MOMENT

for it in your life. So, although I'm obsessive with work, I set time aside for this sport.

There's this comment my Mom made when my life was always busy, running from one meeting to the next, thinking only about work and the next project. I hadn't had breakfast, and was about to leave for work. I was late, of course. And then, Mom, who studied Latin, stopped me and asked me: '***Roberto, do you know where the [Spanish] term for business [negocio] comes from? From Latin. It's nec and ocium, and together they mean [no idleness]. To generate new businesses, you need idle moments that will allow you to come up with good ideas. Relax and keep calm, and then find new ways of being productive. That's where business comes from***'. Who would have thought that after my cancer her words would come true?

I have worked non-stop since I was 20. I threw myself into the rat race at a very young age, and on purpose. It was my choice, and I did it because I wanted to make a difference at home. Instead of choosing to work in the family business, or in any company in which my Dad had influence, I chose to find out what I was able to do in the business world.

Having a brilliant, renowned, and assertive man for a father is a challenge. When I was little, I was nicknamed *Tábano* [Horsefly], because I've always tried to do things my way, and I can be a real nuisance if I have to be, until I achieve my goal. And so, from the very moment I entered university, my goal was to be independent. To build my own business; and to do everything possible for that business to flourish as a result of my effort and hard work. Just like my Dad, obviously. In fact, building a company from scratch would be one of the ways in which I sought to get closer to him; not through every-day chat about work, but rather through common interests.

In 2004, when we were 20, my friend José Masihy –Pepe– and I created *Touch*, an events production company that evolved into sales and marketing, and that started with a capital of less than US$1,000 and a lot of optimism and hard work. In time, *Touch* took off and is now a company with a valuable team of over 50 employees, which gives work to over 1,000 youngsters every weekend. After all these years, we feel that we've built a good business and that we have done well. We aren't playing at being businessmen, we are businessmen.

Pepe and I know each other very well. We love each other, we trust each other, we complement each other. We are truly friends. Workmates, but also pals in life. In this cancer story, Pepe ended up playing a very relevant role, always letting me lean on him, always there for me, as though he were part of my own family. I guess that is because he really is.

With *Touch*, we discovered professional satisfaction and acknowledgement. We became entrepreneurs. Several media outlets interviewed us, and our client base grew. So much so, that we ended up getting large-scale companies as part of that client base.

But it wasn't easy at first. We had the ideas and the stamina, but nobody seemed to believe in us. Pepe and I know how hard it was to launch this company. We were just a couple of kids, so at first very few people were willing to take a bet on us and on *Touch*. At the beginning of that first summer, when we were just creating the company, without any clients, after having made a few contacts that hadn't gone anywhere, we suddenly got a call from *Watt's*.

Pepe had done his first internship as business administrator in that company. They wanted him to negotiate a motocross event for them in the seaside city of *La Serena*. Pepe did it really well, and so next thing we knew he was being told:

–You need to create a summer team for the Motocross event, and hand out 2,000 *Ice Fruts* daily. And they'd better be ice-cold!

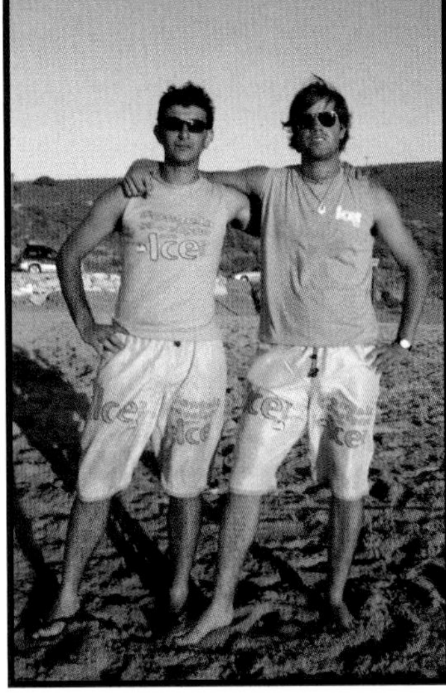

MY FIRST COMPANY: TOGETHER WITH PEPE MASIHY, MY BEST FRIEND AND BUSINESS PARTNER, WITH THE TEAM WE CREATED IN *TOUCH* FOR *LA SERENA*, IN THE SUMMER OF 2005. THE COLD CART WAS THE SPRINGBOARD TO OUR SUCCESS.

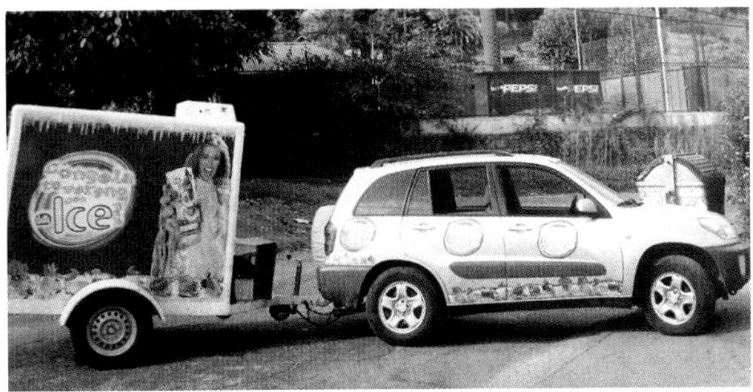

It was January, and we had 20 days to make it all happen. We designed a cooling cart to keep the drinks ice-cold, and that was our differentiating element. Pepe sent *Watt's* the budget, and they approved it. We got a summer team together by turning to friends from our Business School at Adolfo Ibáñez, where Pepe and I studied, and from other universities. And we jumped in!

At the beginning my Dad disliked the idea of *Touch*. I guess he thought of us as just 2 college guys looking to hit on the models that worked at the events we were organising, rather than 2 guys with serious goals (and he wasn't that far from the truth, to be honest).

WITH MY BUSINESS PARTNERS FOR *TARINGA*, VERY PROUD OF OUR FIT, IN A PICTURE THAT APPEARED IN THE CHILEAN ISSUE OF *¡HOLA!* MAGAZINE.

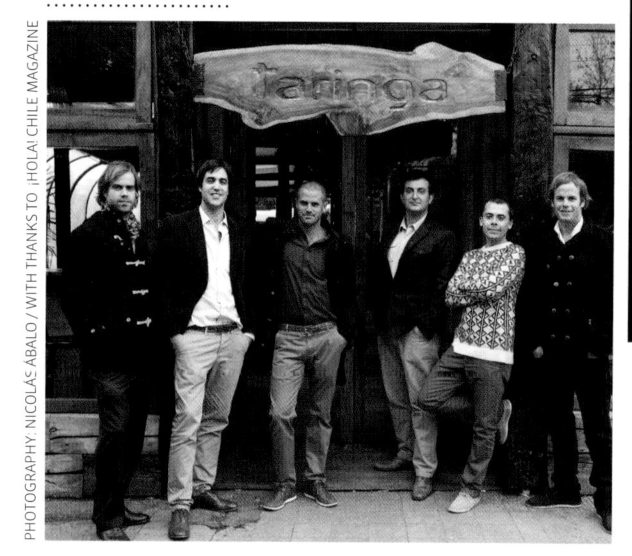

PHOTOGRAPHY: NICOLÁS ÁBALO / WITH THANKS TO ¡HOLA! CHILE MAGAZINE

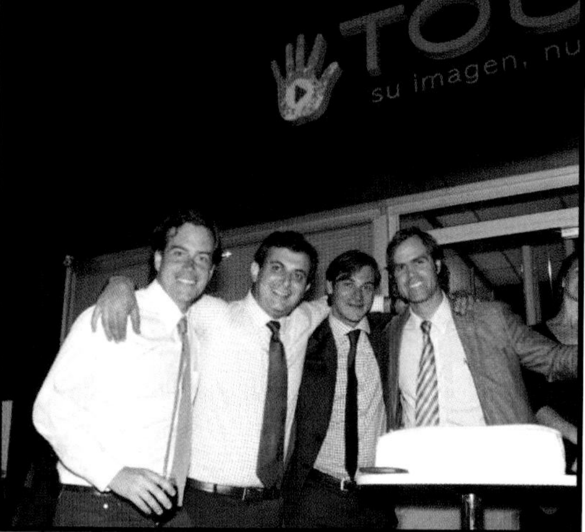

IN 2007, WE INVENTED THE CONCEPT OF CAPTADORES [*PROPELLERS*]: UNIVERSITY STUDENTS THAT DRIVE MASS CONSUMPTION PRODUCTS IN SUPERMARKETS. THAT RECIPE WOULD TAKE US, *TOUCH'S* 4 PARTNERS, TO CELEBRATE 10 YEARS OF THE COMPANY IN 2014. IN THE PICTURE ON THE RIGHT: ANTONIO MONCKEBERG, PEPE MASIHY, IGNACIO ROJAS, AND I.

As for me, I had the feeling he would have much rather have had me by his side in one of his companies. Much rather have me take part in a company in which I could also get professional experience and expertise. He was always hinting at the very tempting idea that the greater the commitment, the greater the benefits we'd get. I know how my old man operates. How efficient and obsessive he can be when it comes to his job. And I know myself, too. That mixture would have been dynamite. Successful? Yeah, sure. But I wanted independence. I wanted to build my own stuff. To take a real risk with this project that Pepe and I had started.

When we began, I had to ask my Dad for help, because we didn't even have a space to call our own in which to set up an office. He lent us a storage place above his own office, which was enough to plant the first roots of our small company. And that's where it all began, where we first bet on this opportunity. My dad, never fully convinced, kept a watchful eye on us. I am 100% sure that he chose that storage space to help us in this first business venture of ours, but also to be near me and keep a handle on my comings and goings. In time, I would realize that he also wanted to be aware of any needs I might have, because my old man is who he is: A generous guy.

Nowadays I know he takes my job seriously. My sister Antonia confirmed that at first my folks didn't fully believe in *Touch*, but today it's obvious that they support me. They attended, front row, our rollout. They've seen how we've grown into a powerful team driven by the mobile event staff that are central to our concept. I think I wouldn't be wrong in saying that *Touch* makes them proud. In fact, I'd insist: They both love the fact that I became a businessman following in my dad's footsteps. They are also aware that, as parents, they must have given me a lot for me to have been able to set up my own business.

I suspect that the change in the way they saw all of this took place in 2010, before my cancer, when we gave a presentation about *Touch* to my Dad. A serious and professional presentation. We showed him earnings, estimates, and actual figures. That's how he learned about what we'd done in our short and intense history, and how we planned to move forward. That day, Dad spontaneously said "Roberto, you're doing a great job. Keep up the good work full throttle." Wow. That was a moment full of relief and pride. It sent shivers down my spine. I felt it like a huge support, a show of trust. A loving gesture. From father to son.

The truth is, back then, I was always full throttle. I worked like a mad man, spending every minute of the day at *Touch*, and my evenings at *Taringa*, the restaurant and bar we had opened with my brother Sebastián, our cousin Jeremy, Pepe, and my friend and schoolmate Joselo. The place is always crowded. Many people go to it every day of the week, and it works in terms of business. All of us partners strive to make sure it's always a happening place, and for it to be a 'good journey' for our clients (which is our bar's slogan). There, I could unwind and enjoy myself; it was a break and –okay I'll admit it– that the bar was always full of beautiful women, was also a plus. Crazy.

With Pepe and some other friends we also set up *Top Roll* at the same time. It was a sushi-cart company that sold at different universities with the differentiating feature of selling the sushi roll as a whole, so that it could be hand held, not sliced in edible pieces. Sort of like a wrap. We were doing well, until we lost our focus: We set up a delivery service just as the market in Santiago was getting saturated with that kind of service, and we forgot the cart. It was a nightmare. We ended up selling *Top Roll* at a loss.

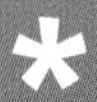

I'd spend the entire day at *Touch*, and then I'd run to *Taringa*. My friends used to tell me that something would happen to me if I kept that up.

My friends often told me to slow down, to take my foot off the pedal and chill out a bit. They said that if I kept up that pace, something would happen to me. One of them even warned me:

–Careful, Roberto, you're gonna end up getting cancer.

I didn't stop, though. Because it's in my nature to keep walking. It's a distinctive feature in our family, because the Ibáñezes just don't stop.

They work and work, and whenever they go on holiday, it's hard for them to really enjoy the break. Our nervous energy and restless brains take over. I know what I'm talking about, it's also hard for me to take a break. I believe myself to be a good salesman, intense and obsessive, I'd even say I'm a workaholic. It wasn't in my nature to take a break, let alone set boundaries, and even nowadays, whenever I set my mind to something, I go all the way. Like this book, for example.

I work intensely because I want *Touch* and the remaining projects I take part in to grow strong and that, in the process, those who work with us can also benefit. If the people on your team aren't as committed as you are, you're not doing a good job as a businessman. Without incentives, people have no motivation, and rightly so. According to my Dad, I have an impressive capacity to focus, and surprising stamina. He says I'm stubborn, and that whenever I set my mind to something, no one can move me from that goal until I achieve it. It's true.

Despite the pace of the life I was leading, I knew that not everything had to be work. I always had in mind this idea of being a non-stereotypical businessman. I wouldn't be the successful dude that has a disastrous home with a shipwreck of a family. I dreamt, and keep dreaming, of having a family.

The résumé by 2010 was this: I had already created 3 companies (one of them a failure), I had lived overseas, I knew about depression, I had to live with my sensitivity, had had 2 long-lasting romantic relationships, loved risky sports, and managed to avoid the typical disenchantment everyone sometimes feels in ways that were far from creative. Parties, much too much work, and sports.

My life was a mixture of an entanglement of love affairs, partying, a certain amount of longing or sadness that was sometimes hard to handle, and the happiness I found in my family, my dogs, and kitesurfing. Plus, the challenges and satisfactions I got through *Touch*. And that was it. Nothing special. Very far from an interesting life and from the idea of writing a book. Until...

* Towards the end of 2010, this weird thing appeared on my right arm. A protruding skin-colored mole that resembled an ugly flesh mushroom.

Towards the end of 2010, this weird thing appeared on my right arm. A protruding skin-colored mole that looked a bit like an ugly little flesh mushroom that I used to cover with a band aid, so that nobody would see it.

As it seemed a bit weird to me, just for my own peace of mind, I got an appointment with a dermatologist. She said it was nothing. That I shouldn't worry, and that I should come back in March if I wanted to get it removed for aesthetic reasons. She didn't say much more about the flesh mushroom on my arm. And I didn't worry, because she didn't convey any worry herself that might have made me think something could go wrong.

One afternoon that summer, I was at home, working at my computer, and I wasn't wearing a T-shirt. My Mom noticed the mole and asked whether I'd gone to have it checked. Focused on what I was doing, and without paying much attention to her, I muttered: 'Yeah, about a month ago. The doc said there's nothing to worry about.' Reassured, she proposed we get rid of it with a nail clipper, which she'd done with one of her sisters when younger. I gave it a thought. 'Why not?'. But then I remembered a friend of mine who, in the middle of a party at a house in *Pucón* which we'd rented with a group of friends one summer, had had the same procedure done by us. He bled so much we had been forced to cauterize it with a match. The mere memory of it made me reject my Mom's offer.

If we were talking about a movie script this would be the turning point, the dramatic twist in the tale that changes the main character's narrative arc and sets them on a new journey. With me being the main character, not paying much attention to this flesh-mushroom on my arm...

I was 27 years old, and I just thought: 'Damn! That's one ugly mole!' Full stop. ■

I KNEW VERY LITTLE ABOUT SUN EXPOSURE WITHOUT SUITABLE BARRIERS. THIS IS ONE OF THE ONLY 3 PICTURES I HAVE IN WHICH THE BUDDING MELANOMA CAN BE SEEN. MY DAD AND I DIDN'T KNOW AT THE TIME WHAT WE WERE ABOUT TO ENDURE.

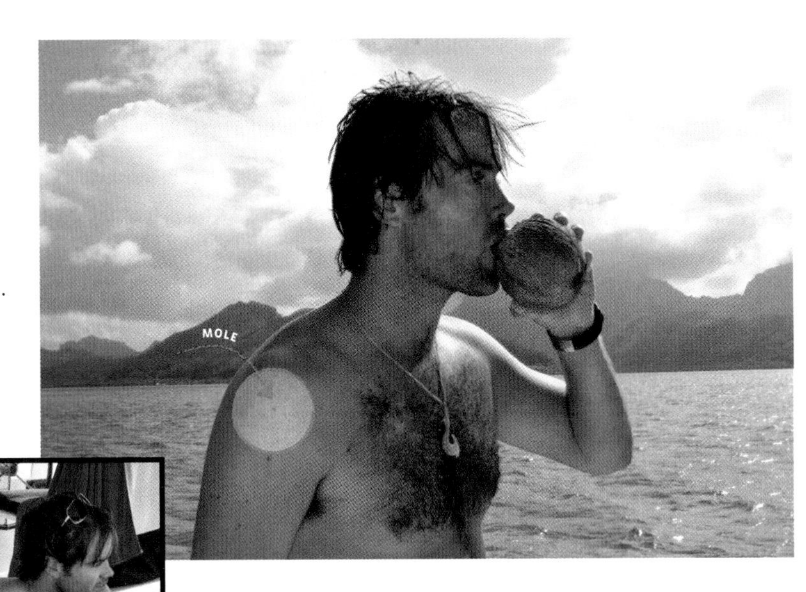

2. Kaboom!

After April 27, 2011, nothing would ever be the same. The emotional earthquake that shook my life and that of my family would have a huge impact the magnitude of which we came to assess only later.

Towards the end of March 2011, I went to the hospital and the dermatologist removed the infamous mole. She suggested she remove, as well, 2 other suspicious moles she had detected on my back. She sent the 2 of them for a biopsy, and told me she would include the one I didn't like in that package, too. As far as I was concerned it was all standard procedure, nothing to worry about. After all, that's what the doctor had said, hadn't she?

I called her mid-April to ask about the biopsy results for my 3 moles, and she said that the 2 on my back were fine. 'Right, so...what about the one on my arm?', I asked, super calmly. 'We're not sure', she replied, calmly as well. She then explained something about epithelial cells and some sort of staining. She could have been speaking Chinese, for all it meant to me. She said that the biopsy had to be stained, and that in order to do so I had to pay a little extra. After our conversation, the doctor wrote to me immediately: *Roberto, I'd like to know if we could talk about the biopsy over an email. Please let me know a.s.a.p. The pathologist found epithelial (skin) cells, but with a heterogeneous aspect (different from one another), and now is concerned about it being a healthy mole. To be sure, he needs to go ahead with some special staining of the biopsy.*

I didn't freak out. I asked Isabel Valdés, my Dad's personal assistant, to help me out with this. She tried to do so, but at the pathologist's office they told her it was something I had to do myself. Completely unconcerned, I let 2 weeks go by. But, as it turns out, it was my dermatologist herself who decided to take matters into her own hands.

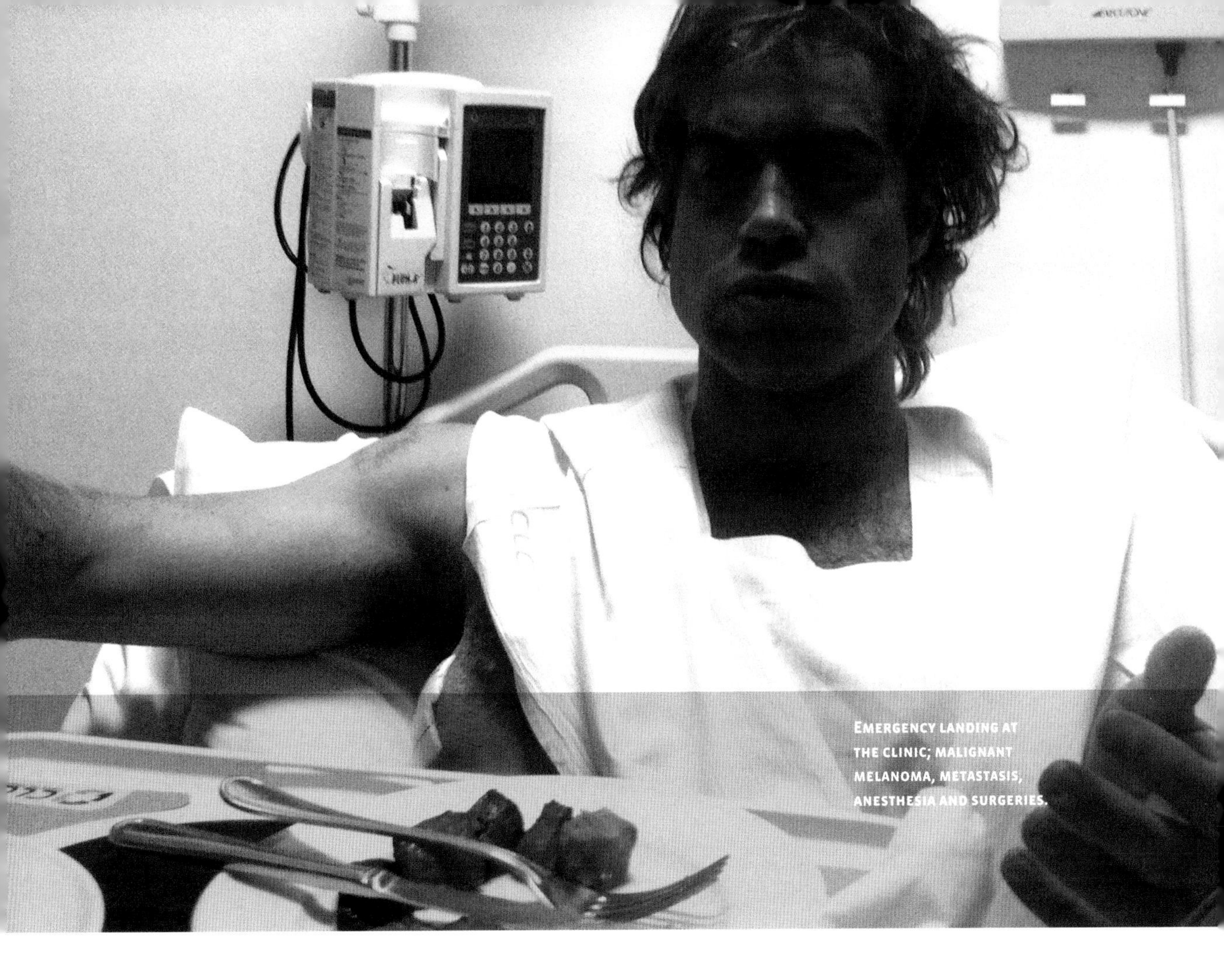

EMERGENCY LANDING AT THE CLINIC; MALIGNANT MELANOMA, METASTASIS, ANESTHESIA AND SURGERIES.

It was April 27. I remember it as though it were yesterday. A lunch party had been organized at home for the people of the Santiago Municipal Theatre. There were many guests, photographers, and journalists. Suddenly, I heard my cell ring. It was my dermatologist. 'Hi Roberto, are you by yourself?' To be honest, I thought it strange that she'd ask that, but didn't give it much thought and just walked away from the crowd. She then said, in a serious voice: 'Roberto, you have a melanoma'. A melanoma. The word meant nothing to me. Up until then I simply didn't know what that was, let alone how serious and lethal it could be. I asked her what that was exactly, but she avoided a direct answer and suggested instead we meet in her office. Yet, I insisted: 'What the hell is a melanoma?' It was only then that she answered directly: 'It's a type of skin cancer that, depending on its progress, can be lethal'.

Amelanotic melanoma. That's what it was. Strange, because melanomas normally appear as moles of a darker pigmentation, and mine was skin-colored. But that's something I learned much later. That day, I ended the call without understanding a word of what we'd just discussed. I went upstairs, walked into my bedroom, and sat on the bed. It was a silent moment. Silent and slow. As though that moment belonged to someone else, as though it wasn't happening to me. I cried, but it couldn't have been more than a few seconds; and then I asked myself: 'Why am I crying if there's nothing wrong with me?' *There's nothing wrong with me.* I repeated that sentence several times in my mind. *There's nothing wrong with me.* I di-

PHOTOGRAPHY: *EL MERCURIO*.

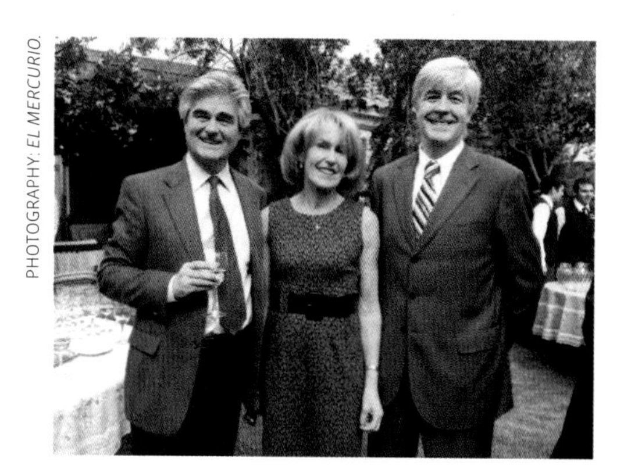

THIS PICTURE WAS TAKEN ON THE SAME DAY I WAS INFORMED OF MY DIAGNOSIS, DURING THE LUNCHEON FOR THE CORPORATION OF FRIENDS OF THE MUNICIPAL THEATER, WHICH MY MOM THROWS EVERY YEAR AT OUR PLACE (MY PLACE AT THE TIME). FEATURED: FERNANDO KREIS, HEATHER ATKINSON, AND SANTIAGO QUER.

alled my Dad, who was attending a board meeting at Walmart. My family has a policy that I really cherish. Dad, even if super busy, always –no exceptions– answers when we phone him. He answered right away, and I gave him a summary of that brief conversation I'd held with the doctor: mole + biopsy results + melanoma + lethal.

During that phone call, which was the first of many but which was the most confusing one as I tried to make sense of the news I'd received, I cried a little. But my Dad put a lid on it: 'Nothing's going to happen. I'll call you in a little while.' And so I thought it was nothing to worry about, because he'd taken it calmly...

But I was wrong. Twenty minutes later, he, who a short while before had been presiding over a board meeting, called me to say he was already at the hospital with the doctor, and that I should meet them there. 'We need to find out what this thing is,' he said. So I left for *Clínica Las Condes.*

The 'thing' was 1.5 mm thick, and we had to make sure it hadn't metastasized, because that was the worst-case scenario. By then it wasn't an ugly mole anymore, they were talking to me about skin cancer, about malignant melanoma, about metastasis. Far too much information in a very short while. All of them words I had never paid attention to, and the actual meaning of which I still didn't understand. Had I jumped outside my body and looked at the scene, I would have seen myself sitting at that desk, next to my Dad who was asking many questions and writing everything down, across from the doctor, who kept answering all those questions and looking at him, with a very serious expression in her face. What was the next step? Was there a next step?

The doctor, supported by Dr. Carlos Regonessi, of that same hospital and a cancer specialist who is friends with my parents, sent me to an oncological surgeon. A few hours later, we were headed for the office of Dr. Gustavo Vial. I noticed my Dad's attitude: He walked with his back straight, sure of himself, calm. He was facing a problem, and he was going to solve it. I had nothing to worry about. My Dad was facing a crisis, and he would make everything right. I managed to catch a glimpse of his disbelief that this was happening to me, his son, but I also noticed he felt the need to always act in the most rational and logical way, without wasting any time. He is a hands-on guy; with immediate reaction: with him there's no putting things off, and from the very first meeting with my dermatologist that's how I saw him acting. It took him 3 days to internalize what was happening. And when he did, he had a pragmatic approach.

The logical approach he felt he had to adopt as head of the family, so that we could organize ourselves and act. That is how I interpreted his attitude that day.

To be honest, I had no way of imagining the emotional earthquake my old man lived through when he found out about my diagnosis. It was only a long time later, –three years later to be precise– during a lengthy, deep and emotionally charged phone conversation that we had after a lot of water had flowed under the bridge, as he drove to Puerto Montt and crossed over to Castro, did I find out what a huge impact the news of my melanoma had had on him. "Nothing ever went back to being what it used to be," he commented over the phone, in a conversation that was at time interrupted due to interference, and with a voice that let me hear how much it moved him just to remember those first moments, when he'd just learned about the diagnosis. "At the time, Roberto, I just thought of protecting you from everything: from the melanoma, from despair, from fear, from uncertainty. I was going to feel all of that for you, so that you could live life without that burden. I'd take care of looking for the necessary information to understand where were you regarding the illness. I was your Dad and I wasn't about to let anything happen to you!", he said. I was moved, when I realized that, even after so many years, I'd never finish getting to know my father, and that surprises such as this are gifts life is giving me. Why had we never talked like that before, with such intensity, putting all our feelings out in the open? Never mind: this books deals precisely with cancer being a very long process during which successive events take place that, whether small or big, end up transforming us.

That conversation changed everything, and so I decided to rewrite most of what follows in this book. Because I needed to include, along with my perspective –which is conveyed throughout this book– that of my Dad's, my family's, and that of some of the doctors who played a vital role in all of this. 'What's important about this book is that it should be honest. It should include all points of view. So that everyone reading can understand the tunnels that they may go through,' suggested my old man. And he was absolutely right.

> * They were talking to me about skin cancer, about malignant melanoma, about metastasis. Far too much information in a very short while.

So, when we were sitting across the table from Dr. Vial, I felt they were talking as though I wasn't there, as though I was incapable of understanding, let alone making a decision. I felt like a 5-year-old listening in to a conversation of grownups. And I didn't like it. Come to think about it, I probably wouldn't have contributed much anyway, given how shocked I was. Yet, right there and then, I did not like that feeling of being a fly on the wall.

Wasn't it me who had the melanoma? In retrospect, and after having talked to many patients who have endured similar situations, the truth is I was in no condition to grab hold of the reins, and I needed that rock-solid support from my Dad.

Back then, my Dad was solving things, or trying to solve things, amid the turmoil he himself was going through. But to me, it seemed as though he had grabbed control of things. It reminded me of what I'd often heard him say regarding the way he tackled fatherhood: that rather than being a friend to his children he should be there to guide, protect and take care of them. And I thought about how much I needed for him to be my friend at that moment. I thought about the support I longed for amid all the chaos following that apparently so complex diagnosis. I also felt like he wasn't giving me the chance to take control of my own crisis.

Today I know he acted as a parent. He told me so himself. I haven't had kids, yet, but I'm able to see that his protective instinct was his way of armor-plating me from bad news. My folks, amid the shipwreck it all seemed to be, realized they had to protect me from all of the negative information out there. And there is, in fact, a lot of it about melanoma. I can only imagine how unbearable it must be for a father or a mother to hear that there is a death risk, even if negligible, for a child of theirs. In my case, at least, busy as I was dealing with my own hardships, from the diarrhea I endured to my romantic mishaps of the moment, I wasn't even capable of really taking the risk on board, and just couldn't get past the anger my father's attitude provoked in me. Nowadays I know one ought to be very careful with anger, because it blocks both good and bad things, and it hinders good decision-making. If you give in to anger you can really regret it. Anger can be stopped. I did.

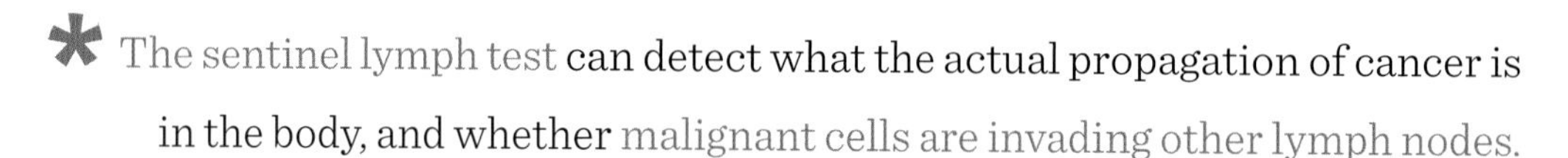

Nevertheless, during that first visit to Dr. Vial, I got a grip of the basics: the malignant melanoma diagnosis had been confirmed and I had to have surgery to remove every bit of skin surrounding the mole that might have been compromised. I also needed to have a test run on the sentinel lymph node in my right armpit. What the heck was that? No idea. I learned afterwards that it was a test that can detect how far an illness has spread, since the sentinel lymph node is the one that sends the warning signal if something is going wrong in that part of the body. Thus, I'd get to find out if malignant cells had invaded any of the lymph nodes in my arm. If so, it would be a sign of metastasis...that the cancer had already spread.

Vial calmed us down by adding that, given the characteristics of the mole, the most likely scenario was one of no metastasis. He gave that option a 70% chance. The second possibility meant I went straight from Stage-I cancer, in which I presumably was, to Stage III, with the worst prognosis (please check the chart on p. 65). But I still had a long way to go before I began to understand what all of those terms and percentages meant. I still had to learn the cancer lingo.

After learning that I would have to admit myself to hospital a few days later and have surgery, I continued to be confused. Dad kept assuring me *this* would be solved (the cancer, the doubts, the fear, and a hundred other things), as though it were all up to him. I realized he was conveying to me that he was on a mission. And right then, in the context of everything that was happening, with a terrifying biopsy at hand, instead of feeling secure and trusting him, I sort of wanted to get back at him.

I had chosen to become an entrepreneur, taken risks on my own project, and set up my own business, and I also wanted to be in charge of my cancer, I wanted to be the one to drive initiatives. It was MY sickness, MY territory. My Dad was invading MY space. And that pissed me off. Still, I just couldn't express any of this. The shock had jammed my emotions somewhere way down my throat. The only certainty I had was that he was there, by my side, to face that huge wave that was coming towards me, and that he was showing me that I had to trust him. He was taking charge, because my life was at stake. I was unable to welcome his support; I didn't know how to.

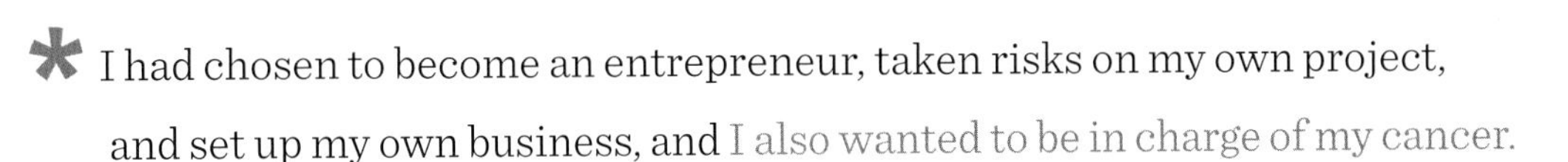
* I had chosen to become an entrepreneur, taken risks on my own project, and set up my own business, and I also wanted to be in charge of my cancer.

I didn't know, either, of the conversation he had with Nicolás, his brother, and when he recalled it during our long conversation 3 years later, and after everything had happened, my voice shook just as his must have shaken back then: Not even 2 hours had gone by, and he had already spoken to Dr. Vial 5 times to gather all the information he could, to understand what my situation was. So he rang Nicolás, who knew nothing about what was going on. I can imagine the conversation: Nicolás might have been offhand, aloof even, maybe. However he reacted, he didn't seem to get how my old man was feeling. And that really sent my Dad overboard and he asked "Don't you get it? Roberto might be dying!". Until he told me about that conversation with his brother, I had never thought my Dad had even contemplated the possibility of me dying. That's when I understood what he'd been doing: he'd protected me with all his might so that I wouldn't feel the anguish that had him fighting for air. That left its imprint in me, and continues to be a reminder that is leading us both to an ever better relationship.

Now that I am better balanced on both my feet, so to speak, I see it like this: When it's you that is sick, you don't want anyone bossing you around, telling you what to do. And back then, I didn't want my father to become the CEO of *Roberto's Cancer Co.*, dictating what the next steps would be. But in reality that's of course not what he was doing... I was so into myself and into what I was going through, that I lost track of my family. I was incapable of empathizing with those around me, let alone with their anguish and fears. Most likely, my other worries seemed back then much more important than that infamous melanoma. And all of that piled up and triggered a lot of anger. It was that simple.

How relevant individual perspectives are. How important it is to truly listen to others...

I saw my Dad tackling my cancer as one more of his huge challenges, and living it as though it were a battle-front he'd been called to contain. All of that despite the stress and anguish that sometimes took hold of him. "I knew I had to get a grip of myself. Keep my head cool. Act rationally; with courage. Because if I fell... well, it'd be complicated. There's things I never told you, or which maybe I changed a little. Still, I chose to protect you, and your Mom and your siblings decided to weather the storm in order not to lose our North. What we can take from all of this is that we lived through the process as a family, and each of us undertook the role assigned". "Roberto, in my case, your cancer left a mark that'll last a lifetime, and so now I look at things from a different angle," he said a short while ago. I was speechless. Mulled that over quite a bit.

I now appreciate deeply his efforts to gather all that information, him working day in, day out to understand my cancer and find solutions. His executive abilities were worth gold-dust throughout my process, and it was acknowledged by Dr. Vial. But I was blind to all of that back then. In a very healing conversation I had with Dr. Vial on everything that had happened during those confusing days that followed my being diagnosed, he let me in on his own perspective. And that enabled me to rethink many of the things I lived through back then and which I'll recount here.

After that afternoon spent at Dr. Vial's, I returned home, to a short truce before the surgery. I was still confused, so it's hard for me to remember exactly what happened during those days. I know I told my Mom. She'd seen the mole, but hadn't thought it serious. Yet, now I know she had a sort of premonition. About 2 months before the diagnosis she told a friend of hers she was worried about me. 'I don't know what is wrong with Roberto, but something's going on with him. He's suffering from diarrhea. He doesn't look well. He has this weird look in his eyes...'

My siblings learned the news from my parents. None of them really understood the magnitude of a melanoma. To them, it was some kind of cancerous mole, they didn't fully grasp the actual implications. When I told them I had to undergo surgery to remove it and check whether there was metastasis in the lymph nodes, and that if that happened the outlook was far from good, I know they worried, that they were sad. But they disregarded it, because they knew no one with melanoma and knew nothing about the perils of this kind of cancer. Plus, as my parents and I were betting on the 70% chance of survival Dr. Vial mentioned, they thought it would surely all be alright. They never once guessed it was something that could kill me. Neither did I, really. It's hard to believe, but even though they told me about the dangers back then, I didn't really take it on board.

* My siblings never imagined this was something of which I could die. Neither did I, really. It's hard to believe, but although they told me so, I never fully internalized it.

I didn't talk it over with my friends, and didn't google anything, either, to find out what a melanoma was really about. I stayed with what I'd been told during the doctors' appointments. I acted like an idiot, really, I disregarded it completely. Something in me simply blocked information. I wasn't accepting my cancer. At some point during those days, we went to a family wedding, and I realized my parents were very much in tune with what was going on. Even if we weren't talking about it, during that difficult time of waiting without really knowing how things would turn out. That was a strange night, but a very special one, too. Many of the people there knew what was going on, so they approached me; it was one of the first times I had to face the world as someone sick. My folks were extra caring, close to me, and although I noticed how scared they were, I felt them trying to connect both with themselves and with me.

And so my Dad began to try and understand, through every possible means, what was it that was really happening to me. He began to study what my melanoma was, and to gather as much information as possible, in order to make better decisions. It took him 5 days to read everything he could get hold of on the subject. He began researching whether surgery was necessary. He watched videos, met with doctors. He interviewed patients. And worked tirelessly 24/7. Loreto Besa was one of the people he interviewed. She was an acquaintance of my sister-in-law, my brother Tomas's wife, and the conversation with her was a real contribution. My Dad took notes, *verbatim*, just as he did during all the conversations he held on account of my melanoma:

MY DAD'S NOTES DURING AN INTERVIEW WITH LORETO BESA, ALSO A MELANOMA PATIENT.

- 3 Melanoma surgeries (back, leg, and eye).
- Surgery by Gustavo Vial – excellent – the best!
- "He's wonderful, very thorough, very serene".
- Arm is a super safe place, because there is no organ near it.
- Back melanoma: they removed 5 nodes. Had ramifications.
- They reached the Sentinel lymph nodes.
- It wasn't necessary to get in touch with the U.S.
- Gustavo made sure to remove everything necessary.
- Apparently nowadays it's quite **common** and **highly treatable.**
- Technology, with the Sentinel node, is wonderful.
  Shows up every symptom there might be in the body.
- "Let me convey to you all my calmness, I'm **perfectly** well! With 3 surgeries."
- "Mine has been a fantastic experience!"

By the way, Loreto also shares all of her tips in the last part of this book.

After having gathered all that data and processed it down to the tiniest detail, my father, supported by my siblings and my mother, concluded surgery was necessary. He also concluded it could be performed in Chile, and that it was urgent to do it right away. There wasn't a moment to waste.

Between that Wednesday of the diagnosis, and the following Tuesday, which was the day of my surgery, I led a normal life. I was overwhelmed by the initial impact, but supposed that by removing my melanoma and that sentinel lymph node, everything would be fine. And so, I went to work as usual, partied a little, and practiced sports. People around me seemed to fully trust that 70% that I, comfortably, told them about whenever they asked.

I now realize I had no idea what it really meant to be diagnosed with cancer. Maybe I just didn't want to see it. In fact, on the day of my surgery, my folks gave me an iPad, and I thought: "What the hell! I'm not sick, I'm not staying in bed. I don't need an iPad". I wasn't afraid of the surgeries, I had already had 3 in my life: two on my nose and one on my hip. I wasn't afraid of needles, either, given I'd suffered at least 4 tonsillitis episodes a year since I was 12 years old. One more needle seemed like nothing at all. My surgery took place on May 3rd, 2011. That day I got up really early, and saw my Dad was up, and wearing a suit and tie, as though he was attending a business meeting. That got to me. I don't know, maybe I was too tense. The sight of a father in a formal suit to take his son to the hospital so that he could get cancer surgery... it hit me. Maybe it's a very unfair thought, but the truth is that what I saw was the business man, and not the Dad I needed by my side and that I now have. I felt like telling him to lose the tie, but I didn't. Now I know that all of these feelings of anger are part of the process that cancer patients endure. Especially at the beginning. I really hope those reading this pay attention to these tiny details, because later on... you'll find they make a difference.

* On the day of my surgery, my folks gave me an iPad, and I thought: "What the hell! I'm not sick, I'm not staying in bed. I don't need this device". I just didn't get it.

Criticizing my old man because of his formal attire on the day of my surgery was pretty unfair, to be honest. It was his automatic way of showing he cared. Plus, I later found out through my sister that his role back then had been paramount. She'd seen how he'd reacted and what he'd done; I hadn't. I just couldn't see it. Antonia says Dad never even mentioned being tired, though his haggard face said otherwise. She knew he was suffering inside. And that he was under a huge amount of stress. Antonia is the only one who can tell when Dad is on the verge of tears, or when he's feeling affected by something. Yet, he never cried. At least not in front of her. And in front of me he was nothing but a tower of strength. My sister believes that was good for me, because she also knows that having your Dad near instills a huge sense of security. He's the kind of guy that looks you in the eye and is convincing when he says everything will be alright. That nothing will happen to you. That you should leave everything to him. Yet, this time, my Dad did ask her for help. She told me he'd gone to her and told her he trusted her strong and rational nature. And that he needed her to help him take care of Mom. "We cannot let the family crumble, Antonia, we cannot collapse," she remembers him saying.

In my ignorance, the only thing I knew before entering the OR was that I had 2 options. The first one entailed surgery being brief: They'd remove the skin surrounding the mole, would test the sentinel lymph node, it'd turn out to be negative, and I'd be off to recovery. The second one was the dangerous one: For the test on the sentinel lymph node to turn out to be positive and for it to show one or several nodes to be compromised. That would mean a 4-hour surgery, plus the chance of there being metastasis. ***One hour before the operation, I asked my family to leave me alone with Doctor Vial, so that he would explain to me in detail, for the first time, the surgery and its consequences.***

Looking back on it, I guess those weren't easy days for him, either. My Dad was so stressed out that he kept putting pressure on the doc. He wouldn't allow Doc Vial to tell me anything without him having listened to it first. Always in an effort to protect me.

As Doc Vial only now told me, back then he gave me all the time in the world to let the surgery I was about to face to sink in. Because that's what he always does. As an oncological surgeon he believes himself to be a partner to his patient. He tries to explain all the implications. And to make sure that the patient understands. "But, naturally, I also tell them what I would do," he said. And that's exactly what he did during that pre-surgery conversation. The doctor explained to me that, from a psychological perspective, whenever patients do not mentally incorporate whatever the specialist is informing him or her, that has a name. It's denial. Clearly, I was one of those patients in utter denial. Luckily enough, my family was much more in synch with the matter than I was.

Without them, the story would have been quite different. Back then, I still went about things with a shallower perspective. I just focused on the high likelihood of my cancer not having metastasized, and kept going. I didn't give myself the space to talk things over or to confront the possibility of a metastasis. As I had to not long after. ***And this is a an important piece of advice that I can offer those faced with a cancer diagnosis r: It's of paramount importance to give your family some time. Once a month. Once a week. Whatever. But talk. About everything. Masks off.*** My Dad owned up to it: there were times that he faked it. He pretended he wasn't in distress, when

* The doctor explained that, from a psychological point of view, denial is the phenomenon of patients not internalizing and assuming what the specialist is telling them.

in fact he was very much so. And he did so only to save me from hardship. Come to think of it, I wish I had hugged him back them... I wish I'd known how everyone was feeling. But the cancer wouldn't let us. That was our time to talk about things. We postponed it. I sincerely hope others start sooner.

When I left for the OR, I cried. I broke down when saying good-bye to my family. I took a glance at the clock on the wall. Half past eleven in the morning. I thought that if everything went well, by the time I woke up it'd be 1 or 2 o'clock in the afternoon. Before I was rolled in, I looked at my Mom. She was in tears. So I said: *Shit happens.* She's a mighty companion in my life. And given she's Scottish, we speak English to each other. We have our special way of communicating. After I told her that, and through the tears, we laughed. And that's the mood in which I entered the OR.

Out there, in the hall, my whole family waited. I later learned that Tomás, who'd caught up with the meaning of the term melanoma, explained to Sebastián how serious the issue was. He'd watched videos, had read, had asked. And he already knew that if I happened to have a metastasis in any of my organs, it could end up being deadly. Tomás was the first to talk to him about survival chances. It was only then that Sebastián realized what was going on. That's when he freaked out. When he thought: "Oh my! Roberto might die." That's when he really felt the sadness. A lot of sadness. For me, for my Dad, for my Mom. That's when he promised himself he'd fight with my Dad against that melanoma.

Before that conversation with Tomás, Sebastián thought it was merely a matter of removing the skin where the mole had been, covering it with a Band-Aid, and that would be it. That was the best-case scenario. But things changed in a matter of seconds. After 2 hours, the doctor walked out and announced he had removed the sentinel lymph node, and that it was infiltrated. The melanoma had metastasized. Kaboom!, according to Sebastián. Everyone became nervous. My illness had taken on a new dimension.

> * My operation had turned into that dreaded second possibility. My family was terrified. And inside the OR, I had no idea of what was going on.

I also found out that, for my folks, that was a devastating moment. At least one lymph node was compromised. That meant the cancer had entered the lymphatic system. That it wasn't encapsulated. The doctor returned to the OR and removed the 22 lymph nodes in my armpit. He removed everything. My surgery had turned into that dreaded and distressing second possibility. My family was terrified. And inside that OR, I had no idea of what was going on.

When I woke up the first thing I wondered was what time it was. Doctor Luis Fernando Coz, the father of one of my very best friends, was by my side. He replied it was 5 in the afternoon. I calculated and knew right away something had gone wrong. I felt the weight of his words and immediately positioned myself in that new situation. Had there been no results then? So it hadn't just been a case of removing the tissue and that was it? I couldn't believe it. I was still under the effects of the anesthesia. Drowsy. But even so, I felt the tension in the air. The result of the surgery wasn't what we'd all been expecting.

Pain was an unwelcome arrival. It was a deeply-set pain. Indescribable. A pain that prevented me from moving my arm. I despaired. It felt as though they had ripped it off at the shoulder. Sebastián and my Dad were already there, by my side. My brother says that as soon as I opened my eyes, he took one of my hands, while my Dad held the other one; and that I asked how everything had gone. "How did I do?" They confirmed that the test on the sentinel lymph nodes had not resulted in good news, that there were 2 infiltrated nodes. Microscopically, yet infiltrated. I cried. My Dad cried. And so did Sebastián.

Immediately afterwards, pain paralyzed me. Despite the nurses telling me they administered the highest possible dosage of morphine, the pain was unbearable. I was weak, I couldn't move my arm. The surgery had gone all wrong. I could not

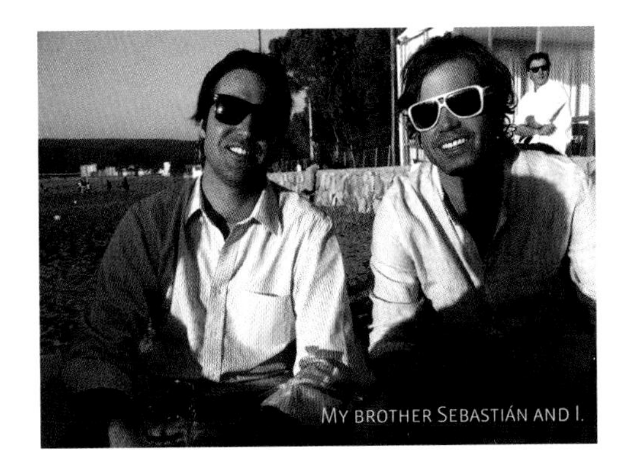
My brother Sebastián and I.

stop crying. Then, suddenly, I felt Sebastián's hand on my cheek. A warm, loving, hand. "Roberto, chill," he said. My brother was there, supporting me, trying to give me some peace. He seemed like an angel to me, watching over me, and so, despite the pain and the fear, I felt I wasn't alone.

That was a very emotional moment for Sebastián. For years, we had been constantly at each other's throats. Very competitive. We were far from being the typical chummy brothers that party together. It was the total opposite. Up until a while before my cancer, we had a distant relationship. Afterwards, we became a little closer. We opened up Taringa along with our business part-

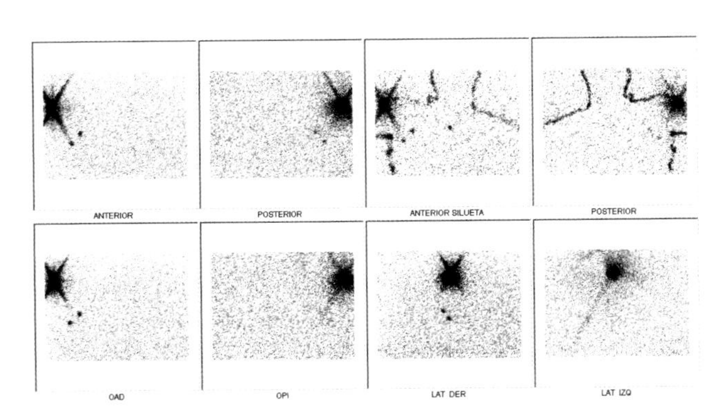

Metastasized melanoma in the sentinel lymph nodes in my right armpit; May 2011.

ners and a bond was born. However, even though we were more in synch, neither of us was very prone to displays of affection. Now I know that the unforgettable act of touching my cheek with his hand sprang from deep inside. Sebastián felt sad and helpless when he saw me, lying there, in tears, drowsy and in pain. ***The message was* We are a family, we are here to take care of you, we are right by your side.** Then I felt my Dad's hand on my other cheek. My Dad, worried, just as terrified as I was, was there, looking after me. Both of them were there to stay.

"I don't understand why you and your brother don't get along. You have so much in common. You are so alike!", insisted Pepe, my business partner, who is also friends with Sebastián. And he was quite right. The truth is that we're mending our relationship even now, and it seems as though we love and support each other more and more with each passing day. I will never forget that night we were partying in a nightclub at the beach, dancing side by side, and we hugged the way brothers do, right there in the middle of the dance floor. That was after my cancer; a moment of reconnection on this path of building a closer relationship.

Sebastián stayed with me that first night. Antonia during the second one. Her main role was to look after my Mom. We didn't talk about the cancer, because to be honest that wasn't what worried me. What really worried me was what was happening around me, in my family. I like that feeling of knowing my siblings were looking after me. It felt good. After so much pain, I finally managed to sleep. But the nightmare was far from over. When I woke up Doctor Vial explained to me, in detail, what had happened. Indeed, there were 2 infiltrated lymph nodes, one of them with a micro-metastasis, the other with a macro-metastasis. On top of that, during surgery they had brushed past my long thoracic nerve, which innervates the muscles in the scapula (the shoulder blade) and enables controlling it. I couldn't believe it. "Don't worry," said the doctor. "It's a nerve that's hardly ever used. Only when practicing sports that require some muscular effort on the shoulder, like swimming or tennis." The doctor didn't know I was into sports, and that I needed my arm to be strong and work properly. I asked him what the next step was. He replied it would be fixed through another surgery, one he wouldn't perform himself. And he assured me of a 60% chance of success. They would remove a part of the sural nerve in my calf to replace the damaged one through a graft.

My Dad was all for that surgery. Obviously, I also agreed with the idea; I wanted to recover the mobility in my arm. Sebastián was the one to convince me about the surgery being a good idea. "Let them remove part of the nerve on your left leg, because everything is happening on your right side," he suggested. I did as he told me.

***** The first night after that surgery, I spent it in the company of my brother Sebastián. I liked how it felt to have my siblings taking care of me.

I underwent surgery the next day. They warned me about a very slow and painful recovery, but I couldn't care less (how could I, after everything that had happened?). It was 4 more hours in an OR.

When I woke up from that second surgery, they gave me *Propofol,* an anesthetic agent known as *truth serum.* It's known to trigger several reactions: sadness, anger, anguish. In my case, I became a no-holds-barred truth teller; deep in a sort of euphoria. When the nurse asked how I felt, I let her have it: "Fine. Perfect, you b...! I have a Foley up my dick, they've just removed a nerve from my leg to graft it into my shoulder...How do you think I feel?! I feel awesome! And have the doctor come! I'm gonna put a Foley up his butt..!"

Twenty minutes of that.

After that, in walked my uncle Nicolás, who loves to sail. Right away, I begged him for a yacht. "Just a little yacht for this poor convalescent soul! That's nothing to you! C'mon! Open up that wallet!" Later, it was my Dad's partner, Jorge Gutiérrez, who had to deal with me. He is shorter than I am. And I shot: "Hey, shorty! Come here, d'ya know what smegma is?" It was insane. I even told him his wife was attractive. The pain-specialist had to bear with my complimenting her breasts, and I invited her to *Taringa.* "I am married," she replied, in a very professional tone. "So what?! I'm not a jealous guy!". I crossed every line thanks to that *Propofol,* but after shocking everyone, at least I made them laugh. I had them laughing out loud, in tears. Until a spark of reality got through to me, and I said: "F...! I have cancer. That's just shitty."

After I left that episode behind, Doctor Vial explained to me that, according to the instructions from the surgeon who grafted my nerve, exercising would complicate the recovery, because the nerve could detach from its place. In the end, I recovered 60% of the enervation. That surgery left a scar I see every day. I lost skin sensitivity, I have less muscle capacity, sometimes my shoulder blade simply shoots out, and I feel a sort of tingling... or prickling sensation in my left leg, as though I had it half anesthetized. From my current perspective, and after having talked it over openly with Doctor Vial, they are minimal consequences in the face of the huge challenge faced while completely cleaning the area infiltrated by the melanoma. And he never once hesitated in telling me he'd brushed that nerve, which is right next to the area he cleaned. He hid nothing, and he repaired it right away.

This much I can infer: I was so stunned with the dizzying developments, that my family, especially my father, set up a permanent communication with Doctor Vial, and a natural channel developed through which to exchange information. I felt left out a couple of times, but I didn't do much, either, to be part of those conversations. The level of concentration was such that my Dad would jump

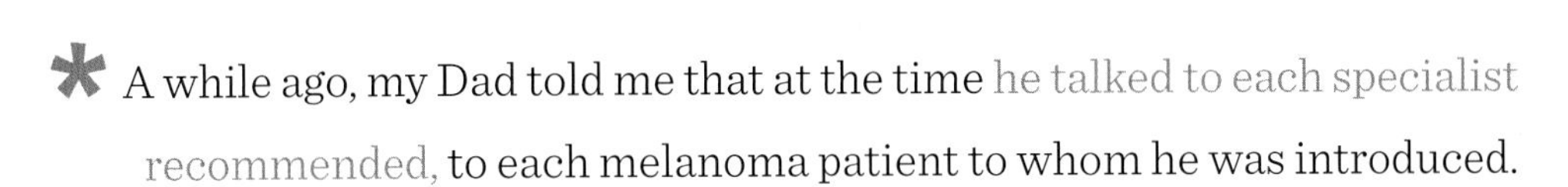

After my first surgery, the pain was such that it felt as though they'd yanked off my arm. By then I still had not internalized the true implications of the melanoma and its metastasis. Hence the laughing face of disbelief.

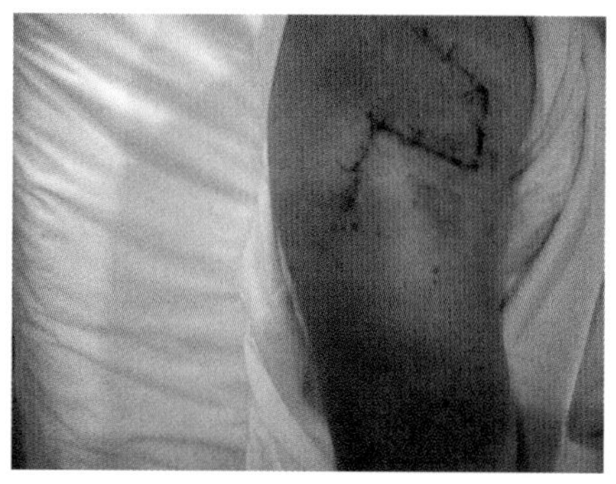

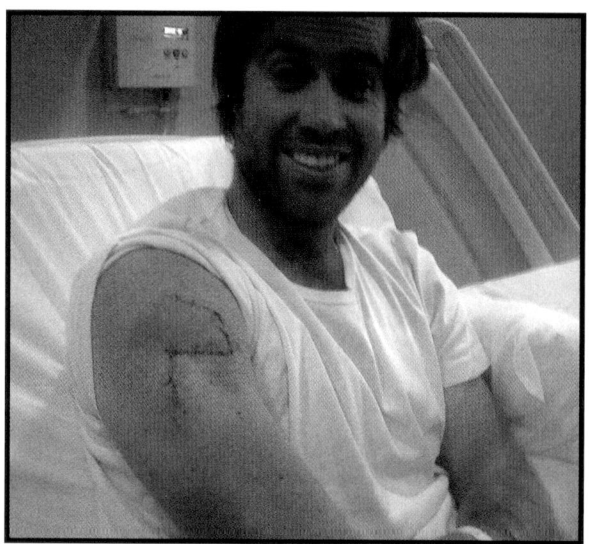

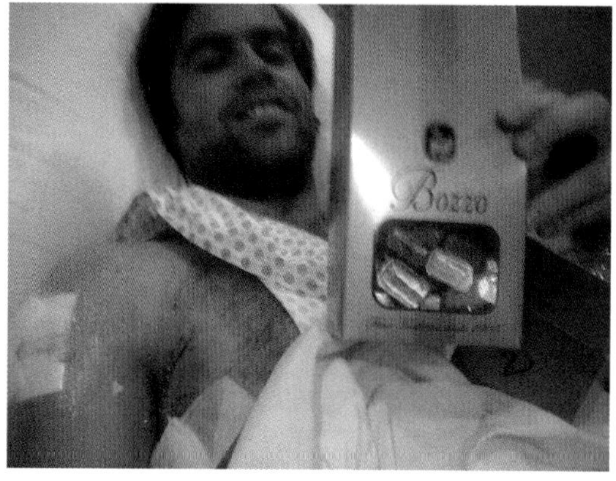

off his chair whenever not directly informed about something, I guess not to sideline me, but rather to gather all the necessary information to continue making decisions. "I wasn't in a position to take my foot off the accelerator, I met with every specialist recommended, I interviewed every melanoma patient or former melanoma patient to whom I was introduced," he told me recently. Learning this firsthand makes me think my Dad and I are much more similar than we think: to tackle this book, I acted just like him; I had in-depth interviews with doctors and people connected in some way to cancer, and I filled its pages with almost a hundred personal accounts that share people's tips.

And I must say, I am thankful for having fallen into the hands of Gustavo Vial, who even now answers all my calls (and they aren't few), and clarifies all my doubts without a moment's hesitation. "The biggest step is complete," I remember him saying after the surgery. Those words filled me with optimism and confidence.

While I was in hospital, I received many, but MANY visits from friends. I'd say 350 people over 4 days. I felt like a rock star. The nurses were impressed; they didn't understand how I had the stamina to welcome one person after the other. The room, the halls, the waiting room, were all packed with friends. I was exhausted, true, but how was I supposed to say no to those people, if each one of them had taken the time to come and see me? To go through the hassle of getting to the hospital, finding a free parking space (no mean feat), and finding their way up to my room? I am so thankful to each and every one of them. I would have loved to have a guest book to read over and over afterwards. But it never crossed my mind at the time. ***I now know many patients do so, and it seems like a great suggestion.***

At the time, Pepe was always there. He'd camp out every day in my hospital room to keep me company, and he simply was there. He held me, so to speak, he was permanently there, supporting me. Afterwards, he told me he had tried to respect my need to be alone –he knows well enough how much I value having my own space–, but that he also tried to be very present, so that I would realize I wasn't alone. Having Pepe there all the time, he and his computer... it was awesome. He'd sometimes go down to the cafeteria, so that I could talk to doctors or my folks, but he was always there. Damn! He was like a girlfriend, come to think about it! Hahahaha! We laugh when we remember he would pace up and down the room in sweat pants and sneakers, as comfy as possible, acting as a host to guests whenever there was a crowd.

It's weird. Clinically, you have been declared sick, physically impaired if you will, but you don't feel sick. People ask and you answer pleasantly and in detail, everything they want to know. You have a throng paying attention to you, worried about you, ready to address your every need. You talk about cancer with ease, as though you weren't starring in that movie, as if it were an anecdote. Someone else's anecdote. "Yeah, here we are. With cancer. Everything's A OK, I feel fine. And you? How are you doing?" You can talk, joke, turn to black humor so that you can laugh the drama off for a while. You are filled with a special adrenaline. As though something in you were disassociated from reality. Despite feeling tired, I could have welcomed even more guests. I could have laughed even harder. As though nothing in that patient's file were true. Except for the pain in my arm, which reminded me every so often that that stay in hospital wasn't due to a sprain. Seeing people from so many different areas of my life moved me. There were friends from my bicycling world, who would start planning with me the next outings. Then there was my kiting group; and my former schoolmates, who had been alerted by José Coz, my friend since junior school. There were the people from *Touch,* who painted signs full of well-meaning and positive messages. It was a stream of good vibes that did me good. And Pepe; the ever-present Pepe. Mentioning the business now and again so that I'd understand that things were going smoothly while I was out of the picture.

 While I was in the hospital, many, many friends visited me. About 350 people over 4 days; I felt like a *rock star.*

Maybe all of that happens because the distraction is necessary. Because one needs to avoid the possibility of feeling alone. So that you don't have time to think and imagine things. I don't know, it's strange, because you get used to being important for so many people. But then it all vanishes. Obviously. Everyone has his or her own life and their own burdens to carry around. But you miss it. You miss that attention, that loving care, those conversations with those guests who are worried about you. Yes, all those people willing to keep you company and listen to you, helps you dodge what you are going through. It helps you escape from all of that for a brief moment, even if you are talking about your own sickness. It's odd; you talk to others about how sick you are, but you dread going through that insight on your own.

One of the things that most cheered me up was learning what Uke thought of it all. Uke, Eduardo Pérez de Castro, is a friend from the kite world, a sportsman just like me, a friend from good weekends spent together in *Matanzas*. He was there at the hospital, keeping my family company during the surgery, and he later told me he'd seen my Dad become the heart of the family, devoting all his time to my sickness, and that his attitude had affected everyone, even my friends. My Dad made them part of it all, was considerate to them, and explained the situation to them in detail again and again.

It's true: after all of that, the structure of my family's interactions changed forever. Without ever making a big deal of it, we began to spend much more time together. Lunches, activities, weekends at the beach, fishing trips down South. Not as an obligation, but out of love. That unspoken change made life better for all of us. Uke is absolutely right.

Not that I thought about this while I was in the hospital. This awareness would only come about later. Back then I was still in that rebellious stage, that first step so typical in mourning: rebelling against fate, against the random occurrence that changes your life without any warning whatsoever, and that, somewhere along the line, will force you to reflect on what to do, now that the jigsaw puzzle of life has fallen to the floor and the pieces lie scattered everywhere.

There was time enough for these thoughts. One of the last nights I spent in the hospital I insisted that my family go home and rest, and I stayed on my own, watching a movie called *127 Hours*. It's the real story of an American climber who decides to go out on his own and, unluckily, gets his arm trapped under a rock after a rockslide. Five days go by until he decides to cut his arm off with a penknife with a very blunt edge. The movie shows in retrospective many of the thoughts that climber had. He recalls decisions he regretted, and thinks about what he'll do if he survives. He does not think about his job or the car he's just bought, or anything like that. His thoughts revolve around his family, his friends, the joys of life, and love. When the movie was over, I turned on the light in my room at *Clínica Las Condes*, opened my laptop, and wrote a few emails apologizing to a few people who, because of my ego, I'd mistreated. I also decided there and then that the first thing I'd do once I left the hospital was to buy, with my savings, some land in *Matanzas* –a seaside spot at which I'd been kite surfing for some years, and that I'd build myself a little house there. At its entrance, it'd have a big sign that would read *House of Joy, La casa de la alegría.*

During the days I was in the hospital, some of my friends didn't show up. I'm not one to hold

* Dad cancelled all activities linked to the companies, and devoted his entire time to understanding my sickness and looking for a solution.

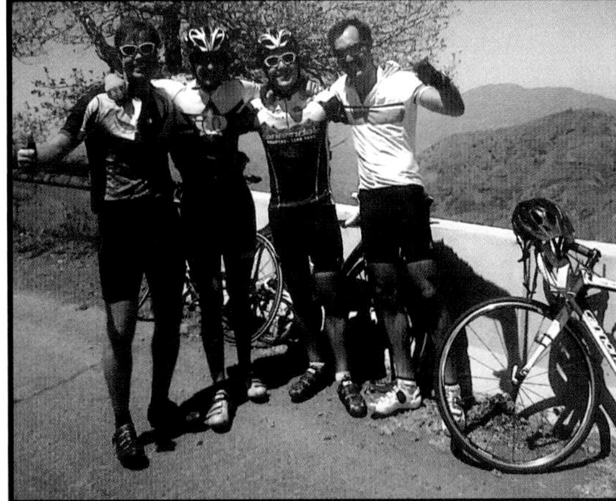

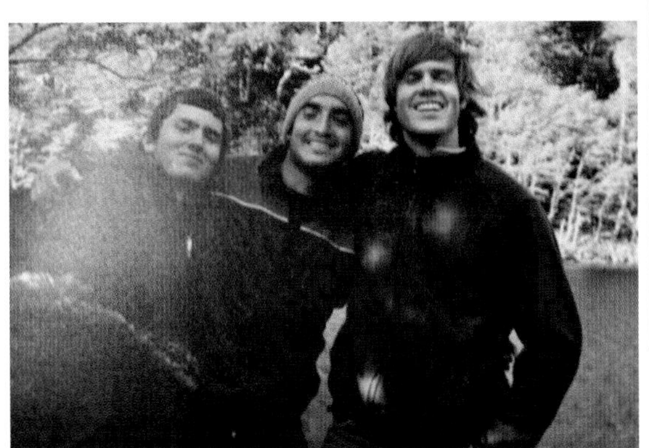

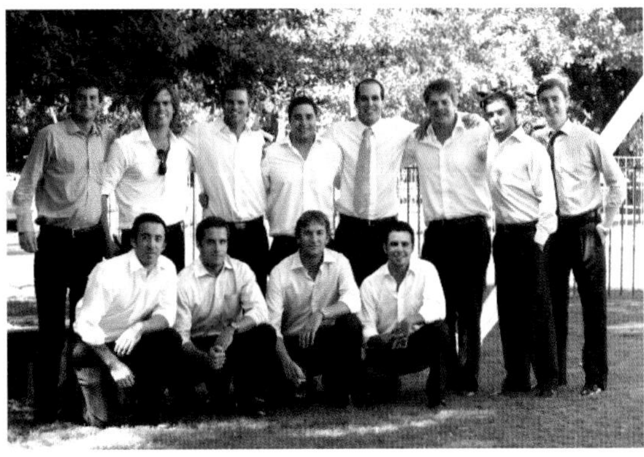

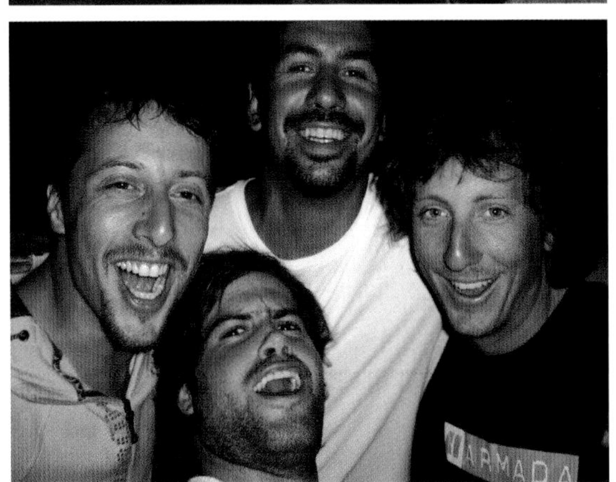

It was very moving to see people from everywhere visiting me while in hospital: my friends from the bicycling world, my kitesurfing group, my schoolmates, the people from Touch. Good vibes flowing and doing me good.

grudges. They sure had their reasons. I don't feel, and never felt, angry at them. Many of them called me regularly afterwards and said they didn't know what to do, whether to visit me or not. They thought they might be a nuisance. Maybe they weren't confident enough. I understand. It's not easy to deal with the idea of someone they had always seen extra-active to be suddenly seriously ill. ***But I can say this: It's better to listen to a friend talking awkwardly, than not hearing from him or her at all.***

As I got ready to go home, I didn't know that my Dad had continued to battle in the war against my illness. The post-surgery recovery was in progress, I'd be discharged, and would have to go back into the world. How would I face things from that moment on? I had no idea. I knew I had to be in bed because my arm kept hurting like hell. During that time, and without my knowing, my Dad and Sebastián had contacted Pepe and José Coz, and had commissioned them with coordinating with my friends to keep them near, for them not to leave me alone, for them to visit me and distract me.

In medical terms, the information was that I had had all the lymph nodes of my right arm pit removed, and that 2 of them had been contaminated. The probability of the melanoma having metastasized in another organ was of 30%. There was a 70% chance of the illness having simply come to a stop. In other words, those 2 infiltrated lymph nodes didn't necessarily mean a propagation of cancer to the rest of my body.

So my Dad, in record time, coordinated meetings and visits to the best oncologists and dermatologists in the United States and, also, learned about the subject with as many specialists as possible in the different private and public hospitals in Chile. His was a marathon. He set all other activities aside, told his secretary he was unavailable to anyone and everyone. He delegated all business responsibilities to his business partner, and let it be known that he was unavailable because he was busy –body and soul– learning about and gathering information to do with my illness.

Sebastián remembers perfectly how my family "went to war". My Dad was the leader, but according to my brother, he was a studious, obsessive, sensitive, and such a perfectionist that he was almost obnoxious. Sebastián says he was in such a state of concentration that he became unbearable, because he didn't want anything to escape him. He also says he realized there is a loving dimension to my Dad that moved him –my brother– and pushed him to work harder.

My old man compiled a huge file with all the information he'd gathered. Pages and pages of research, opinions of Chilean doctors, contact data from doctors in the U.S., cancer research hubs in Europe, treatments and their pros and cons.

* I opened my laptop, and wrote a few emails apologizing to a few people who, because of my ego, I'd mistreated.

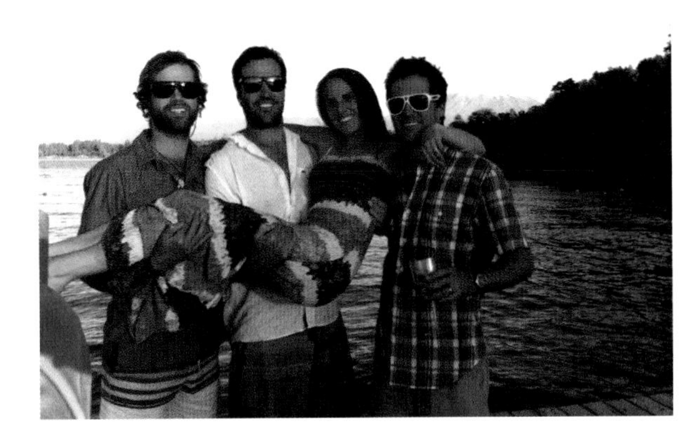

Along with my siblings, Sebastián, Antonia, and Tomás, during the celebration of Antonia's civil wedding, in the Summer of 2014. Each of them has had a paramount role in my healing process.

* At a family level, everyone assumed his or her duty. My Mom's was to keep the family together. My sister's job was to keep my mom company and distract.

Pages and pages of notes, sketches, and percentages, dates of meetings with Chilean doctors, names of people who had suffered a melanoma, specialists to visit if in the States –an option he proposed, but that I chose to postpone, because I wasn't ready to travel when I first left the hospital.

Within the family everyone took on their role. My Mom recalls hers was to keep the family united, the house running. She filled it with flowers, she played hostess to every friend who visited to learn how things were going. She'd call Pepe, whose duty was to always have a friend by my side. Antonia would back her up in all of this, and her friends never left her alone. At the time I didn't know it, but as she divided flowers into vases my Mom would cry, thinking of the possibility of my dying. Antonia was strong and, just as she'd promised my Dad, never left my Mom's side. She devoted herself to distracting Mom, talking to her, being there for her. What I do know is that, since my sister couldn't cry in front of my Mom, she'd do it on her own, once she went to bed.

Tomás also had his role: he was the one to sort of armor-plate me. Everything had gone so quickly, and a way had to be found to break hard and painful news to me. An "emotionally healthy" way, in the words of my brother. I had to have a good attitude in the face of my sickness. If I crumbled, everything could get worse.

Tomás later told me he'd seen my parents very affected by all of it, even in tears at the beginning, when the news was like a bucket of cold water on their heads. He says my Dad would refer to the *tsunami*. That was a shock. It's harsh to realize that you can be the epicenter of profound movements in your family structure. My brother is amazing: a hands-on guy, practical, determined. Which is why it doesn't surprise me what a rock-solid support he was to the whole family, right from the beginning. He made a slogan of Doctor Coz's words: "We're taking the road of the healthy, not the sick". Throughout it all, he kept everyone's spirits up.

Tomás stopped going to work while I was in the hospital, and he set himself to work along with Sebastián and my Dad. He would take his laptop with him, research the net, check videos from speakers on melanoma, compare, confirm, rule out. All of that while at the same time dealing with the risky pregnancy that his wife, Caro, was enduring.

For his part, Sebastián went with my Dad to the meetings with doctors and interviews with patients that had gone through the same experience. Many friends got in touch either with my Dad or Tomás, to give them information and, so, a network was born. That's how they confirmed that chemotherapy does no good in the case of a melanoma, and that neither does radiotherapy. Also, that there is no effective procedure against this type of cancer. It was a time of hectic work for everyone. And one of enormous uncertainty. Sebastián says they didn't know where to start.

* Many friends got in touch with my father to supply him with information, and thus it was that the support network was born. It was a time of hectic work for everyone.

CUADRO

Probability of metastasis depends on::

METÁSTASIS	**ROBERTO**
Size	1.5 mm
Micro / Macro	it's micro – that's good
Mitotic index	Low
Ulceration	No
Regression or not	We still don't know
N° of compromised lymph nodes	3 or less would be +/- the same as 1
Spitzoid	A little better (chance of metastasis)
Study of cells:	Will define metastasis capacity.
More accurate assessments on the way (quickly)	

THIS WAS ONE OF THE CHARTS MY DAD AND 2 BROTHERS PUT TOGETHER WITH MY MEDICAL DATA AND THE INFORMATION THEY WERE ABLE TO GATHER.

They received tons of information that had to be organized and hierarchized. Would it be better to get treated in Chile or abroad? If outside Chile, what would be the best option? The cancer center in Australia, the one in Houston, or maybe the one in New York?

This family battle against melanoma generated a list of doctors and centers around the world that dealt with the illness. They contacted them, but it wasn't easy. They were renowned doctors in their countries, leading figures in their field, in high demand. Doctors that wouldn't even return calls. Yet, tenacious as he is, my Dad sent over 600 emails, and managed to get on the phone with everyone he was trying to contact. During that stage, the role of Isabel Valdés, his secretary, was essential. She helped with unbelievable perseverance, getting contacts on the phone and by email. Isabel, whom I adore, had also suffered from melanoma in situ (that did not metastasize) some years ago. She's known me since I was a boy, and she's very close to the family. So she was an enthusiastic and devoted participant in the tasks my Dad commissioned her with.

Sebastián and my Dad compiled a medical file with all the information on my melanoma, and sent it to each of the doctors in the U.S. that had been recommended to them. Finally, they put together the schedule for a clinical tour, planning to travel as soon as I felt strong enough and emotionally ready. In this task, they received a lot of help from the Chilean oncologist Benjamín Paz, from the Hospital City of Hope in Los Angeles, California, who kept coming up as a recommendation from family acquaintances. Mario Valdivia, another friend of my Dad's and a former board member in some of my family's companies, was also a big help. Mario had lived in Boston and understood the American medical system. According to Mario, the way in which my Dad tackled this mission helped him channel his worries about me and the anxiety that my cancer produced in him. That is why he devoted himself to the task. He says there was no way he could have seen him sitting at a board meeting, since to do so would have taken his attention from the illness. My Dad was getting his Master's in melanoma.

 My brother Sebastián and my Dad organized our clinical tour, starting from a long list of doctors and centers around the world that treat this illness.

For her part, my Mom felt –and still does– a lot of rage for what happened to me. She'd seen that mole long before it was removed, she'd commented on its ugliness, and had for some time thought that there might be something wrong with me, but she never connected the dots. Who could have? My mother and I have always communicated well with each other. As she puts it, we are very much alike in the way we see life. She is very sensitive, and talking about the cancer made us both suffer. So we avoided the topic. Still, I always felt her company and her devoted and loving care. ■

3. (Post-surgery)

Off with the tie

In personal terms, the stage that followed that of the surgery was one of the most complex throughout this process. Beginning to understand that my attitude effected those around me was a difficult realization.

I **lived through the post-surgery** period in a bewildered state: They removed lymph nodes I never even saw, and everyone around me looked at me with worried expressions, when just 2 weeks before I'd been perfectly well! I had left the hospital, but didn't know what to do or where to start. So I just thought: 'What the hell... I'm going back to work!' I still hadn't internalized what had happened.

I hadn't yet fully understood what a malignant melanoma was when doctors and my family had already started talking about what to do and the way to go now. I listened, yes, but I couldn't make much sense of it. Information wasn't making its way into my mind as quickly as the cancer had gone into my lymph nodes. I needed time, space, hours to think about it!

My Mom started her own research, and received lots of information from her friends and acquaintances. One day, she got home and said that it might be good for me to meet some Loreto Agurto woman, who'd had the same cancer as me. She insinuated that talking to her might be really helpful. "No, thanks," I replied.

To be honest, I was in no mood for meetings with, and advice from, strangers. Plus, I imagined that anybody in my situation would only be talking religion and faith and whatnot. It's not as if I don't believe in God, but the idea of that kind of advice seemed superfluous at the time.

In the middle of all that general confusion what surfaced was a very strange selfishness. I was just starting to envisage what I was going to do and I was slowly trying to accept my situation. I didn't

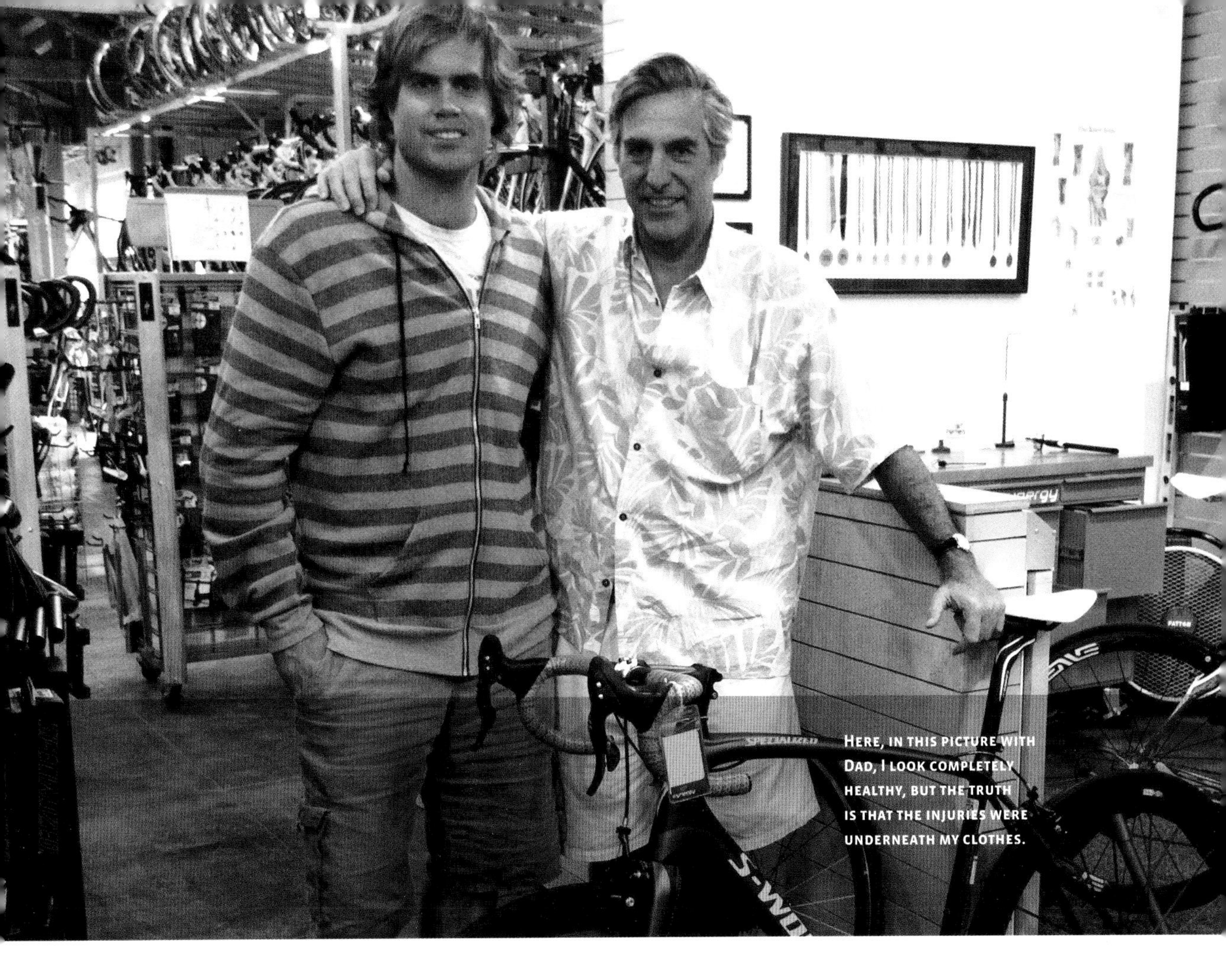

HERE, IN THIS PICTURE WITH DAD, I LOOK COMPLETELY HEALTHY, BUT THE TRUTH IS THAT THE INJURIES WERE UNDERNEATH MY CLOTHES.

want to be bombarded with information. I didn't want questions from my family. I needed to move at my own pace, even if it was slow and selfish.

Of course that slow rhythm of mine drove my folks crazy. But I wanted to be the one to make decisions. On my own. It was a tense period for everyone. I would have loved back then to have gotten hold of this book, to understand how hard it is to internalize the illness when you've got cancer; to learn about the stages in the process and use them to your benefit. I like that Doctor Vial told me it never crossed his mind to disregard my opinion: I was informed about everything that he discovered. However, at the same time, Dad, Sebastián, and Tomás seemed more interested in the development of disease than I was. And they kept attacking the doctor every so often. "I didn't want to marginalize any of them, because I realized their intention was to support you, to do things as best they could. To not make any mistakes in the decisions that were being made. I respected that attitude. It was your family. They love you," he told me when we had that heart-to-heart conversation.

Still shaken by everything that had happened –and so quickly–, I just didn't take the post-surgery recovery too seriously. I was so enraged that I kept saying really dumb things. Without meaning to, I kept hurting those around me. For instance, Sebastián had for a long time been planning a surfing trip to Indonesia with his friends. Yet, he cancelled it to keep me company and to be there, along with Dad, for anything I might need. One day, while talking to him, I said, in a very derogative manner, without even realizing it:

"Be honest: you didn't go to Indonesia 'cause it's been ages since you stood on a board and you're fat." Sebastián felt really bad about that, and he obviously got mad at me. But he didn't say a word to me. He just took it on the chin and swallowed hard. He understood. I didn't. Through the interviews he gave for this book, it's only now that I realize the reasons behind his decision. And I now understand when he says I hadn't yet gauged what that cancer really meant to my family.

It really took me a long time to understand that cancer isn't a disease or condition that only affects the patient. It radiates throughout the entire family. I only understood that, and many other things, thanks to the opinions and experience –wisdom even– of many individuals who endured cancer, who accompanied their parent or their child in the process. I held long conversations and interviews with them. Their words enlightened my personal process and, at the same time, gave a very special value to this book, which, of course, isn't only mine. It belongs to all of those who took part in it by sharing their unique and intimate perspectives.

Through all those I interviewed, I discovered that sometimes patients can be very selfish. That they become very egotistical and lose perspective of the big picture. Especially in terms of the effects of their cancer on those around them. Learning that it wasn't only me who reacted like that was quite a relief. One of the people I interviewed was journalist **Amaro Gómez Pablos,** who accompanied his first wife, Pilar Ruiz, along the difficult path of colon cancer. He opened my eyes and made me think of my family and the bomb that went off in our living-room. This is part of the transcript of that conversation:

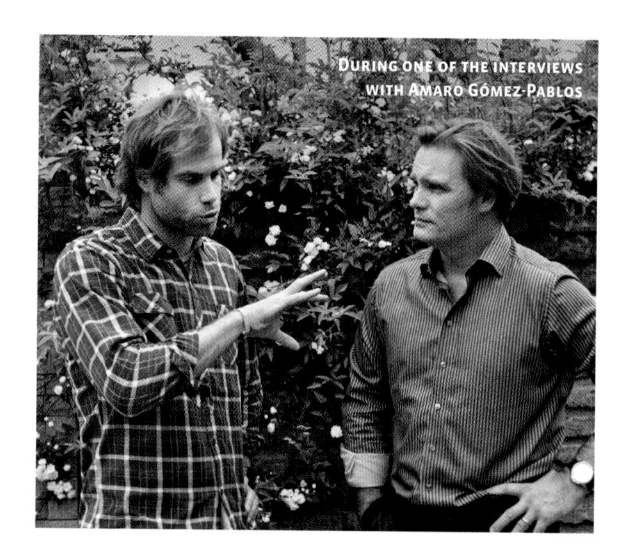

During one of the interviews with Amaro Gómez-Pablos

–What does it mean to be the husband of a woman who is going through cancer?

–Given what happens as a couple and as a husband, I'd say I also had cancer. I didn't suffer from it, but I somehow entered that cancer mindset, and I realized everything becomes urgent. When you love someone with cancer, that concept of having to live the here-and-now –which is basically an ideal– becomes your daily praxis. And it's beautiful, because from that being a sort of picture... it becomes a reality.

–Did you guys utter the word cancer?

–There is a dual purpose, and one which appears to be a contradiction. It's about reconciling 2 opposite poles. It's challenging the cancer sentence to try and eradicate it, while at the same time learning to live with it. Integrating it, so as not to avoid the term.

It's about uttering 'cancer' while looking the person you love in the eye without feeling condemned and fighting to survive. ■

Amaro's words helped me to begin to realize that when a family member has cancer, everyone everyone in the family suffers with them. He made me realize that cancer is a very experience-based illness, whether the prognosis is good or bad. And Amaro faced it, as a husband, with that advice of making it a fully-lived-through experience. "People with cancer generate respect, and that respect triggers a change in their family and in the environment surrounding that person. Because it's waging an enormous battle, one that leaves many scars," he also said. And it made so much sense.

Helping me get acquainted with the reality that the family of a cancer patient lives, the experience of **Gonzalo Muñoz,** co-founder of *Triciclos,* was a big contribution. He and I met at the Aconcagua Summit, an event he organized. Yet, I only learned about his experience with cancer when I was gathering the testimonies for this book. Gonzalo and his wife, Teresa, were faced with the leukemia of their youngest daughter, Rosario, when she was 2 years old. Gonzalo talked to me, among other things, about how hard it is to have a sick daughter, and also about the fears instilled by what his elder 2 daughters might have felt:

–What was it that triggered the greatest fear regarding your 2 other daughters?

–One day, while driving, this image burst into my mind. It was Magdalena, my eldest, who at the time was 7 years old. I pictured her at 20 years old, sitting across from a shrink, telling him: "My life changed when I was 7. My parents abandoned me, they devoted themselves to my little sister's cancer, and I was tossed aside, their 18th priority, if that. My life since then has been one of complete loneliness. And it's been one f... up after the other." In that fantasy, I was a ghost, and I kept telling her: "Baby we'd have done the same for you." Then, in my mind, the shrink said to her: "That's what you perceive, but that's not necessarily what happened. We will need 150 sessions of psychotherapy just to discover it." ■

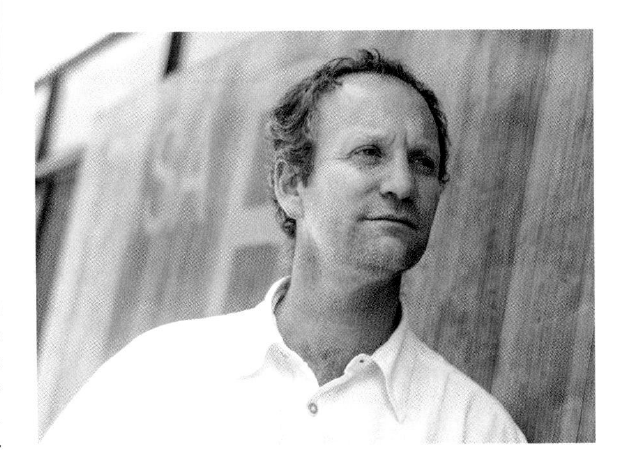

GONZALO MUÑOZ, WHOM I INTERVIEWED, DECIDED TO WRITE A BOOK ABOUT HIS EXPERIENCE AS THE FATHER OF A GIRL WITH CANCER.

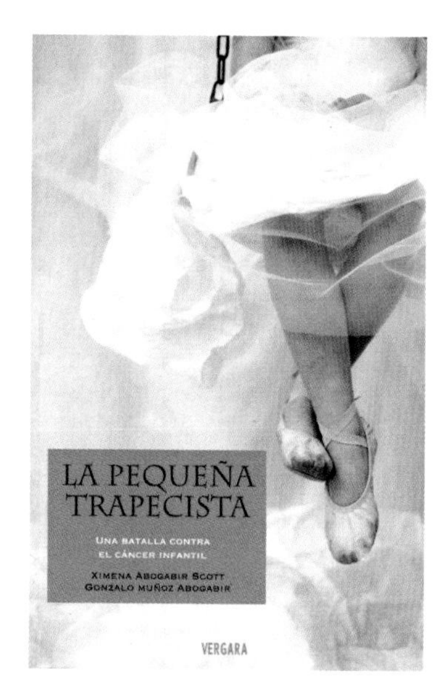

THE STORY OF ROSARIO MUÑOZ, WRITTEN BY HER DAD AND HER GRANDMOTHER

After that, Gonzalo decided to write a book so that his daughters could learn how Rosario's cancer had had an impact on all of them. He wrote the first notes, but soon his mother, journalist Ximena Abogabir, took over and documented through photographs, memories, and drawings, the effort the whole family had made. *That book, La pequeña trapecista [The Little Trapezist], includes the emails Gonzalo used to send to his extended family and friends, and many of the responses he got from them, besides the account by Ximena herself who, with that journalistic rigor of hers, describes the process, which lasted, overall, 5 long years.* With that, Gonzalo managed to get his family to pay attention to all 3 girls, and not just Rosario. He also managed to get daily life to run parallel to the cancer path they were on. "I just hope it saved me the 150 sessions with a shrink," Gonzalo said to me humorously.

> * Upon learning about my cancer, my Mom followed the advice, and researched alternative treatments, always fueled by her endless wish to see me happier.

Cancer really spreads fast towards the support network, the family, and friends. It's not simple for them, and I guess it can also be quite awkward. No one really knows how to interact with someone who's just been diagnosed and how to be a help and not a hindrance on the way.

After the huge number of visits and the support I received during the days I was in hospital, my mother remembers people continued to come to me, with prayers, images of the Virgin Mary, little religious medallions, magic *potions* or prescriptions. She thinks all of that exhausted me, but to be honest it wasn't tiredness I felt... I felt like I was somewhere else, disconnected, with the "Pause" button permanently pressed. Not understanding. Not willing to understand yet. None of this could be happening to me...

Mom didn't sit still at the news of my cancer. She started looking for answers. She followed advice. She researched alternative treatments. I can see in all of that her ever-present and endless wish to see me happier than she felt I was. Mom has since told me how helpful it was for her to me able to open up to people about what was happening to me.

To tell her friends what was going on, because she felt fantastic and heartfelt support. She received a lot of help from her friends. Friends who kept her company, others who sent her images of the Virgin Mary, and religious medallions. She's told me she learned something from each of them, and that thanks to all of them she discovered that no human being is an island. Simple things, said with love and care, which left their imprint. My mother is such an adorable woman, so generous, some people describe her as a true angel... she never lacked support, or company.

When I went home, Mom told me about her discoveries, about people who could help me in parallel with traditional medicine. Once, she took me to the office of a renowned *iridologist*, an eye-healer, from *Viña del Mar* who had also been recommended to me by a friend while I had been in hospital. We had been told it was very hard to reach him, because he doesn't always receive new patients. But we were lucky and got an appointment. During the appointment, he told us I had bacteria in my stomach that had weakened my system. The bacteria had entered my system through food, and I was supposed to follow a treatment with homeopathic drops. His words made sense to me. I had spent years with stomach problems so, ever optimistic, I started taking the drops right away, what harm could it do?

Meanwhile, Dad and my brothers were planning the medical trip to the U.S. and I was again afraid. The prospect of a journey to search for answers didn't calm me down at all. On the contrary, it triggered my permanent and obsessive mechanism of never-ending questions. How were we to interact with doctors there? I sort of hated the idea that was emerging... that of me going with them –my family– rather than them going with me. I wanted to understand, to participate. To star in that show, if you will. Because, I was already the person in the spotlight. I hadn't yet truly internalized the possibility of my own death. I supported the trip. Wanted to go on it. But since I wasn't in control, I couldn't define whether it was what should be done, or if there was another possible path. Some time later, I read what Dad had written in his notes. Had I read it back then, maybe my mood would have been altogether different. Or maybe I wouldn't have believed it. Who knows. I was in the middle of a very complex stage in the cancer process. *My advice is, I insist, to talk inside the family circle and to let everything about the illness be aired.*

Between us we'll find the strength if the news is hard to swallow. Or very hard. This is a lesson that we, the Ibáñez-Atkinson family, learned. This is what Dad wrote down in his notes:

Roberto must participate throughout the process, and he must be part of the team. He must live the entire experience.

At the same time Dad was investigating cutting edge clinical trials on melanoma; where they did them, what the trials consisted of. A clinical trial is research with voluntary patients to determine, for example, if a certain drug is harmless and efficient to treat a disease. Bottom line, it's a road to identifying pharmacological treatments that give results, within certain safety parameters. The rules for these clinical trials are very strict and are provided by the United States Food and Drug Administration (FDA). ***For further info on the ones currently under way, go to clinicaltrials.gov.***

Once his *mega report* was ready, Dad came to some conclusions on the best places and doctors to visit in the U.S., and the scope of the clinical trials –when they were started, how long they lasted, how they worked–, in order to explore the possibility of me being included in one. He thus prepared what would be our "roadmap" in the U.S. It's a binder that includes notes, drawings, and reminders for himself, such as this one:.

Finally, Dad came up with a shortlist of 3 American cancer research centers. All of them prestigious and fully recommended: The Dana Farber Cancer Institute and the Massachusetts General Hospital Cancer Center, both in Boston; plus the Los Angeles Clinic, in California. I know how hard it is to get an appointment with the doctor you want in Chile, especially for the day and time you'd be comfortable with. That's why Dad's work was amazing. In 10 days, he managed to get 11 very renowned and busy doctors from 3 prestigious centers or hospitals to receive us at their offices. When somebody asks how Dad got that, he answers without any hesitation: "working". That's Dad in a nutshell: simply brilliant.

Still, I also believe he achieved this because at the time he was working with Wallmart. In the U.S., Walmart has an important division dealing with employees' health and wellbeing. They had contacts in cancer centers, and they helped him ensure that doctors would see us during our trip. This is, in fact, another reason why I wanted to

THESE ARE SOME OF THE TASKS DAD WROTE DOWN BEFORE WE TRAVELLED

- Contact Dr. X.
- Tomorrow: meeting with work committee along with Roberto.
- Contacting Houston. Urgent.
- Daily schedule.
- Contact 3 clinics. Call
- Watch videos.

write this book: Dad managed to get in touch with those doctors, but I know that is an exception. *This is why I am sharing here everything they told me, strictly based on the exhaustive records Dad compiled, and on my own recollections.* Sometimes, after a doctor's appointment, I'd leave more confused than when I'd gone in. Sometimes with double the questions, or fears. Yet, I also felt some relief and a certain amount of confidence, or ease. Dad made sure he took notes and highlighted the most useful tips. True, they specifically focus on my melanoma, but many of the suggestions I got are of vast and general application, and can be useful to more than one person. At the time I was pretty much resigned to fate, so I accepted the proposal: I would travel to the U.S. with my parents, Sebastian, and Mario Valdivia. However, I decided it would be me who would ask the doctors about each and every doubt I might have. Call it past experience: I know for a fact that when it comes to my family, the best way to bring something up isn't by establishing conditions, so I chose to –very sincerely– thank them for what they had done for me. Just before we got on the plane, I sent them an email. In the subject I wrote: *Off with the tie.*

Mommy, Dad, Seba, and Mario:

I would like to thank you in advance for the mind-set and willingness you have shown in joining me on this trip. The truth is... this "off with the tie" vibe we get from the emails we've recently exchanged, is just how I imagined things would be. I believe the doctors and specialists we are visiting will get this, and that I will, therefore, be able to get the most out of what they'll tell me. And in the process, we will be well informed as to where we stand.

I feel very calm, and I'm going fully willing to listen and learn.

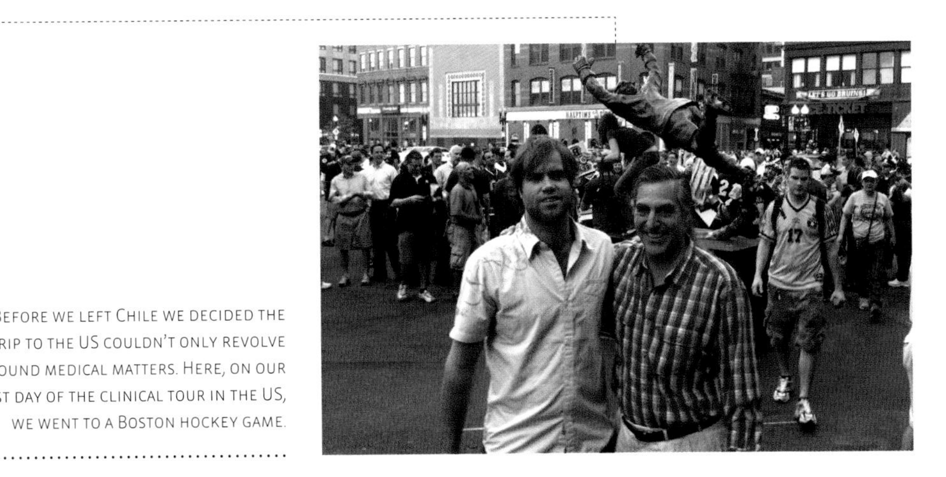

Before we left Chile we decided the trip to the US couldn't only revolve around medical matters. Here, on our first day of the clinical tour in the US, we went to a Boston hockey game.

While carrying out their exhaustive research, my parents had come across a name that had nothing to do with allopathic medicine: Mark Mincolla.

Mincolla is a naturalist doctor from Cohasset, near Boston, who treats diseases starting from the angle of people's diet. He has a perspective about being healthy that ended up setting the *before* and *after* standards of my recovery process. Iván Mimica, a friend of my parents in Chile, had recommended Mark. I will talk about Iván later, since his approach to food influences the way I eat even today.

Mario recounts that before our trip began, one of the things that most stressed them out (him, Dad and Sebastián), was that, from L.A., Benjamín Paz seriously recommended that I participate in a clinical trial for *Ipilimumab*.

Ipilimumab is a drug belonging to a class of medication called monoclonal antibodies, which act by helping the body to delay or stop the growth of cancerous cells, and it's used to treat melanoma that has disseminated in the body.

What didn't convince Dad was that, in a trial, some patients try the allegedly effective new drug while others receive placebos; I could be one of the latter patients.

Paz sent the papers anyway, since the trial was about to close its registrations, and he was hopeful because of the recommendations he had received from specialists in California.

But in the end, with all the pressure I felt, I decided not to take part in the trial. It wasn't a decision taken lightly; I thought about it a lot and leaned on Dad for advice. He consulted several of his medical sources and acquaintances. *Ipilimumab* is mostly recommended for Stage-IV cancer patients, I was in Stage III, according to the scale that measures the progress of cancer in the body. To be honest, it just didn't seem necessary or justified; the risk was too high and the benefit unclear. I would have had to stay in the U.S. for several months –throughout the duration of the clinical trial– and I pictured myself, alone, in a hotel room. I was convalescing, and it wasn't in my best interest to be away from my family. Having taken part in that would have been an unnecessary trauma, another stone to add to the heavy bag I was already carrying, so to speak, and one which, as enthusiastic and passionate as I am, was getting heavier and heavier by the day.

Sebastian agreed. He didn't believe clinical trials were the way, either. He thought it might not work out. A high percentage of the people participating receive placebos, so as to have a control group. You might get the new drug... Or you might not. And it may also well be the case that the drug doesn't work. Plus, the side effects of this drug knock you out, they leave you wasted. This on top of something I only learned later when a doctor in Los Angeles told me that several patients had died of diarrhea during the trials. I had been suffering from an awful diarrhea for a couple of years by

* My parents came across a name that had nothing to do with allopathic medicine: Mark Mincolla, a naturopathic doctor who would mark a *before* and *after* in my process.

then... *Ipilimumab* is the last option in the face of an advanced and aggressive melanoma.

Once the decision was made, Dad asked Mario to deliver the samples of my biopsies to a pathologist at the Memorial Sloan-Kettering Cancer Center in New York, in order to validate the results of the exams and biopsies undertaken in Chile. That way, the doctors we were consulting would have them available. There'd be no need to go there. Dad spoke to the super-specialist on the phone.

Pathologist Álvaro Ibarra, from *Clínica Las Condes*, helped us with this. Although it's unusual for a pathologist to speak directly with a patient – let alone with his family– he met with Dad and explained to him in detail the results of my biopsy. He gave him the *tacos* (the cross sections of my biopsy placed in wax) so that they could be checked at the medical centers we visited. This was key. I know the pathologist made an exception and I thank him for that. His was an optimistic report, according to the opinion of experts in melanoma surgery, such as doctor Gustavo Vial.

Stages in *Cancer*

The stage or status refers to the extension of cancer. It helps in understanding the seriousness of the disease and the survival rates, so as to determine the best treatment plan, and to identify the clinical studies that may be an option for the patient. The universally accepted system is the TNM classification, where T refers to the size and extent of the tumor. N refers to the number of nearby lymph nodes, and M refers to whether the cancer has metastasized. The TNM system helps describing cancer in detail. Also, for many cancers, TNM combinations are grouped together in 5 less detailed stages or statuses: 0, I, II, III, and IV, associated to the prognosis of the disease.

Stage	**What does it mean**
Stage 0	There are abnormal cells present, but they haven't disseminated to the nearby tissue.
Stage I, Stage II, and Stage III	There is cancer present. The higher the number of the Stage (I, II or III), the bigger the tumor, and the more extended it's to the nearby tissue.
Stage IV	Cancer has disseminated to distant parts of the body.

Source: cancer.org

We set off for the United States towards the end of May 2011. Dad took his "road map" with him -all the information gathered and crosschecked, dates, appointments, questions, doubts- so that on our return we could determine *which treatment I should follow to combat the feared resurgence of a melanoma. One of the most pressing questions that needed answering dealt with Interferon, since it's one of the few treatments that seemed to work for a cancer like mine. Interferon* is an immuno-modulating substance that helps the immune system act over cancerous cells. It doesn't get rid of cancer. In simple terms, it's a substance called *cytokine,* which we all produce when faced with a viral infection; a protein secreted by the cells in the presence of viral infection. Its mission is to protect the cell from infection. The immune system activates itself when it detects the presence of *Interferon.* It produces a generalized inflammatory response in the body. That's why you feel so bad after you are injected with it. It's as though you were injected a virus to then generate the symptoms of a strong cold.

Obtaining conclusive information on *Interferon* was essential. Dad had asked around about this substance; had questioned doctors and patients in Chile alike. Although some recommended its use, opinions were divided. We would also ask about the PET CT, a key control exam in patients diagnosed with cancer. It's run to detect the stage of the disease or if there is metastasis. It's also used to assess the results of therapies. There were several paths: You could get it every 3 months, every 6 months, on a yearly basis, or not at all. The PET CT is a very invasive exam; you are injected a type of radioactive contrast liquid filled with glucose in order to detect the areas that are swollen in your body. *

* *Interferon* produces an inflammatory response from the body, so that it attacks the cancerous cells. Despite some doctors having recommended it, opinions were divided.

We had no way of knowing what would happen, but at least I was finally able to feel some ease: *I would start confirming data and ruling out possibilities. Now my family and I would have a much clearer big picture.* ■

* *Please check the impact of glucose and refined sugar on the body in the chapter* You Are What You Eat (Page 170).

- *All evidence of cancer was removed, and around the scar was only healthy tissue, with nothing being spread further. It's very unlikely for something to have remained between the original location and the lymph node. All 'skin' cuts are negative.*
- ***19 lymph nodes, all of them negative for tumor.***
- *'Highest' node, negative.*

=> 20 negative nodes.

NOTE 1: *Probability here for cancer to flow through the blood is really low.*

NOTE 2: *Normally, the paths are:*

- *From the exterior part of the original location to the Sentinel node.*
- *From the Sentinel node to the other nodes.*
- *From the other nodes to the other organs.*

ASUNTO: Sending information requested.

Dear Bethany,

I have asked my secretary, Isabel Valdés, to send you an attachment with the information requested on my son Roberto F. Ibanez:

1) Medical Record
2) Medical Report
3) Pathology Report
4) PET – CT Report
5) MRI Report

I will carry with me the PET-CT images contained in a CD. Please mail me at with any comments or further requirements.

Yours sincerely,
Felipe Ibanez

SR. ROBERTO IBAÑEZ ATKINSON

1 TACO Nº105198 (taco blanco)
20 TACOS NºS11-2184 (tacos verdes)

26 LAMINAS HE (color rosado-azul)
10 INMUNOHISTOQUIMICAS (láminas pálidas, algunas con color café oscuro)
(en total son 36 láminas de vidrio).

I STILL GET EMOTIONAL WHEN I SEE HOW PROFESSIONAL MY PARENTS AND SIBLINGS WERE WHEN IT CAME TO GATHERING AND ORGANIZING THE INFORMATION THEY FOUND, SO THAT THEY'D UNDERSTAND MY DISEASE, AND DOING EVERYTHING IN THEIR POWER TO HEAL ME. THIS MATERIAL IS JUST A SMALL SHRED OF EVIDENCE OF WHAT THEY WERE ABLE TO GATHER

4. *Touring* US Hospitals

Not everyone who's ill can travel abroad for medical answers. I hope what I found may help others. I learned a lot, arrived at my own conclusions about my disease and, above all, I discovered that food can heal.

Two destinations were clear: Boston and Los Angeles. As I learned later, this journey was necessary for my father because it would determine what the chances were of my being healthy. And also what the chances were of having cancer after my surgery. In a nutshell: the chance that I'd survive. Life or death. He didn't mistrust Chilean diagnoses, but he felt that, as qualified as they were, he couldn't leave his son's life in the hands of 2 people. He said that to every Chilean doctor whom he consulted. Chile wasn't enough for him, he wanted to get in touch with every person he considered useful for his goal. Dad is unstoppable when he sets his mind to something.

The day we arrived in Boston we rested for a while and I went with Sebastian, Mario and my father to an ice hockey final. One of the teams competing was Boston, so we rooted for them. Mom stayed at the hotel. It's odd, we were on this "medical mission", but this was definitely one of the most relaxed trips we've ever been on as a family. They were all really attentive and worried about me. Dad asked for my opinion, what I thought about things. This lowered my anxiety levels and made me feel in charge of what was going on. The *Off with the Tie* email was working!

Mario was in charge of entertainment on the trip. We moved around together in a van he drove. Once the agenda of the day was completed, Mario took care to get us to "*Cancer* mode OFF". When we got off "work", we had a good time, chatting about anything but cancer.

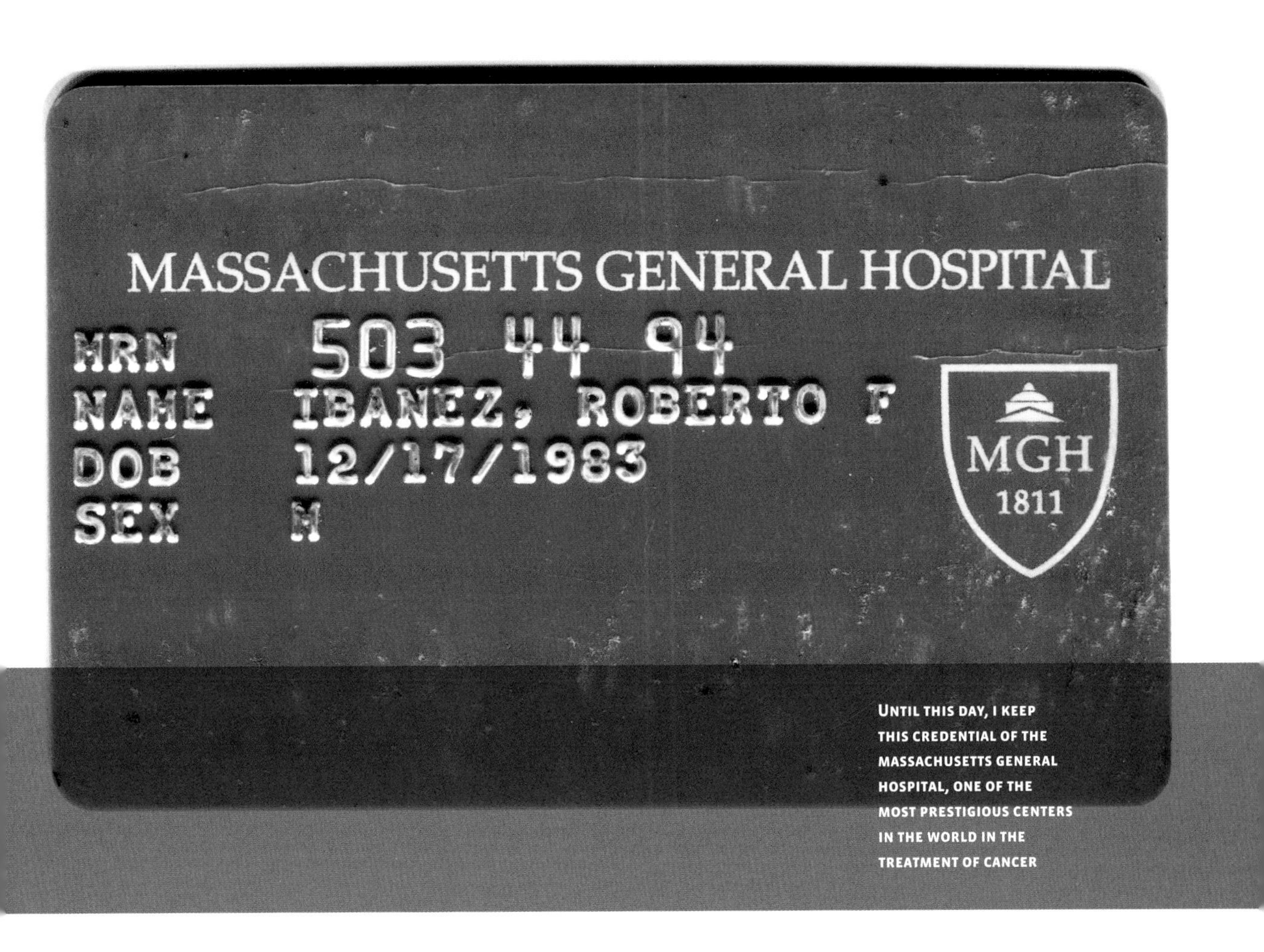

UNTIL THIS DAY, I KEEP THIS CREDENTIAL OF THE MASSACHUSETTS GENERAL HOSPITAL, ONE OF THE MOST PRESTIGIOUS CENTERS IN THE WORLD IN THE TREATMENT OF CANCER

The first day of the tour, we were visiting Mark Mincolla, the food and nutrition expert that Iván Mimica had recommended. Mincolla turned out to be a *guru*, and visiting him was a decisive move. In Sebastián's words, he convinced us all that the path to follow was naturopathic medicine. That I had to recompose my body, regain balance, and be healthy again in order to reassemble my defenses. I'd say he convinced us. Before we met him, my mother was the only one to have some faith in Mark.

When I went into his office in the Santi Holistic Center, enlivened with Hindu music and incense, I didn't come across the archetype of the white bearded, tunic-or-the-like type of man I'd imagined. He was dressed formally, but not *'doctorish'*, if you will. He talked slowly, and it was impossible not to just be quiet and listen to him. Sebastián remembers him as profound, nice, and captivating. In his office, he asked how long I had been on antidepressants, and why was I on them. He also wanted to know when my stomachaches had begun, where exactly it hurt, if I'd had any sort of surgery and, if so, when. In a sort of bliss, I answered his every question. Strangely enough, I felt really comfortable.

It was then that Mincolla told me something that stayed forever in my mind: "You have an enormous charisma and a spectacular strength to move forward on the day-to-day, which is the hardest thing to do and what knocks most people down. The problems are your worries from the past and those about the future. If you can face those I strongly believe you will become a person with a beautiful long term view".

I 100% identified with what he told me. I woke up every day and wanted to see the good things in life, be happy, move forward. But unfortunately for some time now I'd been ill-at-ease.

Mincolla listened to me attentively, and then gave me his diagnosis. He said that at some point I had lost balance, that my defenses were seriously reduced, and that the few left had been focused on fighting illnesses for a long time. According to him, my body had been fighting for far too long; it was stressed out. My uncomfortable chronic diarrhea came immediately to mind. For Mincolla, it all made sense, although I should emphasize here that one thing wasn't necessarily a consequence of the other. The diarrhea was a warning sign as to how badly I had been taking care of my body, but not a cause or manifestation of the melanoma.

Specifically regarding my cancer, he told us that he saw it as a fungus, an inflammatory disease of the body. His opinion on *Interferon* was lapidary: "It is crazy to destroy the body in order to cure it." He made absolute sense.

I wasn't convinced that the *Interferon* was a valid choice for me. Doctor Vial, my oncologist, had specified that it was the only medication providing a degree of certainty – from 7% to 15%

* According to Mark Mincolla, my body had been fighting for quite a while. It was stressed out. I immediately thought of my so very uncomfortable chronical diarrhea.

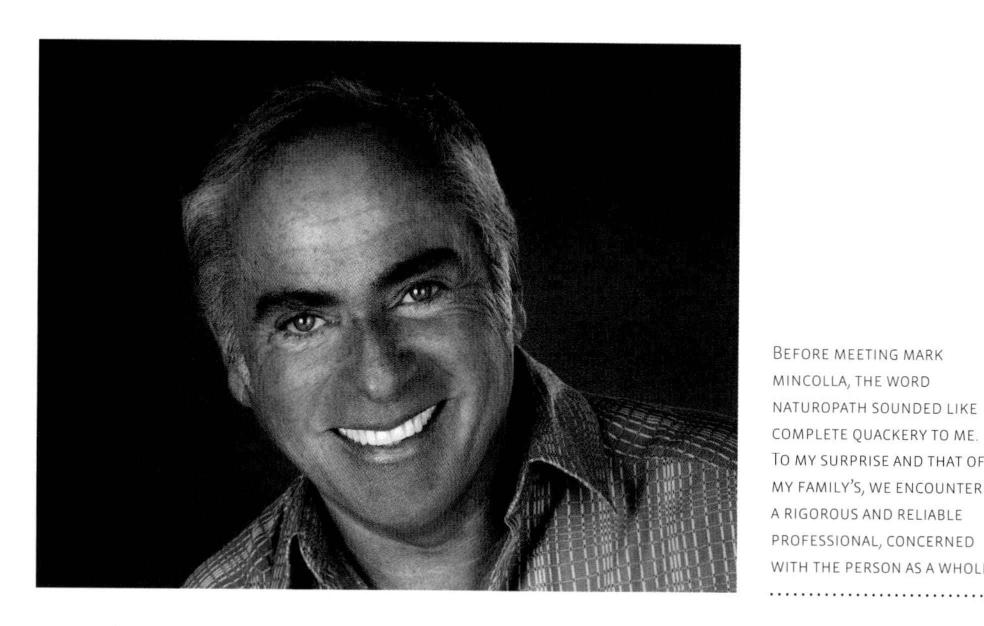

BEFORE MEETING MARK MINCOLLA, THE WORD NATUROPATH SOUNDED LIKE COMPLETE QUACKERY TO ME. TO MY SURPRISE AND THAT OF MY FAMILY'S, WE ENCOUNTERED A RIGOROUS AND RELIABLE PROFESSIONAL, CONCERNED WITH THE PERSON AS A WHOLE.

effectiveness – but he didn't recommend it as treatment, since not much was gained. He was emphatic: Interferon may delay cancer for some months, or some years, in the best-case scenario, but not cure it. This on top of the fact that many of the doctors and patients we consulted with, and who have tested Interferon, underscored its adverse effects regarding quality of life.

Mincolla then presented me with a list of practically all existing foods, before subjecting me to a very curious test that, as he explained to us, is a combination of tools of ancient Chinese medicine with modern research in nutrition. He started to go over the foods one by one. He stood before me, pressed my stomach with one finger and said: 'Close your eyes and extend your left arm to the height of your shoulder' (it would have been impossible for me to do so with the right arm, for the pain and the scar of the surgery). With his hand pressing against my extended arm, he would name the foods. *Apple*, for example. If my arm didn't resist the pressure of his hand, he would murmur: 'This food is bad for you'. In order to find out how bad it was, he would again press his hand against my arm, and assess its resistance. When he said *'banana'*, my arm sort of collapsed. Sebastian was flabbergasted. He knows I never eat bananas, because I feel horrible afterwards. He continued with other foods, and he pin pointed one by one those usually giving me a hard time; besides many others that, according to me, didn't. We were all impressed. Mom, who has always been very intuitive, believed he was right about everything. Mincolla explained afterwards that this Electromagnetic Muscle Test is based on the fact that the nervous system *knows*, so to speak, the bar code of your energy, and your muscles tend to weaken upon the mere mention of a food that doesn't fit such code. That's why my arm kept falling when certain foods were mentioned.

Just as the *iridologist* had done back in Chile, Mincolla detected that I had a bacterial imbalance in my stomach and body. He didn't speak about the medical issue, he only recommended that I follow a diet. According to him, regular medicine artificially interferes with processes. It treats effects and not causes, while he focuses on the cause. But sure, if you have a malignant melanoma, you have to treat its effects, and Mincolla understood that in my case I had to do both: diet and treatment.

> * Mincolla detected a bacterial imbalance in my stomach.
> If I wanted to get better, I had to make a radical change in my diet.

Mincolla explained that I had to make a radical change in my diet, which would mean a great sacrifice from me if I wanted to get better overall. He added that if I followed his instructions, my diarrhea could be dealt with forever. This was the first time I ever heard somebody say that with complete confidence! Among the thousands of forbidden foods that he named, I

Food chart with color code

Alkaline foods   Neutral foods   Acid foods

Acid foods that turn into alkaline ones whenever there is a stable pH.

Animal protein

- Beef
- Chicken +1
- Clam
- Cod
- Crab +1
- Egg white -2
- Yolk -2
- Sea Bass +7
- Southern Ray's Bream +7
- Sole +9
- Ham -6
- Lamb -10
- Liver
- Lobster +1
- Pork
- Salmon +1
- Sardine
- Prawns +1
- Shrimp +1
- Octopus +1
- Tuna +1
- Turkey +7

Dairy and its substitutes

- Cheese
- Rice milk
- Rice cheese
- Cow milk
- Yoghurt
- Almond milk
- Soy milk
- Soy cheese
- Soy yoghurt

Legumes

- Beans
- Black beans +1
- White beans +1
- Soy sprouts / Tofu
- Lentils +1
- Chickpeas
- *Pinto* beans

Nuts and seeds

- Almonds
- Cashew nuts
- Macadamia nuts
- Peanuts
- Nuts
- Pistachio
- Sesame
- Pumpkin
- Sunflower

Fats

- Avocado
- Butter
- Coconut
- Cream
- Margarine
- Ghee
- Vegetable oil
- Olive oil

Vegetables with low starch content

- Arugula
- Asparagus
- Brussel sprouts
- Cabbage
- Khale
- Cucumber
- Cauliflower
- Celery
- Chinese cabbage
- Eggplant
- Endives
- Lettuce
- Iceberg lettuce
- Hydroponic lettuce
- Garlic
- Green beans
- Turnip
- Leek
- Mushrooms
- Onion
- Parsley
- Cilantro
- Basil
- Radish
- Chive
- Sprouts
- Chard
- Watercress
- Zucchini

Vegetables with high starch content

- Artichoke
- Beetroot
- Carrot
- Chestnuts
- Corn
- Lima beans
- Peas
- Potatoes
- Pumpkin
- Sweet potato

Grain produce

- Amaranth
- Barley
- Buckwheat
- Milet
- Quinoa
- Oats
- Rice
- Brown rice
- Rye
- Wheat
- Spelt

Sugars

- Barley malt
- Sugar
- Brown sugar
- Honey
- Maple syrup
- Rice syrup
- White bread
- Cane sugar
- Stevia
- Yeast

Acid fruits

- Grapefruit
- Kumquat
- Kiwi
- Lemon
- Lime
- Orange
- Pineapple
- Strawberry
- Tomato

Sub-acid fruit

- Apple
- Apricot
- Blackberry
- Blueberry
- Cherry
- Grape
- Mango
- Peach
- Nectarine
- Papaya
- Pear
- Plum
- Raspberry
- Mandarin

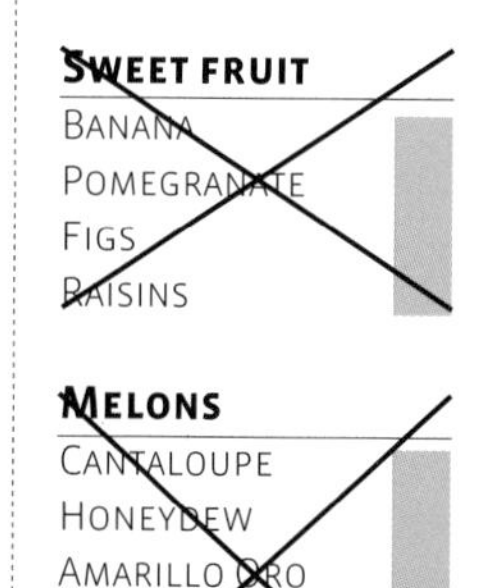

* This is the table of acid and alkaline foods that Mincolla prescribed to me and that still guides my diet. The general guideline is very simple, for each gram of acid food you eat, you have to compensate it with four grams of alkaline food. In my case, the foods in yellow were those that were best for me at that time, according to Mark's test. Food marked in red instead, did no good to me, and all food crossed out was forbidden. This table is repeated without colors in chapter "You are what you eat", in order for everyone to use it as a guide.

identified several of them right away. From now on, no more sugars, no more junk food; no more red meat, and no more booze. I would have to say goodbye to all of that since my body was poisoned. And what about my life? The parties, the barbeques, my friends? From then on *my thing* would be special food, ultra-healthy, a change for everyone at my house... no milk, no wheat. Never again processed foods. Phew! There was so much that was restricted, and so little I could eat. But how could I continue to feed myself off things my body supposedly rejected?

Along with all of that, he prescribed that I should sleep well, practice sports, continue to work, and be disciplined in what I ate. ***"You have the power", he told me. "Clean your body and your mind".***

When we left the doctor's office, we were absolutely convinced that we hadn't wasted our time. Mincolla's explanations seemed pretty coherent. I left with a list of what I could and couldn't eat. And, obviously, there were a lot more forbidden foods than permitted ones. I couldn't eat pork, or any corn, or mushrooms. All things we often ate at home. Rice would have to be brown and the chicken organic. That was what I retained in my mind. How the hell was I supposed to do all that? I thought about my plans to move out of home and in with friends. How would I get around it if every day I needed special food? Most shocking of all was that Mincolla didn't propose a temporary change in my diet. If I wanted to remain healthy it would have to be for the rest of my life. Another idea that had to sink in. Things weren't looking so easy for me. The visit to Mincolla gave us hours of conversation.

The second day started with a meeting at the Massachusetts General Hospital Cancer Center. We were welcomed by dermatologist James Click who, after a physical, gave me guidelines to take care of myself: 45 SPF sunscreen as a minimum, taking 1,000 mg of Vitamin D per day (since I cannot be exposed to the sun), annual ophthalmologic exam (because the melanoma can reappear in the eye), monthly personal check of the skin, and with a dermatologist every 3 to 5 months during the following 6 years. Doctor Click warned me: "People who have had melanoma may produce a second one. The thing is to detect it on time". Damn!

After that meeting, we met with doctor Hensin Tsao, also a dermatologist and top expert in melanoma at the same hospital, recommended by Patricio Vives, a Chilean pediatrician living in Boston for the past 40 years. An almost unreachable eminence if it hadn't been for Dad's invincible perseverance. Like Click, Tsao already knew the result of my exams. I've since learned that my mother complained and was very frustrated and angry at not being able to come with us to doctor Tsao's office. Mario says they thought it would be best because it would be a moment of great

* No more junk food. Mo more red meats. No more booze.
I would have to let go of all of that. Because my body was poisoned.

stress for her. I'm sure that Sebastián and my Dad didn't want to subject my Mom's feelings to such pressure.

As I see it, though, a decision like this one is a matter of personal choice. She should have been the one to make that decision. It is good to live through the bad things to later enjoy the good ones. Remembering the bad things you went through makes you stronger. One ought to *live* the sorrows since, as I see it, that is a learning experience. Besides, it's different to *live* them than to be *told about* them. I would have let Mom be with us every step of the way.

Doctor Tsao was very kind. He listened carefully to all of our questions, and made an effort to address our doubts.

I haven't said this yet, but my melanoma was a spitz-type tumor, and he explained that this had a better prognosis. However, he warned me that I couldn't stop worrying. He also said that young patients with this type of melanoma respond much better than adults. In fact, he commented, there's a school of oncological doctors that think this type of melanoma may not be cancerous.

One piece of advice he gave me during the appointment – and that I would hear of later from other specialists – is that I had to analyze all choices, and only then make a decision. And to then not look back. He also reminded me about something I believe to be so true, and that I tended to forget amid the mess of events: 'Roberto, today you are healthy'.

But the most amazing thing of all, was that this guru of melanomas changed the percentages and improved my statistics. He told me that, according to the results of my biopsy and the type of melanoma, the probabilities of the cancer spreading to the rest of my body were 20%. It was very big news, since I now had an 80% chance of the cancer chapter being completely closed, and not a 70% chance, as I'd been told in Chile.

* The visit with American dermatologist Hensin Tsao improved my statistics: The chance of my cancer spreading was 20%, not 30%.

Even so, that 20% made my stomach ache. Each passing minute, I concretely understood more of what was happening. Each figure, each medical term I learned, each treatment he mentioned, *plugged* me, so to speak, into my fragile reality. That 20% instilled respect. Cancer was still there. Intimidating. Restricted to a percentage that ruined my life perspective. I tried to be optimistic and stay with that 80%. It was hard. So at the time I found it easier just not to think about it.

The doctor gave me a complete physical. Head to toe. He checked my moles and told me something I already knew: That I had exposed myself too much to the sun. That is why he recommended that a dermatologist in Chile carry out a check-up every 3 to 6 months, because, through a simple checkup, you can detect a melanoma on time. Before it has a chance to become really dangerous. This is how later on, in Chile, I met a doctor that has been a fundamental support: dermatologist Francis Palisson, who I'll talk about later.

With Tsao, we again talked about the famous *Interferon*, a very sensitive subject for me and my family, because it is the only treatment that one can follow in the event of a melanoma. Tsao recommended it, but he suggested that there was also the option of not doing anything, and that in fact I had to consider that it had not been tested on spitz-type melanoma that I had. He ended up by saying that the PET CT exam, which indicates whether a tumor is localized or has disseminated, was irrelevant.

I left this eminent doctor with mixed feelings. I would have wanted him to say, *take the Interferon!* or, *do not, on any account, follow that treatment!* But hey, the medical tour was about me making decisions. I thought it was going to be simpler to take the lead on this matter, and Tsao's words didn't help. Luckily, though, that 80% was slowly injecting optimism into my overwhelmed mind.

That same day, in the afternoon, we had to see an oncologist who is a specialist in *Interferon*, doctor Donald Lawrence, from the Melanoma unit of the same hospital. He said I had to think of my melanoma as a real one, even if it was a spitz-type melanoma (in other words, he wasn't about to go soft on it as Tsao had done). And he added that its treatment doesn't have a simple, nor an obvious, answer.

Then he said that doing nothing was as good a decision as any, and that he'd respect me if that was what I decided to do. But, he added, he thought I should seriously consider using the drug, because it could reduce a potential metastasis by 10%, according to the research he had. He highlighted that benefits are modest, that it has annoying side-effects, and that it doesn't cure melanoma –although some could consider themselves cured if there is no metastasis. He insisted: *Interferon* could make a difference in my case, but that I had to take into consideration my chronic diarrhea. I told him I am a very active person,

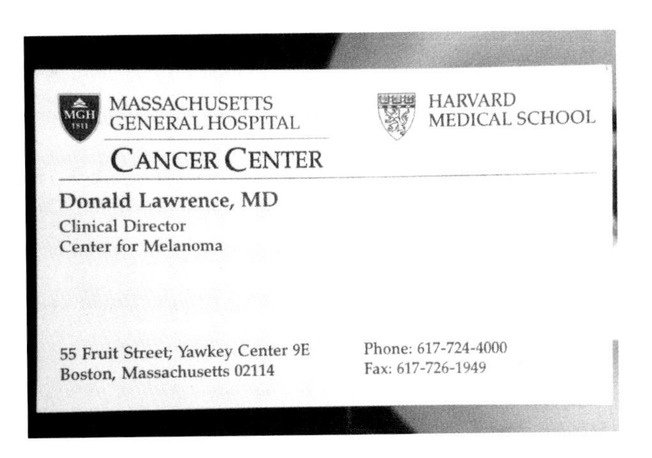

Doctor Donald Lawrence's business card. He was one of the doctors I met in Boston.

that I practice sports and that from that point of view, *Interferon* was no good for me, given the negative effects on quality of life.

According to Lawrence, using *Interferon* for a year might be overwhelming, but he noted that the first 4 weeks of intensive treatment are the most relevant: "Set your mind to it: You do it for the first 4 weeks and then get on with your life. I would do that. You have virtually 100% chance of feeling well after finishing the treatment".

–Will *Interferon* help?–, I asked.

–Until now, research says it doesn't help.

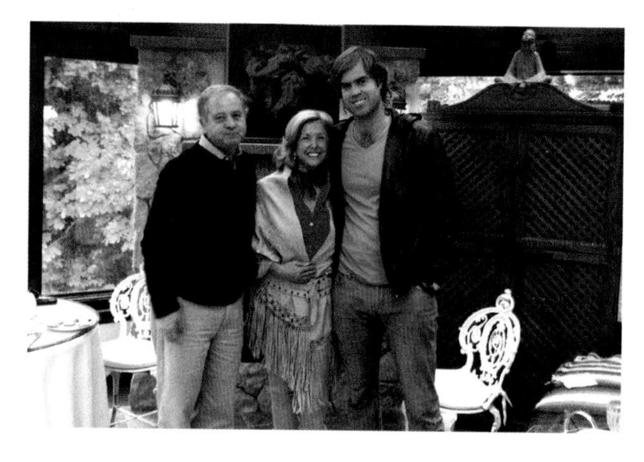

WITH MARIO VALDIVIA AND REBECA RÍOS, THE WIFE OF CHILEAN DOCTOR PATRICIO VIVES, BASED IN BOSTON, WHO HELPED US SPEED UP THE MEDICAL CONTACTS, GAVE ME EXCELLENT ADVICE, AND EGGED ME ON.

Curious answer, to say the least. It seemed impossible to find out the truth about the famous drug. For Lawrence, the consequences of a metastasis are so serious that it was worth at this stage exploring all options, *Interferon* included.

On the frequency of the control exams (PET CT), he told me that it depended on each person's philosophy. He recommended I get them every 6 months, but that there are those who prefer to do so every 3 months, and others that prefer not to take them at all. He warned me: other apparently abnormal things that could worry me may appear in these exams. But he added that, most likely, they wouldn't be linked to a melanoma. ***He told me to trust my doctors for the correct interpretation of the exams.*** And he emphasized that in 5 years-time, i.e. in 2016, the outlook would have completely changed, since the drugs used on Stage IV patients would be able to be used on stage III patients. "Things are moving fast", was his encouraging message.

Despite this doctor supposedly being a specialist, he didn't offer any certainties. He insisted I had to do it, but he didn't give me a clear answer, guidelines, or concrete results. He didn't even mention his experience with patients. He only repeated that I had to do it. Honestly, every new piece of information left me in an even greater state of confusion.

What I considered the *turning point* was the visit, that same Friday, to Doctor Choi, a famous gastroenterologist in Boston. I wanted to consult him about my diarrhea. He said it was chronic, that I wasn't going to die because of it and that it wouldn't get any worse. That it would most likely go away alone. He said this type of diarrhea is a functional digestive disorder, and that it usually occurs in young people with anxiety or stress. Once these factors are kept at bay, it might disappear. He prescribed the obvious: reducing booze, increasing water and fiber intake in my diet, and taking a medication that, according to him, would slow down the work of my colon. I would have to take it for a long time, despite one of its side-effects being the feeling of my mouth being very dry. Then I realized how absentminded I was as I'd been prescribed it in Chile and was in fact already taking it.

Between all the visits to the doctor's offices, one day we went to visit the northern beaches of Boston, and had lunch with doctor Patricio Vives and his wife. The two of us had some time alone during a drive we took up to his house in the suburbs. We talked and he asked questions related to my thoughts about what was happening to me. We addressed the subject of my options and *Interferon*. We got along from the get go, and meeting him and listening to him helped me make my decision. The pieces of the puzzle signaled –red lights and all– that *Interferon* wasn't necessarily the only, or the best, choice.

That same afternoon I received a very caring email from him:

"Dear Roberto,
It was very nice meeting you. You have enviable drive and tenacity. I know you are going through hard times, but the picture will become clear. I was impressed by your courage and originality to start your new group (he referred to Touch) *that, after these years, no one doubts was a good move.*
It's the same at these crossroads you are living. I wish you luck and for you be able to choose the best path in order to have a serene future.
Think several years ahead, and not about the immediate future. This will help you decide.
I enclose a comment by Teddy Roosevelt, a great American President:

"It isn't the critic who counts; not the man who points out how the strong man stumbles, or where the doer of deeds could have done them better. The credit belongs to the man who is actually in the arena, whose face is marred by dust and sweat and blood; who strives valiantly; who errs, who comes short again and again, because there is no effort without error and shortcoming; but who does actually strive to do the deeds; who knows great enthusiasms, the great devotions; who spends himself in a worthy cause; who at the best knows in the end the triumph of high achievement, and who at the worst, if he fails, at least fails while daring greatly, so that his place shall never be with those cold and timid souls who neither know victory nor defeat".

Big hug,
Pato

Back in Boston we focused on the Dana Farber Cancer Institute, one of the centers with global experience in immunotherapy for melanoma. We wanted to talk to a specialist who had been recommended to us, but he wasn't in town for the week. So, we were welcomed by doctor Angie Tsiaras. She didn't say anything very different from what we'd already heard. She told me that the possibility of my being completely healthy oscillated between 75% and 90%. She gave me concrete indications: 50 SPF sunscreen every two hours, use of special anti UV t-shirts, feeling my lymph nodes. She recommended PET every 3 to 4 months during the first 2 years, every 8 months until the fourth year, and from the fifth year onwards, every 12 months. She also told me that spitz-type melanoma was more benign, but that it had to be treated as normal melanoma. ***Also, she told me it was mandatory that I check all my moles at home, including those on my back, because of the probability of developing a new melanoma. She added that every 3 months I had to check up with a dermatologist.*** On *Interferon,* she told me that it is a controversial therapy. That there is medication that helps palliate its side-effects, and that it might postpone for a year the reappearance of a potential new melanoma.

Later, we went to see Doctor Nageatte Ibrahim, who told us that the surgical treatment performed in Chile had been suitable for micrometastases like mine. She specified it was in an A-III stage of melanoma. The stage refers to the reach of the nodes to the cancerous cells; i.e., whether cancerous cells in the lymph nodes can be seen with a microscope and if the primary tumor is ulcerated (that the epidermis or the external layer of the tumor isn't intact). I was in A-III stage (after there is B and C). IV is what comes afterwards, the worst stage.

On *Interferon,* she said that in 15% of the cases it postpones for 8 months the reappearance of melanoma and that the chances of it not working were higher than of it working. Contrary to what I'd been told, she was categorical when explaining to me that one month of *Interferon* didn't make any difference, that younger patients tolerate it better and that she recommended a minimum treatment of 3 months and maximum of 6 months with this drug. But she also suggested I focus on being healthy and do everything to achieve that. I said to her:

–I want to feel good and I am in the process of a healthier life. My decision for now is not to take *Interferon.*

Then she commented that there was evidence that Vitamin D did a lot against melanoma. I have to say that this recommendation –given to me before– is the only one I didn't follow from the beginning, but only from 2013. I didn't do so, because Mark Mincolla indicated specific food from which to obtain it.

* I told Doctor Nageatte Ibrahim that I was in the process of achieving a healthier lifestyle and that, for the time being, I have decided not to take *Interferon.*

As I had followed my new radically restricted diet without taking calcium supplements, when I fell off my bike and took a bone-density test, it showed that I was in the lowest segment of the normal range of calcium. That's when I met Doctor Mario Sandoval, whom I will tell you about later. He ran my tests and Iván Mimica completed his treatment with Vitamin D, which makes calcium affix to the bones easier.

Exhausted, we went to the oncological surgeon James Cusak, who got straight to the point: *Interferon* isn't good; there are no strong indications of its benefits.

In fact, according to Cusak, it may kill a patient. "Remain healthy, exercise, and reduce stress. Taking care of your immune system is a very good idea." He also suggested that once I made a decision about my treatment, I should follow it. I liked him.

The last stop of the medical tour was Los Angeles. There, we went to see oncologist Omid Hamid, of the Los Angeles Clinic, who from the beginning warned me that the use of *Interferon* may aggravate depression. He attributed a 3% of the benefits to this medication. He said it was bad that I had 2 nodes infiltrated, but the good news was that it had been a micro-metastasis; my melanoma didn't measure more than 1,5 mm, wasn't ulcerated, and it was spitz-type. The latter improved the prognosis and probabilities. He advised me to follow the therapy with the least side-effects "You have a microscopic disease in a slightly aggressive melanoma". If I decided to take *Interferon*, he recommended a full year.

I asked:

–Doctor, if you were me, what would you do?

–*Interferon* doesn't give a clear answer so I would have to think it through a lot. I suggest you do things that don't affect you and that adapt to your current life style.

I liked his clarity. Slowly I was untangling the skein of crossed-information. He told me that the one-month clinical trial of *Ipilimumab* wasn't useful at all, and that a natural way to face my melanoma was to reduce the levels of stress, a healthy diet and lifestyle, and Vitamin D. He told me that the alternative of natural medicine was a good path. He supported the diet that Mark Mincolla proposed. I felt immediately in sync with this doctor. In fact, it was he who had invited me to the clinical trial of the *Ipilimumab*, but as soon as he read my medical chart, he assured me that if I had chronic diarrhea this drug isn't practicable. He had known patients who had died due to the diarrhea caused by the drug. I felt a chill down my spine, and it didn't stop because, right away, Hamid explained bluntly that if I was within the 20% of patients whose melanoma makes metastasis in another organ besides the nodes, I had 5 years left, at the most. It was hard to hear, since that 20% that Doctor Tsao told me in Boston was seeming less terrible... but Hamid

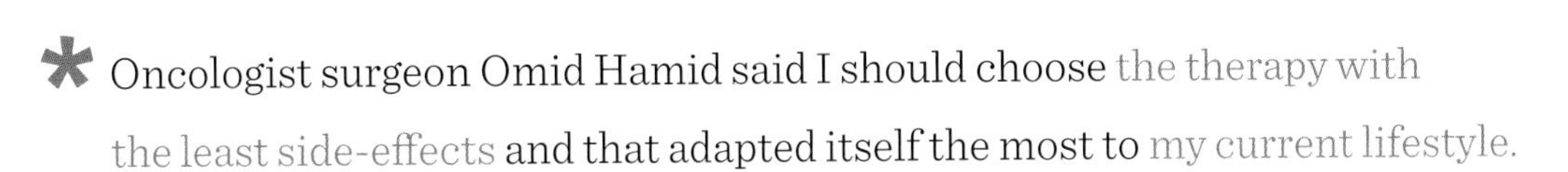

was straight-forward: If the melanoma came back in another organ, it would be a death sentence. He was one of the first people to make me see how dangerous my cancer was. And then, like a slap in the face, I saw it all. For the first time I could gauge the potential tragic consequences of the melanoma. In a sort of dizzying flashback, I relived everything that had happened to me from the time I answered the call of the dermatologist in my garden, and then I realized that my family had understood my vulnerability much earlier than I did.

That night we had dinner with Doctor Benjamín Paz and his wife, an encounter that made quite an impression on me. He made me concen-

* I understood that I had to deal emotionally with cancer days and cancer moments, emotional states affecting many patients.

trate on the positive side of Tsao's figures: I had a 75%-80% chance that the disease wasn't recurrent, and he highlighted that I was 100% free from the disease. In his opinion, my goal had to be for my immune system to defend me from an eventual recurrence. His prescription for this was simple: to live a good life together with an exhaustive analysis of my moles and clinical check-ups. "If there was any recurrence, this would manifest in clinically detectable nodes that may be removed. The body sends signals when there is a problem!" He recommended the PET every 6 months, not more often, because there is no connection with these exams and the survival rate. He repeated that *Interferon* is useless and that he doesn't recommend it to any of his patients. According to him, it has been proven that it doesn't increase the survival rate, and that that's what matters. It delays the time in which the melanoma manifests itself, but the survival rate is the same. He instructed for me to avoid situations in which the immune system gets weak, such as excess alcohol, diseases, surgeries, stress, and excessive fatigue. Cigarettes, alcohol... That's why every doctor had asked me: *Do you drink? Do you smoke? Do you take drugs?* That night, Doctor Paz shared with me a secret I already sensed: There is no experience that isn't worth living, there is no wrong decision.

It was a conversation I won't forget. We talked in depth about what he calls cancer days and cancer moments, emotional states that he has repeatedly seen in his patients. He told me I had to be patient. Everything he said was so useful to me, that when I got to the hotel I wrote down every one of his words so as not to forget them. "Suddenly you meet someone or you see something that reminds you of the fear and the pain, and you relive the anguish of the days of your disease. You have to accept them. You have to assume that that isn't a good day and that it is going to pass. Those flashbacks occur all the time and usually last a few seconds, but they can also last days. The important thing is to learn to deal with them and live them as positively as you can. They are a part of you, they are important and intense, but they go away".

He generously shared 10 very useful tips for anyone who is living through cancer and that reflect the spirit of this book. This is why I reproduce them in this book.

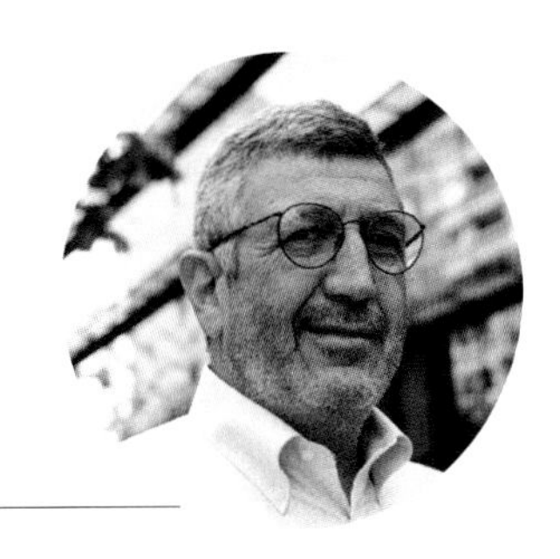

Tips from Benjamín Paz

1. *Every experience in life is a good experience. Good things come out of everything. From this point of view* ***there are no wrong decisions.***

2. There are some experiences that shift your perspective on the world. Cancer is one of those experiences. Remember that nobody looks at the world from the same perspective. Therefore, there are as many points of view as people in this world.

3. *As Bill Gates' father wrote: "You have to plunge into life, you cannot be a bystander".*

4. *You have to worry about living a good life. You have to be happy in life. I will repeat it:* ***only live well.***

5. At this precise moment, you are 100% healthy. You cannot give the tumor any chance. You have to live a healthy life.

6. *Luck is on your side, not the tumor's.*

7. *You will have cancer days and cancer moments. Take all the time you need to think. Also tell your loved ones how you feel; this will help them get in-sync with you, understand you and understand how to react when those moments happen.*

8. *When a person says "I don't feel well", the immune system is working on something. It doesn't matter if it is psychological or physical, it's working anyway. Then, protect your immune system. This is for me one of the most important things.*

9. Sleep at least eight hours a day. When the body and the immune system regenerate the best is when you sleep well. Less than eight hours is like you didn't sleep at all.

10. *Have a good breakfast and a healthy lunch. Those are the two most important meals of the day. Remember to stop what you are doing and sit at a table. Don't do two things at the same time. As you get old you will understand better what I am saying.*

Our medical tour wasn't over yet, we had the last specialist to visit. We went to the office of a Catalan doctor, Antoni Ribas, a young celebrity in the research field of melanoma. He told us that from the over 100 studies there are on *Interferon,* only 3 show positive results. From the remaining ones, many of them mention that they harm patients more than they benefit them. One of its big risks is the depression it may trigger. "The benefit is very low and if there are additional risks, it isn't worth taking it. Roberto, you have made the right choice." It was encouraging to hear him congratulate me that way, although naturally a great part of those congratulations were addressed to my parents. Ribas had all his hope in the future: according to him the mutation that makes the cancerous cell grow had already been found. "Lead a normal life" he said when we said goodbye.

Before we came back to Chile I had decided I wouldn't use *Interferon.* After everything I had heard, the most sensible thing to do was to rule it out, as well as all that was invasive to the body, including clinical trials. I would get the PET CT every 3 months at the beginning, every 6 months as of the second year, and every 12 months as of the fourth year, and until the 10th anniversary from the time that I was diagnosed.

I would follow Mincolla's indications to a T. I would make a change in my diet in order to detox. ***I chose to prioritize my quality of life, and in that, my old man was fully supportive.*** Immediately, at his unstoppable rhythm, he proposed that we seriously investigate the autoimmune vaccine for melanoma created by a team at *Universidad de Chile,* about which he had read a story in newspaper *La Tercera* shortly before we travelled to Boston, and of which he'd asked almost every doctor we visited. In fact, he had already made the first inquiries, and when considering the possibility of this treatment, all of them commented *a priori* and without more information than that supplied by my dad, that they thought it harmless and a good opportunity.

***** The *Celebraciones con Sentido* Foundation is a way to pay it forward, to feel that I am alive and contribute to those in need.

About the vaccine I would inform myself later, once I returned to Chile. My hyper-exposed brain wasn't able to handle one more ounce of information.

After all the conversations with oncologists and dermatologists, that had my head in a spin and completely connected with my melanoma, the first thing I asked myself was where did I want to be if I was one of those 20% of patients with a second melanoma. Did I want to be alone or with someone? With a family of my own? With a woman with whom to dream a future together? Then I was filled with doubts and when I placed myself in the worst case scenario, I wondered what legacy I would like to leave when I died. My first thought was spontaneous: A family and many children.

Tendencias

LA TERCERA Domingo 15 de mayo de 2011

Nueva terapia ha permitido sobrevivir a 35 pacientes con cáncer avanzado

- Los pacientes respondieron a la terapia y han logrado una sobrevida superior a cuatro años. El promedio con melanoma avanzado es 11 meses.
- El tratamiento fue creado por especialistas del laboratorio de Inmunología Tumoral de la U. de Chile.

INMUNOTERAPIA CELULAR

La terapia consiste en activar una respuesta del propio sistema inmune en contra de las células cancerígenas.

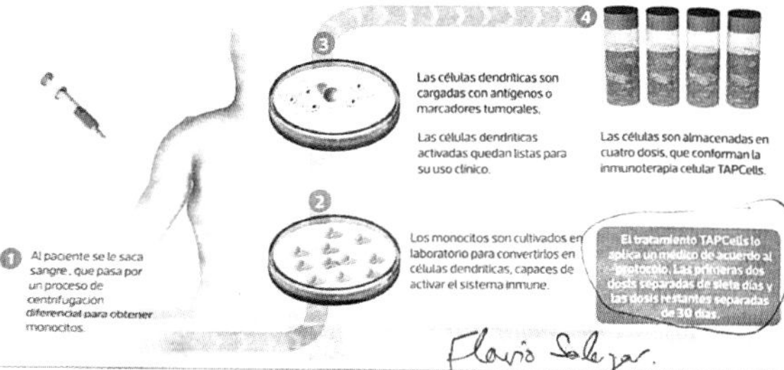

FUENTE: Oncobiomed

LA TERCERA

▸▸ Oscar San Martín se sometió al tratamiento en 2006. Hoy no presenta recaídas. FOTO: RICHARD ULLOA

LAS FRASES

"Este es un caso excepcional. El parece curado de su enfermedad...".

"Las bioterapias van a ser usadas en 20 años más en todos los cánceres".

Mercedes López, *médico inmunólogo U. de Chile.*

José Miguel Jaque

Oscar San Martín (58) culpa a su trabajo. Como jefe de obras de una constructora, pasaba todo el día bajo el sol. Un día de 1997, pidió a su mujer que le viera una molestia en la espalda: un lunar del porte de un ojo y de color rojizo le provocaba picazón y sangramiento. El diagnóstico no fue bueno: melanoma, el tipo de cáncer a la piel más agresivo.

La extirpación del lunar mediante cirugía le devolvió a gotas la tranquilidad. Pero nueve años después, dos bultos en la axila izquierda le jugaron una nueva mala pasada. "En el melanoma, como en otros cánceres, las células pueden migrar hacia otros lugares distintos del tejido de origen. En este caso, lo hicieron a los ganglios linfáticos", explica Mercedes López, médico inmunólogo del Instituto de Ciencias Biomédicas de la U. de Chile que trató a San Martín. La noticia le tumbó el ánimo a Oscar. Hasta que un doctor le comentó que el Laboratorio de Inmunología Tumoral del Instituto de Ciencias Biomédicas y la empresa biotecnológica Oncobiomed estaban reclutando pacientes para probar un tratamiento de inmunoterapia, que consiste en fortalecer el propio sistema inmune entrenando células específicas para atacar el tumor **(ver infografía)**. No es cualquier terapia: los resultados de los estudios clínicos la posicionan como uno de los tratamientos más prometedores en melanoma y que está ad portas de entrar a la fase 3 de la Food and Drug Administration (FDA), organismo que certifica medicamentos de Estados Unidos.

Oscar aceptó ser "conejillo de indias". "Yo hacía todo lo que fuera por mi salud", cuenta. Se trata de una característica de los pacientes que presentan un cáncer avanzado. "Uno se aferra a lo que sea por seguir viviendo porque tiene una mochila. En mi caso, mi familia".

El pronóstico no era alentador: su cáncer estaba casi en etapa 4, donde casi el 90% de los pacientes recae a los cinco años. Pero contrario a todas las posibilidades, Oscar no ha recaído pasado ya ese tiempo. "Este es un caso excepcional. El parece curado de su enfermedad... aunque en melanoma nunca se sabe", dice la doctora López.

San Martín es uno de los pacientes que se han visto beneficiados con este tratamiento, creado por el equipo de la U. de Chile que dirige el Dr. Flavio Salazar, que fue probado con pacientes con melanoma maligno avanzado. La sobrevida promedio de estas personas no pasa los 11 meses. "Cualquier intervención o droga que se aplique a estos pacientes no supera ese periodo", explica Carlos Saffie, biotecnólogo de la U. de Chile. Pero la realidad es otra con este tratamiento: el 60% de ellos respondió a la terapia y 35 de los 121 pacientes tratados sobrepasaron los cuatro años de sobrevida con cáncer en etapa 4. El análisis de los resultados indica que los pacientes que responden a la terapia reducen en un 72% el riesgo de muerte en relación con los pacientes que no responden al tratamiento. "De los tratamientos que existen en el mercado, este es el que entrega mayor sobrevida a los pacientes que responden a él", asegura Saffie. El trabajo con TAPCells fue publicado en la versión de abril de la revista Clinical Cancer Research.

El registro es alentador y una nueva prueba de cómo la inmunoterapia se levanta como novedosa línea de combate al cáncer. "La era de las bioterapias empezó y no va a parar. Las bioterapias en general -uso de células dendríticas, de anticuerpos monoclonales o la transferencia de linfocitos- van a ser usadas en 20 años más en todos los cánceres, ya sea como tratamiento solo o, lo más probable, combinado con otros tratamientos", explica López. Los números de TAPCells son muy buenos: en marzo pasado, la FDA aprobó un anticuerpo monoclonal -el nombre del fármaco es Yerboy- basado en el mismo principio de inmunoterapia, pero que en lugar de provocar una respuesta específica del sistema inmune, inhibe una proteína para que no apague la activación del sistema inmune. En sus pruebas demostró entregar una sobrevida de hasta 10 meses, a cambio de US$ 120 mil y que genera efectos secundarios.

Gana terreno

Si la inmunoterapia va demostrando ser una buena salida, la pregunta es por qué no se usa, entonces, en el inicio de la enfermedad. "La prueba de terapias en cáncer se hace en etapas avanzadas porque existen otros tratamientos ya establecidos y tienes que 'pelear' con ellos", explica López. Y el mejor escenario para dar esa 'pelea' es un estado avanzado, pues los nuevos tratamientos contra el cáncer tienen que probar dos cosas: que las metástasis disminuyen o desaparecen y que aumenta la sobrevida de los pacientes. "Mientras antes se hacen los estudios, mayor tiempo de seguimiento se requiere para saber si una terapia logra efectos. En un etapa dos de cáncer, por ejemplo, la sobrevida es mucho mayor y el tiempo de seguimiento se alarga demasiado".

En el caso de la terapia TAPCells, ya pasó las fases clínicas 1 y 2 -se probó que no tiene toxicidad y que hay un efecto real de sobrevida en los pacientes. Ahora viene la fase 3, de prueba en un grupo de pacientes más grande, un paso largo, caro (cerca de US$ 18 millones) y necesario para obtener el visto bueno de la FDA. ●

LAS CIFRAS

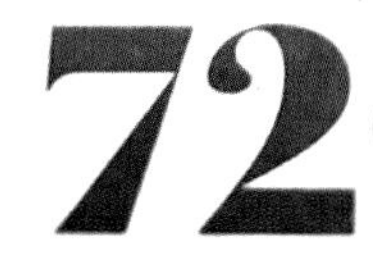

72 por ciento menos de riesgo de muerte tienen los pacientes que responden al tratamiento creado por los científicos de la U. de Chile, en comparación con los pacientes que no responden a esta terapia, según los análisis de los resultados.

200 personas murieron en Chile por cáncer de piel, entre los años 1998 y 2008. La cifra representa el doble que la década anterior.

18 millones de dólares requiere la empresa biotecnológica Oncobiomed para empezar la fase 3 de los estudios clínicos de esta terapia.

"New therapy has permitted 35 patients with advanced cancer to survive"

During my healing process Dad came across this story in newspaper *La Tercera* on an autoimmune vaccine developed by Chilean doctors to fight melanoma and other cancers. A little later I underwent that treatment.

With time, and given the way in which things have turned out, I learned that being close to those you love the most, being a good friend, enjoying life day by day, and even writing a book or creating a foundation, are also a good way of leaving a legacy. You already know it: the book is written and you are reading it. But I also created a foundation. *Touch* organized a birthday party for a renowned entrepreneur, who requested that instead of gifts, his guests should send a contribution to the NGO *América Solidaria.* With this in mind, I came up with the idea of creating a bridge foundation that helped other foundations. That's how *CCS, Celebraciones con Sentido* (celebrations with a meaning) was born: To encourage celebrating something with meaning; to make it fashionable. I created a non-profit board of directors and we began to spread the idea that you could get married or make your birthday party asking your guests that instead of making a gift to you, they donate the equivalent amount of money to one of the foundations supported by us.

Why they would buy a bottle of wine or a last minute gift, if they could help a foundation with which they identified? *Celebraciones con Sentido* makes me happy. It's a way of giving back. Feeling that I'm alive and contributing to those in need.

Given that the melanoma could reappear I felt that I couldn't take my life for granted. So it was impossible for me not to ask myself what I was doing with it. At the time I felt very lonely emotionally, and I guess that's why I held on to relationships without any future. I grabbed something before losing it all. The impact of cancer in my life was like an earthquake: It shook me and made me look at things I had never consciously looked at before. And I decided that life cannot go by without making commitments or taking chances.

My parents stayed in the US for a few more days and I returned to Chile. I began to write my thoughts down, to put on paper what I was feeling. Each line helped me understand myself, to fight my fears, to see life from another point of view, to take a proper look at life and not from the perspective of the hamster-wheel of work I'd submitted myself to in order to validate myself. That trip had been an enormous opportunity and a great learning experience. I decided to write my parents an email, that in some way reflected the change that was happening to me:

"Mummy, Papá!!
(...) We are going to get through all of this, because life is precious and despite my being only 27 years old, I've had to learn various aspects of what it is to live. We have shared so much together in these past few months, and this is a milestone for me. One which is going to mark a great difference for the future.

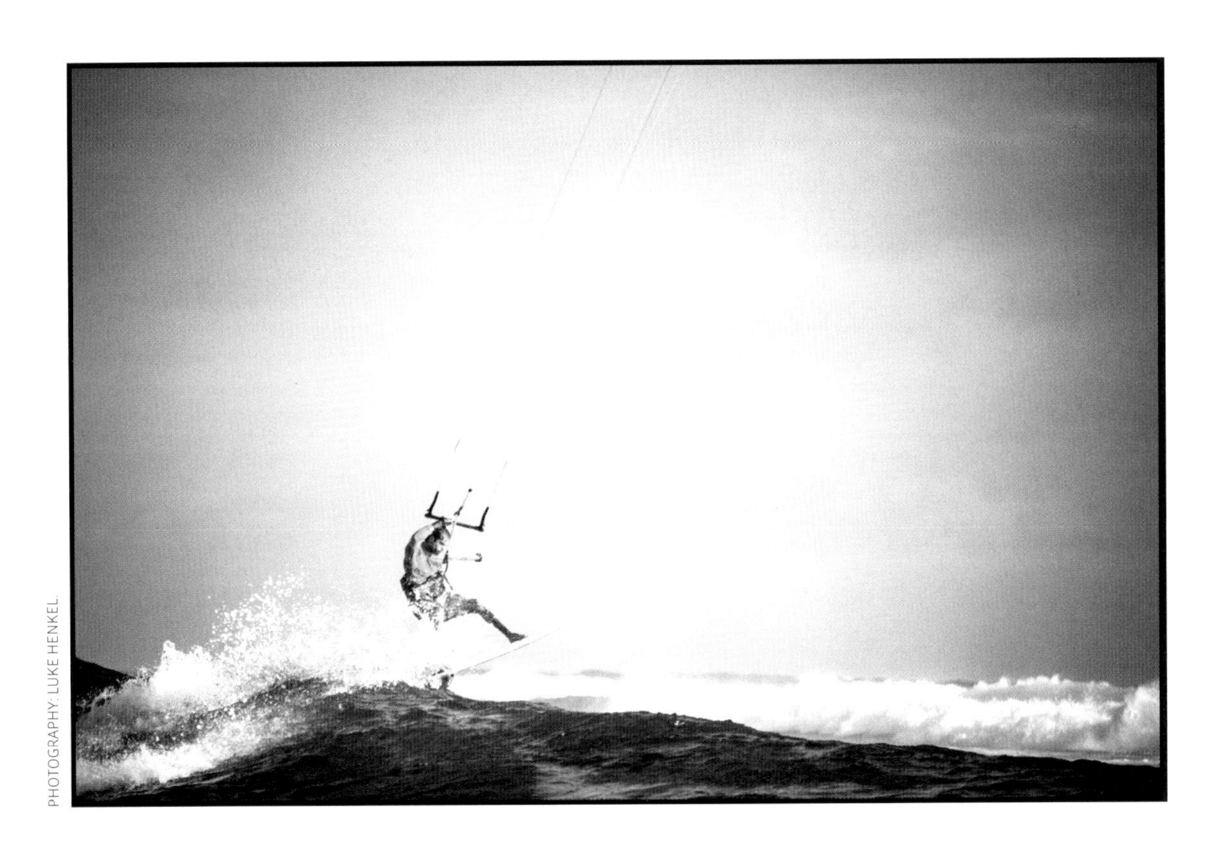

PHOTOGRAPHY: LUKE HENKEL.

WHEN YOU PRACTICE KITE SOMETIMES YOU JUST ONLY ESCAPE WAVES THAT ARE ABOUT TO BREAK OVER YOU. IN THIS STAGE AFTER THE SURGERIES, THE VISIT TO THE US, THE CHANGE IN MY DIET AND THE TREATMENT OF THE AUTOIMMUNE VACCINE, I FELT THAT I COULD PASS MY FIRST WAVE.

5. I will live in the 80%

When you have had cancer, moving forward is an art. This is why the testimony of valuable people you find on the road marks a *before* and *after* in how you face your new reality. As Doctor Coz said, you can choose to walk along the road of the sick, or that of the healthy. I chose the path of the healthy.

Back in Santiago, and after meeting many doctors who were quite cold –surely because they see cases like mine every day– I came across a doctor who surprised me with her warm-heartedness: immunologist Mercedes López. She took the time to answer and explain, one by one, my doubts. Sometimes, the answers to those doubts turned out to be hard blows, as when she explained: "If you had not removed that mole you would be dead today, because malignant melanoma is one of the worst types of cancers". That was the second hard punch I received since my diagnosis. And what a blow it was.

She took care of injecting me with the autoimmune vaccines that Dad had read about in the press, a treatment called TAPCells led by a group of doctors at *Universidad de Chile*, aimed at stopping the eventual reappearance of a melanoma. The vaccine is distributed by Oncobiomed, a biomedical company working with researchers at the university's immunology department. The treatment consists of four doses injected subcutaneously and, for the time being, treatment is not at all affordable for everyone.

Doctor López detailed how this vaccine works: first, the blood of the patient is extracted. Then, at the lab, they transform certain specific cells, called monocytes, into dendritic cells. During that transformation process, monocytes are "fed", so to speak, different types of dead cells that, nevertheless, keep their genetic information. Afterwards, they are reinjected into the patient. Dendritic

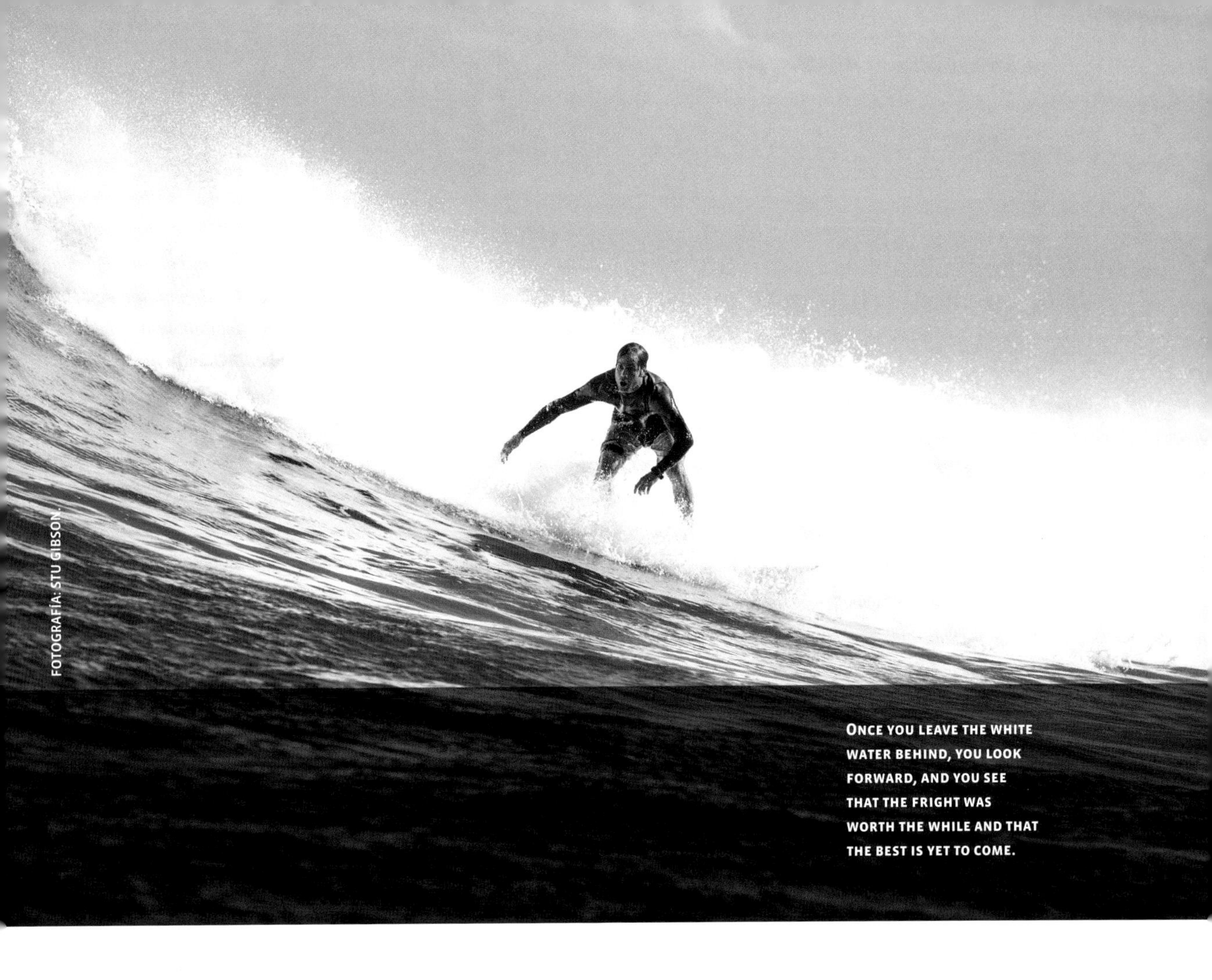

ONCE YOU LEAVE THE WHITE WATER BEHIND, YOU LOOK FORWARD, AND YOU SEE THAT THE FRIGHT WAS WORTH THE WHILE AND THAT THE BEST IS YET TO COME.

cells are specialized cells in our immune system, and their role is to capture and process the antigens –threats formed inside the body as viral or bacterial toxins, or external threats, such as chemicals–, and present them to very concrete lymphocytes in order for them to begin the body's immune response. By then, I knew perfectly well that lymphocytes are the white blood cells in charge of the production of antibodies to fight infections and tumors. ***Learning medical nomenclature is very useful in order not to miss anything from the doctor's explanations.*** *

Bottom line, Doctor López and her team, led by Doctor Flavio Salazar, 'educate' dendritic cells in a lab to trigger a natural response in the patient's body, if they can find some cell similar to those that serve as 'food'. In my case, melanoma cells. They also expect that, when reinjecting the patient, those cells would in turn 'educate' lymphocytes to get rid of the tumor, stop its growth, or make micro metastasis disappear. Put simply, Oncobiomed gives the immune system a sort of crash course in responding to melanoma. I remember Flavio Salazar made me a drawing that clarified many doubts: it was almost like looking at a comic book!

They use the concept of vaccine because the procedure seeks to generate immune memory. When you generate a response against a tumor,

** More on medical nomenclature in chapter 100 Frequently Asked Questions on Cancer (Page 206).*

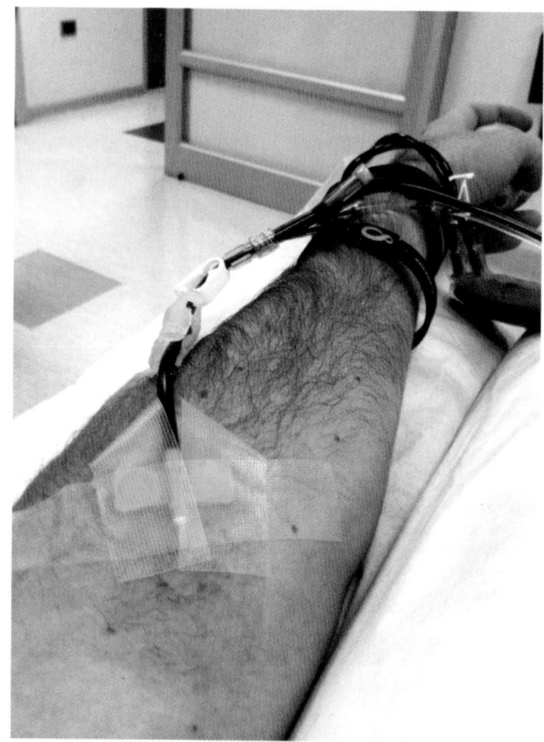

THE AUTOIMMUNE VACCINE IS CREATED FROM YOUR OWN BLOOD; THEY EXTRACT IT, CENTRIFUGE IT, SEPARATE MONOCYTES, CULTIVATE THEM IN THE LAB, AND CONVERT THEM INTO DENDRITIC CELLS THAT ARE LATER CHARGED WITH MELANOMA ANTIGENS. FINALLY, THEY ARE REINJECTED IN 4 DIFFERENT DOSES.

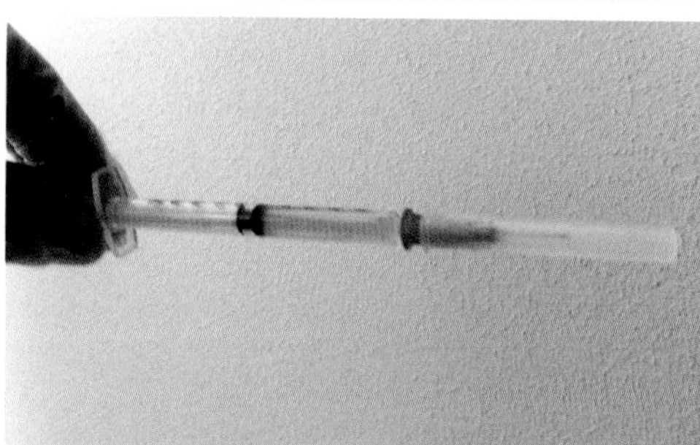

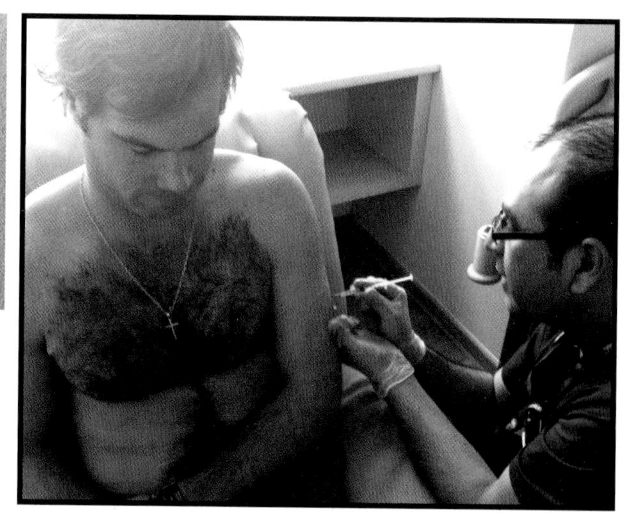

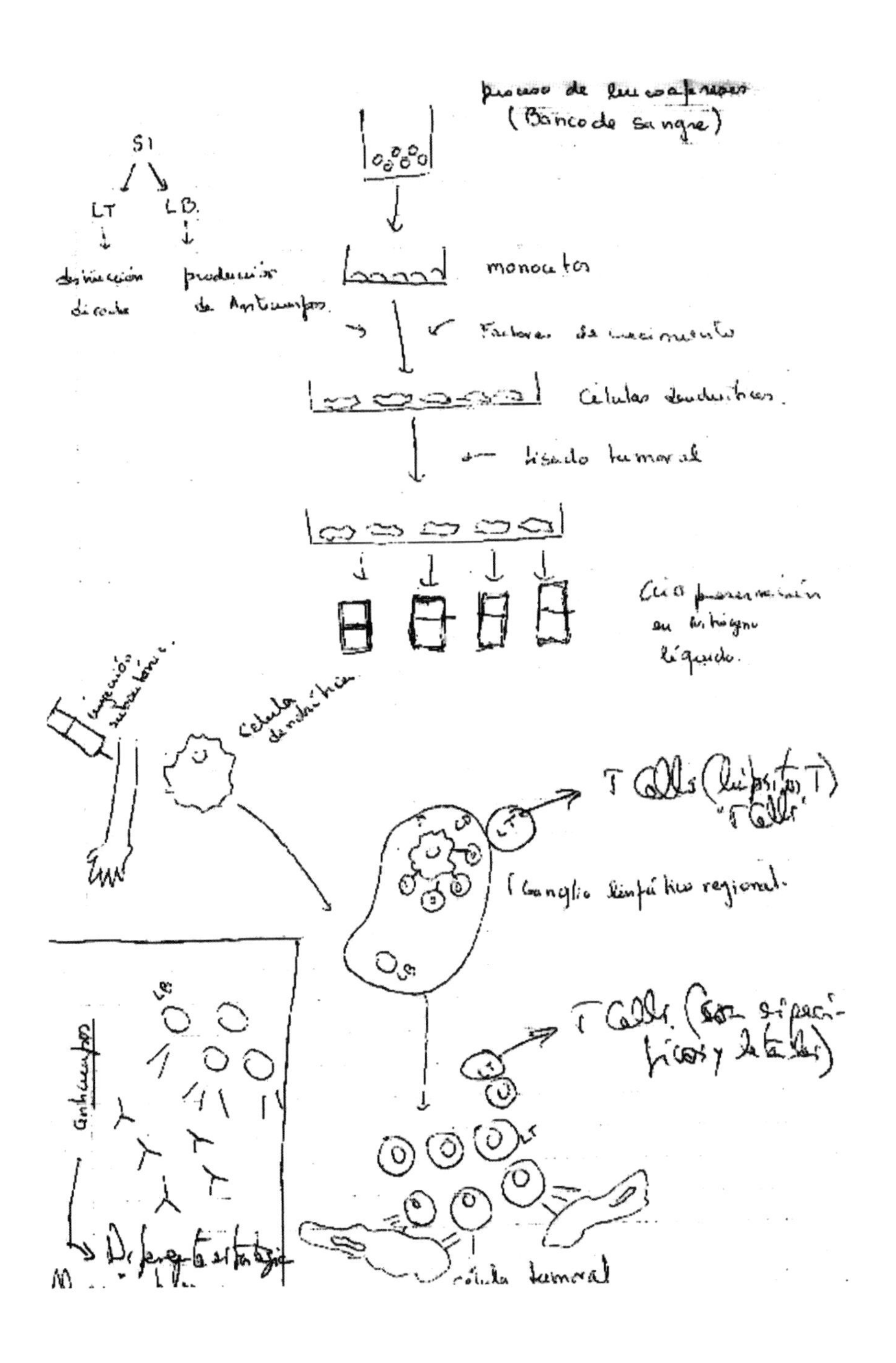

In the interview Dad and I had with Flavio Salazar before injecting the autoimmune vaccine, he explained the whole process to us in a very didactic manner. This is the diagram he drew while Dad and I listened to him.

you always have the possibility of generating autoimmunity. I did not know that it had side effects; in fact, I received all 4 vaccines without being aware of their side effects. When I talked to the doctor for this book, she told me that, as like treatment or medication, it could have side effects. In some patients it causes vitiligo, that is, a depigmentation of the skin in some areas of the body. And in some very extreme cases, it causes alterations of pigments in the iris, or in the adrenal medulla, although she and her team have only seen a few vitiligo reactions. Fortunately, it did not affect me. I mainly focused on their clinical results, because that is what I was looking for: results. From the many patients treated (I was something like patient No. 200), several of them were in an advanced stage of the disease and, even so, over 60% of them responded immunologically to the therapy. According to what Doctor Mercedes López told us, thanks to the vaccine they have lived longer (twice as long as expected), and the progression of their disease has been significantly slower. In some cases, they have even seen the regression of the tumor.

* As Doctor López told us, patients treated with the autoimmune vaccine have lived twice as long as expected.

In July 2011, I had the first dose of the vaccine at the chemotherapy center of *Clínica Las Condes*, and the truth is that I was not prepared to see other patients that were undergoing chemo at the time. Many of them had lost hair and waited, with a catheter in their arms, for the doses to enter their blood. It was shocking. Denial returned. Why was I there if my *thing* was the vaccine and not chemo? What if I was not *sick-sick*? It left me pretty shaken up. I even cried. It was one of those moments when you once again confront the disease. It was one of those cancer moments about which doctor Benjamín Paz had spoken to me in Los Angeles. One of those when you feel the stigma of being sick and are forced to face certain limitations.

Constanza Larraín is the daughter of the late magician Fernando Larraín, and I met her one day at *Taringa*, through mutual friends. Talking to her was fascinating, since she showed me the other side of the coin: A daughter being by her father's side during the last 2 years of his life, after a long fight against prostate cancer. She came back from Barcelona to Santiago to be with him. And among the countless anecdotes she shared with me – Coni has a sense of humor similar to her father's when facing even the hardest side of life– she told me that her father had a rough time accepting these limitations.

–What limitations affected him the most?

–What really complicated his life towards the end was the wheelchair. Sometimes he wanted to leave his apartment, but the chair limited him. When I would finally convince him, we would stroll around, and if he saw an old man sitting on a bench with a nurse, he would ask, "I'm more fucked up than he is, aren't I?" Whenever he could, he took it with humor. I also saw him cry from sorrow at the sight of his wheelchair, and never before had I seen him break down.

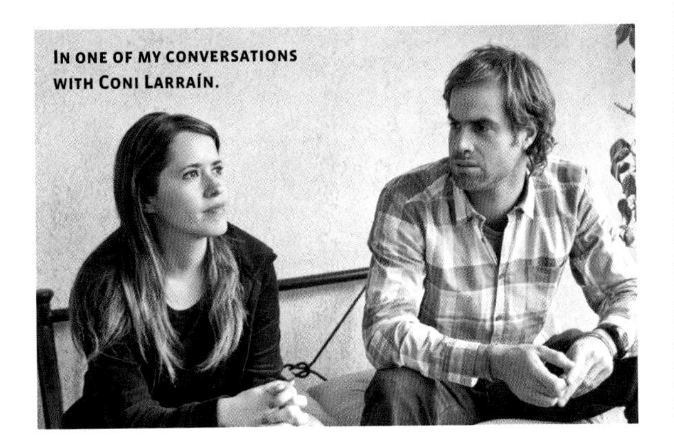

In one of my conversations with Coni Larraín.

–I can imagine that his ability to laugh was helpful to get out of those emotional states.

–Once, we were alone at home, right after a lunch with friends during which he'd had some wine, and he fell down. The medication he took made him intolerant to wine. I could not lift him up, so I lay down on the floor beside him and we began to talk. "Can you see how terribly limiting this is?", he asked me. After an hour I told my father we couldn't stay on the floor forever, so I dragged him to the bed, and placed him there. It was hard. My father was laughing loudly because of what I was doing. ***Laughter always saved us.*** ■

Finally, the vaccine and the drops from the iridologist were the only things I did, besides changing my diet according to Mincolla's indications. He told me that if I followed them, in 8 months the diarrheas would decrease. Amazingly, on the ninth month... they were gone! After years of torture, the diarrhea disappeared! This was paramount for me, since food and my new diet are even now essential in the changes I made in my life. In a nutshell, they meant a special organization at home from the very beginning. A change in the shopping list, but also a change in *me*, feeding myself in a healthier and more responsible way made me feel lighter both physically and emotionally. In fact, I lost 12 kilos (27 pounds).

Sheer willpower was not enough to keep up the changes. The help and support from my family was paramount throughout. Besides healthy food, order was really important. I have to eat four times a day, without skipping any meals, in order to nurture my body with balance. For example, at breakfast I could not eat just fruit and run to work, I had to sit at the table and eat a plate of oatmeal with strawberries and drops of stevia, plus a couple of rice cookies with turkey ham and avocado. I said goodbye to bread, got rid of white flours, and opened the door to rice flour. You can read about this in the chapter *You Are What You Eat*. This didn't mean I stopped eating tasty things, like cake, because you can also bake all kinds of tasty foods with different types of flours or milks and other things, as I have discovered.

That's how my life progressed. I took care of my body, as Mincolla had told me to, but the world kept spinning, and I went back to work, stepping on the brake whenever I remembered that I was still in a process, whose ending was still unclear. My business partner, Pepe, together with Antonio Monckeberg, at the time CEO at *Touch*, and Ignacio Rojas, Country Manager for *Touch* in Peru, were always very respectful of my schedule and, I will always be grateful to them for that. They never put pressure on me, either to reduce my workload or expecting me to perform as I had done previously. They knew how to give me my space, and honestly, the diet issue had me very busy in the first few months. Diana Strauss, whom I met because she had melanoma and we shared experiences, is a woman who has persisted in a profoundly healthy diet. ***Her worries have led her to have her own vegetable garden to eat consciously.*** She follows Mark Mincolla's philosophy regarding her diet. She discovered his books after removing a melanoma from her thigh, that begun as a bluish mole. She was 24 years old at the time. Luckily, her melanoma was encapsulated. Meeting her was impressive, because she had made Mincolla's words a reality: change in food is forever. "It was an experience that helped me build my life. Although I had a special sensitivity from the time I was a child, after cancer I decided to live according to nature and the laws of creation. Eating with awareness is part of that," she commented.

That same year, 2011, two months and a half after I was diagnosed with melanoma, my family and friends organized a party at home and, taking advantage of the Chilean national soccer team playing in the Americas Cup the day of the gathering, we named the party *Celebrate Life*. Pepe and several work mates at *Touch* took care of production: they set up a tent, stands, and a big screen. I was enthusiastic and suggested inviting all those who'd helped me and joined me on my path through cancer. I invited them to celebrate life, and I even took care of little details. I wrote a letter to my neighbors telling them I had cancer surgery and that since things were successful for the time being, I wanted to celebrate:

Having faith in cancer being completely gone, and knowing ***life*** *is something worth fighting for, today I have invited all those who cared for me during my illness, to watch the soccer game and then to continue celebrating life. We are having music, a barbeque, impersonators, and a cool vibe. I would like to ask for your understanding on this occasion.*

Excerpt of the letter I wrote to my neighbors the day we held Celebrate Life, so as to party without any problems.

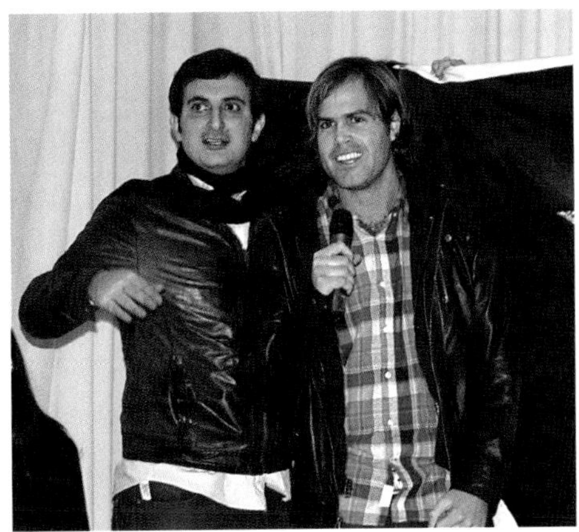

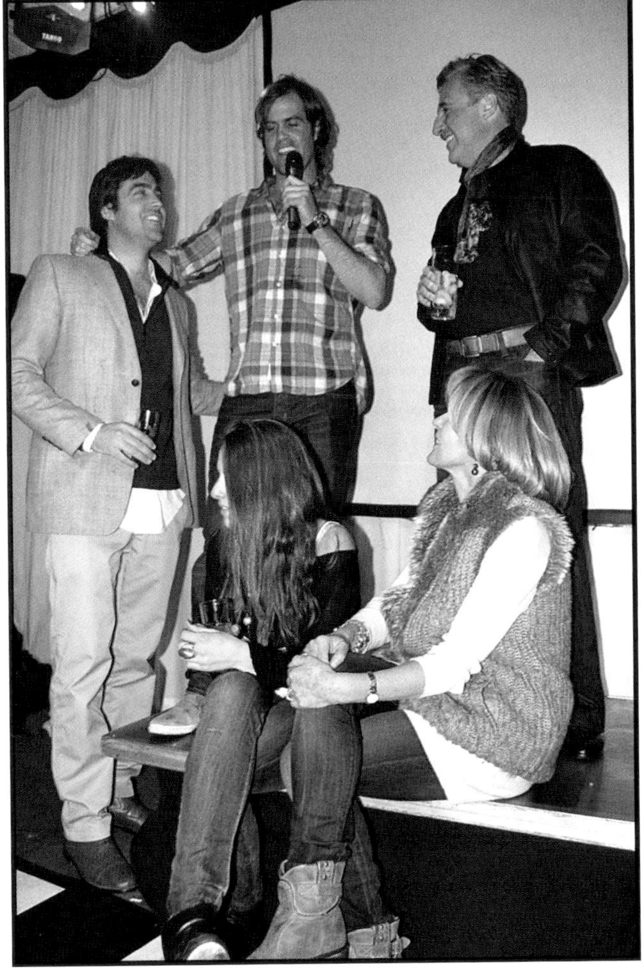

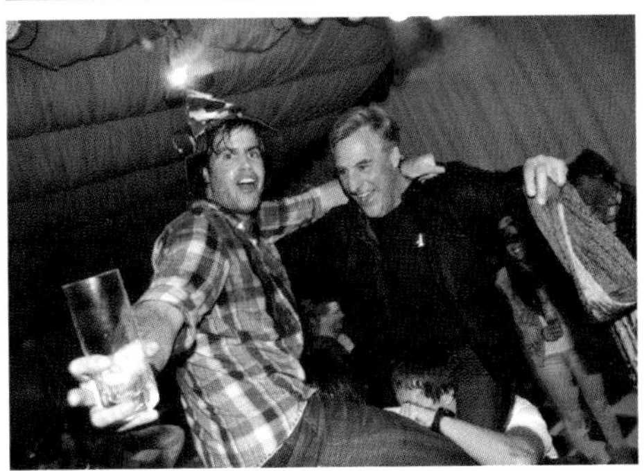

MY FAMILY AND FRIENDS THREW A PARTY AT MY PLACE TO CELEBRATE LIFE AND KEEP WALKING THROUGH THE PATH OF THE HEALTHY AFTER TWO AND A HALF MONTHS OF THE DIAGNOSIS OF MY MELANOMA.

Now that I think about it, it was perhaps odd to organize the party. I'd just returned from the US medical tour and nothing was completely settled. It was a good party, but the celebration was about me being healthy, when actually we didn't know what was still to come. It was still a long haul. At that time, I had not read yet *El Mundo Amarillo* (*The Yellow World*) by Spanish author Albert Espinosa. He wrote about what he learned over the 10 years he had cancer (between 13 and 23), life-long lessons he still uses today. One of them is celebrating. He said everything is a reason to celebrate. That is why he had a farewell party for his leg a few days before it was amputated. Luckily I will never forget that each day hides a chance to celebrate. With meaning, of course.

After the party, Mom insisted I had to meet the woman that had had melanoma, Loreto Agurto, but I refused. "No, no, no", I would tell her. Not interested. But fate is fate –as I told you in the prologue– and I ended up meeting her by chance, in a hospital waiting room. She recognized me because a few days earlier I had been in the social life pages of a magazine. Today I feel that running into Loreto was like meeting an angel. Despite how odd it was to be talking to her in that waiting room, her honest attitude and open way of talking won me over. I remember her smile, conveying only sweetness. It was obvious she only wanted to help me, and I remember that, for the first time since everything had started, I felt I was with a peer, with somebody who had gone through what I had, and who was smiling and happy. It was so magical that I smiled, too.

> * When I first met Loreto Agurto, I felt I was with a peer, someone who'd lived the same I had, and that made me smile, happy.

As in this picture, I met Loreto: cheerful, charismatic and charming.

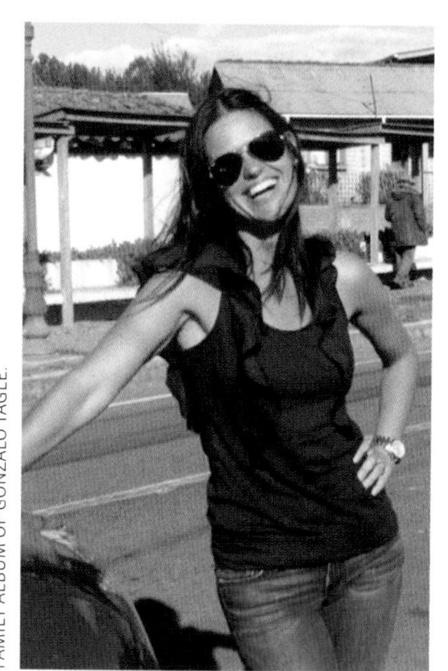

Family album of Gonzalo Tagle.

Meeting her, listening to her, and understanding her convinced me: I had to make a 180-degree-change. She told me that since her cancer diagnosis she had decided to live every day as it came, and leave her ego aside. She had learned to say no, and was closer to those she loved the most. Her attitude touched me deeply. That was what I wanted for my life! And I vowed to myself to live in the same way.

It was thanks to Loreto that I wrote this book. I wanted to leave a written legacy, just as she had shared her fresh and lucid view on cancer with me. I was annoyed with myself that it should have taken such a hard and painful experience to make me see how I could change myself and live my life as she had suggested. So I decided, and told Loreto, that I would write this book.

During one of our lunches together I asked her if she was happy. She answered "I'm much happier now, with melanoma, than ever before". Her answer hit home. Right there and then, I decided to start guiding my life by the by the idea of being happy, even with cancer as a concrete presence in my life.

It has also made me look at myself better and others from a new perspective. I wrote about the change, and about *Cholo Ibáñez* –a nickname given to me by my friend Davor when I was 17 and had dated a Peruvian girl and then a Bolivian girl right afterwards– and his euphoria, versus *Roberto Ibáñez*. I wanted to focus on being *Roberto*. I threw out letters from old girlfriends, and photos that linked me to a less-happy past. Although I'm not religious I took off the Easter Island pendant I always wore around my neck, and bought a small silver cross. Later I replaced this with charm in the shape of a little Fijian turtle that better represents the deep sense of calm

> * I wanted to focus on *Roberto*. That is why I tossed away old letters and pictures, all related to the anguish of the past.

I now feel. When my dog Mora died, I buried her together with the turtle necklace. Like I wrote in the prologue, I'm happy that this book is published today, 6 years after the initial diagnosis, and not 4 years ago, when I was living cancer at its worst.

Loreto had injected me with special energy. I began writing and put together a 3-page text about how to let go of one's ego, and to live a better, lighter life. I sent it to a newspaper and to a magazine, but it seemed as though no one was interested. They replied that my text didn't have any scientific content, that it was pure emotion. And they were right. I'd written it from the heart, as a way of unburdening my sadness, and of following through with this impulse I had to share what I had discovered. Maybe it wasn't publishable material, but it was honest, and as I see it, it had special value.

In that text, I wrote exactly how I felt. Cancer had triggered an internal process and awakened tons of insights.

In this text I sent to the media I wrote: ***"cancer was a blessing, one of the best things to ever happen to me in my short life. You may think I'm crazy, but it's true."*** Without cancer I would not have had the chance to get to know myself, nor the time to think or understand that there is always somebody that may need a shoulder to lean on. Why this change? Because I wanted to be a better person.

That hastily-written text also echoed what I felt was also about how I felt about Santiago, the main character of *El Alquimista* (*The Alchemist*) by Paulo Coelho. When I read that book, I identified with him: Santiago used to live thinking that something better was always about to happen and that he owed it to himself to keep looking until he found the perfect balance. What I didn't understand then –and I do now– is that life's perfect balance is the right-here-and-now, and that adventures come on their own. There is no perfect woman, friend, parent, or partner. Everyone has a beautiful side to them, and less beautiful aspects that make them human.

 Because I'm obsessive, I decided if my column was not published I was going to look for a way to publish it on my own as a book.

Then I thought about my family and what cancer meant to them. This disease is not exclusively mine. We were all affected by melanoma. I thought about the unconditional support from my friends, the good times we had together, also the mistakes, the harm that I may have caused someone in the past, the heartbreaks. I know about breakups, losing trust, carelessness, and lack of understanding. I have started to slowly realize that, if there is love, things can be fixed. That's why in my text I'd written: "One has to simply be humble, be able to stop seeking happiness to realize happiness is right in front of you, and that you can find it without trying so hard; just by admiring the person close to you, listening to them, understanding their worries, their interests and anxieties, just as that person may admire and understand you."

Because I'm obsessive, I decided that if my text was not published, then I would look for a way to publish it on my own, as a book. Once this idea was set in my mind, I understood the overpowering urge moving my father to research melanoma. It quickly became urgent and important to me to do it. Cancer wasn't something I'd had in my life for very long, but how many people were lucky enough to have the kind of access to information that I had? Very few, probably. The best way to put the project together was to gather all the data and the life experiences, contacting people directly or indirectly related with this disease, and turning those testimonies into a book. Fired up, I began to dedicate time to the project. My sister didn't understand, and said: "Roberto, writing a book? On cancer?" It just didn't add up for her, but when I told her the project came from Loreto's advice, of living life simply letting go of one's ego, and being happy, she understood me better. I explained that was the cornerstone –in my opinion the "big tip"– and that I intended to gather more tips like that one, from people who work with cancer, or had gone through similar experiences to mine, and from families who had endured its effects firsthand. In the end Antonia's comment was that to leave this sort of "witness statement" of what we'd been through, and to invite others to participate and share it, was a generous act.

How was I not going to be motivated to put together the information my family had gathered with so much effort? I'm lucky, I have a dad that led the family into battle for me, determined to learn everything there is to know about possible treatments for melanoma. I'm also lucky because my family has the resources to make contacts, to travel anywhere in the world and pay doctors' fees and medical procedures. That's not everyone's reality, and that was obvious to me. I had to write this book.

As we became friends, **Loreto Agurto** and I talked on the phone and exchanged emails. From the very beginning, her generosity was overwhelming, she only wanted to pass on and share what had taken her months, or years, to discover about her melanoma. I always felt her unconditional support and positive energy. Listening to her only increased my desire to write, to share this experience, to communicate. This is why I want to share part of an interview with her for this book, in which she told me the story of her melanoma and her way of coping.

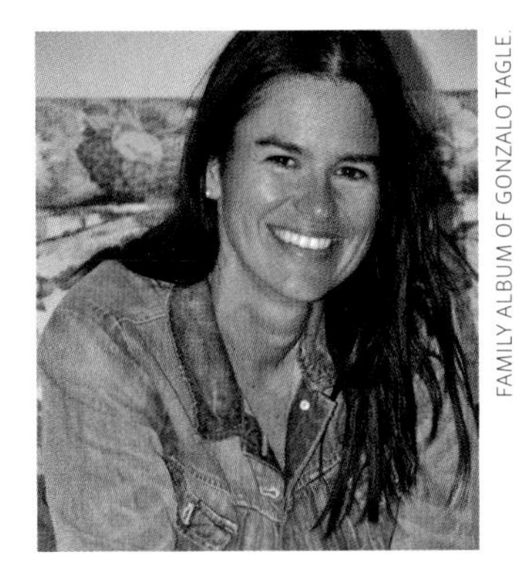

FAMILY ALBUM OF GONZALO TAGLE.

–Loreto, how did everything start?

– I had an in situ melanoma in my leg, which was removed; and that was that. In 2008, another one appeared on my scalp. I have so little hair that in the summer my scalp is always sunburnt and then peels off. One day I found partly loose skin where my hair parts. A rugged piece of scalp that never fell. My husband told me to go to the doctor because it looked ugly. I went to the same dermatologist who detected my first melanoma, and I quickly realized that matters were complicated, because he started to sweat. An oncologist removed the mole the next day. They took a long time to give me the result of my biopsy. It is all a very blurry. And then, I went to see a surgeon at another hospital to get a second opinion. He told me I had to undergo surgery. It turns out it was an infiltrated melanoma. The lymph nodes and part of neck tissue were removed. I had to undergo a second surgery in 2011, because there was metastasis in my lung. The exams showed that the lymph nodes were infiltrated and muscles in my neck and shoulder were removed. I had so many questions... I was pregnant with my third child, and the second one had just started school.

Loreto Agurto

–Did you see a good side to it?

–People are very caring, one has no idea. After surgery I couldn't receive many visitors, because I felt horrible, so I left a notebook outside for visitors to write to me. It's filled with so many beautiful things! Melanoma is a shitty disease, but it has let me see the other side of the coin: being loved by so many people.

–How do you live with the feeling of being sick?

–People often get nervous when they run into me, because I look good, I don't have a "sick" face. I forget I have cancer: if your family sees you look good, they won't allow you to fall. I have 3 children, so I don't stop. But I advise everyone to let themselves be taken care of. One tends to feel powerful; you can do everything! Until your body says "no more". Then, you have to ask for help, and allow yourself to receive it. It would be great if no one had to live through a disease in order to remember that we have only one life to live. I still have not given myself permission to cry, but for now, I have many things: a wonderful husband, unconditional friends, and an incredible family.

–is there one aspect of cancer that is the most difficult to you?

–When I go to *Arturo López Pérez* foundation to get control tests, I see bald kids and moms in despair. Then you feel sick. I'm full of scars because of the surgeries, and for some time I tried to hide them. One day I was in Buenos Aires trying on a dress and I told the sales assistant: "Not this one, because you can see the scar on my back". She asked me what was going on, and I told her my story. Then she said to me: "wear it proudly, your scars are those of battles won." It changed my perception. She showed me her hand and it was burned. She had had an accident when she was little. "They wanted to remove it, but I said no, because it is a part of me", she said.

–Did you tell your children what was going on?

–It's important to tell them what is going on. Maybe not everything, because my children are too small still, but tell them that you are going to be away for a couple of days and they are not going to see you. One day outside my children's school a person shouted "When does your chemo start?", and I was with the kids! My daughter at first asked me if it was my birthday, because she saw I received chocolates and flowers and was surrounded by people.

–How do you keep your spirits up?

–I give myself bubble baths, manicures, I pamper myself. I have my own space without regrets. I let myself be in a bad mood. I decided I cannot manipulate my mood: if one day I'm sad, then that's just the way I feel. ■

At the time, I also told Loreto to send me a list with her tips, and I asked that she write them thinking about their use for patients with cancer and their families. Over the next few days she sent me her notes, which I share below. In her email she particularly emphasized her attitude to the disease, with words I still remember: "I always kept my spirits high, even in the worst situations. Symptoms never affected me. I always thank God that this melanoma happened to me and not my children, my husband, my parents or siblings. That would have destroyed me."

Tips from Loreto Agurto

1. *Surround yourself with people that make you feel good.*

2. Stop worrying about the little things.

3. *Take into consideration the treatment the patient wants to follow. I preferred to undergo surgery rather than a drug treatment.*

4. Conduct tests rigorously every 3 months.

5. Have a spiritual and an earthly guide to whom to pour your heart out.

6. *Don't have pending issues with anyone.*

7. *Autoimmune vaccine against melanoma (www.oncobiomed.cl).*

8. *Ritestart 4life Vitamines (www.4liferitestart.com).*

9. *Having a "guest book" for when you don't feel like seeing visitors.*

FAMILY ALBUM OF GONZALO TAGLE.

* In her email, she she particularly emphasized her attitude to the disease, with words I still remember: "I always kept my spirits high, even in the worst situations".

One of the first consequences of the change I undertook was that I purchased a plot of land in *Matanzas*, a beautiful beach south west of Santiago, just 2 hours away. We went with my parents, Sebastián, and Caro (now Sebastián's wife) to choose it. We stayed at a hotel by the sea, we surfed, took the dogs with us, and I went stand-up paddling for the first time after the surgery. It was a healing weekend for everybody. We enjoyed it so much that we even took a few days off work. It was perfect. I quickly started to build the house I had had in mind since I was at the clinic. That was my first personal project. I could kite surf, be with my friends, have my own space, something like my first home where, in the future, I could go with my own family. From the moment the house was ready it has brought me only joy. I relax there, I do whatever I want, I live my independence with happiness, taking care of the garden and making things work. I connect with the sea, the best psychologist in the world. And just as I had envisaged it, at the entrance of the house I placed the board that reads "House of Joy."

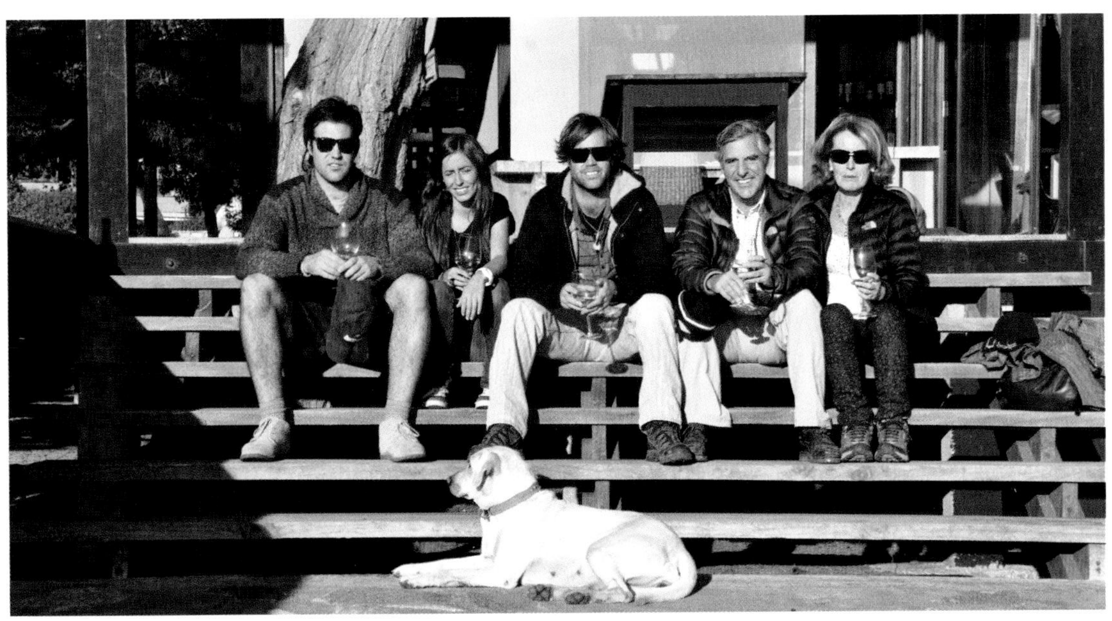

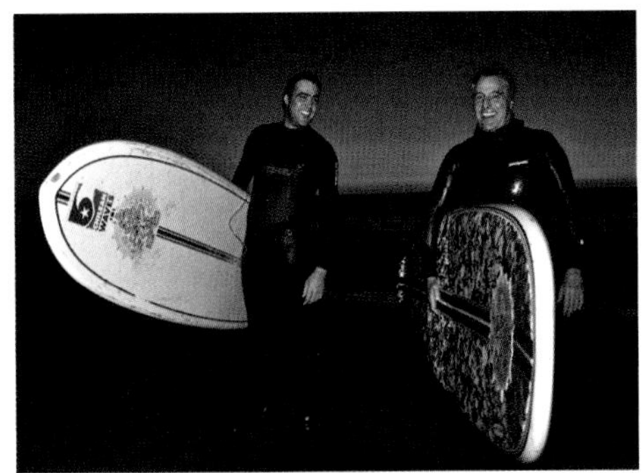

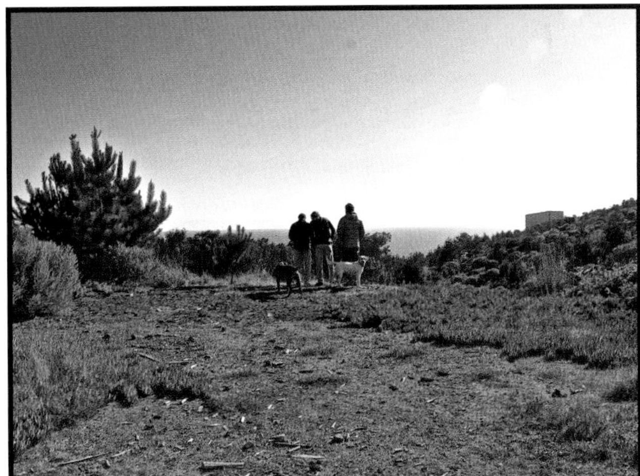

I HAVE BEEN GOING TO *MATANZAS* SINCE 2007. I ALWAYS SAID I WOULD BUY A PLOT OF LAND, BECAUSE THE SEA AND NATURE REPRESENT MY LIFESTYLE, BUT I I DIDN'T HAVE THE COURAGE TO DO IT UNTIL I HAD CANCER AND WAS IN HOSPITAL, AND REALIZED I COULD NOT WAIT ANY LONGER. WHEN I LEFT HOSPITAL, THE FIRST THING I DID WAS BUY THE LAND. MY FAMILY CAME WITH ME TO CHOOSE IT, THEN I BUILT A HOUSE THAT I CALLED *HOUSE OF JOY*, AND FROM THEN ON I HAVE THOROUGHLY ENJOYED IT.

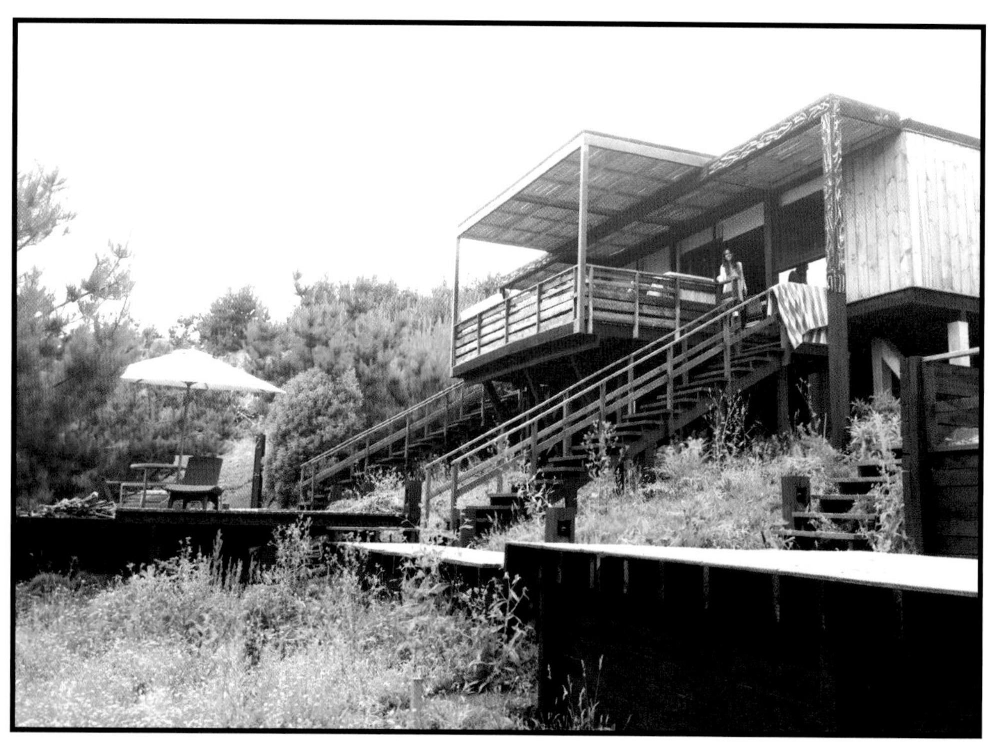

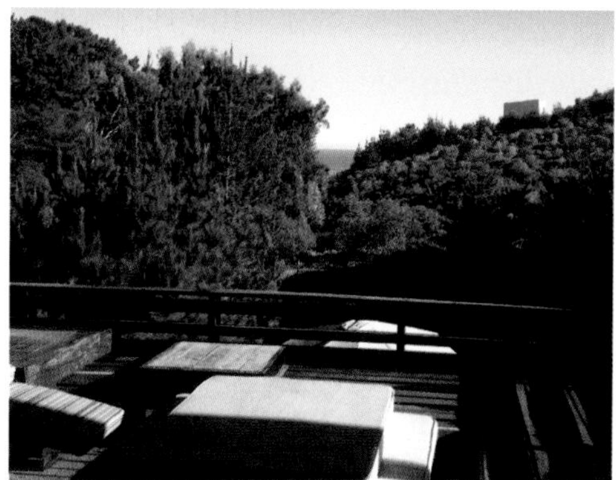

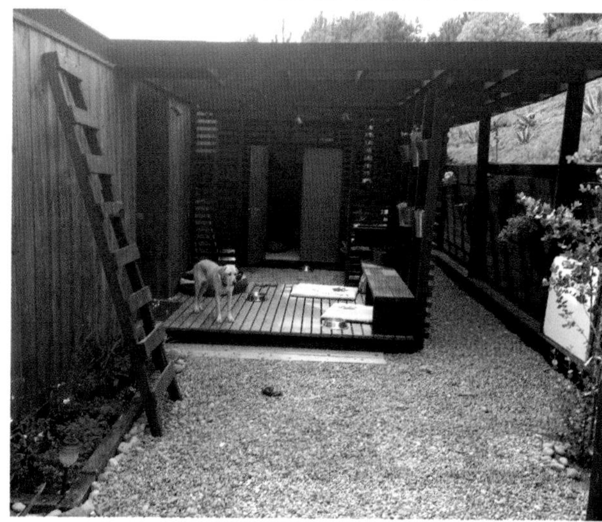

MY HOUSE IN *MATANZAS*,
HOUSE OF JOY.

Along with this, ***I decided to focus on the 80% chances of living, and sweep the dark 20% under the rug, forgotten.*** It was not an automatic change; it grew slowly after the initial shock. *"I'm ok, I'm ok."* I told myself over several months.

But no, I was not OK.

We all lived that initial shock, and from that point onwards, between the *before* and *after* cancer, our story began. Mine started with a phone call, some random day, to be told about the ambiguous result of a biopsy. It could catch you under any circumstances, in different stages of life, at any age. **Carmen Hodgson,** sister of a colleague from *Touch*, was diagnosed with Ewing sarcoma in the iliac muscle in 2001, at the age of 15. Today she is fully recovered. I had a very emotional interview with her, in which she remembered some of the moments from during her illness. She went to the hospital because of a "lump" she discovered on her waist. When she saw doctors going through encyclopedias and the Internet, she realized that it was more serious than she had thought it would be. It was a malignant tumor and she immediately underwent surgery.

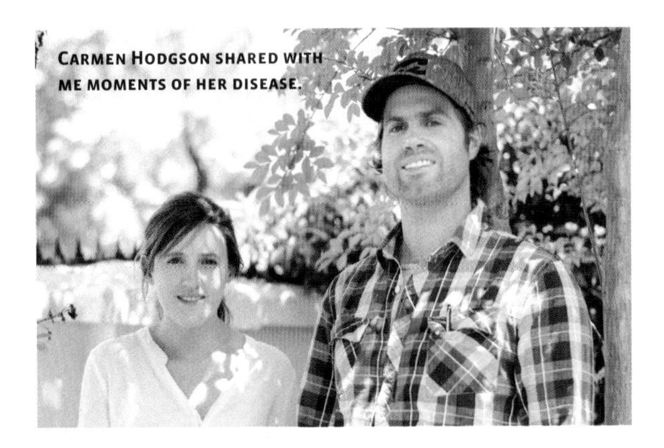
Carmen Hodgson shared with me moments of her disease.

–What do you remember of the first moments of your disease?

–I went through every emotion: fear, sadness, rage, anguish, and even happiness. It was a whole year of treatment, but it was not traumatic, maybe because I was too young. I always thought, how do I get out of this? When they told me I had to undergo 24 chemotherapy sessions, I was counting down. 23, 22... I had all the information: the oncologist told me that the sick person was me, and that I could ask whatever I wanted.

–Did you ask if you were going to die?

–No, because I knew I was not going to die. When I had the chemo, I only thought I was going to win the battle inside my body. I'd imagine everything I'd do once it was over. Chemo was terrible. I threw up a lot, I could not lift my body, and the discomfort was unbearable. I got so thin that the doctor told me if I did not gain weight, I wouldn't be able to take the following chemo. ***With practically no strength, I held on to the future and never gave up. I thought it was a cycle, and that after feeling bad I necessarily had to feel good again.*** ■

Carmen told me that at a certain point she stopped looking at herself in the mirror and didn't purchase pants, simply to avoid having to look at her thinness. When she woke up, she counted the hairs on her pillow. She said that her hair falling out affected her more than the discomfort of the nausea from the chemo, since it was a testimony to her illness. She was at a stage in life where how you look is extremely important. With her simplicity and coolness, I imagine her shaving her head and then wearing a wig of natural hair, as she did.

Like Carmen, **Carlos Ferrer** also had cancer when he was a teen. I have been with him many times, because he photographed extreme sports, and I knew he had cancer, but had no idea he had had it twice. The first time was in one testicle, when he was 20, and then at 30, in the other testicle. It was amazing to hear that despite the adverse scenario, thanks to the good decisions they made, he is now the father of twins, Angel and Amelia. Carlos felt pain in one of his testicles and thought he must have hit it. He went to the emergency room to get something for the pain before going to the beach. His friends were waiting in the car. He had some tests, and when Carlos told the doctor he was in a hurry, he said "Carlos, you will have to stay so tell your friends to go. It would be good to call your parents, because you have a tumor." Carlos was in shock.

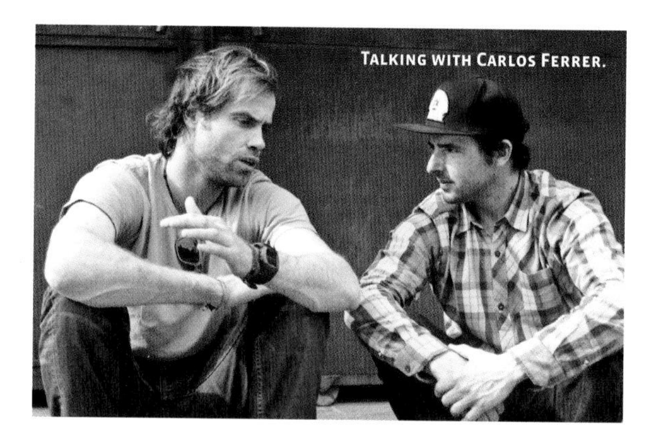

TALKING WITH CARLOS FERRER.

–What did this cancer mean to you?

–I thought I was going to die. I had my testicle removed in Chile and had a silicon implant to hide the surgery. Afterwards, I was in Houston for two weeks with my dad, in order to validate the process. I slowly realized that cancer does not always mean death. ***At the time I did not think about the possibility of not being able to have children. I was a teen, but some friends of my dad's suggested we freeze my sperm.***

–And emotionally? Did you make changes in your life?

–I grew as a human being. Before, I was a bratty teen. Always fighting everyone. Today I value life very much, and each day I appreciate it more, because I can see my children grow. At 20 I discovered life can't be taken for granted. I did not want to die, so I started to take care of my friends and loving people.

–Were you depressed when they discovered the second cancer?

–No. because it wasn't as invasive as the first one. I didn't even need chemotherapy, only checkups. But I had my other testicle removed, so today I don't produce sperm. Every 3 months I have to inject myself with testosterone, which is useful for ejaculation, my mood, and hair growth. ■

You can feel the happiness in Carlos and his wife, Javiera, who was his girlfriend when he was 20. After a breakup, they got back together and then got married. They are now proud parents, which you can tell.

But, what happens when the initial shock is due to someone you love having cancer? I talked about this with **Patricia Marchesse,** a friend of my mother's. In 1990, her eldest son, Tomás, then 4 years old, was diagnosed with lymphoblastic leukemia. At first she was overwhelmed by fear and doubt; she felt powerless and lost, until she was able to take some decisions that made her stronger and changed how she could confront the horrific reality. Tomás died at the age of 11, and although almost 20 years have passed, she remembers by heart everything that happened. Below, I transcribed some fragments of our long conversation, which coincided with the death of my unforgettable dog, a Rhodesian Ridgeback called *Maasai*. I empathized with Patty through my tears.

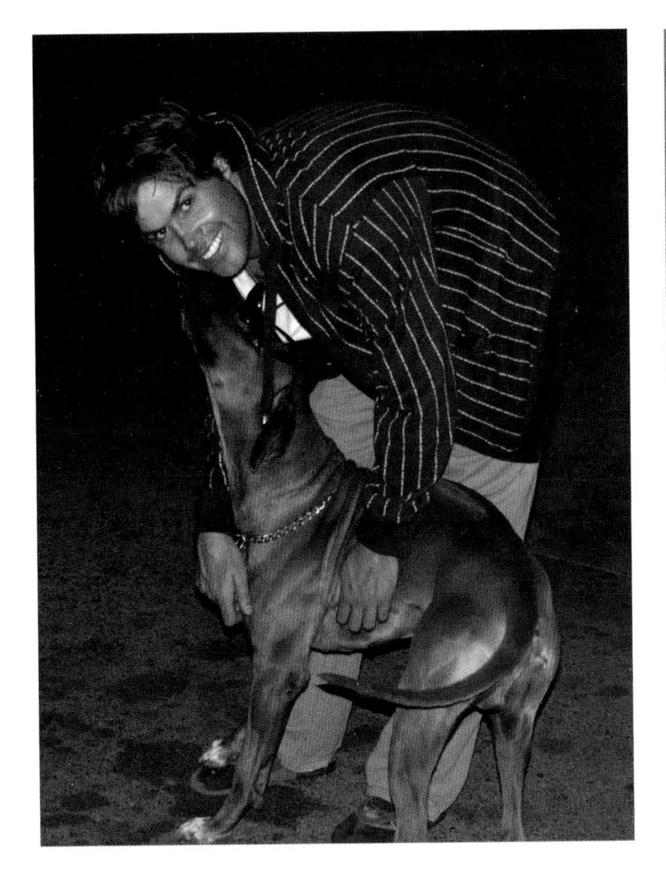

* What happens when the initial shock is due to someone you love having cancer? I talked about this with Patricia Marchesse, whose son was diagnosed with lymphoblastic leukemia at the age of four.

I INTERVIEWED PATRICIA MARCHESSE THE DAY MY DOG *MAASAI* DIED. SHE TOLD ME OF THE STRUGGLE WITH CANCER OF HER SON TOMÁS, WHO DIED AT THE AGE OF 11, AND WE CONNECTED IN A VERY SPECIAL WAY.

–How did you learn of Tomás's illness?
–We took Tomás to the emergency room, because they called us from his kindergarten saying that he wouldn't stop crying because he had swallowed the cap of a pen. At the emergency room they assured us he would get rid of the cap by himself, but when this didn't happen we took him to see his pediatrician. He examined him and noted his lymph nodes were swollen. A couple of hours later we knew he had leukemia.

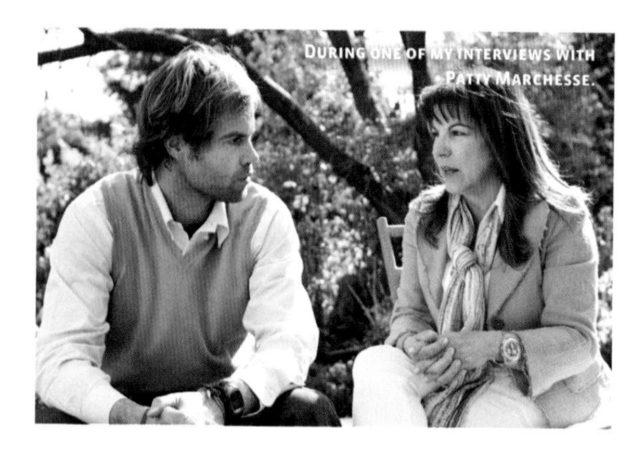
DURING ONE OF MY INTERVIEWS WITH PATTY MARCHESSE.

–What was your attitude when you received the news?
–I cried and cried. When I stopped, I dried my tears and started fighting. For the next 7 years I didn't once stop fighting. It was hard work along with my family and the doctors, but especially with Tomás. He wanted to live and subjected himself to the worse torments you can imagine to achieve this. Shortly after he was diagnosed, and when we believed things were going well, they told us the cancer had mutated to myeloblastic leukemia, much more aggressive and requiring a bone marrow transplant that was not performed in Chile in the 90s. His youngest sister, Camila, who at the time was only a year old, gave her bone marrow to her brother. She was the only compatible family member.

–Did you know Tomás could die?
–Tomás taught us a lot. The strength, courage and bravery of this kid was incredible. Eleven months after the transplant, which meant spending four months in Germany, in a bubble, without touching anyone, he relapsed. He was 8 years old and I had to talk to him. "We are not OK", I told him. He asked crying, "Was all that for nothing?" "Honey, we are not doing anything you don't want to. You are going to help us decide", "Mom, I want to live". I could not cry. I had to fight the leukemia. ■

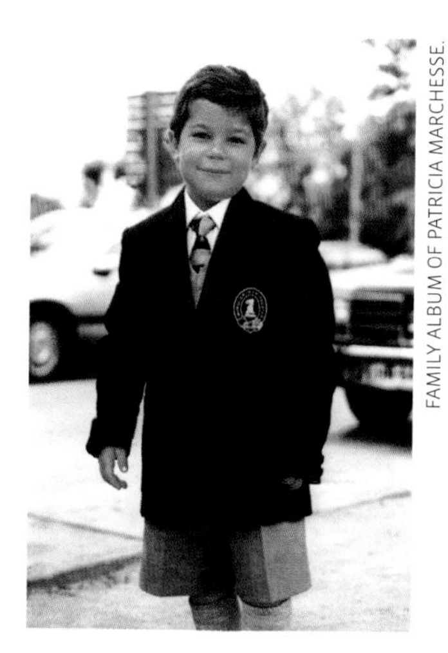
FAMILY ALBUM OF PATRICIA MARCHESSE.

TOMÁS HARTLEY, SON OF PATRICIA MARCHESSE.

At *Celebraciones con Sentido* I worked with **Alejandra Méndez,** a vital, cool, fun and positive woman. Human nature is so unfathomable that when meeting her, it was hard to imagine she had gone through such a dark tunnel, without ever letting go of her son Pablo's hand. Or of her husband's, **Pablo Allard.** We met one night to speak about the *clear cells* cancer detected in Pablo, when he was 2 years old and they were living in Boston. When I wrote this book, Pablo was already 16, and in that conversation I had with his mother he learned a lot about his own experience - things he'd forgotten or never known. I was impressed by his ability to listen to a story that most people would rather forget about, and how he mentioned specific things and volunteered information that even surprised his parents.

Pablo's cancer is rare, and statistics and research scarce. It has a low survival rate. At the age of 2, he had a melon-sized tumor removed from his liver, which generated metastasis in his bone marrow. At the age of 4 he had another tumor, of 0.5 kilos (1.1 pounds), removed from his brain, and at 6, yet another one from his thyroid. His parents dealt with each relapse with strength and determination, and they arrived at important conclusions through the experience, learning how to live and how to fight for life. Ale and Pablo always talked to their son truthfully. They didn't even avoid the word death. The following is a small part of what we talked about that night:

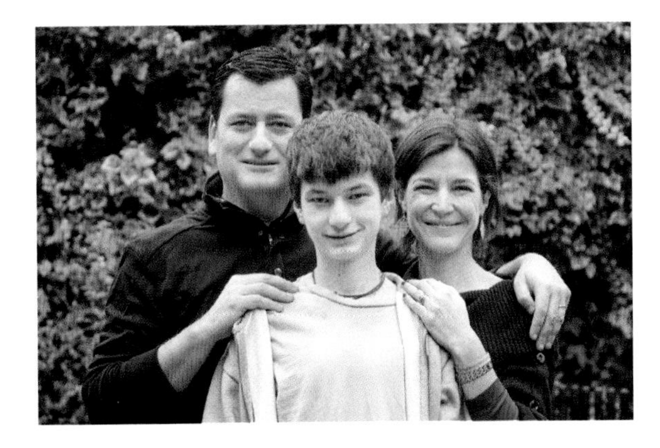

-Did you talk to Pablo of his chances of dying?

-We never lied. If he asked, we answered. Especially after he turned 6 years old, when he could understand certain things.

-What did you answer?

-If he asked, "Am I going to die?", we told him "we don't know, but we are going to do everything we possibly can for you not to die." We never lied. If he asked, "Mom, are they going to put a needle in my arm?", I would say, "Yes son", "Will it hurt?", "It probably will". Our only certainty was that we had to tell him the truth. "Is the needle going into my arm again?", "Yes, honey, again". We wanted him to always believe us, to trust us, so when we told him it wouldn't hurt, or they wouldn't put a needle in his arm, he would also believe us. "Yes, it is going to hurt, but we are going to be with you and we are counting to 10 together." We invented techniques, took deep breaths, held his hand. We never fell apart in front of him, or showed him our fear. We always protected him from other people's negative energy. Pablo still remembers his great Hot Wheels collection. Each time he got a needle, we gave him a new one. ■

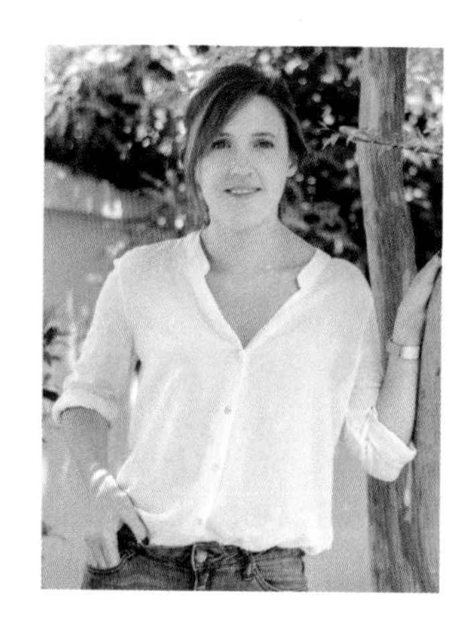

It was hard listening to the testimonies. But everyone I interviewed taught me something, and at the end of this journey I came out stronger, renewed, different. When I asked **Carmen Hodgson** about her conclusions after the disease, she told me that everything was worth living, and that she would not change her story one bit:

–Have you ever wished you hadn't had cancer?

–No. ***Cancer opened my eyes, and that's why it has never been traumatic to talk about it. It gave me the possibility to get closer to people that maybe I would have never had the chance of meeting.*** When I attended radiotherapy, after the chemo cycles, I always ran into this man. One day he talked to me: "I told my daughter you were going through the same thing I am, and she sent you this." It was a watch. I was so excited! Cancer gave me wisdom, although at the beginning I felt so much anger. I was angry to think that I was going through cancer and was a little girl and had never done anything wrong. When I assimilated that if it wasn't me it could have been one of my brothers or my parents, I'd rather have it be me than them. It is much worse to have the situation beyond your control that under your control. It was really worth living it.

This concurs with the theory I had, in that things have to be lived personally, and that it is better to have the personal experience than having other people tell you about it.

–Not even when you think about all the pain it meant?

–***The pain is the first thing you forget.*** I remember the experience, not the pain. In fact, the cancer was not the worst. I had surgery to take the tumor out, to put the catheter in place for the chemo medicine, and then afterwards to take the catheter out. Later came more chemotherapy and radiotherapy; I had surgery on an ovary that had stopped working due to the treatment, and then a whole year later I had to have surgery on my spine. I only retain the experience, not the pain. ■

Without the melanoma I would never have met these people and heard their stories; I was privileged to witness their strength and determination, and also to feel the changes that these meetings brought about in me. It sounds obvious, but you're not the same person once you've been through cancer. This was really clear with **Patty Marchesse.** She chose to give meaning to what happened. It's amazing how, after so much pain and loss, she can focus on the good stuff and transform the negative into positive. I asked her straight-up what she felt, she had learned:

* I would never have met these people and heard their stories; I was privileged to witness their strength and determination, and also to feel the changes that these meetings brought about in me.

–What good things have you been able to take from Tomás' leukemia?

–I grew enormously. I think today I'm a woman that feels and suffers with everybody, more empathetic, generous. I hope it does not sound arrogant, because I say it as humbly as I can. I'm proud I was brave enough to take on this fight. I remember that at the cemetery I asked God to take me with Tomás, and today I look at my daughters that are 27 and 22 years old and I realize how happy I am to be alive. Once, in the middle of the storm, in one of Tomás' relapses, I felt guilty about neglecting the girls, and a doctor stopped me and said: "Patricia, the guilt can be fixed later." And I thought "what a cold guy". But he was right. Tomás was in extreme danger, he could die at any moment. If I'd not been at his side I'd have regretted it later, so I had no choice but to stay. I forgave myself many things and the girls did, too. ■

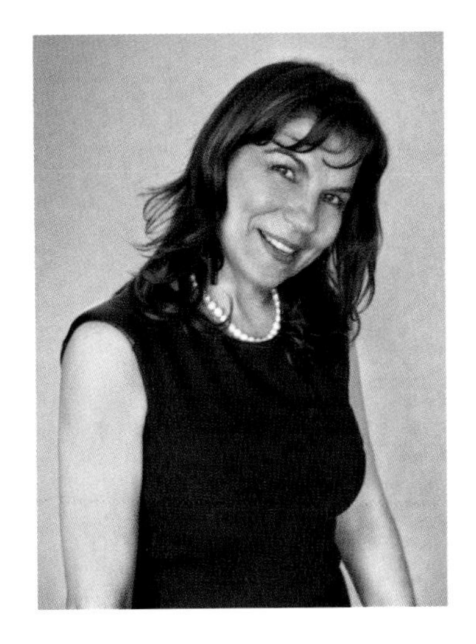

Something similar happened to **Carlos Ferrer** after his testicular cancer:

–What was the greatest personal change you faced through your diagnosis?

–I grew up a lot. I became sensitive. My attitude to things changed. Now, for me, life is sport, nature and family, not ambition. My cancer also strongly affected my friends, and thanks to it we all changed, we all improved. I've had the chance to talk to teenagers who are going through the same thing I did. ***They call me to ask me about the silicon prosthesis, that obviously is one of the biggest fears at 20. I say that the plastic testicle is fun and that they won't have any problem, but I also speak to them about the emotions in the process that they are beginning to live.*** ■

The list of my interviews was getting longer and longer, and all of them gave me invaluable support. The stories didn't always have happy endings, but every experience I heard about taught me something. **Diana Strauss,** for example, had thought a lot about the origin of her melanoma. She was at peace with the explanation she had come to accept:

–Diana, do you think you have come to understand the cause of your melanoma?

–For a long time I thought I had had cancer because I had gone through some hard times, always having fear as a recurrent emotion. I felt that melanoma, which is a wound in the skin, the organ protecting and separating me from the world, appeared because I was not able to defend myself.

–Do you still think that?

–Not anymore. There was a moment when the anger I felt through thinking like that just overwhelmed me, I threw a tantrum and started yelling. In that moment something switched gears in me. And I'm grateful that that happened before the tumor could develop a metastasis which would have meant an even worse, more dramatic change. You have to translate change into your everyday life, and it's not always easy to do that until you've lived a border-line experience like having cancer.

–You are now focused on food to stay healthy.

–I'm convinced that a strong immune system keeps you strong and healthy. ***I think cancer is a deep wound that doesn't let you go, but it is also a huge chance of opening your eyes to life, and to become more aware of things, to be awake.*** I now build my life my way: I eat what is good for me and surround myself with people that are good for me, too. ■

I was impressed because –although I don't directly admit it– I, too, have placed the responsibility for my problems on other people. And it's powerful to hear someone else say the same thing. For me, cancer has been a huge pain, but also a gift: an adverse situation that has given me the chance to restart relationships, to heal wounds from the past, to change my attitude. I can talk about cancer from the time it appeared on my arm, but its origin isn't so clear. Did it appear because of my lifestyle? Due to my sorrows? From sun-exposure? From keeping emotions bottled up inside? Because of the way I ate? I don't know. And I wouldn't dare answer that. Although there is an idea circulating that you make yourself sick, the variables influencing an illness are too many, and with time, the way I look at the inner meaning of cancer has changed.

When I think back to the time this book was a project, I remember I needed to run away and find the space to forget what I was going through. Between the end of 2011 and the beginning of 2012 I entered the very tempting game of escapism. For people who are sick, as I was at the time, this is a possibility. I was disorganized, all over the place, I was into relationships with no future, I looked for certainties in the wrong people. I boosted my ego in order to protect myself, because you get tired even of your own sensitivity, you don't want to suffer anymore. When would this sadness leave me in peace? I was a mess, I stopped following my diet, and my emotions were all over the place.

* Between the end of 2011 and the beginning of 2012 I entered the very tempting game of escapism. For sick people, like me at the time, it is a possibility.

Mornings were terrible, I felt an awful anguish, my mind didn't stop, my obsessions were at their peak. When would I stop questioning things? *Cancer days and cancer moments*, those days during which cancer images were there like intermittent flashbacks. I was not as accompanied as before, people moved on, friends went back to their routines. I got phone calls, but I didn't have that permanent reinforcement of when they took turns to talk to me about other subjects and to make me laugh. It's not that they changed, I did. Cancer altered the order of things, and the direction my life was taking. Suddenly I was standing on this new side of the road, with my family always watching over me. I was afraid, but now I had a huge need to overcome it.

Caro, my sister-in-law, told me that I never stopped surprising her. For this book we had her opinion too, because she had a very important role. While Tomás was fully supportive with my father in his endless search for information, she was going through a very hard pregnancy. "I saw him sad, of course, he had a rough time during 2011, but he was always surrounded by friends, he's very sociable, he's a leader –I'm still impressed when I remember how many people came to see him in hospital, he would have filled a whole stadium– and now he's intent on putting this book together. I really don't know where he got his strength from. Roberto gave me a good lesson, because he is a person who enjoys life, he is positive and special; I see him becoming an ever more fulfilled person as time goes by." That was what she told me for this book.

Her words remind me of the value of a strong family that accompanies you in a way that you may never feel again in your life. I would feel it again some time later when my dear dog Mora suddenly died during a trip to the south. My parents and siblings were with me when I buried her in *Matanzas*, by the sea.

Carmen Hodgson, who was almost a child when she lived through cancer, felt that strength in her own way.

–What did you hold on to in order to move on? Was there a psychologist with you?

– I didn't have a psychologist. My family was, and still is, my psychologist. We became close, I was their number one priority. I never had to comfort my mother, never saw my father crying. They always had my back. I think it was harder on them than it was for me, and I also leaned on God. ***When I underwent surgeries my parents waited outside the OR, but no one was with me inside, when I was unconscious. I trusted God.*** ■

In my case, I went to see a psychologist. I had needed her before, and it was impossible for me to act as though I could do this all by myself. The psychologist gave me a support that was different to that my family offered me. Family is pure love, care, and constant preoccupation. ***"Family and love feed you", Patty Marchesse told me. That's what kept her strong when her son was ill.***

–When did that love strengthen you?

–When I faced fears that paralyzed me. If I hadn't felt that love for Tomás, I would not have had the strength to react the way I did. Sometimes I felt the world would come to an end, and I only made it because of love. Love in its purest form, when you only think of him and yourself no longer exist. It's only giving, giving and giving. ***When my husband said goodbye to Tomás, he told him something I have never forgotten, and which proves what I'm saying. "Tommy, every parent dreams of their children taking after them, but from now on, I will dream about taking after you."*** ■

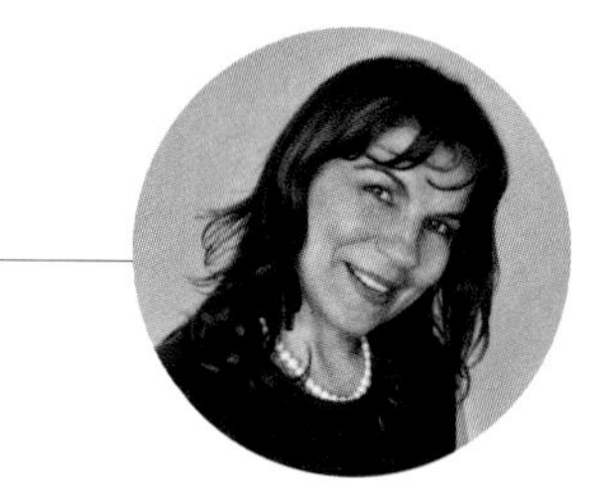

Gonzalo Muñoz knows how different things could have been had his family not supported him as they did. Just after his daughter Rosario's leukaemia diagnosis many friends came to see them, but two close friends stayed away. Gonzalo found it particularly odd given that both of them had, when they were little, had siblings with cancer. The absence of one of the friends, whose sister had survived, especially surprised them. But when that friend did eventually turn up, Gonzalo understood something:

–What happened during that visit?

–I was shocked by the expression on his face when he looked at Rosario. He's normally such a cheerful person, but it was as though he'd been disfigured. He was reliving his childhood pain, the rage and feeling of parental abandonment without understanding why. Seeing my friend's face at that moment made me realize what my other daughters might be feeling, and from that moment on we took care to build a solid family network of support around ourselves. ■

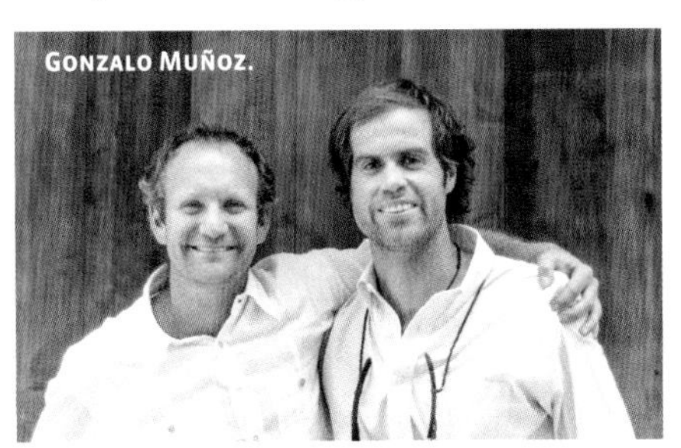
GONZALO MUÑOZ.

The way cancer got into Gonzalo's life was so ferocious, that before Rosario's disease was fully at bay, he made the decision of quitting his successful and well-paid job, and to the astonishment of his boss he set up a company that would put his skills at the service of important causes. That's how he founded Triciclos, a Recycle Hub network that also provides environmental education spaces. "A company appraising human capital beyond financial capital," he explained to me.

Of Teresa, his wife, he says: "I feel I have the best wife in the world. I admire her capacity to cope, she was almost my only certainty when I took the risk to create *Triciclos* with some friends." Today, she works in the foundation *Nuestros Hijos*, which assists children from lower-income backgrounds that suffer from cancer.

–It seems as though you all changed...

–Let me put it this way: today, when I look at Rosario, my daughter, who was terminally ill, I only think of the word love. Then, I ask myself how I keep this sensitivity inside me, to continue giving, to connect better with people, to live life without feeling I'm already as good as I can be, to be a nice person and to laugh as much as possible. Rosario's illness was the worst, but thanks to her, I now ask myself those questions every day. ■

However, the energy devoted to taking care of someone who's ill, the denial, and the circle of love in the family, sometimes has costs for parents focusing their attention on the sick sibling. In our conversation, Patricia recognized that once it was all over, she had to take care of pending issues from the time she had focused solely on Tomás' treatment. This was her answer:

–I imagine that your husband and you had no time to ask yourselves as a couple...

–We were 2 racehorses, because it was an intense treatment. One did the day shift and the other the night shift. If I fell he moved on; if he was down, I stood up and we managed. We were the best parents in the entire world for Tomás. But our relationship suffered along the way. We had to work on it after it was over. ■

Antonia, my sister, also sees in me some of that optimism my sister-in-law talks about, the drive that lives alongside my sensitivity. She remembers that when I underwent surgery I asked doctors when I would be kite surfing again. They answered that maybe in 3 months, but a month and a half later I was already on the board again, despite the pain in my arm and all that I had gone through. As my Dad says, that's typical of me: if I want something I chase it until I get it. "A pain in the neck"... he he he!

However, sometimes that drive was just not enough to dodge the waves that frequently and unexpectedly arrived. One day I felt a discomfort in one of my testicles. I was like this for a while, because a patient waits a little bit while begging in silence that the symptoms will pass. The discomfort didn't disappear and I went to get an ultrasound. I went alone, since I felt I did not have to be escorted, supported, and guided all the time. Also because I don't like company at those moments. The person with you gets nervous, I get

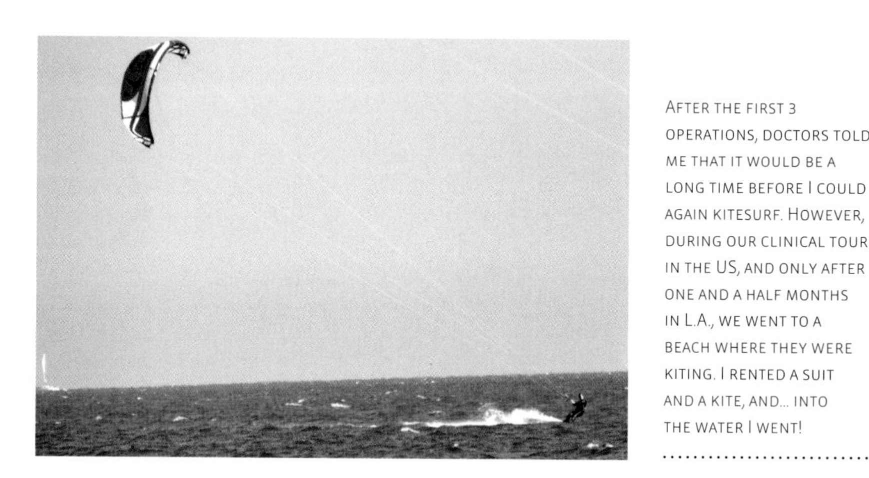

After the first 3 operations, doctors told me that it would be a long time before I could again kitesurf. However, during our clinical tour in the US, and only after one and a half months in L.A., we went to a beach where they were kiting. I rented a suit and a kite, and... into the water I went!

more nervous and feel invaded, so I prefer to do it quickly and forget about it. But I was wrong. That day before going in for the exam, I ran into a schoolteacher, Miss Margarita, who I knew had been fighting cancer for a long time. She was with her daughter, who was a classmate of mine. When I said hello, she hugged me and started to cry. I thought she'd just had some bad news. No. She was crying out of happiness, because finally her cancer had gone away. When she left, my shield fell apart and I couldn't stop crying. I called Dad and told him everything, that I should not have come alone. He came quickly and together we heard the doctor say that the exam did not show anything, that everything was good. Hearing that, and feeling supported because Dad was there with me, for me, I didn't cry. I was able to be happy, because I had his support.

I've thought a lot about why I went there on my own, and I'd have loved to have interviewed Miss Margarita for this book. She'd been so happy with the all-clear. Tragically though, soon afterwards the cancer came back with a vengeance and before I had a chance to contact her she passed away. That's cancer for you; it hits hard and sometimes those waves are *tsunamis*. ■

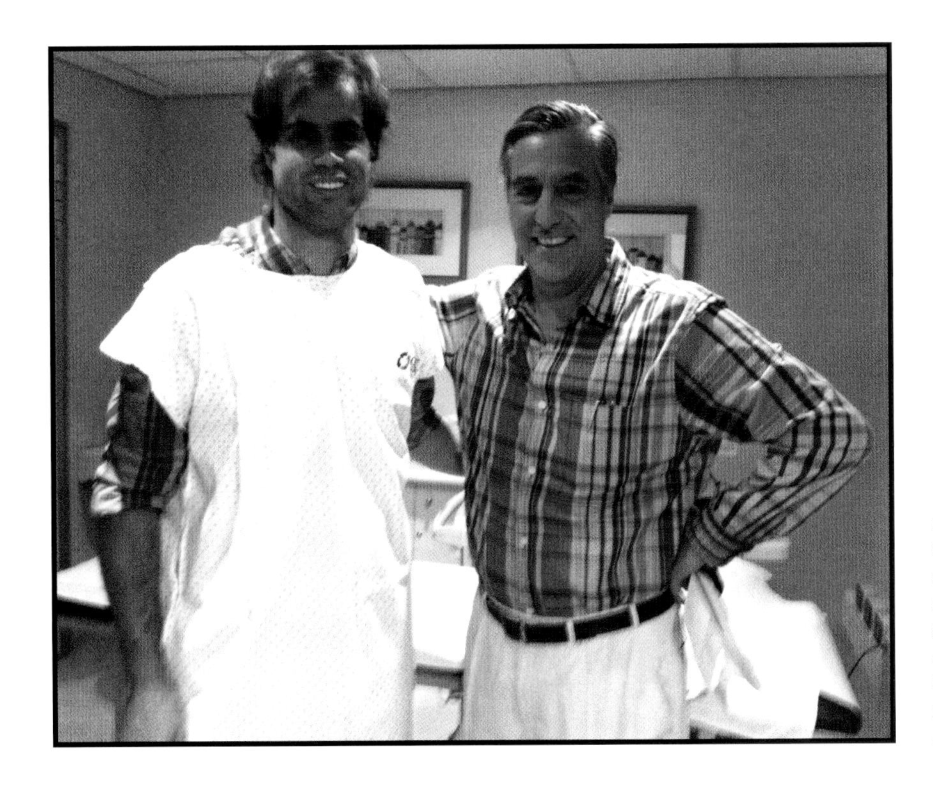

I learned that being with someone, in this case my father, during a medical consultation, or an exam, gives you a necessary support. Especially when the issue is cancer.

6. *Cancer mode* ON

Sometimes turning *Cancer Mode* ON is healthy, because you put on hold the worries that tend to fill our days. You can forget responsibilities and demands, without having to give anyone explanations. Period.

Being "ill" implies a special condition, especially if your illness is cancer. I call it turning the *Cancer Mode* ON. Without having ever asked for it, you have a certificate excusing you from many responsibilities and giving you a space to live the cancer moments when you just don't want to deal with the daily issues of life; those that come from your job, your friends, or your family. Personally, I consider it to be a very useful tool, and that people with cancer should use it whenever they feel tired of everything and they don't want (or do want) to do something, no questions asked. ***Having cancer gives you the freedom to use Cancer Mode ON. The important thing is to use it suitably and carefully.***

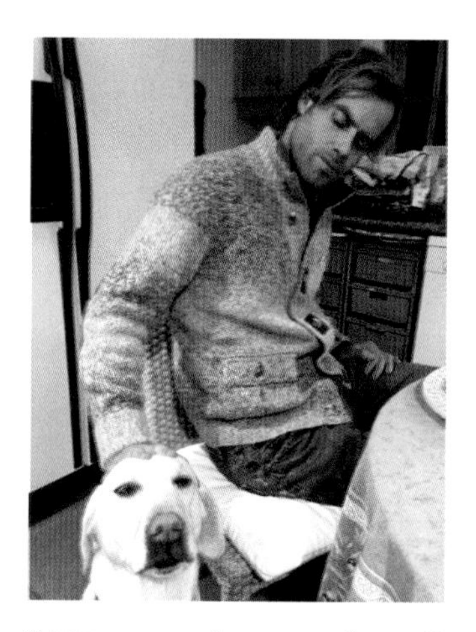

Many times when I turned my *Cancer Mode* ON, I took the time to relax and to do things I wouldn't normally do. Here, I let my dog Paloma into the kitchen to cuddle her. Mom took this picture of us.

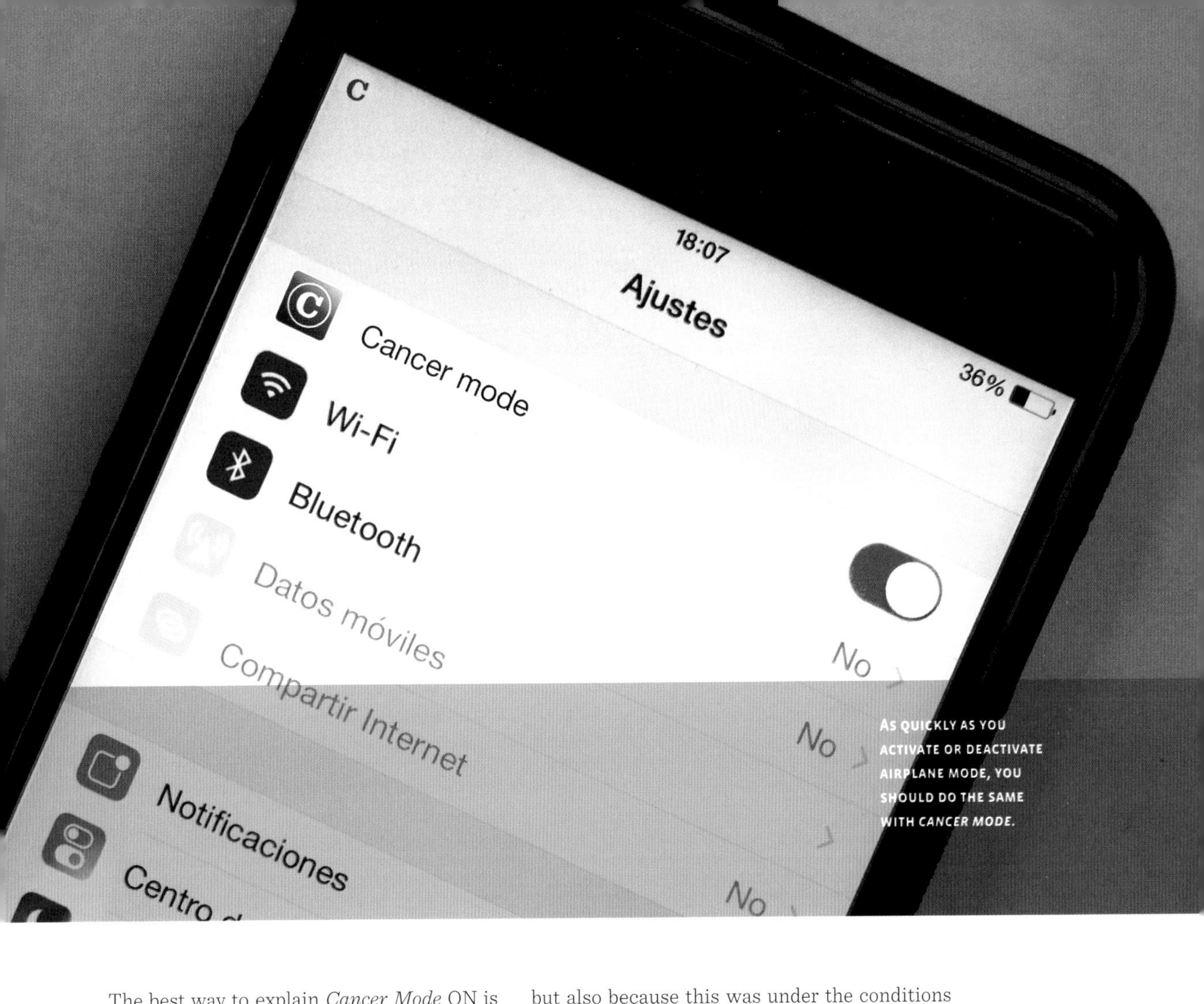

As quickly as you activate or deactivate airplane mode, you should do the same with *cancer mode*.

The best way to explain *Cancer Mode* ON is when you are in the hospital. Surely, more than one person reading this book must have been in a hospital room for at least a day. In the hospital you can let yourself off the hook - others can take over for a while. No questions asked. Another good thing about being in thc hospital (and it's not easy to let go of this once you're out again!) is that everyone worries about you, and without asking for it you've suddenly become the center of attention. Warning: this can be addictive, unhealthy even. But to be honest it can also be really useful when you just want to switch off and turn away from the world.

Ale Méndez lived the forced confinement in hospital intensely. Not only because of the many months she accompanied her son Pablo, but also because this was under the conditions of total isolation due to the two bone marrow transplants that he'd undergone. Both times they had to be 6 weeks inside a bubble, completely isolated from the outside world. It all happened in Boston. They were there when the cancer began, and as they had insurance covering the expenses, with each relapse they went back to the same center.

–Ale, it must have been hard being far away from the people you love. That was one of the main reasons that I didn't take part in the clinical trials.

–Actually, being far away meant we avoided something that would have been hard for us: dealing with the constant flow of visitors and the sad faces and pitying voices that people inevitably adopt in these situations. The social pressure of people is overwhelming, tiring and contagious. In Boston it was only us, the Allard Méndez family, and in a way that safeguarded us, a bit like in the movie *Life is Beautiful*. When Pablito lost his hair, Pablo shaved his head. We hung the poster of the Brazilian soccer player Ronaldo in his room, he went around bald wearing his soccer shoes and he swore all soccer players were like him.

Pablo totally agrees: *"Our motto was* work, *don't think. I'm telling you something: Pablo's illness didn't take away the happiness of being completely together. From the 20 years we have been married with Ale, we have never been happier as a couple and as a family than when we were fighting this together."*

Ale says her husband is right: "It was beautiful, although difficult to understand if you have not lived the experience. You focus, as a marriage and as a family. We had to be alone in the U.S., and that is why I could fully focus. I was at the hospital all day long, without any other worry on my mind. No home, work, friends, visitors, nothing. I would wear whatever I wanted to, and I could have the luxury of reading stories, painting, or watching TV with my son. I never had that luxury again; the world stopped. No guests to attend to, no emails to send. My mother was in charge of Max, my 1-year old son, and I could focus on Pablito. When I returned home, the way I relaxed was with Max. He gave me the energy I needed. ■

Nowadays, they have left *Cancer Mode* ON behind, and the five of them are in *living mode on*, enjoying every second. There's nothing closer to pure happiness than a weekend in which the 5 of them are together. Pablo, Alejandra and their 3 sons: Pablito, Max and Antonio. Together they feel strong, happy, normal. That's what they told me. But they didn't have to; you can tell.

Carmen Hodgson lived *Cancer Mode* ON in a way similar to mine. We connected when we talked about this, because it is true that it has an unhealthy and hard-to-define element to it, because only someone who has known it, can feel it. It is non-transferable, as Ale Méndez says. That was what Carmen and I talked about:

–Haven't you sometimes missed your time in the hospital?

–What I'm about to say is weird, but about once a year I want to be there. My mother thinks I have lost my mind; how could I want to be sick! However, it's not that. It's like escaping.

–I have that feeling, too. When you go into hospital you leave petty worries behind.

–Exactly. Everyone would be worrying about me. It's the comfy side of the illness. Really! Everything revolved around me.

Schoolmates from high school were there with flowers, even friends I met at parties. My friends took turns so I wouldn't ever be alone. There were times people were in and out, but those 2 secs of conversation took me out of that world. As though I was being beamed away. I actually miss that feeling sometimes. ■

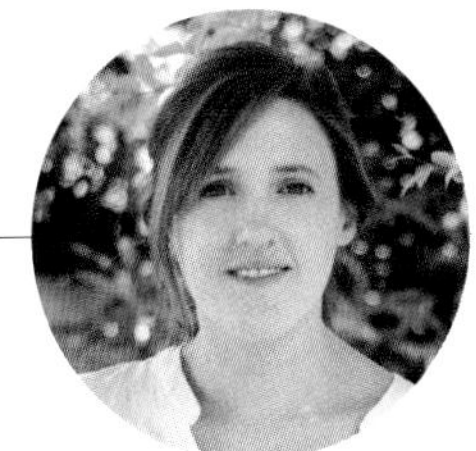

When I interviewed **Diana Strauss** we talked about this, but she lived it very differently. She saw the other side of the coin:

–Did you ever feel comfortable while in hospital, without having to think about your disease, because the doctors and nurses did that for you?
– I hate being in the hospital. I feel that real things are happening outside and that I'm missing them. While in the hospital, I lived for results –waiting for various tests to be run on me on a daily basis– things being injected into me. I kept trying to read the expression on the doctor's face to see how things were going, nurses would not listen to me... I don't want to be back in the hospital ever. That's why I strengthen my immune system with the healthiest food possible. ■

After that stressful episode in the hospital, waiting for results, I discovered that there are other situations in which it's better to have someone by your side. Once, I went alone to *Matanzas*. I felt sad, a little tired of everything. It was one of those cancer moments. It was early morning on a Friday when I turned my *Cancer Mode* ON. I called work, let them know I was not coming in, I took my dogs with me, and I left. Believe me, there is nothing worse than driving two and a half hours in a moment of despair. Hideous.

In those moments of loneliness and sadness, when everything seems to fall apart, think about the *what for* that **Amaro Gómez-Pablos** talked about when I interviewed him. Unfortunately when I took that long and lonely drive to *Matanzas* I hadn't met him yet, hadn't heard anyone talk about things in the way he would.

* The best way to explain *Cancer Mode ON* is when you are in the hospital. Surely, more than one person reading this book must have been in a hospital room for at least a day. In the hospital you can let yourself off the hook - others can take over for a while. No questions asked.

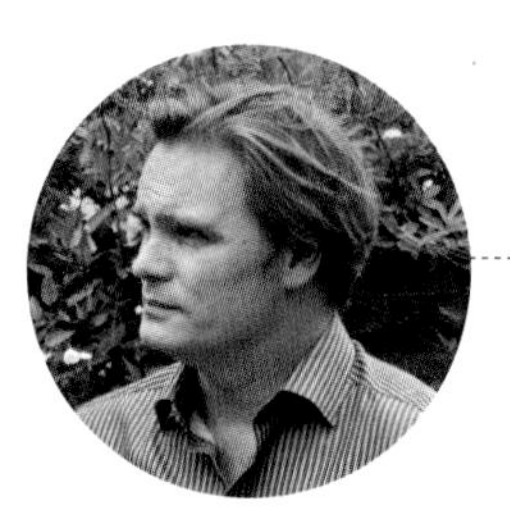

He showed me that being stuck in the *"why"* –especially in the *"why me"*– was not worth it. This positive turn left me highly motivated.

–Amaro. How did you manage not to ask yourself time and time again, *why me*?

–I thought of the great Austrian psychiatrist Viktor Frankl, Holocaust survivor who wrote a famous book, *Man's Search for Meaning*, where he writes that even in the most extreme situations of suffering, you can find a reason to live. A *"what for?"*. *If you only ask the* why *of your disease, you spiral downwards and there is no way out. In turn, if you ask yourself* "what for?" *– what do I live for – you begin a process of questioning.* You have an illness inside you, but also a question that drives you to find why you are here, where you are going, why you want to continue living. What for. Pilar, my wife, asked for help, when confronted with things that seemed to attack her femininity –the hair stuck in the shower, for instance– and between chemo and chemo when she felt strong, she focused on the *what for*.

–What do you mean? What did she do?

–We went searching for pictures. That's how we called it. We went looking for beautiful things. Pilar was an adventurous woman. We had the opportunity to travel together, in order for her to see the beauty in the world. Afterwards she would rest and we would revisit our trips through the pictures. This is what is worth the most and what you remember and –above all– what pushes you on, to keep fighting to live. Between one chemotherapy and another, we did everything we could to have memorable moments, getaways –nearby or distant ones, depending on the possibilities–, and took the mandatory picture. Then, during chemo, while she was being bombarded with chemicals, we would look at those pictures; we talked, laughed... it was a breath of fresh air. Pilar was really fond of the opera. As a child, her father narrated opera plots instead of reading stories to her. Watching *Madame Butterfly* in dim light to a full house, I saw a tear running down her face. "Are you ok? Are you in pain?" I asked. She held my hand. "I feel no pain", she answered. "It's a temporary sorrow. There's so much beauty out there and it makes me sad not living long enough to see it." This was the aesthetics of a hard, fragile, and very beautiful life. Pilar found her *"what for"*. ■

What was my *what for*? Being positive? Healing? Writing my book? Consolidating *Celebraciones con Sentido*? That seems to make sense. These and many other reasons were, and still are, my *what for*. It is the only way to focus on life and enjoy the beauty Pilar spoke about. **Gonzalo Muñoz** told me the following:

> *"Look at life, not death. The first reaction when facing cancer is feeling that death is around the corner. You set aside the idea of life being among us, every day, with or without the disease, with all its frailty and, mainly, its briefness. That's why you have to live life to the fullest".*

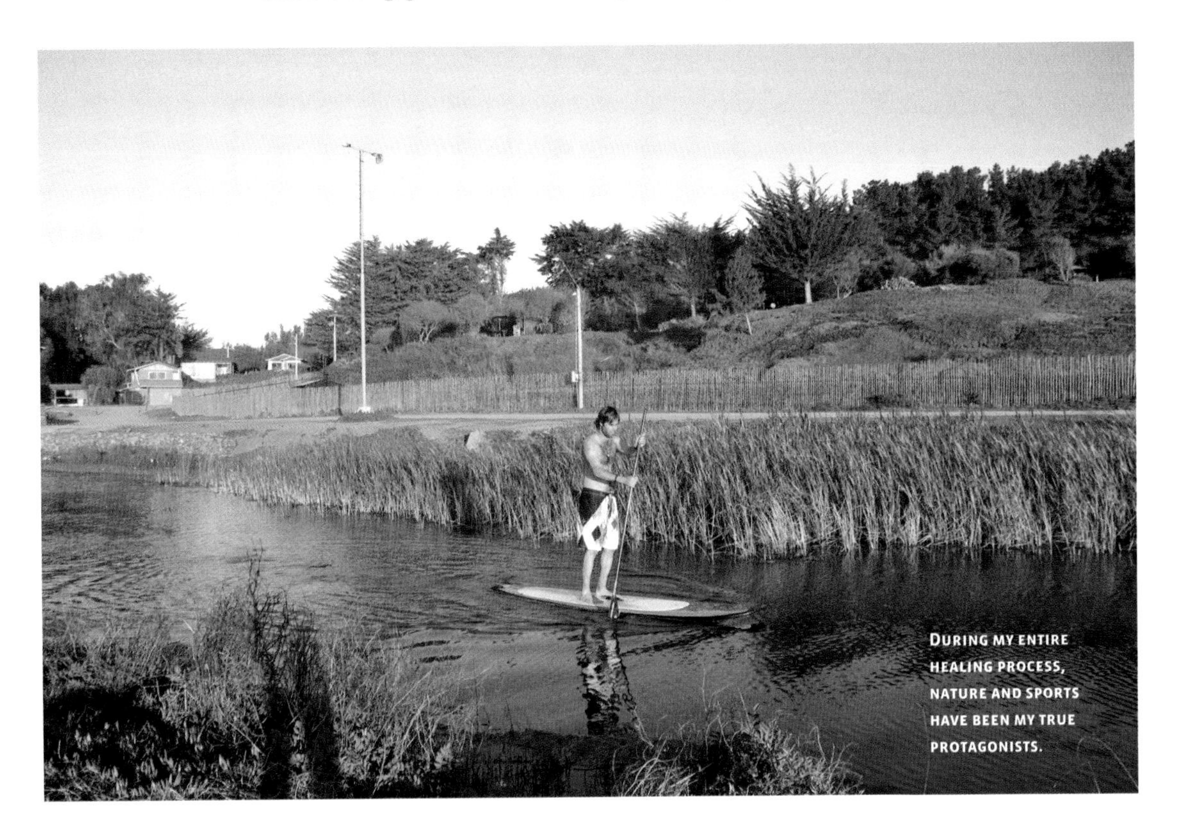

DURING MY ENTIRE HEALING PROCESS, NATURE AND SPORTS HAVE BEEN MY TRUE PROTAGONISTS.

When you have cancer, relapses are terrifying. They are like a ghost that's always there, haunting you. I sometimes pretend it has vanished, that it does not exist, until something happens and causes an emergency. As it did in February, while I was on vacation in *Panguipulli*, with my family. I love going to the lake; especially, when my brothers and I get together at my parents' house. It reminds me of the environment of the bungalows in *Tunquelén* from my childhood summers in *Pucón*. I am filled with energy. One morning, after showering, while I was drying my armpit I noticed a small bulge a little below the scar left by the nodule dissection. I remembered doctor Vial's words:

On the same night I arrived in Santiago, Doctor Vial received us at his house. He detected an inflamed node and suggested taking an ultrasound. There was a possibility the melanoma had metastasized. I panicked and felt a deep sorrow. I couldn't bare the idea of starting all over again: the hospital, the doctors, the exams, the pain. The loneliness, anguish and... not fear, but terror.

I got an ultrasound. I let my parents know that I would have the results back soon. Antonia told me she was shaking just thinking of the possibility of the swelling meaning I had metastases. I also shook.

* "I shook, because the idea of dying and not being able to enjoy the new and good things that were happening to my family, friends and me tormented me."

"If you ever feel any hard bumps in that area come to see me right away." I said nothing for a day, and prayed at night for that strange swelling I'd found to disappear. The following day, it was obviously still there. I approached Sebastián and told him: "Seba, feel this." He did and was immediately concerned. He reacted the way I didn't want him to. Under no circumstance did I feel like hopping on the plane to Santiago, to see Doctor Vial, and for him to tell me the cancer had metastasized. Not now! Not in the middle of Summer. But Sebastián and I travelled to Santiago. *I had learned those trips are not the kind you take alone.* We didn't speak. At all. Did we avoid doing so? Probably. But what were we supposed to say? I by far preferred feeling his company and empathy, then contemplating together the possibilities.

After the doctor confirmed I had nothing to be worried about, I suddenly relaxed and started crying. I released the anguish I had kept inside, the shitty feeling of having to go down to the hospital, seeing the worried faces, feeling enclosed within those white walls and smelling that hideous smell that resembled bathroom disinfectant.

I cried because I didn't want cancer to return.

I shook, because the idea of dying and not being able to enjoy the new and good things that were happening to my family, friends and me... tormented me.

That whole process gave me the chance to look at the big picture, of looking "through the window." The world was a much bigger and more complex place than I had ever imagined it to be, and to understand it I had to stop focusing on myself and leave selfishness aside. I understood this, one day at a time, and liked the feeling. I didn't want to lose it!

I texted my parents telling them everything was ok. According to Antonia, when my parents read it they felt a great weight was taken off their shoulders. They hugged, thanked God and the Holy Virgin, and that night they celebrated. We were adopting a new style, there was no possibility we would now lose sight of the essentials.

day towards the end of March, almost a year after my first surgery, I was admitted again into the hospital. I approached the center of outpatient procedures and was told my name was not on their list. It was very strange... The doctor had assured me it would be a quick procedure. I went to General Admissions, was assigned a room and then, in the waiting room, the anesthesiologist told me they were going to give me general anesthesia.

Why? Had there been a change of plans that I hadn't been informed about? She explained

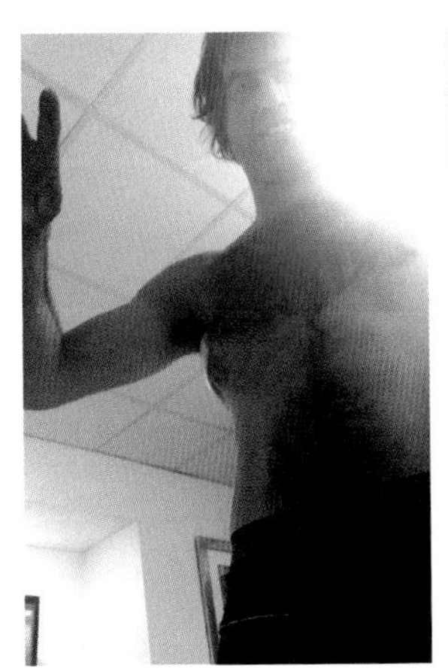

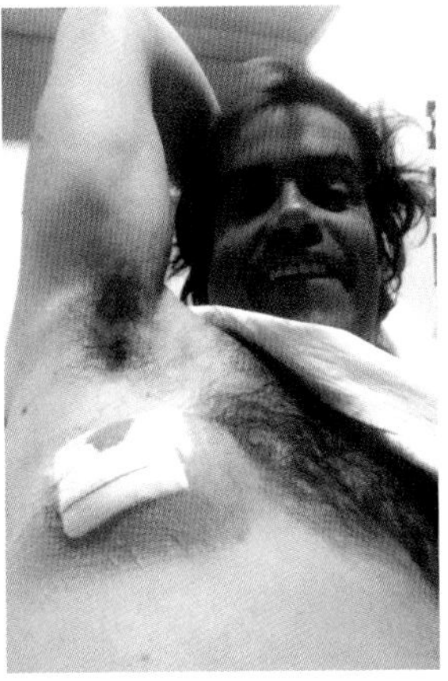

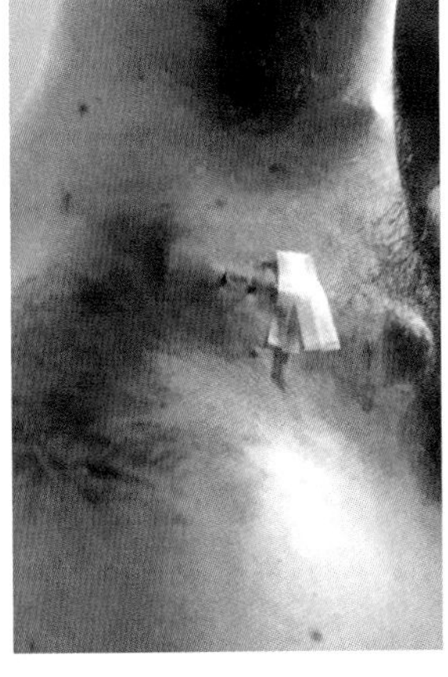

You never know how the body will react after surgery. Sometimes a process may worsen and, as a cancer patient, you need to be mentally prepared and fight till the end.

Anyway, I still needed to undergo surgery. The bump in my arm was not serious, but the doctor warned that if the swelling didn't go away in 3 months, it would have to be removed. I was already reluctant to accept first opinions, so I talked about this with Doctor Mercedes López, whom I trusted and still trust a lot. She recommended undergoing surgery, because it was the best way to make the swelling disappear.

I waited two months for the node inflammation to go down. But it did not go away. One Mon-

the area of the arm I had to be operated on was complicated because it was irrigated by blood vessels and so the best option was general anesthesia. Confused and angry, I asked to talk to Doctor Vial, who did not change the type of anesthesia, but instead did everything he could to calm me down.

I had undergone 3 painful surgeries the previous year, I had limited mobility, was confined to a hospital bed, with a catheter inserted into my urethra, my nodes had been removed, one of my nerves had been damaged, and another one was removed to fix it. I had an inflamed node, I was going to undergo outpatient surgery and it turned out I needed general anesthesia for the surgery. When would all this end?

I must literally be a bad patient, because I don't have the patience sick people are supposed to have when facing "unexpected" post-surgery events. While I was recovering from surgery, I started bruising in the area of the surgery. It ended up looking like a boob again! And, above all, I would have to stay in hospital. Isn't life meant to be simpler when things are going right?

*"According to doctor Vial, it is reasonable to spend the maximum time possible in the pre-surgical stage, to talk in depth and show all the consequences."

Every so often, uncertainty prevented me from breathing properly. Trying to speak from behind the shield that protects us from weakness, I told Mom once again: *Shit happens!* Shit happens, I know, but it was happening to me.

I talked about that episode later on with Doctor Vial during a conversation we had for this book. I told him how bad I'd felt. I spoke about how confused I'd felt back then, and he empathized with me, and was really honest. He told me there was a lot of work to be done in order to improve doctor-patient communication. "Patients often don't remember what their doctors explain because they're, obviously, nervous. On other occasions, and although most of us are extraordinarily meticulous, we forget to mention some things," the doctor said.

He feels that doctors should spend as long as is necessary with patients before a surgery, to discuss all the issues and possible consequences, to talk through what the patient expects and how the specialist should react to different situations. "The ideal is to go into the OR with a relationship of deep trust between doctor and patient, knowing the decisions are made by the patient. However, many times, these conversations end up being insufficient due to the lack of time. And, sometimes, patients are not in the best state of mind to know what they want. It is important for doctors to provide some time. I usually emphasize the urgency when treatment shouldn't be deferred, but I try not to pressure people, and I aim for a patient to know as much as possible about the process they are undergoing and what they are dealing with.

Based on that experience, I repeatedly asked the people I interviewed about the space they had to make decisions and take control of the situation. **Gonzalo Muñoz** went through a very positive experience and I was relieved to hear it.

–Could you make decisions or did doctors just inform you of the procedures?

–We were lucky enough to meet Doctor Milena Villarroel; she was on call when we were told Rosario had cancer, and we continued the process with her. That was essential. She always considered us as parents and people, she explained every detail of the case. Every time we faced a new step, the 3 of us took decisions together. This doctor set her professional ego completely aside –even though she is an eminent doctor–. When matters got rough, she consulted other specialists. She opened up new roads, but knew we were the ones who would make the final decisions. Doctors usually pretend they know the truth; however, she adopted an apprentice attitude, not that of a teacher, as if she was learning from Rosario and us. She accompanied us all along the path. ■

Drago Gluscevic surrendered to his doctor. He trusted him simply because he felt they clicked from the very beginning. His story is chilling. I had heard it because I'm friends with his children and him. Eight years ago he faced a Non Hodgkin lymphoma and, while he was fighting against cancer with chemotherapy, his wife was diagnosed with breast cancer and his business partner –and lifetime friend– was diagnosed with lung cancer. All at the same time. It's unbelievable.

–Why did you feel you *clicked* with your doctor? Was he the first oncologist you visited?

–No, first I visited a very polite and professional doctor, but for whom I felt nothing. I didn't feel he was the one. I believe that if you don't trust your doctor, you will be checking his instructions with others. A friend recommended seeing another oncologist and I immediately clicked with him. He is one of those doctors who laughs with you, spends more time attending you when needed, and gives you a hug at the end of the appointment. Maybe we developed that relation because, at the very beginning, he told me something that encouraged me during the treatment: "Do you know something, Drago? I am sure you will defeat the disease. You're not the type of patient who becomes mute when I say the word cancer and fight alone. And, also, you don't smoke." He gave me lots of tools and asked me how I felt and what I wanted to do at every stage. He listened to my intuition. ■

Drago and Susana, his wife, are no longer at risk. Although recently he detected a carcinoma on his face as a big pimple, on the rim of his eye, it was removed. On the other hand, his partner and lifelong friend died in 2011. His cancer was really aggressive. Drago was beside him right up up to the end, even when nothing more could be done.

It is hard to imagine a patient tired of fighting against the disease and losing optimism, but obviously, sometimes the body is exhausted. Most likely, I just don't want to imagine it. *As* **Patty Marchesse** *told me, cancer patients have the right to get tired.* She gives a lot of her time providing support to families that endure the pain of having a child with cancer, listens to lots of sad stories, and provides her unique optimism, but she gave me a straight answer when I asked about that tiredness.

–When can a patient give up?

–If a person doesn't want to fight, it's their choice. It's their life. *When a patient gives up, they need to be respected just as someone who is fighting needs to be provided willing support.* ■

I find it hard to imagine a patient so tired of everything that he or she has nothing more to dream about.

I remember talking about this with Amaro. After his testimonial, I started accepting it's also valid to take a break for a while and stop running, making an effort, trying. This is hard for the people who love you to accept, it's sometimes even perplexing, but at the end of the day it's you who is suffering from the disease, and that's it.

–Did Pilar fight until the end or did she get exhausted? How did you approach the subject with her?

–It's a very complicated subject for couples. How do you give her that space she needs as is absolutely her right, to give up? That very delicate and intuitive balance: you sometimes need to be supportive and push forward, and sometimes you need to understand this only causes pain. One needs to develop some sensitivity to accompany her with her will to live and to support her when she wants to exercise her right to rest; because fighting gets one tired. I paved her way. ■

Being sick is hateful. You have half the energy, lack the thousands of answers and are not capable of asking questions. You're afraid, tired, want to go back in time and regain the life you used to have, as if this was a bad movie and you only needed to change channels. But it's not that simple.

Loreto Agurto couldn't tolerate being looked at as a sick person. She said this to me time and again. Her husband, **Gonzalo Tagle,** confirmed it. I didn't know Gonzalo and it meant the world to me talking to him about Loreto –Lolo, as she was called at home– because it helped me to approach her in a different way. She was no longer with us, but her vital and wild spirit was quickly felt between us. I hope Gonzalo knows how grateful I am for our meeting. In the conversation we had, I asked him how things had happened. I needed to know, wanted to reenact her last days to feel as close to her as I wasn't at the time, but didn't know whether Gonzalo would open up and talk to me about it. He didn't have to, we weren't friends. That's why his generous and willing disposition overwhelmed me. He listened, and laid my doubts to rest. I later write about his attitude as the husband of a woman with cancer and the legacy she left. Reasonably, Gonzalo prefers leaving the rest of our conversation in private.

–Loreto hated being looked at as a sick person. Do you agree?

–Lolo wanted to continue living; so she avoided visible signs of the illness appearing on her body. She set her mind on her children and family not seeing her suffer and on not being treated as a sick person. She kept her melanomas a secret. I can assure you that most of the people who went to her farewell mass –even work mates– didn't know why she had died.

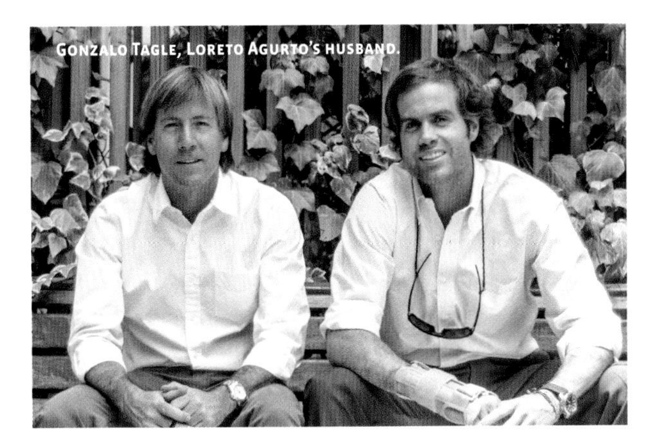
GONZALO TAGLE, LORETO AGURTO'S HUSBAND.

Cancer helped her lead her life more intensely, and she lived as though she was healthy all along, until the last day. She didn't suffer cancer. Apart from surgeries to remove her melanomas, she was always well.

–As her husband, how did you face her disease?

–We devoted our time to living happily and avoided everything bad. Since was detected the first melanoma on her leg, Lolo taught me to face life looking at the bright side. To see the glass half-full. She showed me that the only way to be happy was by making us happy. She died when we were coming home from a trip. We had travelled alone to celebrate her birthday in Miami. When we returned, she suffered a stroke. And I always perceived in her eyes that her only aim was that neither me, nor our children, had a bad time. She wanted us to continue being happy, as she had taught us to be. ■

Talking to Gonzalo was fantastic. It was enlightening. I made use of that time to tell him about the circumstances in which I learned about Loreto's death. It happened a day before I underwent surgery to have the node that had surprised me in *Panguipulli* removed, a few months before. But I didn't know that day. I had surgery on a Monday, and on Thursday, still on my way to recovery, I went to work. That afternoon, on my way home, a friend called me while I was using my hands-free car kit: "Roberto, I'm sitting beside your future wife." He was obviously trying to introduce me to a girl, so following this Chilean custom, I asked for her name. I only heard her surname, Agurto, and immediately thought about Loreto, her joy, her wise words, and I liked where this was going. "Are you related to Loreto Agurto?" I asked her. "Loreto?" she answered. She didn't speak for a while and then continued: "She died on Sunday. Yes."

That's all she said.

I wanted for it to be a lie. I hung up the phone and started crying. Loreto had died and nobody had told me! Why didn't I learn the news when it had happened? How had nobody told me, knowing how important she was to me? A very deep loneliness invaded me. My parents knew. They knew when I was going into surgery. I felt stupid, hadn't imagined the seriousness of her melanoma, she looked radiant and happy during our lunches, with a bright future ahead of her. A few months before, she had been hospitalized for a lung metastasis. We'd spoken, and she'd told me everything had gone fine. She had assured me it had. I now realize that, with her kindness and generosity, Loreto didn't want me to know. She conveyed that optimism of hers until the very last minute.

Loreto had died on Sunday, right before my surgery. Mom learned about it at the exact same moment I was bitterly complaining about my surgery being under general anesthesia. A friend of hers called to give her the bad news, and Antonia said she felt she had to keep it to herself. They all assessed the situation and decided to prevent me from suffering at the time, considering how upset I had been about the general anesthesia.

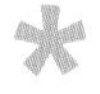 My parents decided not to tell me about Loreto's death at that moment. I walk a mile in their shoes, they wanted to take care, support and provide trust to me.

Today I know that, neither Dad nor Mom wanted to tell me about Loreto's death, just to protect me. I have to walk a mile in their shoes to understand that decision. They wanted to take care of me, to support me and make me feel confident, and as Dad told me when, 3 years later, we talked about my being diagnosed: ***"We all see only one side of a story. Sometimes, some things are hidden to avoid hurting others and to make the burden lighter. Finding the right time for some things was hard."*** And delivering such sad news in the condition I was in was not good. I have said this before, I believe that it is better experiencing than being told about some things, because of morbid curiosity, but because I really believe one needs to be surrounded by those you really love always, even when you die.

My soul hurt; it's one of the few things that still make me angry when I think about it. Loreto Agurto had been a transcendental woman throughout my disease. She'd given my melanoma a meaning. She had left a bright imprint on my life –that's how I felt at the time–, and I wasn't able to say goodbye to her. I can now understand that my parents didn't realize the depth of the friendship we had cultivated, because I hadn't shared with them –or even with my brothers– the discoveries I made through her.

Loreto was an amazing discovery and, self-absorbed as I was in my own process, I didn't speak about it. Had I done so, I know my parents would have made another decision, but at the time they weren't aware of our connection. Today, as I have already mentioned, I believe in the importance of having a monthly or weekly family moment to share what happens to you, however trivial an occurrence may seem. To talk and share news, and give each other space for fear and need is the best way to keep the family rock-solid. I would have loved for my family to get to know Loreto the way I did.

Gonzalo Tagle told me something I was already aware of: Loreto had died without leaving anything pending; she was completely at peace.

Sometime later, I learned that Loreto's mom, Loreto Fuentes, was going to be in Santiago. She lives in *Yerbas Buenas*, a town near *Linares*, and since Loreto's death I had been wanting to talk to her. There was a sensitive and sentimental side to my feelings and my sadness since her death, which it wouldn't have been right to share with Gonzalo.

We arranged a meeting at a coffee shop near *Touch's* former offices. I can't remember whether I waited for her or if it was the other way round, but as soon as we sat down and I looked at her, before she even uttered a word, I started crying uncontrollably. I was mourning and I wasn't able to share that with anybody. Who would have understood my sorrow? Just her. Just as Loreto had done when we first met, her mother hugged me and stood by my side. She told me many cool things about *Lolo*, or *La Negra* as they called her. And together we remembered a woman who –although I had known her for a very short time– had left a big impression on me. I told her about our magical encounter in the waiting room at the breast radiological center, and talked about the path I had followed since that moment, which had led me to be sitting in front of her that day.

When I finished my coffee, I was no longer sitting beside a stranger, but in front of a mother and lifelong friend, whom I didn't want to let go.

Despite this comforting meeting, I feel something is still pending with Loreto. And this has only boosted my desire to publish this book, to speak about her legacy and her unquenchable optimism, which may be useful for many people; and also, as a very personal way of saying goodbye.

Despite having been together only few times, I consider Loreto Fuentes, Loreto Agurto's mother, a good friend.

A few months after meeting with Loreto's mom, at the beginning of 2013, I was in *Panguipulli* again. A year had passed since the last time I had gotten on a plane to visit Doctor Vial because of the new node in my armpit. One morning, I woke up and felt no fear, anger, or uncertainty. It was a good day, and I had a few of those during my cancer.

So I wrote a list of things I would like to do. They look like commandments, but are not. I just wanted to put down in words how I felt at the time. It was therapeutic and I recommend it. This list may feel stubborn, weird or even make no sense, but... Who cares! Here I go.

THE LIST

1. Do whatever I feel like doing.
2. Miss Loreto. Believe in an angel.
3. Life changes. One grows up, learns, and is grateful to be happy in those moments when the past and the future don't matter, rage disappears, and the only thing that matters is the here and now.
4. Be calm. Acknowledge anxieties and prioritize them: Don't assume they're all the same.
5. Be responsible towards what I like. Be irresponsible with, or forget, what I don't like.
6. Look at the sky and breathe. Look at the sky and be surprised. Look at the sky and be at ease.
7. Don't expect anything from others. Don't expect anything from me.
8. Cuddle my dogs, love them and be loved back.
9. Dive into the lake, enjoy the water and my space.
10. Don't envy your neighbor. Strengthen my state.
11. Be aware of my flaws and find the will to improve.
12. Love my family. Be more tolerant.
13. Love my friends.
14. Drive slowly. Run when necessary. Watch the rest of the time.
15. Be happy with what I've accomplished. Be happy to be just sitting here.
16. Cook and eat tasty food. Drink wine.
17. Cast obsessions aside. Loosen up and let things happen.
18. Be honest, open and transparent.
19. Love and want to be loved.

20 Surround myself with people that make me feel good and stay away from people who don't.
21 Act without giving anyone any explanations. Act without giving myself an explanation.
22 Practice sports.
23 Laugh, alone and with others.
24 Wear the same clothes for 3 consecutive days.
25 Don't worry about hair loss.
26 Share.
27 Know I am happy alone, but I am happier when those that love me and who I love are close.
28 Don't label people.
29 Read more.
30 Watch a silly series. Learn to be silly.
31 Don't wear a tie.
32 Remember that wealth is related to friends and not money.
33 Let others control the situation. Keep quiet.
34 Sleep without feeling guilty.
35 Have the keys that matter to me on my key-chain. Keys from the house at the beach, my toys' warehouse (where I store my kite, bicycles, boards), the spare tire and the truck where I carry my dogs.
36 Eat blueberries, eat *maqui* berry.
37 Have a drink. Invite others for a drink.
38 Take a nap.
39 Recover from injuries.
40 Don't surf the web.
41 Don't look at my phone when I wake up. Don't look at my phone while on vacation, leave it at home and, if necessary, use somebody else's.
42 Don't look at my scars in the mirror.
43 Don't get medical exams if I don't want to.
44 If I have energy, go out and party.
45 If I'm sleepy go to bed.
46 Use sunscreen.
47 Write a book. Share what I've learned with someone who may find it useful.

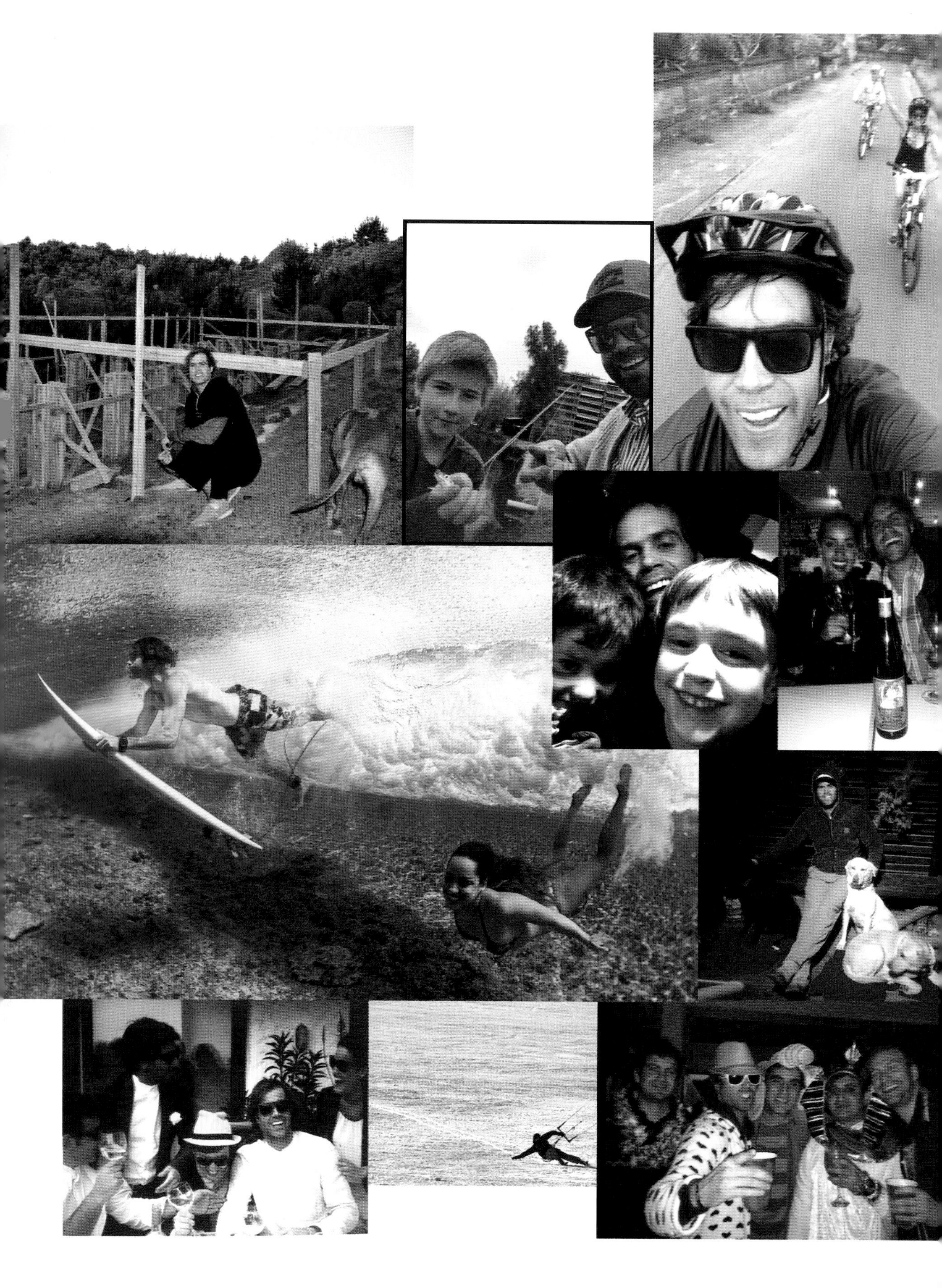

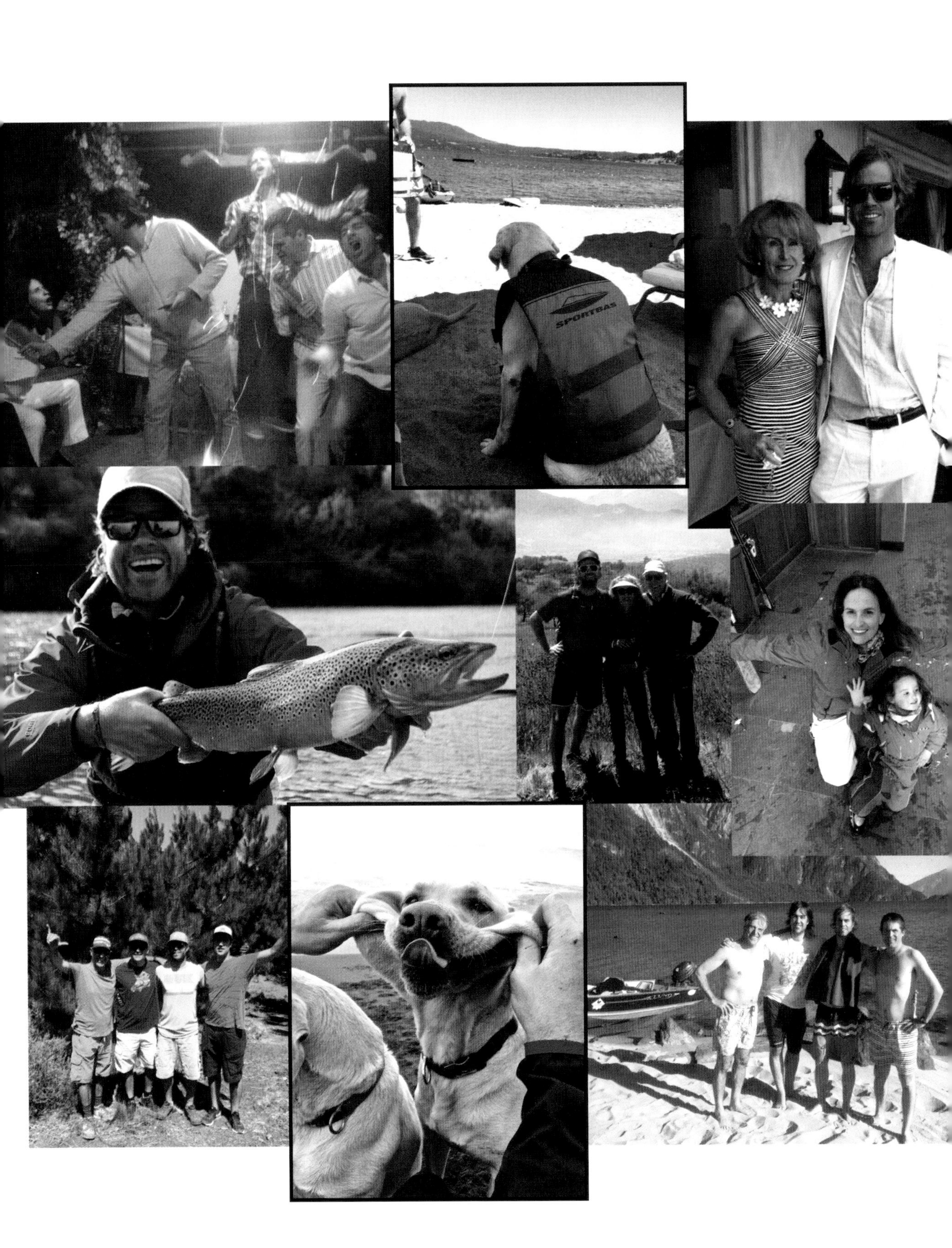
SPORTBAS

7. The spot in my lung

Before being definitely discharged, each test result, each skin bulge, each headache came with an uncomfortable drum roll... Can anybody live like this? There isn't a recipe, but I now know it can be done. At some point, the drum roll comes to an end.

Loreto used to say melanoma is a cancer that does not call a truce. She was most certainly right. With other types of cancer, after 5 years without a relapse you can forget about it forever. However, melanoma may always reappear. That's why keeping calm and trusting ones luck 100% is difficult. Some people, like **Guillermo Acuña,** achieve it. I got to know *Memo* through Iván Mimica; he had also started on the path to recovery through diet after suffering from an eye melanoma. When we met to talk for this book, I was surprised. I had not even thought about the topics that spun around in his mind. He made me think, and I was left trying to understand his point of view. *Memo* is married and has 5 children, and reading about how he currently faces life is worth it.

–How do you face PET CT tests, those that detect if cancerous cells have reappeared in your body?

–I don't get those tests taken. I told the ocular oncologist who treats me that I was going to go down the road of changing my diet, and that he should please avoid asking me to take those tests. I don't want to be irradiated. I don't want to be invaded. If I'm going down the road of cell regeneration through diet and quality of life, I can't submit my body to the stress that might exhaust it as it tries to defend me from radiation. My father died from lung cancer and went through every possible radiation treatment to try and cure the cancer. I saw him ruined.

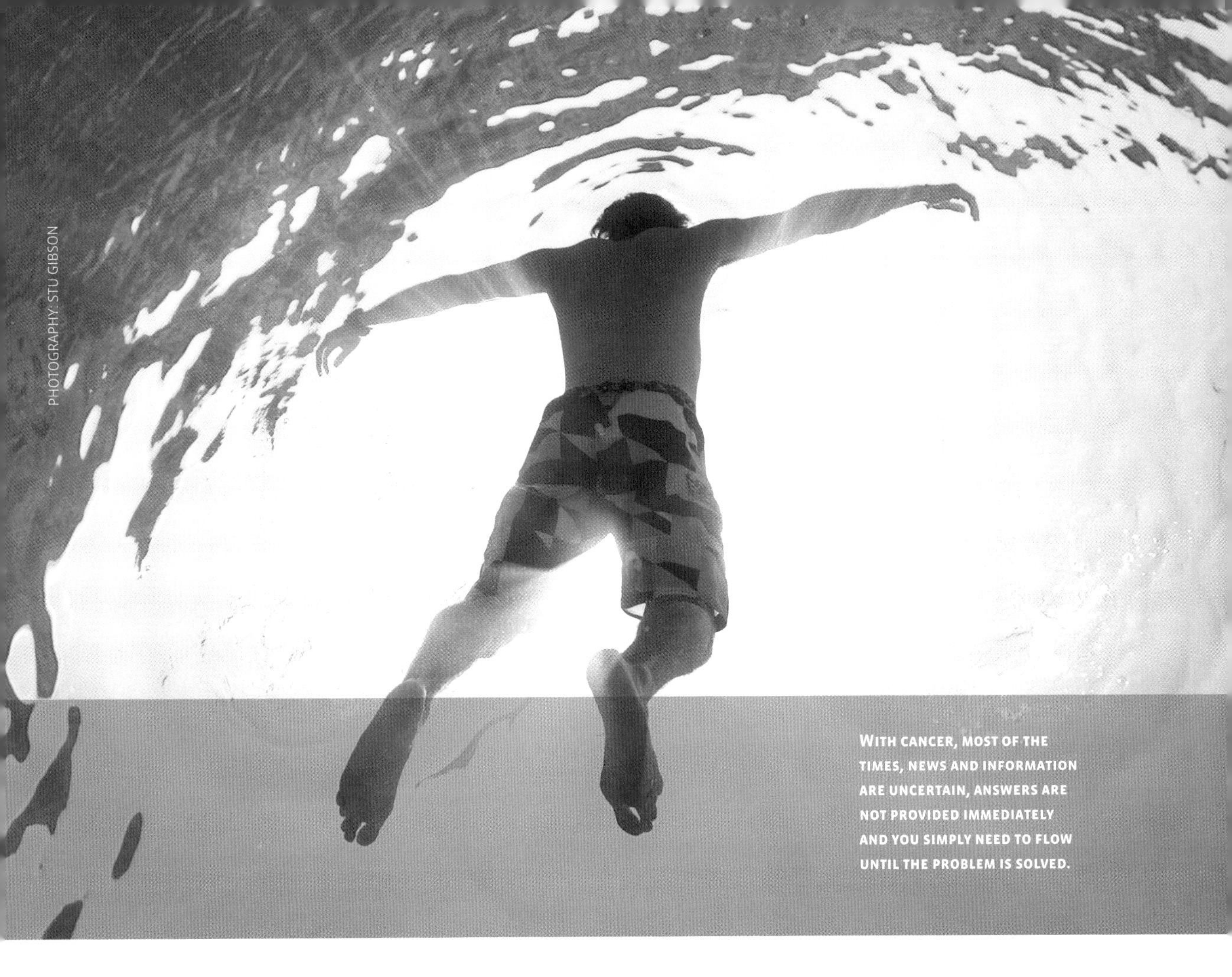

PHOTOGRAPHY: STU GIBSON

WITH CANCER, MOST OF THE TIMES, NEWS AND INFORMATION ARE UNCERTAIN, ANSWERS ARE NOT PROVIDED IMMEDIATELY AND YOU SIMPLY NEED TO FLOW UNTIL THE PROBLEM IS SOLVED.

–Did you make the decision on your own or with your wife's support?

–On my own. It's my body. It's my problem and it's me who has to face it. And I'm facing it. *Look, it's really this simple: wellbeing has no expiration date, but if you decree that the future will be like this or like that, you break down. On the other hand, if you live one day at a time, you destroy the* expectations *variable.* That's what I do. I'm reorganizing my energy. I can't misuse it if my aim is to recover through cell regeneration.

–And what if you feel melanoma symptoms once again, such as nausea and loss of sight?

–I can't be sure yet, but I believe I'd follow

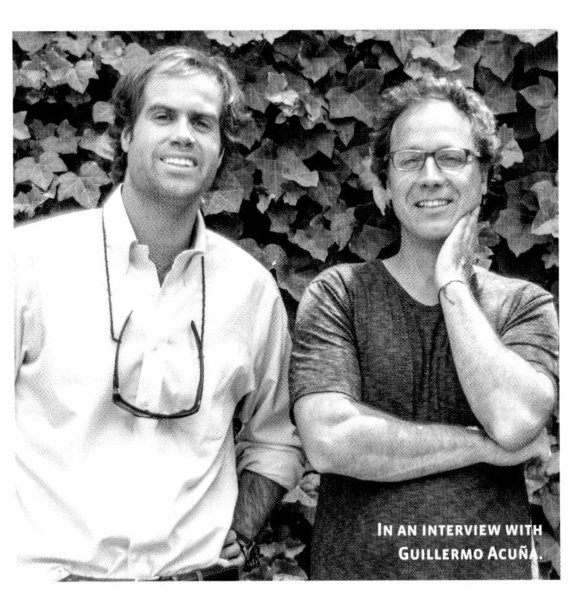

IN AN INTERVIEW WITH GUILLERMO ACUÑA.

all the techniques provided by allopathic medicine, except for frying. By *frying* I mean chemotherapy and radiotherapy. I went through a fry, but a localized and precise one in the eye. They used the ray only in one place, and I was not completely burnt. I think I've already had a taste of death. *If it arrives, I won't fight back, because I am fighting now by eating properly, by changing my everyday lifestyle. Ultimately, the body is an impressive and unique lab, and the only thing you need to do to help it work properly is to understand it.* I would undergo minimally invasive surgical procedures.

–Do you give your decision of not fighting against death a spiritual dimension?

–That's the issue. I believe death is a stage. If I die, I will continue existing, my body is not the end of me. The journey is scary, but that's it. It's about casting fear aside. ■

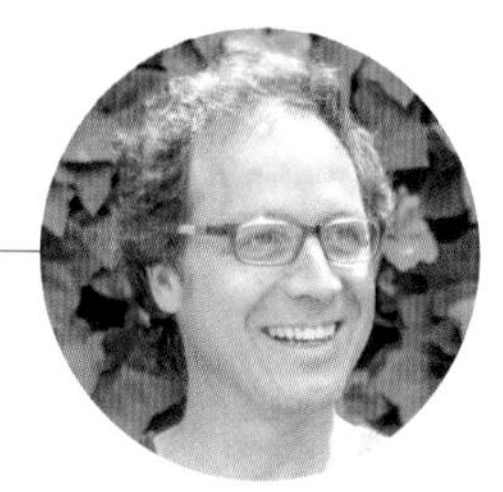

Memo's certainty had an impact on me. I have never doubted the validity of tests, and I'm sure I wouldn't dare to. I know they are invasive and poison the body, but they give me confidence within the context of such uncertainty.

I'm not able to take the risk *Memo* took and not get check-ups. I admire him for this. I don't like to to have radioactive liquid injected into my body. I believe it stresses it out. But still, I haven't questioned it. I believe tests are one of the few empiric evidences I need to make sure I'm healthy.

In fact, in June 2012, the result of my PET CT showed a spot in my lung. Doctor Vial called me to tell me. Usually, results are provided within a few days, but by then our doctor-patient relationship was really strong. Besides, my family's efficiency and proactivity had impressed Doc Vial, who already knew we were on high alert for everything related to my health. This is why he used to call me, and still does, as soon as he checked the images, some hours after the tests. Waiting for those calls is heartbreaking: you're in a full cancer day and your *cancer mode* is completely ON. That day, I was on my own at the office's parking lot when I received the call. After listening, I got scared. I might even say *terrified.* It was really hard receiving Vial's information; I would have preferred to have been with someone else. I desperately needed to hug someone. I didn't want to call my parents, nor did I want to worry them or make them come looking for me. I called Florencia, one of my best friends, who was working with me at *Touch* at the time. I needed someone to lend an ear. I was relieved to be able to count on her. I hope she knows how much her company calmed me down.

After a while, Doctor Vial called to ask whether he could talk about the results with my Dad. I appreciated his sensitivity. Before, I would have been on the defensive, but I could tell him calmly and firmly now: "I'd rather you didn't." I went back home, and when I arrived I told my parents myself. For the second time since the cancer journey had started, I was the one giving the news. First, when I called Dad and interrupted his meeting with the Board of Directors, and now that bad news had returned. Later, I got a call from Sebastián –he was in London– who wanted to know how I was doing after the tests. I told him and, while I was talking, I started crying. A vision of life without doing what I wanted to sprang to mind. It was the first thing I felt. As I wrote at the beginning of this book, one person's reality is different to another's. Being 28 years old, single, and having no children, that was my reality. A spot on my lung could mean surgery again, having a piece of lung removed, the impossibility of going into the water again, riding a wave or riding a bike with my dogs running by my side, practicing sports... living! Sebastián mentioned he would come back to Chile to be by my side, but I asked him not to. He truly understands what sports, life in the outdoors, weekends in *Matanzas*, and my dogs, mean to me. We share lots of things.

I told my parents that, in the future, everything we did regarding the spot or whatever was cancer-related was going to be led by me. I did this full of the confidence I'd lacked during the first stage, when I didn't know where I was standing, let alone what to do. But that stage of my life was over. My parents told me, lovingly and full of empathy, not to worry and that we would deal with this together. And I truly felt completely backed up. After that short, and rather intense, conversation, I went out with Flo, Pepe and Cata –his wife– to exorcize the results of the test.

On the way to the restaurant, I thought I should have invited Sebastián. Besides I should have definitely thanked my parents for all they had done for me during that year and a half, especially Dad. So I decided to thank Dad in a special way. He loves the jackets I use in winter, so the next day, I went to the store and bought 2 identical ones –one for him and another one for me– so we had matching clothes, something he has always liked. I also bought him a scarf. At home I told him: "Dad, I've got a present. This is my way of saying thank you for everything you've done." It made him super happy.

Apparently, I'm not the only one for whom being grateful took some time. **Coni Larraín** told me in her family they're always joking, but don't really express their love. This changed with the cancer, at least between herself and her dad.

 A spot in the lung could mean yet another surgery, the impossibility to go into the water again, practice sports, or even live!

–Were you able to tell your dad you loved him?
–My dad wasn't demonstrative; he was brought up like that. We obviously loved each other, a lot, we loved sitting around chatting and drinking wine, but the way we chose to express our mutual love was special, with gags, jokes and so on. ***I had never told him "I love you" in words, until he was admitted into the hospital. And after that I said it every day.*** When he returned, he started being affectionate, as he had never been before. He said: "Can you do me a favor, if it doesn't bother you? Can you hold my hand?" I wondered how many times before he had felt like hugging me and hadn't done so because of his upbringing. I'm really grateful he allowed himself to be more loving in the end. ■

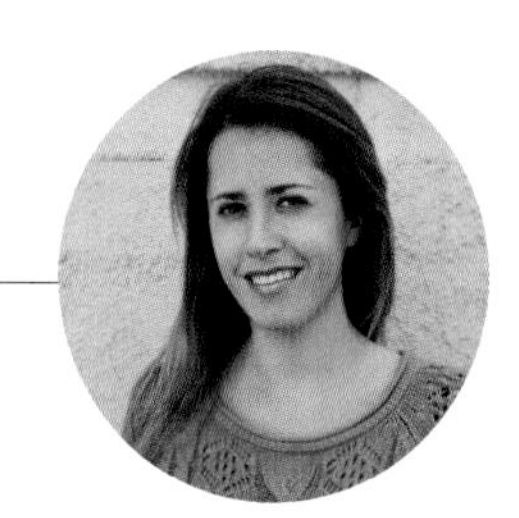

If something like this cancer happens to me again ***I know exactly what I would do: thank, thank and thank from the very beginning.*** I won't stop: families are essential in this process. I confirmed it when interviewing so many people who, like me, experienced the fear, rage and whirlpool of extreme loneliness, until they discovered the support of those who really love them. **Drago Gluscevic** talked about the importance of highlighting, thanking and suggesting family support. Throughout the disease and treatments, he and his wife took care of each other. Both of their cancers were completely unexpected and destabilizing, but they had their networks. Their 4 children were their constant source of support.

–What happened in your family when both your wife and you were fighting cancer?
–Picture it. On the first days I woke up at night and told myself that it was all a nightmare, we weren't going through that, it wasn't true. Couldn't be. But I was sick. And then Susana as well! When our children saw us sick they grew up a lot, we told them we were privileged as such great obstacles are only placed before those who can overcome them. Our children saw how we fought back. They went with me to my sessions –Susana didn't need it–, they held my hand, made me laugh, hugged me. Those were tough times, but I somehow remember them with affection. We celebrated the last session with *pisco sour* for everyone in the room: for nurses, doctors, and anyone who came by. It was a party, because it was the end of chemo. ***And since then, we have eradicated the word cancer from our home. Positive thinking!*** ■

Listening to Drago's story only made me more convinced of the value of family and the networks one has.

Doctors Vial and Paz agreed that the spot in my lung could just be the scar of a cold, but there was no way of knowing immediately. I would have to wait 3 months to see whether it disappeared; or if it got bigger. Doctor Mercedes López warned me that if the spot meant melanoma had moved to my lung, this would situate me at Stage IV of cancer. I would go directly from III A to IV, and then we would have to assess new forms of treatment. The 4 existing stages describe how serious a cancer is, and they are based on the size and extension of the original tumor and on whether it has spread in the body or not. In other words, I would fall within the 20% Doctor Hamid talked about in Los Angeles. A limited chance of survival.

I had a thought at that moment and wrote it down. "Death doesn't scare me," and I was deadly serious. What scared me was that the cancer would return and put a stop to the huge changes I felt I was going through.

That spot in my lung triggered my fear and forced me to confront it. I wrote the following on the iPad my parents had given me as a present at the beginning: "The spot on my lung can be compared to when I'm working with a document on my computer and, at the same time, listening to a song on iTunes: work represents my life and the song the spot. From time to time, I focus only on the document and forget about the song and, other times, I am aware of both, but this doesn't stop me from working or listening properly. And sometimes I only listen to the song and forget about work." The spot on my lung was sometimes the music that joined me, at other times, it was a tune that distracted me, and at other moments it was like one of those songs played in the background that nobody really pays attention to.

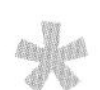
Doctors agreed that the spot could just be the scar from a cold, but there was no way of knowing right away. I'd have to wait for a few months.

I spoke about fear with everyone I interviewed, and they all said things that made sense to me. Made my song continue playing but for a good reason.

Memo *said you can't work with fear. He told me "Remember you're not alone, you're not the only one who has gone through this and that there are many people behind you who have already gone through this. You need to be free from every fear there is."*

The Allards were also afraid. Fear surrounded them. But they didn't succumb to it. Not once. They were a retaining wall which never weakened, not even when facing the worst prognosis.

–Ale, how did you manage your fear when the situation got tough, knowing that Pablito's cancer was really aggressive?

–When everything was against us, everything: statistics, opinions, and even the expressions on the doctors' faces, neither of us, ever, gave up our certainty that Pablo would survive. They probably thought we were insane or just completely lost. Even our own family started wondering: "Well, have you already thought about what you will do? We were advised to travel together, the three of us on a last, farewell, trip. *They told me: "Drop it, let it go." I never did. I'm never going to drop it. Never ever. It went on and on, always another relapse, but we never let go of his hand.* "Ale, stop it, you're going to explode." I have tried to talk about this with people close to me, but it's impossible to convey to them what this abyss means. It is inexplicable. We confronted this abyss and it's too intimate, too intense. But it strengthened our marriage, because it's something I can only share with Pablo. Not with my sisters, whom I adore, nor my friends who, like sisters, would understand me. Only Pablo confronted that abyss with me.

–Pablo, did you live this like your wife did?

–Yes. We faced death and defeated it. We looked fear in the eye and defeated it. I remember like it was yesterday one afternoon that Pablito was really doing badly - he was dying. The doctors' faces said it all. The treating physician entered the room and said something like "We will leave you alone so you can say goodbye." I remembered my rage; I screamed at the doctor and told him I would never say goodbye to my son, because that would mean giving up and stopping fighting. Until you realize that you've defeated it, that it's all behind you, and that life can go on. But we didn't surrender even an inch to death. Not even one. We know death, we fear it, but this fear does not turn us into victims, it keeps us alert and encourages us to make the most of each moment we spend together. ■

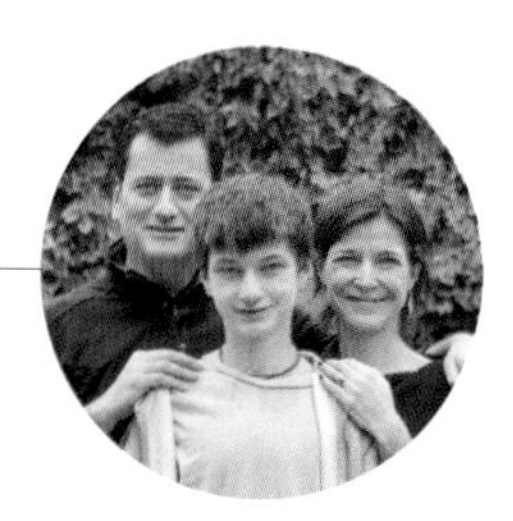

Naturally, I have felt fear. I experienced fear many times during my treatments and subsequent tests. I can still feel it. However, kitesurfing has shown me one can feel many different types of fear. Facing a very big wave I used to think: "Fuck, if it knocks me over and a line catches my leg I won't make it to the surface." I was scared and didn't catch it. Then, out of the water, I wondered why I had been scared if I was used to handling the board after 2 years of practicing the sport. Why? Because it was, and is, legitimate to be scared; everybody feels afraid and what I believe one needs to do is make an effort to control it. Understand the fear, its possible consequences, and accept them. I believe this is the turning point between catching a wave or not. Therefore, from my point of view, I believe *fear is not bad because it's a motor that makes you act and make decisions. The complicated thing is not identifying its origin and not understanding it.* What I fear most is uncertainty. For instance, I can't stand losing control of situations. It paralyzes me. However, when I'm outdoors and feel afraid of the unknown, it's like an engine is ignited and won't stop until I find a solution.

After Doctor Vial gave me the news and I understood I had no chance of resolving my uncertainty, I went to Fiji for two reasons: to try and stop listening to the song, and to improve my kitesurfing technique in a kind of intensive workshop with a group of people I didn't know and who were just looking to improve their skills on the board. Above all, I wanted the necessary time to go by for the next

* Being scared is legitimate, what I need to do is to make an effort to control it. Understand its possible consequences and accept them.

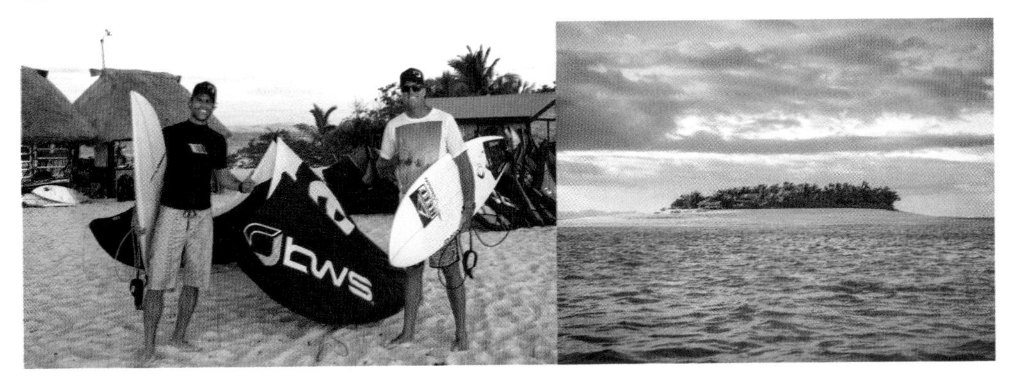

One of the magical places that helped with my healing: Namotu island in Fiji. There I met wave kite surf legend Ben Wilson.

test to confirm or disprove the shadow on my lung.

Amaro has a very clear opinion on fear, and he was categorical, I believe because he has been a war correspondent and, under such circumstances, fear is not a useful tool. *"I don't believe in fear under any circumstances - not when you're facing cancer, or at any other time. It's understandable but you have to do everything you can to get rid of it."*

During the trip to Fiji I heard the song in the background several times and went through bad times, terrible ones, mainly when I was on my own, without the practice group. But there were other times in which I didn't hear it, and I enjoyed the island and its wonders to the full. Unavoidably, when the infamous song appeared in my mind, I wondered why I was feeling like that if I was doing what I had always dreamt of doing –kitesurfing for 18 consecutive days– I foolishly thought it was due to work. I believed I hadn't been able to disconnect from the stress. But no, it was the song playing on loop in my head.

After returning from Fiji, I went to take the dreaded exam: chest scan without contrast. The exam would reveal the origin of the notorious spot on my lung. The test only lasted a few minutes, I was in and out of the hospital in a blink. Doctor Vial would call me after analyzing the results. I went about as if I was not expecting the news, went to buy a wetsuit for kitesurfing, and then... my phone rang. It was the doctor: "Roberto, the spot has disappeared." I punched the fitting room wall out of sheer joy. I cried and thank him. I was truly relieved. I called my parents, who were on a trip, and they celebrated with me. It was September, just before the

> * Then my phone rang. It was doctor Vial: "Roberto, the spot can't be seen, it has disappeared." I punched the fitting room's wall out of pure joy.

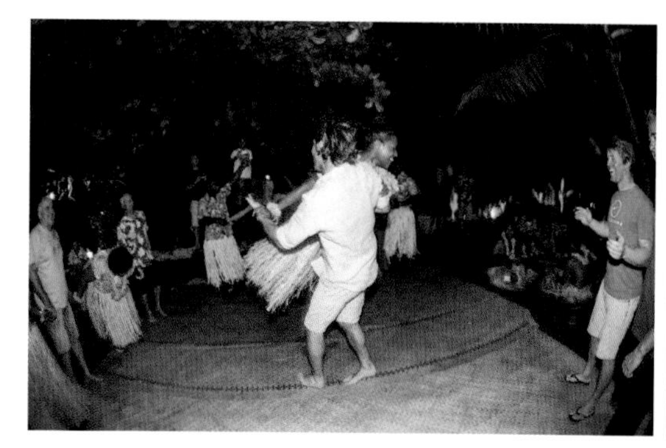

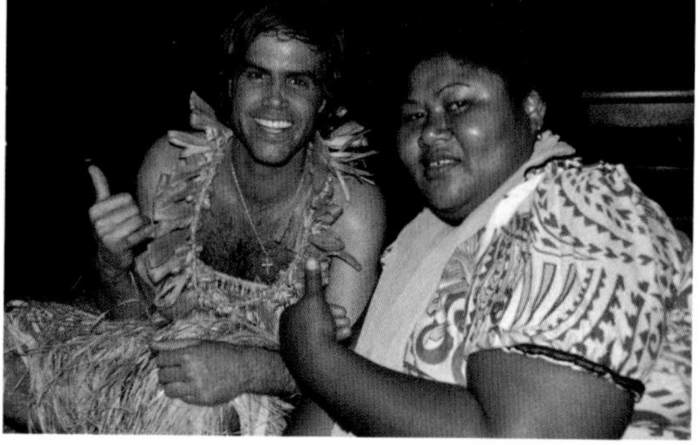

Tribal dance and good friends in Namotu.

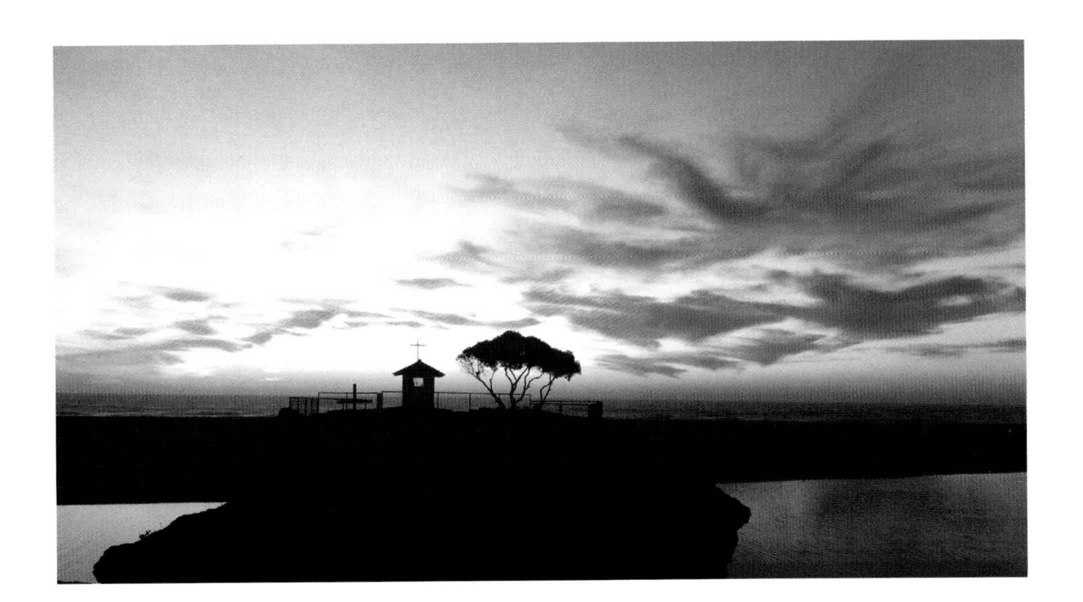

18th (Chile's Independence Day). The news was so emotional and overwhelming that the adrenaline of being alive, of knowing I wouldn't die, lasted a couple of days. The shitty song finally came to an end.

Over the past few days, and also while in Fiji, I'd thought everything was okay apart from maybe some stress at work. But that wasn't it. There had been that song playing in my brain. Until it finally died down, and I realized it had been there.

I went to *Curanipe*, Southern-Central Chile, for the 18th, with school mates, to some very simple wooden bungalows. And as I took a shower, I looked out of the window and thought: "This is all I need."

The spot ended up being not serious. It was probably the scar from a flu, but doctors couldn't tell and I didn't care. So I decided to pour my energy into the changes I felt I was undergoing, because it was working quite well. I thought: "I have to continue living; I can't let uncertainty paralyze me." ■

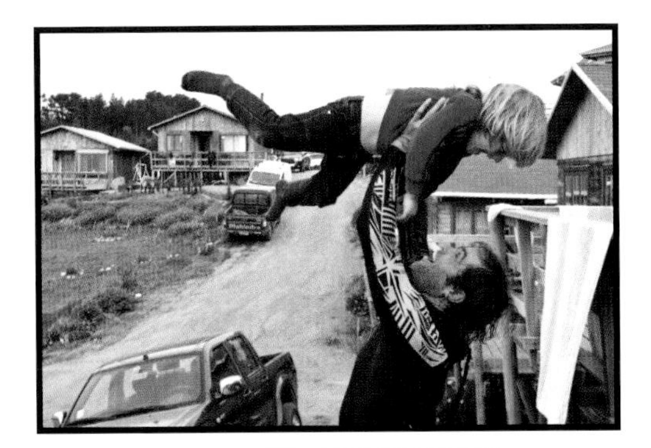

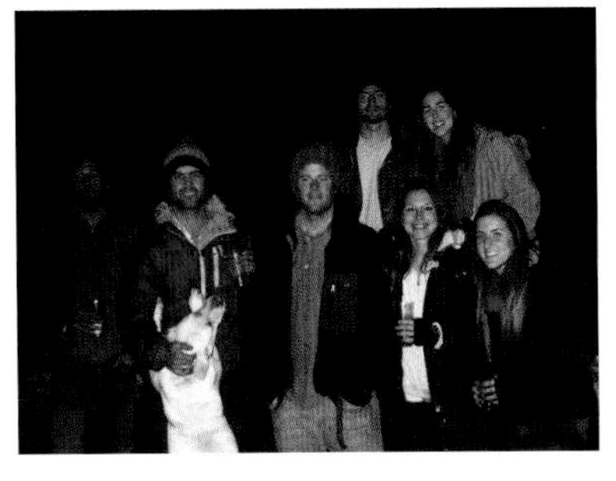

Good news needs to be celebrated. I celebrated the spot on the lung disappearing with my cousin Jeremy and some good friends from school, in *Curanipe*.

8. Cancer mode OFF

I still maintain that cancer is the best thing that has happened to me. It was hard, mainly at the beginning, but I finally understood it. Shocks such as this one make you –and everybody around you– change and, personally, I believe that now, after melanoma, I'm a slightly better person.

I wouldn't exchange these past four years for anything, although it's been a bumpy road and has led to so many contrasting emotions. 'Why?' is a question I believe I will never stop asking myself, and one which I ask myself most days. I guess it's part of human nature. Yet, every time I ask myself why, I remember the *what for*. As I've already said, part of this '*what for*', and maybe one of the most relevant, was the creation of *Fundación Celebraciones con Sentido* (Celebrations with a Purpose Foundation). What for? To return the favor, if you like. To help those in need. In October 2015, we celebrated our third anniversary and, with a huge effort, loads of dedication, and tons of enthusiasm, we have managed to raise over US $230,769.00 through birthdays, wedding parties, and galas –in which those celebrating ask their friends to make a donation in Chilean pesos instead of making them a gift– to support more than 30 organizations and social causes. Within these celebrations, GIVE parties stand out. After Valparaiso's fire in 2014, we wondered how we could help through a celebration. How could we GIVE while partying? We liked the word GIVE (DAR in Spanish) and wanted to create a brand which would not only work for that event, but also in the future. It had to sell tickets and be glamorous. GIVE was born. A party organized by *Celebrations with a Purpose* Foundation in which all the funds raised through ticket sales would be donated to a specific cause.

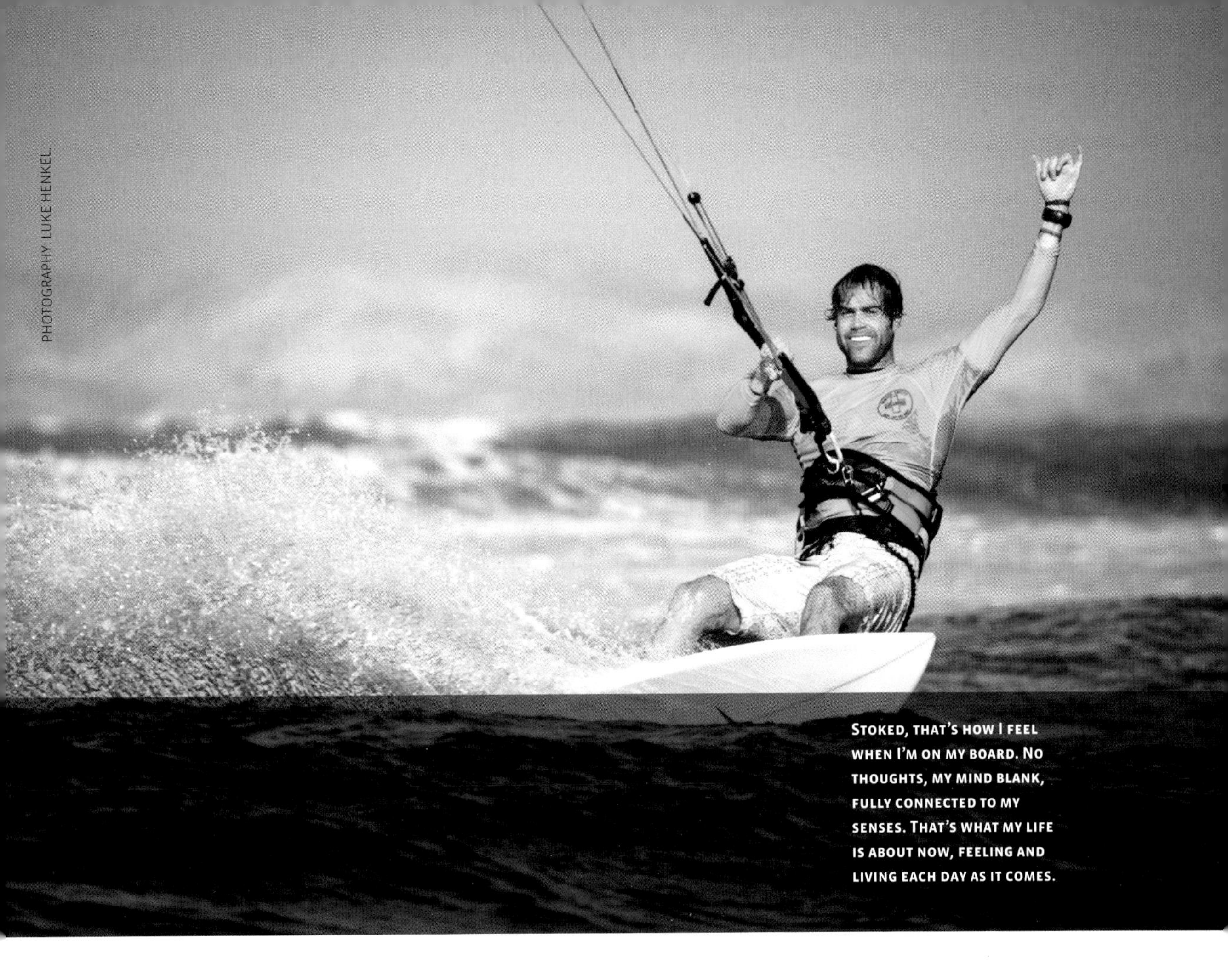

PHOTOGRAPHY: LUKE HENKEL

STOKED, THAT'S HOW I FEEL WHEN I'M ON MY BOARD. NO THOUGHTS, MY MIND BLANK, FULLY CONNECTED TO MY SENSES. THAT'S WHAT MY LIFE IS ABOUT NOW, FEELING AND LIVING EACH DAY AS IT COMES.

Through the first party –Give Valpo–, we raised US 12,020. That went to buy 196 mattresses, which were directly donated to 98 families who had lost everything during the fire. Then, with *Give Norte,* after the disaster caused by the flood in the Chilean III Administrative Region, we raised US 35,164, and took 110,000 liters of water to *Diego de Almagro,* with a direct positive impact on 2,121 families.

Nowadays, there's no questioning that another of my *what fors* is sharing what I do and what I have with those I love the most. Cancer is a very lonely road and, although you might be surrounded by support, at the end of the day the process is a personal, intimate one. And it's difficult to let others in, especially when you feel you're capable of controlling everything.

The truth is you need to learn to accept that not everything is within reach, and that it's impossible to know how things will turn out. So, it's better to walk hand-in-hand with the various possibilities, rather than trying to work against them.

House of Joy, my house in *Matanzas,* my sanctuary –as I call it–, has been my great ally whenever I've needed to relax and, slowly, start sharing again. Thanks to this place that faces the sea, I recovered a little bit of the spirit of my trip to Australia, where I did what I wanted without following a plan. In fact, since I held the house-warming party four years ago, I have always hosted guests. It was conceived for that purpose, and has remained true to its name. As I see it, be-

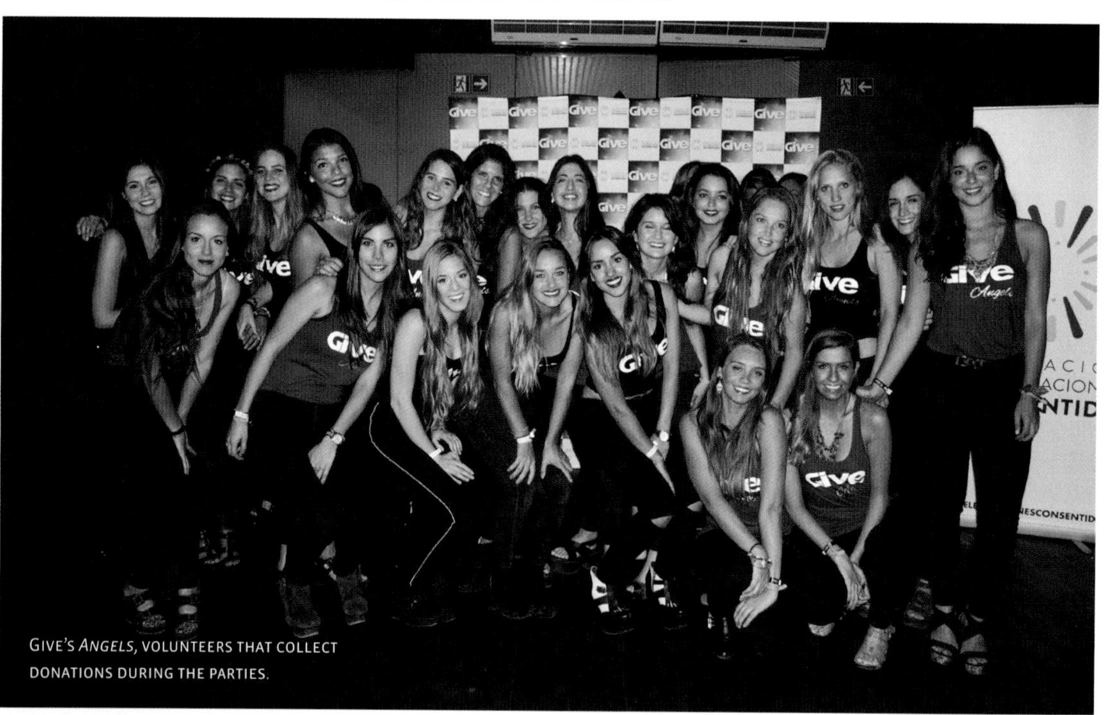

GIVE'S *ANGELS*, VOLUNTEERS THAT COLLECT DONATIONS DURING THE PARTIES.

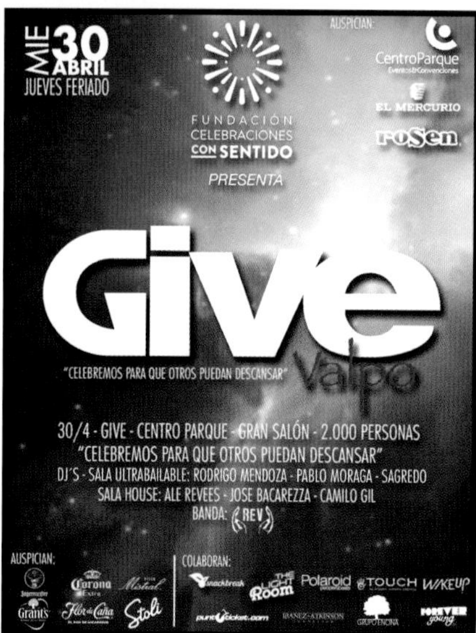

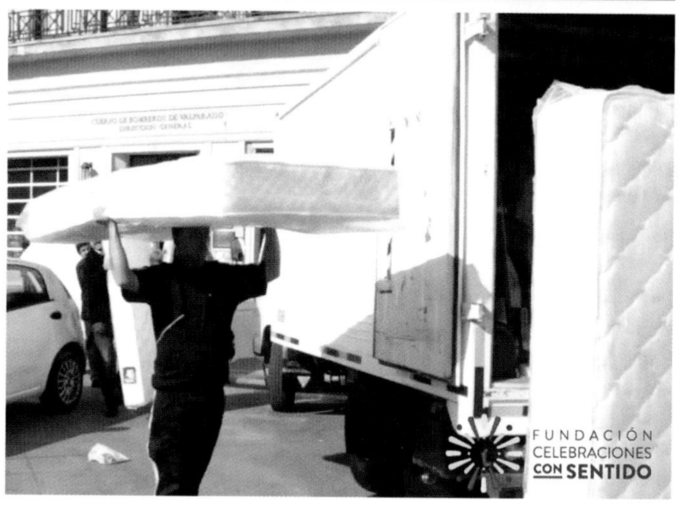

LET'S CELEBRATE SO THAT OTHERS MAY REST. THAT WAS THE SLOGAN FOR THE *GIVE VALPO* PARTY WITH WHICH WE WERE ABLE TO GET 196 MATTRESSES FOR THE VICTIMS OF THE VALPARAISO FIRE.

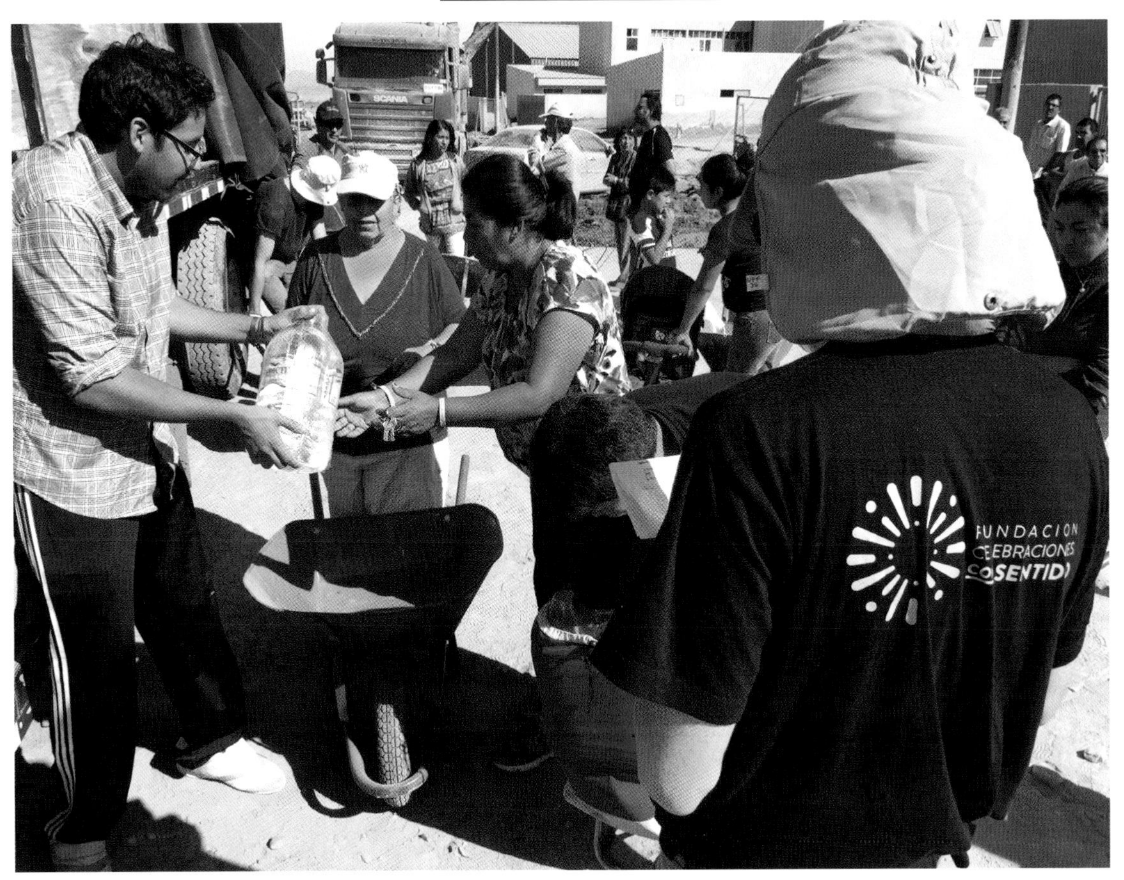

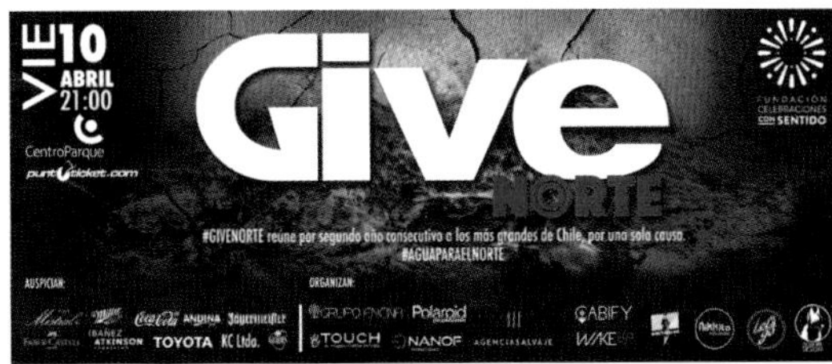

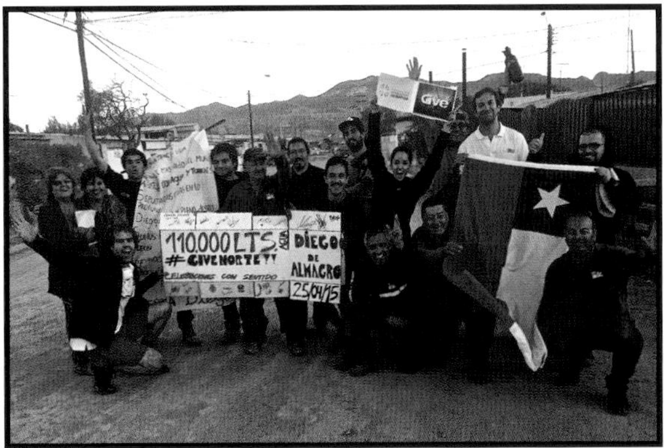

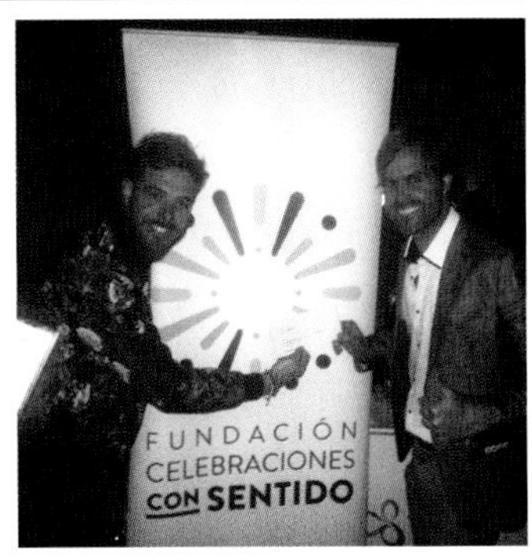

In *Give Norte*, the ticket for the party was equal to a donation in liters of water. The party had a high impact: we gathered more than 110,000 liters of water for 2,121 families.

ing alone is not worth it, I enjoy everything much more when I'm with someone I love beside me: Summers with my family at the riverside; a Sacred Thursday –as we named our monthly First-Thursday get-together– with my school friends; a weekend of kite and surf with my brothers, cousins and friends; a walk in the hills with my dogs; a meeting the Celebrations with a Purpose team, or an annual cancer control at the hospital, with my girlfriend and parents by my side. ***Life is about sharing, helping, allowing yourself to be helped. Laughing, crying, doing a lot or not doing anything at all. Doing something for a cause. Quit that looking backwards! Living the here and now, and looking forward, but without expecting anything.*** As I said at the beginning of this book, I hope to provide some help and lead to something constructive. That's all. ■

* Life is about sharing, helping, allowing oneself to be helped, living the here-and-now, and looking into the future, but without expecting anything.

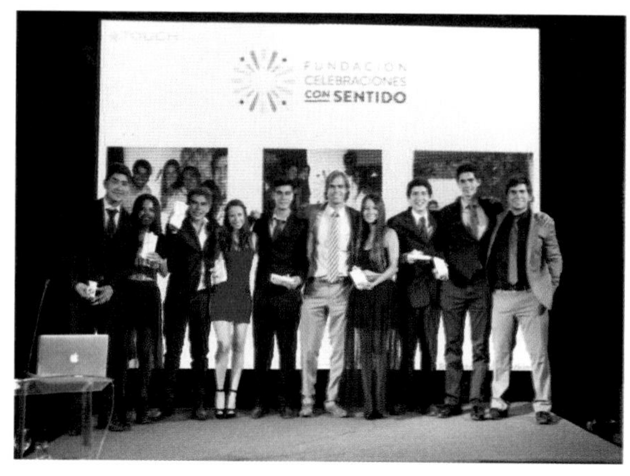

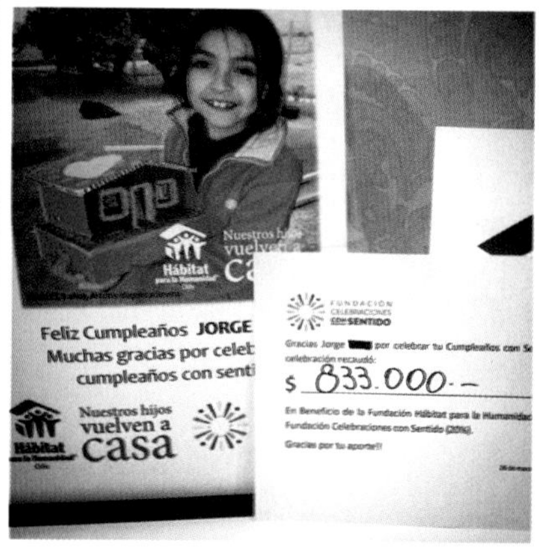

AT *TOUCH* WE HAVE "SCOUTS FOR A PURPOSE", YOUNG STUDENTS WHO WORK AS VOLUNTEERS FOR SPECIAL OCCASIONS AND ARE IN CHARGE OF COLLECTING THE FUNDS DURING DIFFERENT CELEBRATIONS. IN THE PICTURE, THANKS TO THE MOTIVATION OF OUR *SCOUTS FOR A PURPOSE* AND THE GENEROSITY OF THE HOST AND HIS GUESTS, IN JUST ONE AFTERNOON, WE RAISED CLP 833,000 FOR THE ORGANIZATION *NUESTROS HIJOS* VUELVEN A CASA (OUR CHILDREN RETURN HOME).

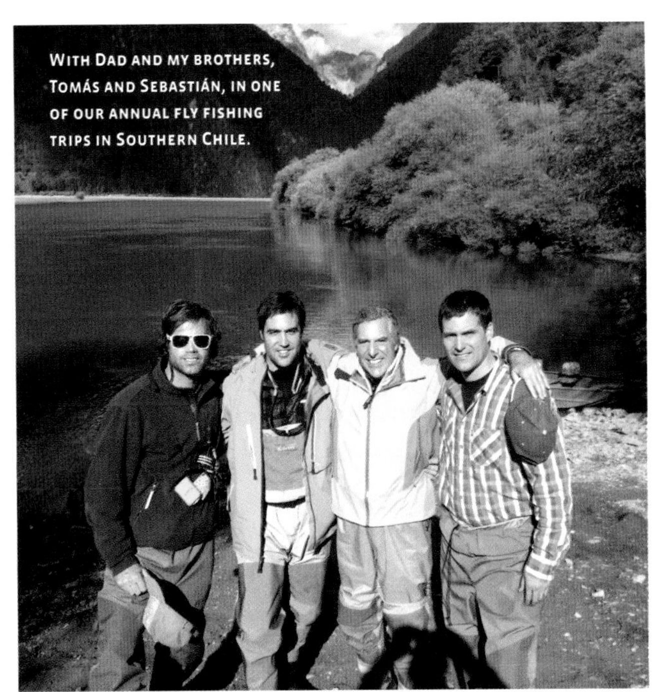

WITH DAD AND MY BROTHERS, TOMÁS AND SEBASTIÁN, IN ONE OF OUR ANNUAL FLY FISHING TRIPS IN SOUTHERN CHILE.

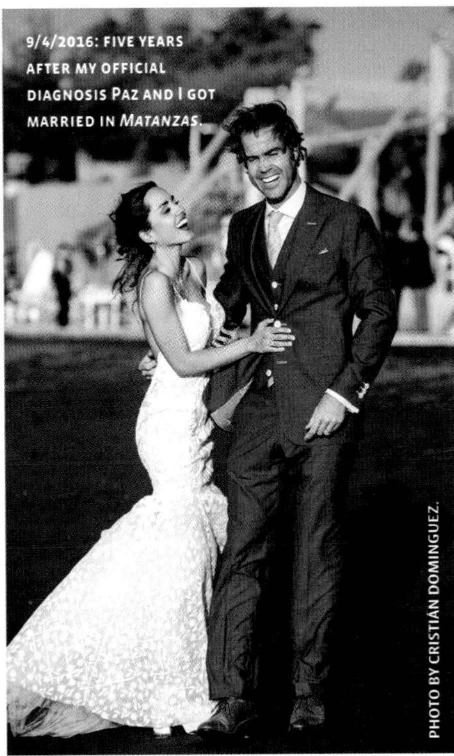

9/4/2016: FIVE YEARS AFTER MY OFFICIAL DIAGNOSIS PAZ AND I GOT MARRIED IN *MATANZAS*.

PHOTO BY CRISTIÁN DOMINGUEZ.

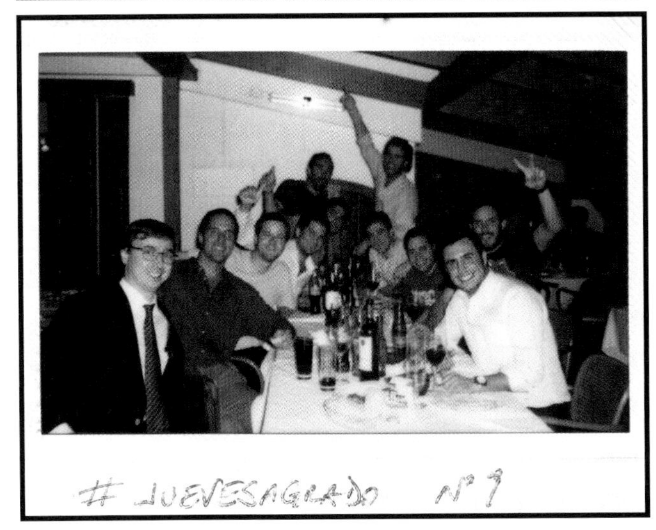

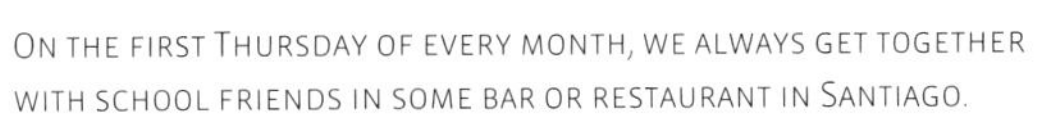

ON THE FIRST THURSDAY OF EVERY MONTH, WE ALWAYS GET TOGETHER WITH SCHOOL FRIENDS IN SOME BAR OR RESTAURANT IN SANTIAGO.

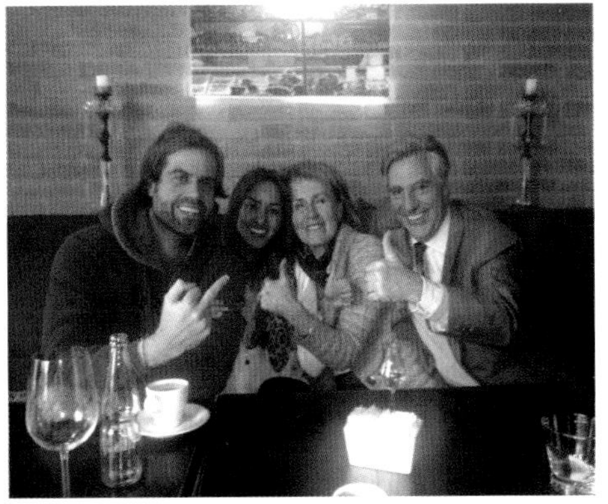

THIS PICTURE WAS TAKEN A MINUTE AFTER I WAS TOLD THAT, FOR THE THIRD CONSECUTIVE YEAR, I WAS FREE FROM CANCER. THAT'S WHY YOU MAY SEE THREE THUMBS UP, FROM DAD, MOM, AND PAZITA, AND MY *GO-F...-YOURSELF*, CANCER! GESTURE.

9. A new way of looking at life

The tower concept

Sometimes all you need to understand life better is to look at it from a different point of view.

With the aim of getting some first-hand different perspectives for this book I interviewed a series of people who had had close personal experiences of cancer. I discovered things I'd never even imagined. Drago Gluscevic, one of the people I interviewed, told me that it's his firm belief that this sort of catastrophe happens to people who are strong enough to get through them and somehow move on. At home my parents always said that crises are positive experiences that make you stronger as a person. *Nowadays I'm sure that living with cancer is something that gives you a different perspective, a change of focus, and a sense of responsibility, which you simply don't have before.*

This book includes over 90 interviews with people who have experienced cancer directly in one way or another: either they're former patients or they're currently in treatment; or a friend, family member, work colleague or somebody close to them has been ill. I also interviewed therapists, doctors and specialists who speak about their knowledge and experiences. They've all confronted the process that has shaken the foundations of their lives, and they generously agreed to share their advice, giving tips on what helped them, the way they took decisions, what they did to overcome fear, and what they held on to. More than one of their suggestions will probably make sense to the reader, connecting them to something that they hadn't thought of before, or helping them see things differently. A

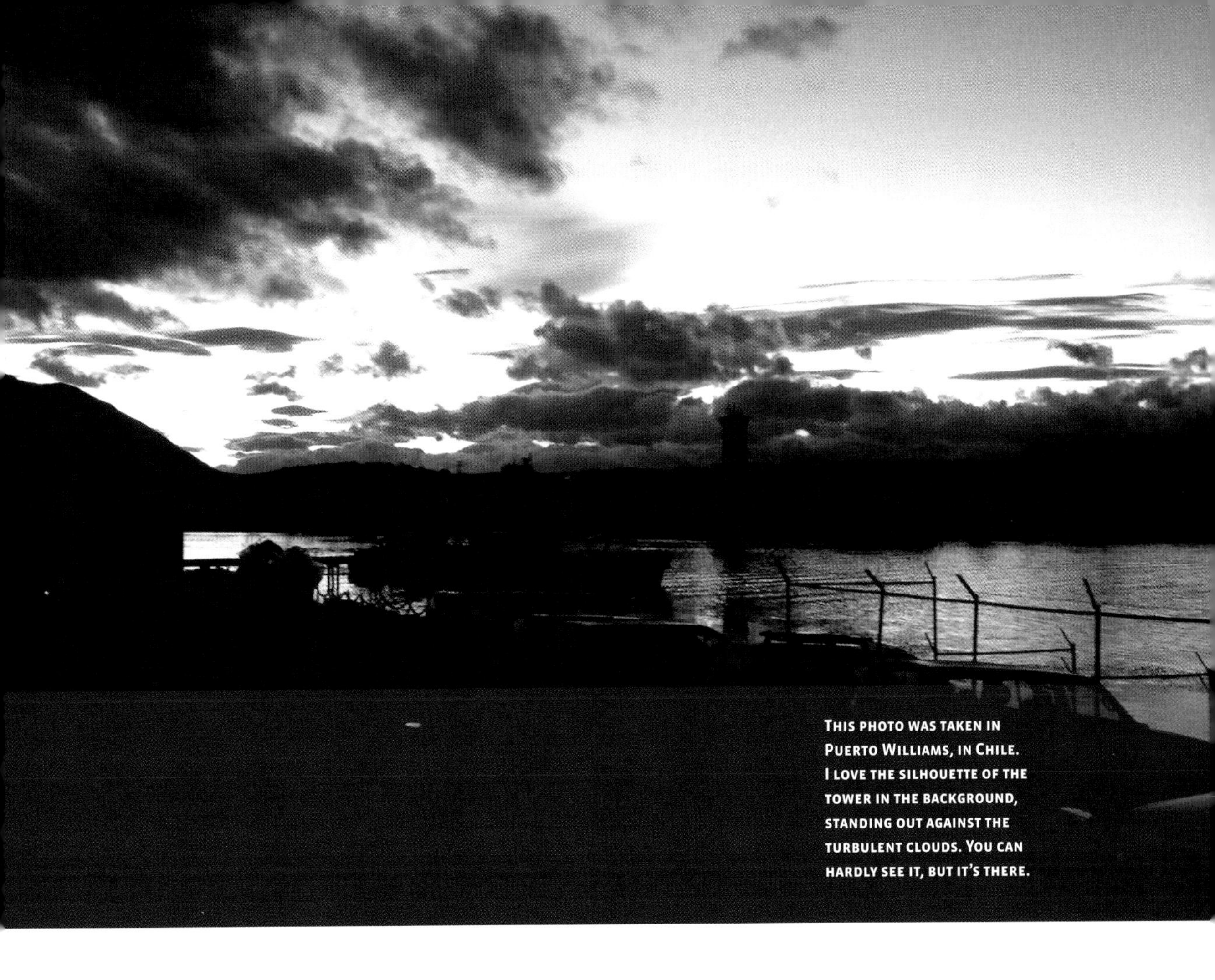

THIS PHOTO WAS TAKEN IN PUERTO WILLIAMS, IN CHILE. I LOVE THE SILHOUETTE OF THE TOWER IN THE BACKGROUND, STANDING OUT AGAINST THE TURBULENT CLOUDS. YOU CAN HARDLY SEE IT, BUT IT'S THERE.

source of relief and hope, a possible way forward; that's what I want this book to give.

I call the process I went through of restructuring my life the Tower Concept. Eight months after my cancer diagnosis, inspired by the Chilean doctor Benjamín Paz whom I'd met in Los Angeles, USA, I started writing about that complete change in perspective that he'd pointed out to me and which so many people mentioned to me later. This is what I wrote down at the time:

Today, after my melanoma diagnosis, I look at life differently. From the moment we're aware of things, very early on in our lives, we climb to the top of a little tower that we've started to build. We can't see all that much from the top of our tower, and what we do see is conditioned and limited by what our parents teach us. As we grow up our tower is in a particular geographical location and usually doesn't move from there. In fact the only thing that changes is that the tower gets higher and higher, which, over time, does change a little bit what we can see from the top of it.

I never really thought about this until after the cancer diagnosis, because people tend to just deal with whatever situation we find ourselves in. Change scares us. We think that life has taken us down one path, and the idea of building a whole new tower from scratch seems a difficult and challenging task.

But from one day to the next I had to move from my old tower onto a neighboring one that I had also built but that had been buried in my subconscious. It's true that the second tower had always been there, but I had to go through a hard experience to find the necessary courage and maturity to move tower and transform my point of view.

Nowadays, from my new tower, I've got a different view: ***the mountains that used to be in the way no longer block my vista, and the river, of which I only ever saw one bend, now appears in its entirety from its source to the estuary as where flows into the sea. My tower isn't only taller, it's also moved.*** In its new location the air at the top is a bit thinner, so I have to breathe calmly, without getting excited, and my challenge is to help any visitor to my tower feel the same sense of peace so that they don't lose consciousness. I can clearly remember the view from the old tower, and if at any moment that memory slips away from me, my subconscious brings it back to me.

I know that everyone who took part in this book with their advice has also had to move towers. I'd like to thank them all from the bottom of my heart, and a particular vote of thanks goes to ***Loreto Agurto, Carla Vidal, Marcela Lorenzini and Luis Silva, who contributed with their experiences and life lessons, and who are no longer with us. They fought to the end and here, in this book, are their moving testimonies.*** ■

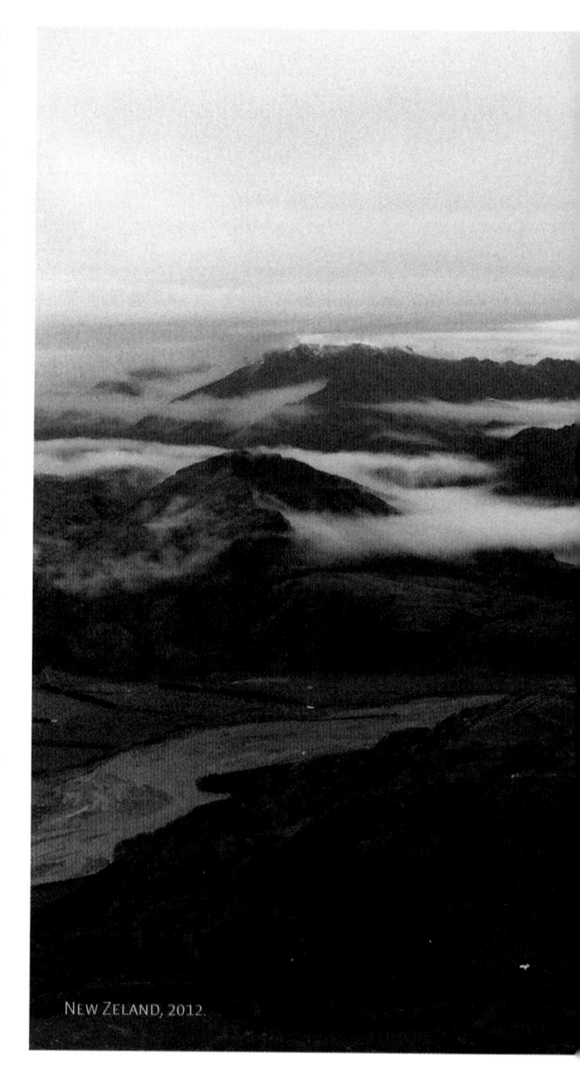

NEW ZELAND, 2012.

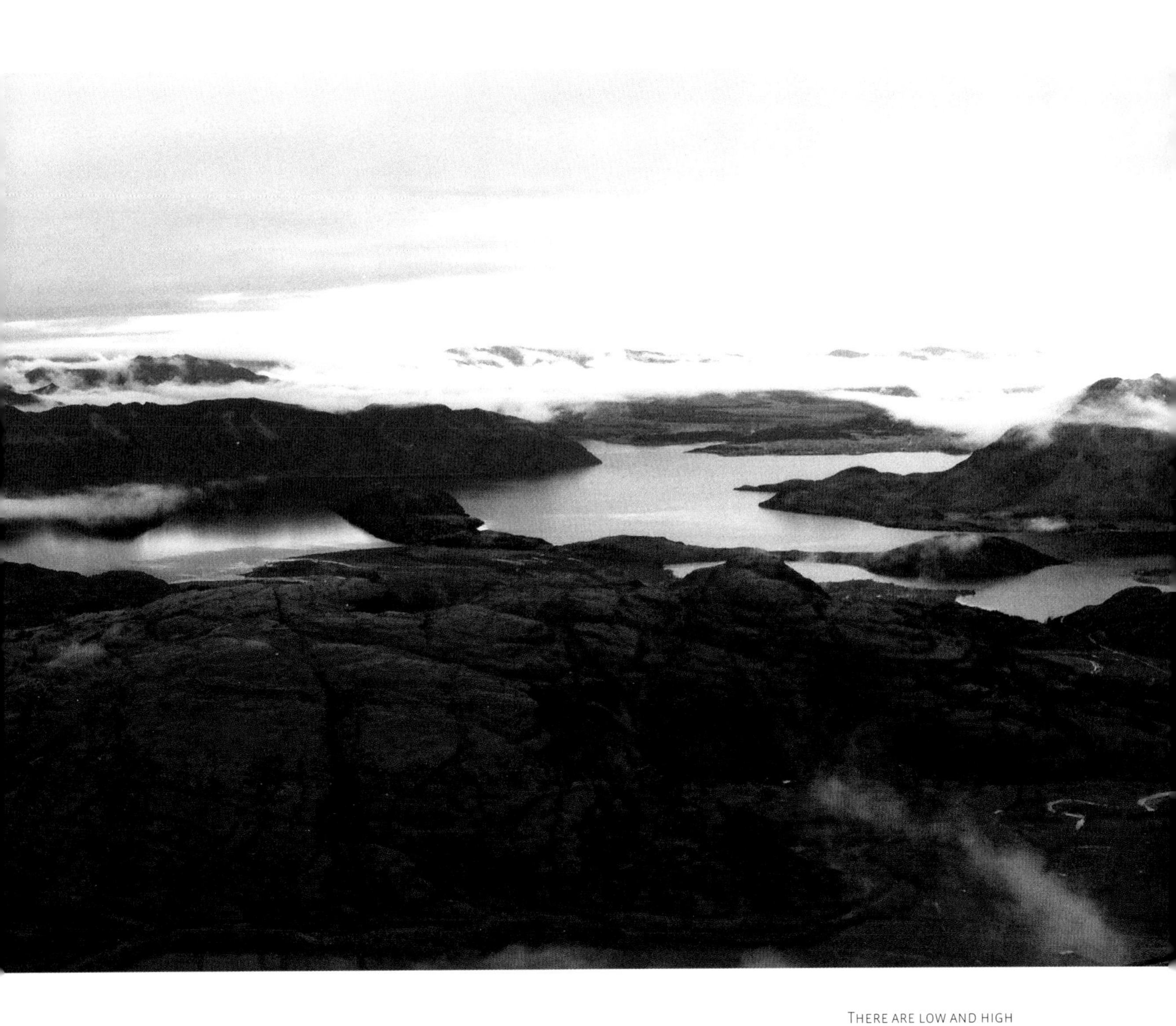

THERE ARE LOW AND HIGH CLOUDS, BUT SOMETIMES WHEN YOU LOOK FROM A DIFFERENT PERSPECTIVE, YOU CAN ALSO SEE THE SUN.

what (the hell) is a MELANOMA

Chapter written in collaboration with dermatologist Francis Palisson and immunologist Mercedes López.

When that April 27th the dermatologist told me on the phone: "Roberto, you have melanoma", I had no idea what it was, nor did I realize its seriousness.

I thought it was skin cancer, something benign, curable, something unimportant. I knew about people who had had it, had undergone surgery and that was that, full stop. However, it was shocking to learn while I was writing this book that when I was diagnosed with melanoma they were actually telling me that I had the most dangerous form of cancer. That I had a deadly cancer that cannot be easily detected unless you are alert and subjected to regular preventative check-ups.

According to the information I gathered from specialists (surgical oncologists, dermatologists, immunologists and medical oncologists) who collaborated on this book, one could say, in general and trying to simplify the seriousness of the problem, that cancer is –to some extent– hereditary. If one has a cell which carries genetic information in its nucleus, 99.99% of the time that cell turns into one that is exactly identical. If you are born with genetic predisposition to a tumor, each of your cells already carries a mutation and each of its transformations makes the following –maybe a cancer– more probable.

I was diagnosed with melanoma when I was 27. What is it? I should probably start with what the dermatologist told me: "It is a type of cancer that, depending on the stage, may be deadly." Melanoma is produced when skin cells called melanocytes develop into malignant tumors. It is a tumor of skin cells, but of cells that multiply very quickly and, therefore, it is very aggressive. Furthermore, its cells are resistant to chemotherapy and radiotherapy; they survive those drug bombs absolutely unperturbed.

Although small, it's a very dangerous tumor and, in fact, according to Doctor* Mercedes López, *it is the worst type of cancer and once it has metastasized beyond the nodes the situation becomes very complex.

Melanocytes are skin cells in charge of producing melanin, the skin, eyes and hair pigment, whose main function is to block radiation from the sun's ultraviolet rays so that it does not harm the DNA of cells exposed to light. Simply put, darker skins do not have more melanocytes than lighter skins, but they do have bigger granules that provide a better protection against radiation. The darker the skin, the more protection it has against solar radiation. My mother is Scottish and my skin is really fair, so I do not have great natural protection.

It is this radiation that leads to transformations in cells that may develop into a melanoma. ***I would really like to make it clear that melanoma is not the same as the most frequent skin cancers. It is much more aggressive.*** The most common type of skin cancer is the basal cell carcinoma which appears as a flesh-colored tumor or a wound that does not heal. Carcinomas bother, become ulcerous and are painful, but the chance they may metastasize is very low.

The name melanoma derives from words *melan* (abbreviation of melanocyte, cell producing pigment called melanin) and *oma* (tumor). When melanocytes group, the usual moles or freckles are formed, which are neither dangerous nor malignant. Complexity arises when melanocytes are transformed and those moles and freckles change their size and look. In my case a flesh-colored mole appeared on my right arm. It was ugly, but it was not a dark mole as melanomas usually are, which made it strange and difficult to detect.

In many of the conversations I had with Doctor **Francis Palisson,** the dermatologist who carries out my check-ups at least every six months, he explained there are different types of tumors, 12 of which are clearly identified, including mine.

Types of melanoma

1. **Amelanotic melanoma.** It's a skin color or reddish color mole, which appears suddenly and has an accelerated growth.

2. **Spitzoid melanoma.** It appears in the form of fusiform cells. Tumors have a characteristic shape under the microscope.

3. **Lentigo maligna melanoma.** It is usually found in older people, in areas of the skin affected by the sun, such as the face, neck or arms. They are abnormal spots in the skin; big, flat, brownish, black-brown or strictly black patches.

4. **Acral lentiginous melanoma.** This is the rarest type of melanoma. It is found in the palms of the hands, soles of the feet or under the nails. It is more commonly found in African Americans, as those are the areas of the body with less pigment (with less melanin).

5. **Superficial spreading melanoma.** It is the most common type of melanoma; it is usually a flat, irregularly-shaped, deep black or black and brown, mole.

6. **Nodular melanoma.** It is one of the most frequent types of melanoma. It usually appears as a prominence in a small area of the skin and becomes of a blackish blue or bluish red tone.

7. **Small cell melanoma.** It is found usually in young people, on their scalp.

8. **Malignant blue nevus.** It is a dark injury formed by pigmented melanocytes located in the mid dermis. They take the form of a shadow, eruption, nodule or plaque with a blue, grey-blue or bluish black tone.

9. **Desmoplastic melanoma.** It is very aggressive. It is an uncommonly encountered type which arises as a normal injury and evolves into a deep, fibrous tumor, with prevalence of fusiform cells.

10. **Ocular melanoma.** It grows in the eye.

11. **Mucosal melanoma.** It may be located on genital, oral or conjunctival mucosa.

12. **Animal-type melanoma.** It is a very unusual type of melanoma which affects mainly African American or Hispanic people.

Mine was an amelanotic melanoma as it had no dark pigmentation, although its shape was abnormal and the skin biopsy determined it was a spitzoid tumor.

For some time I was obsessed with learning how melanomas were formed. And I learned a little. I will try to transmit my knowledge as follows: between the epidermis and the dermis there is a barrier called the basement membrane. Melanocytes are placed over this membrane and, as I already said, ultraviolet radiation is a decisive factor as it can cause changes that allow the proliferation of these cells and the subsequent loss of normal growth control. When this takes place cells go through the basement membrane and invade the dermis, where blood and lymphatic vessels are located. These tumor cells are able to distribute and migrate through blood and lymph vessels like canoes and reach other territories, such as the liver, lungs or brain, tissues where growth control mechanisms are inexistent, in relation to the skin where they cancer. ***This is the reason why these cells are able to grow faster and make metastasis or grow "malignant tumors at a distance".*** When a melanoma makes a metastasis in a lung, this does not mean you have lung cancer; those are other cells of your melanoma that start growing on another organ of your body after flowing through your blood and lymphatic stream, such as in any other type of cancer. ***Cells of a benign tumor cannot adhere to other tissues or survive outside the organ where they first appeared.***

When I started investigating risk factors for this type of cancer I was surprised because there are not only two or three factors, but there is a long list and my case coincided with many items. A key aspect is family history, knowing whether any of your relatives had melanoma, atypical or dysplastic nevus. This was not my case, there was no history of melanoma in my family. Some families have asymmetrical or irregular moles and, therefore it is very important to be alert and check-up.

5 *factors* that influence the development of melanoma

1 SUN EXPOSURE (ULTRAVIOLET RADIATION): The sun is a carcinogen, because of its great capacity to harm the organism and produce cancer. ***Apparently, the earlier one is exposed to ultraviolet radiation in life, the worse it is. Strange it may seem, experts concur that intermittent exposure is potentially more harmful than prolonged exposure.*** In fact, melanomas arise more frequently in areas a person discontinuously exposes to the sun. For instance, the face is always uncovered and it is less frequent for melanomas to arise there than on other body parts which are more protected, because it is constantly exposed to the sun. To some extent this protects us because natural filters are produced. Melanocytes learn. ***It is clear that one must be careful of the sun from early childhood to 17 years of age because in this period the body "stores" ultraviolet radiation.*** Use of highly effective sunscreens is as important as not being exposed to the sun during the peak radiation hours, between 11 in the morning to 4 in the afternoon. **Doctor Palisson** explained it is very strange for a person under 17 to develop melanoma, except

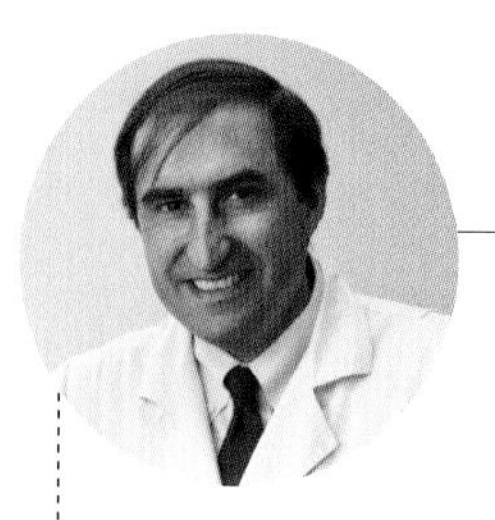

Dr. Francis Palisson

if they have a genetic predisposition or have been frequently exposed to UV radiation.
Melanoma develops when you are grown up and its mortality rate is higher in people under 30. I was diagnosed with melanoma at the age of 27 and, in my case, I have been frequently exposed to the sun since I was young: summers at the beach and lake, practicing water sports, riding on bikes and practicing surf and kite after my 20's. I used sunscreen but wasn't rigorous about it. Sunscreens must be used every day if one is exposed to the sun and every three hours when one is at the beach, mainly after coming out of the water, or in the snow. Although it is comforting to use sunscreen, I started wondering whether I was completely safe and protected this way. And the truth is, not necessarily. There isn't a lot of research carried out to find out if the use of sunscreen is effectively beneficial and studies that have been done are not conclusive; however, experts agree that its use is fundamental. Work performed by the Australian Doctor Adele Green and her team is used as a reference by many of the Chilean specialists I interviewed for this book. One of their studies has an interesting result. She took a sample of 1,600 Australians –Australia is the country with most cases of melanoma in the world– and studied them for 15 years. One group was encouraged to use sunscreen while another was not. Results showed that those who used sunscreen had 50% less chances of developing melanoma at the end of the studied period. Apart from using sunscreen, the best way to be protected from UV radiation and cell alterations is with physical barriers. This is why she recommends ***not being excessively exposed to the sun, to avoid burns, and using hats, parasols or UV protection clothing.*** All filters we place between the sun's radiation and our skin are welcome.
Although nowadays we are more aware, the use of sunscreen is not widespread in Chile. Mainly people of white or very light skin, or those whose relatives had skin cancer and who therefore have increased awareness of the issue tend to use sunscreen in this country. Doctors agree that darker-skinned people tend to be less wary of the sun, unless cancer is present in their genes. In fact, many women buy sunscreens to "tan more". Fatal mistake. When choosing sunscreen, two main aspects must be considered: that it provides protection against UV A and B radiation, and that the level of SPF (sun protection factor) is 50. In relation to skin cancer, you're not looking for 93% protection, but 100% protection. Now I ***ALWAYS*** use sunscreen, before getting in the water at the beach, when I get out, when I'm on the balcony in front of the sea, when riding on a bike and even in the morning before going to the office. ***ALWAYS.*** And never again has my skin become red, nor has it hurt or been sunburned. My skin is the same color in the winter as in the summer: white. Naturally, I am a little bit more tanned in summer, but I always use sunscreen. I get the chills when I see people travelling to the Caribbean in winter and returning with completely sunburned skins. Or those who go skiing and return with small blisters due to excessive sun exposure. They're not protecting their skin, and seem unaware of the risks they're taking.

2 People with many freckles or moles: Someone with many moles always has the propensity to generate melanoma. Specialists also state that freckled people or redheads develop more melanomas than the rest. I have always had freckles and moles, but I never thought this could be a risk factor to cause cancer. ***A normal mole is a benign skin tumor formed of melanocytes that grow in groups. Most adults have between 10 to 40 moles, mainly above their waist, in areas that are exposed to the sun.*** They are located in the scalp, on breasts (for women) or thighs, and these should be examined by a dermatologist. Although normal moles are not cancerous, people with more than 100 of these moles have statistically greater risk of developing melanoma.

3 White skin and light-colored eyes: Skin type is definitely a factor. ***As the sun damages the organism, radiation accumulates; therefore, the more one is exposed to sun the greater the chance of suffering from skin cancer.*** For instance, Australia is the country with the most skin cancer in the world. And this can be understood because it is a country with a large population of light-skinned people who are regularly exposed to UV radiation due to the national passion for water sports.
Dermatologists classify skin tones from 1 to 6 (1 being albino). Obviously, light-skinned people have a higher risk, but those with darker skin, although they have a natural barrier against UV radiation because the granules of their melanin are bigger, may also develop melanoma.

4 Family history: the risk of suffering from melanoma ***is higher if one or more first degree relatives (mother, father, siblings, and descendants) had melanoma.*** Nobody in my family had developed melanoma, but two of my brothers had to remove suspicious-looking moles that had the appearance of melanoma.

5 People between 40 and 50 years of age: there is a very low rate of occurrence of melanoma in children; in fact, the chance of developing one at the age of 15 is around 1 in a million. There are more cases known after the age of 20. The average age of people developing melanoma is between 40 and 50.

To all of the above I would also the importance of the state of mind and the immune system. From the interviews I carried out I arrived at the conclusion that your mind is indissolubly linked to your body. Whether you are sad or happy, this affects your health. ***And, of course, the nutrition factor is key, and I am interested in saying this straight; which is why I dedicate an entire chapter of this book to the subject.*** We are what we eat and if we do not take care of our body we harm it. And then, our body reacts. How? Intoxicating, reducing immunity or with the unexpected development of cancer or any other serious disease, as happened to me. Before suffering from cancer, I didn't pay much attention to schedules and food, I was not worried about eating properly, I had chronic diarrhea and did not listen to my body. If you add up stress or problems, a reduction in defenses is certain.

When melanoma is located in a superficial layer of the skin –in the epidermis– it is said to be *in situ* and there is a good chance it will heal; therefore, an early diagnosis is essential. A melanoma *in situ* has a 100% chance of getting cured. Doctor **Mercedes López** explained that as long as the melanoma does not go beyond the base membrane one is doing well; however, once the cancer passes that membrane, the chances of survival start to decrease: ***the deeper the tumor the greater the chances of metastasis.***

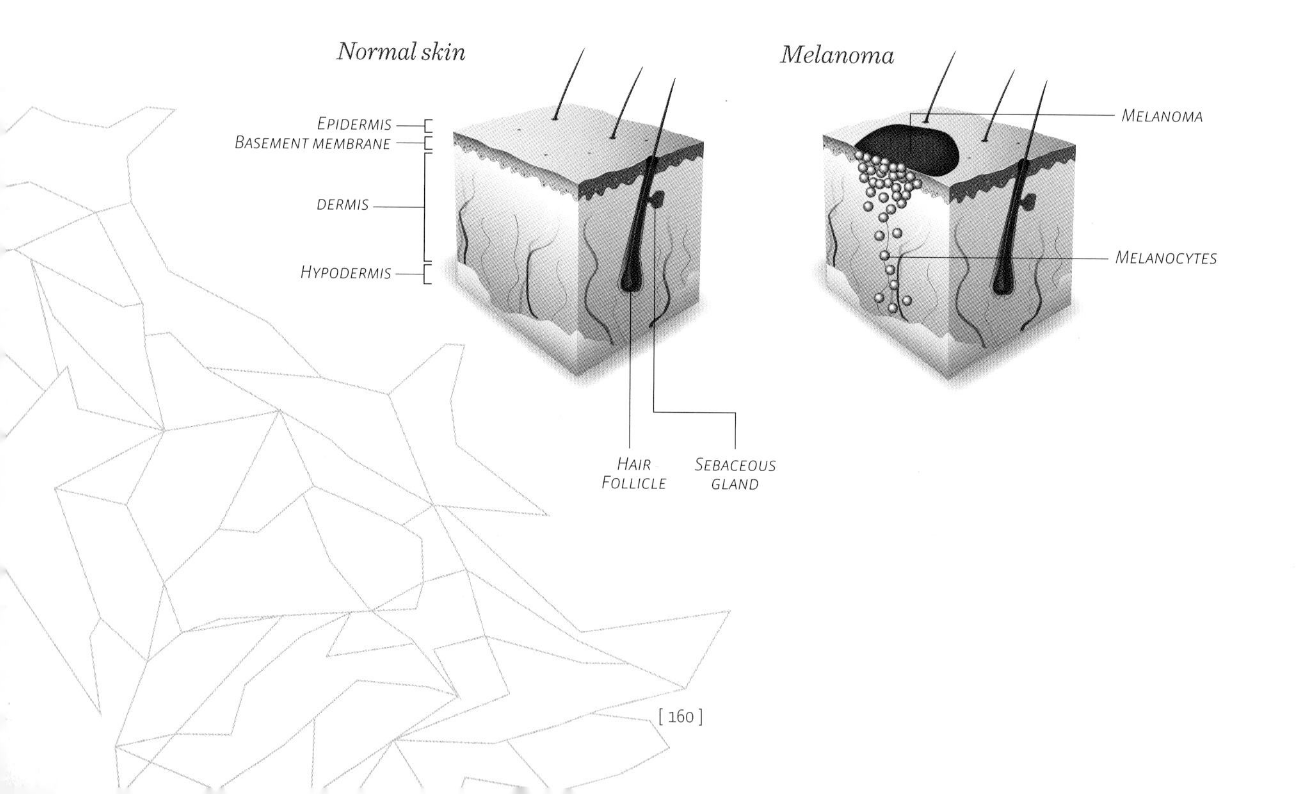

What does metastasis mean? Put simply it is the propagation of the cancerous focus to a different organ, the expansion of the tumor, which is not a new cancer. *In the case of melanoma, the risk is that this is a type of cancer that can metastasize in any part of the organism and can expand quickly.* According to specialists, this speed depends on factors such as the immune system, patient's nutritional status or whether they are exposed to UV radiation, among others. In most cases, if the melanoma metastisizes, it will first affect lymphatic nodes, then the liver, lungs or brain.

If a melanoma is in a stage inferior to 0.5 millimeters of depth, it should normally not compromise the patient's chances of survival. The deeper the melanoma at the time of diagnosis, the higher the percentage of metastasis risk.

My melanoma had a depth of 1.5 millimeters and had metastasized in two nodes. When these were removed any other nodes that could have been affected were also removed. I'm now doing fine and there's only a 20% chance that metastases will appear. As doctors in the United States confirmed.

With this type of cancer, years can go by without there being anything to worry about. Ten to 15 years before one experiences the reoccurrence of the disease, which generally appears in the form of a metastasis. This is not colon cancer or sarcoma when during the subsequent five years there have been no complications, one can be discharged. The melanoma may reappear after a long time or never arise again. I hope I do not receive news about it again. Up to now everything seems to be going well.

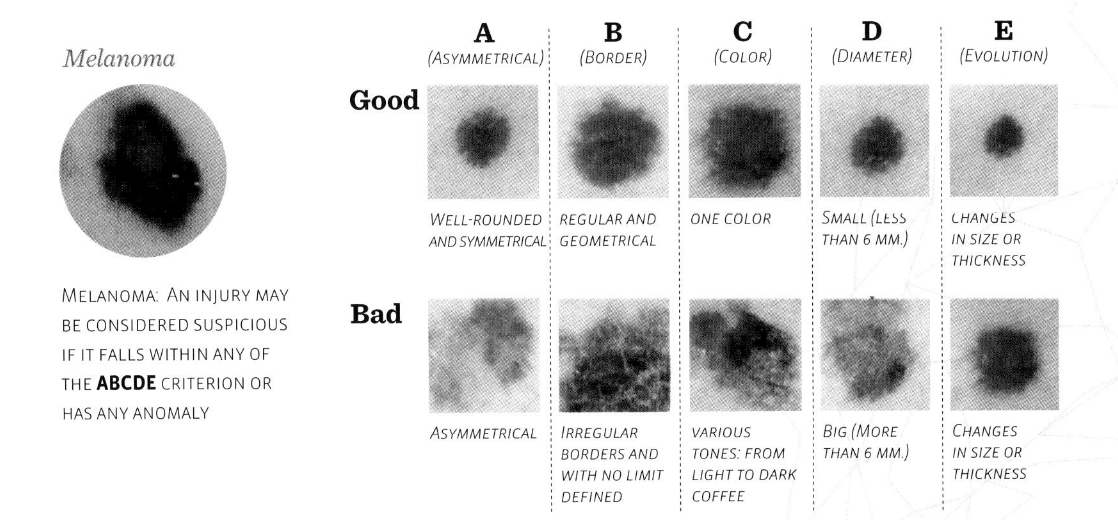

CREDIT OF CHART: MYSKINCHECK.CL, LA ROCHE-POSAY

Worrying questions

Which melanoma has the worst prognosis? Specialists agree it is the one that develops on the scalp because it is an area of late examination and where lymphatic vessels have direct communication with veins; this is called lymphatic-venous anastomoses. Sometimes bad cells go directly to veins and flow to distant points, and this leads to a risk of a greater metastasis. I suffered from local metastasis (nodes in my right armpit), not a distant one, and that made my prognosis better.

How can it be detected?

Doctor Palisson assures that prevention is the safest road. My melanoma was fortunately detected and it was removed on time, so although I had a rough few years, I am today a healthy person.

Every person should undergo a preventative check-up with a dermatologist at least once a year. Check-ups must be made from head to toes because melanomas are hidden in the less visible areas. A superficial examination may affect a prognosis and, therefore, a person's life.

And all of us should be alert to moles that change size or color and that have an irregular border, or itch or bleed. I mention this due to the story I heard from Doctor Palisson. He had a patient with relevant genetic background and a first melanoma *in situ*. The patient (a woman) strictly attended annual check-ups in United States, but on there was one check-up she couldn't make, so she went to see Dr Palisson. Hidden beneath her underwear was an advanced melanoma that took her life less than 8 months later. Fatally, in the US she'd never been asked to fully undress for the examination.

If is detected a suspicious mole what usually happens is that you have it removed and a biopsy is made to dismiss the possibility of it being a melanoma. In the event that it is an invasive melanoma you need to have your sentinel lymph node examined as soon as possible because it is the first one that warns about metastasis. A melanoma is a small tumor that expands fast and which can make metastases through the nodes or blood. It is a relief if the sentinel lymph node is found to be clean. You may have two or three sentinel lymph nodes affected –I had two– and when this happens the advice it to have all nodes in the area removed. "The scar is not important, they all need to be removed", warned Doctor López. This does not mean that after this surgery you will have no lymphatic nodes left in the arm because they are a crucial part of the body's immune system. Not all nodes are removed, a barrier is always left, though –logically– there is higher risk of infection through cuts or viruses in the treated area and prevention as well as care must be maximized.

Facing a melanoma, one needs to act and do it quickly due to it being so aggressive. Experts agree that, although patients need to be given time to assimilate the news, this should be no longer than two weeks. Doctors explained that when a mole or injury is removed, some tumor cells may remain in the body. During scarring many biochemical phenomena take place, which include risks for the patient, such as growth stimulation of blood vessels and more access of cells to the bloodstream. This is why after the biopsy of the mole the initial diagnosis may be modified.

According to Doctor Palisson, bodies are able to provide an immunologic response to some melanomas and destroy them without us even noticing. However, it may have made metastases. Although very infrequent, there are cases in which the body with an invasive melanoma surrounds a malignant mole with a white halo and it disappears. However, metastasis can take place in the years to follow.

I had local metastasis which was completely removed and my organism could stop the process. The first barrier was removed and cancer did not progress. As I already mentioned, I had an 80% chance that all affected cells had been removed when my nodes were removed and 20% chance that some cell remained flowing through my organism. One needs to know that there are microscopic metastases that may remain stable in terms of growth for a long time. ***Therefore, to have a strong immune system it is very important to lead a healthy and balanced life.***

Treatments

What are the treatments for melanoma?

The primary procedure is surgical: The mole is removed together with part of its surrounding area. At this stage of the melanoma, radiotherapy, chemotherapy and immunotherapy provide little help. Melanomas have a biological behavior of high proliferation and low reaction to chemotherapy, as well as low responsiveness to radiotherapy. However, Doctor López explained that chemotherapy may be used in patients on stage IV, the most advanced stage, because the size of the tumor may be reduced and some efficiency obtained. At the terminal stage, this efficiency is understood as some extra months of life as well as providing palliative comfort in reducing pain. At this stage, patients may choose to undergo chemotherapy having survival time in mind, as short as it may be. A melanoma can be considered incurable today if it has entered your organism and is no longer *in situ*. There are alternatives to chemotherapy in order to treat metastatic melanomas with some very specific drugs, such as dacarbazine, temozolomide, paclitaxel, carmustine, cisplatin, carboplatin, vinblastine and others.

THERE ARE ALSO IMMUNOTHERAPIES, such as **INTERFERON** and monoclonal antibodies. This immunotherapy stimulates the patient's immune system to recognize and destroy cancerous cells more efficiently. Different types of immunotherapy can be used to treat patients with advanced melanoma: **IPILIMUMAB,** a monoclonal antibody which is only prescribed for metastatic melanoma in stage IV. It works through cytotoxic T lymphocytes which are part of the immune system in charge of destroying tumors. However, it does not destroy the melanoma, it just increases patients' survival time, although the amount of time is not scientifically confirmed. This is considered case by case.

INTERFERON, on the other hand, is an immunomodulator. This means that antitumor activity of the organism increases. However, this is a controversial treatment. There are doctors that recommend it and others that don't as it has not been scientifically proven that it improves survival and, on the contrary, its secondary effects may affect patients' quality of life: you feel you have the flu, your whole body hurts, you become feverish; in other words, you feel terrible. **INTERFERON** is basically a substance all our cells produce and which turns on or activates our immune system. One of the organism's reaction to a virus or swelling is the production of **INTERFERON** which fights against this external attack. For instance, this is why you become feverish.

I WAS REALLY CLOSE TO TAKING IT, but after travelling to the United States with my family, I decided I would not be submitted to **INTERFERON.** I was not willing to lose quality of life. Furthermore, I did not want to be part of an **IPILIMUBAB** clinical trial where one becomes a guinea pig for drugs and medicine under research. We considered this possibility, but when doctors knew I suffered from chronic diarrhea they recommended not being part of it as diarrhea is one of the possible effects caused by the drug provided in the clinical trial.

I CHOSE TAPCELLS AUTOIMMUNE VACCINE OF ONCOBIOMED, a research center created by specialist doctors from the University of Chile, one of them being Doctor Mercedes López. This is still an expensive vaccine which consists of three doses and is an alternative to treating melanomas such as mine and also prostate cancer. The principle behind this therapy is the stimulation of the immune system: blood is extracted from the sick person and a population of monocytes –a type of white blood cells– is isolated; then, the monocytes are cultivated and stimulated in the lab with tumor cells from different types of cancer so they can fight against them. This process turns them into dendritic cells, ***a type of cell specialized in fighting diseases of the immune system, which are reinjected to provoke a response against malignant tumor cells.*** They are ready to go out and fight after they finish their training in the lab.

This vaccine produces very few secondary effects; in fact, I suffered from none. ***With some very few people it can cause skin vitiligo: Depigmentation appearing as white spots. Vaccine creators have seen less than 4 cases in the more than 200 people they have assisted.***

The vaccine was created by scientists from the University of Chile, led by Doctor Flavio Salazar and tested on patients with advanced malignant melanoma whose average time of survival was not more than 11 months. According to the studies conducted, 60% of patients responded to the treatment with the autoimmune vaccine and 35 out of 121 examined patients survived for more than four years. The complete **TAPCells** research was published in the January 2011 edition of the Clinical Cancer Research journal (medical journal form published by the American Association for Cancer Research) under the title Heat-Shock Induction of Tumor-Derived Danger Signals Mediates Rapid Monocyte Differentiation into Clinically Effective Dendritic Cells (link: http://clincancerres.aacrjournals.org/content/17/8/2474).

Survival time

What is the survival time of a melanoma?

Out of the ten most frequent types of cancers, this is the only one whose cases and mortality rate have increased around the world. In 2008, the World Health Organization (WHO) assessed that its incidence is of 3 cases for every 100,000 inhabitants. According to the WHO, this year 46,372 people died in the world due to melanoma; this equals a mortality rate of 0.7 deaths for every 100,000 inhabitants. According to the [Chilean] Ministry of Health, between the years 2000 and 2010, 1,852 deaths caused by melanoma were registered in Chile.

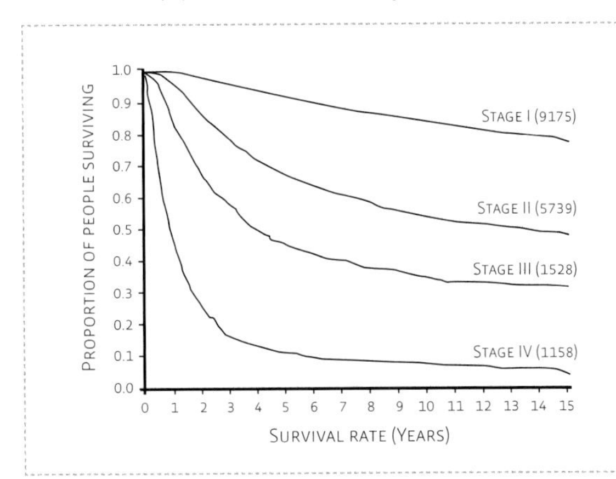

This chart compares the relative survival of up to 15 years for patients with localized melanoma (stages I and II), regional metastasis (stage III) and distant metastasis (stage IV). Numbers in parentheses show the number of patients in the American Joint Committee on Cancer (AJCC) database used to calculate survival rates. There are important differences between the curves."

THE GOOD NEWS IS THAT, although all figures show that in the last 20 years there has been an exponential growth of this disease and of all types of skin cancer due to cumulative effects of ultraviolet radiation, there is a hopeful scenario as early diagnosis has improved. 84% of patients diagnosed with melanoma have the disease localized, 8% are regionally affected and only 4% have distant metastasis.

I WAS PART OF THE 8% and could have ended up dead. I was lucky. ***This is why I always repeat the following: Take care of yourself, be preventive, examine your moles and skin periodically; you need to be healthy and there are tools to achieve this.*** How hard is it to use sunscreen one or five times a day when you are directly exposed to the sun and this will allow you to enjoy that beach, that lake or that pool for many more years? How hard is it to use a hat if it will extend your life? Melanomas are incurable, you may die because they are ferociously lethal. Take care of your children, take care of your family, take care of yourself. The best road is prevention: eat consciously, lead a healthy life and use a good sunscreen. Do not neglect yourself.

Listen to your body; I've said this before, but I want to insist. My immune system was really weakened for at least three years and I ignored the signals it sent me. Although there is no direct connection with the melanoma I developed, I suffered from chronic diarrhea for three years and didn't do anything to cure it; I ignored the signs my body was sending me. Take care of every detail in order not to regret suffering from a serious disease in the future. Don't think twice about it.

So far, the most efficient way to minimize risks of developing melanomas is by using protection against exposure to UV radiation. This is expressed by all specialized sites, it is detailed by the Chilean Ministry of Health, I read it on all serious websites, such as **CANCER.ORG,** the American Cancer Society's website, which is worth checking out as the information provided is really updated. They emphasize that one of the best ways to reduce time of exposure –if you have to be outdoors– is being in the shade. If you will be exposed to the sun, you should follow some compulsory measures to be safe:

a. *Use a long-sleeved t-shirt or shirt.*
b. *Use sunscreen on all areas of your sun-exposed skin.*
c. *Use sunscreen on your lips and verify that the label says it provides protection against UVA and UVB rays, and that the sun protection factor (SPF) is higher than 30.*
d. *It does not end there: you need to use sunscreen every three hours to still be protected.*

When reading this website I understood the difference between two types of rays: UVA make skin cells age and may lead to some DNA damage. They are accountable for wrinkles and they are considered to participate in some skin cancers. UVB may directly damage skin cell's DNA and cause sunburn, as well as most skin cancers.

UV index scale

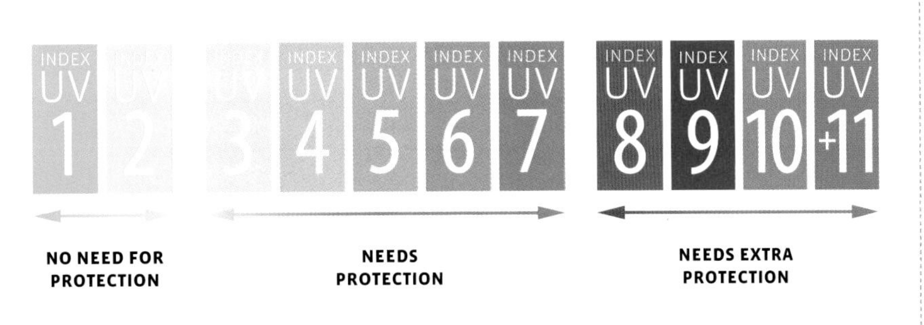

UV INDEX IS THE INDICATOR OF ULTRAVIOLET SOLAR RADIATION INTENSITY ON THE SURFACE OF THE EARTH. THE UV INDEX ALSO STATES THE CAPACITY OF THE UV SOLAR RADIATION FOR CAUSING DAMAGE IN THE SKIN. YOU CAN REVIEW THE RADIATION INDEXES IN CHILEAN NEWSPAPERS AND IN THE WEATHER REPORT IN THE CHILEAN OPEN TV CHANNELS.

Malignant melanoma growth phases

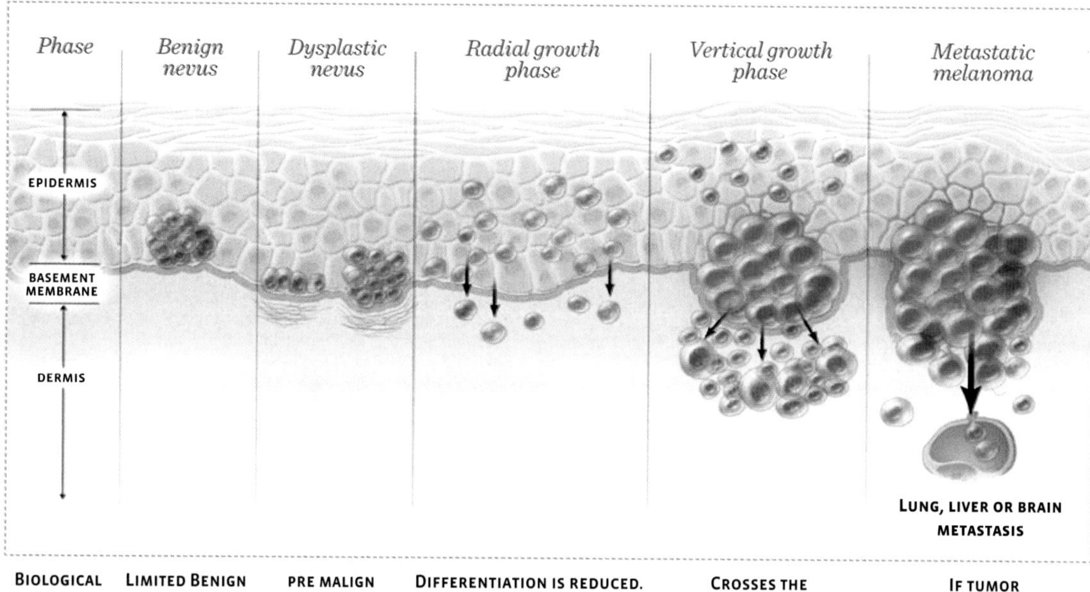

Phase	Benign nevus	Dysplastic nevus	Radial growth phase	Vertical growth phase	Metastatic melanoma
BIOLOGICAL EVENTS	LIMITED BENIGN GROWTH	PRE MALIGN LESIONS MAY COME BACK	DIFFERENTIATION IS REDUCED. UNLIMITED HYPERPLASIA. CLONAL PROLIFERATION	CROSSES THE BASEMENT MEMBRANE, FORMATION OF TUMORS	IF TUMOR DISSOCIATES, IT GROWS IN DISTANT AREAS

CREDIT: ARLO J. MILLER, MARTIN C. MIHM. THE NEW ENGLAND JOURNAL OF MEDICINE 2006

THIS CHART SHOWS THE PARTICULAR STAGES OF THE CLARK MODEL STARTING FROM A BENIGN INJURY TO THE FINAL METASTATIC STAGE. THE CHART ALSO SHOWS CHANGES IN THE TUMOR'S CAPACITY TO PASS FROM THE EPIDERMIS THROUGH THE BASEMENT MEMBRANE AND TO THE DEEPEST DERMIS LAYER.

When you're outdoors: Use a hat and dark sunglasses that offer UV radiation protection. Avoid being fully exposed to the sun between 11 a.m. and 4 p.m. I don't mind repeating this because it is extremely important: during this time of the day UV radiation is particularly ferocious. As correctly expressed on the website cancer.org, rays go through clouds and are reflected in the water, sand, concrete and snow.

And be careful: Genetic mutations increase the risk of developing melanoma and this could be passed from one generation to another. Therefore, if different members from your mother's or father's side of the family have suffered from melanoma, or if a relative has developed more than one melanoma, it is worth your while to be alert for new moles or for those that change their size or color. **Approximately** 10% of all people with melanoma have some family members who have developed this disease. I will personally take care of this subject when I have children. In fact, even though melanomas are mostly developed by adults, they also affect young people and they are one of the most usual cancers among people under 30 (especially among women). I developed melanoma at the age of 27. At the same time, early age has a more favorable prognosis as healthy cells are full of energy.

Cancer.org also recommends practicing sports as one of the ways to prevent any type of cancer and suggests taking an hour a day to walk fast or practice intense exercise, and vigorously exercising for an hour a week if your working activities are moderate. This happens because exercise provides oxygen to cells and cells do not survive without oxygen.

Remember melanomas are malignant tumors that do not die in your body and may kill you! ■

To see world investigation or treatment centers for melanoma, please review **melanoma.org** *and* **melanomainternational.org**

DIET

you are what YOU EAT

Chapter written with the collaboration of Iván Mimica, Mark Mincolla, María Paz Calvo, Doctor Alejandro Stevens and Doctor Mario Sandoval.

Until I was diagnosed with cancer I had no idea of the effect diet can have on our lives. I'd never heard concepts such as "toxicity" or "inflammation" related to what we eat, let alone about our bodies being intoxicated or inflamed with certain foods. I was also unaware of the potentially noxious effects of milk, sugar, gluten, or processed food. I just ate, unaware of the harm I could be causing my body if I did not eat breakfast, or if I ate junk food. I ate whatever and whenever I wanted.

And so I lived believing –naïvely– that I was in control. I didn't even know that eating and nutrition were not the same: "Eating is a voluntary act –in which the senses of touch and sight are involved– as we willingly choose certain food to put in our mouth. Once food is ingested, the physiological mechanism of nutrition begins" explained Doctor Alejandro Stevens, surgeon from the University of Concepción who's currently working in German biological medicine. I also didn't know that 70% of our immune system is located in the digestive system, that we have 100 times more DNA in our microbione than in the cells of our entire body and that our gut manufactures more neurotransmitters than the brain.

Anyways, the melanoma and all its consequences pretty much destroyed any control I thought I had over my diet. When you don't know enough about it you eat what everybody else eats, and you don't follow a regime or special diet: you eat quickly after hours of eating nothing, you skip meals, and without meaning to you fill your body with things that make it hard for it to function properly.

Our body speaks, but most of us do not listen to it. We do not detect the signals, as explicit as they may be. I suffered daily from intermittent diarrhea, and the pain that preceded that used to come up in the most inappropriate moments; and still, I didn't understand... my body was clamoring for attention. I was always stressed out and seldom took care of myself, of my body. I ate without fully understanding nutrition. What did I care? I felt young, healthy, and happy, with energy to spare.

Before all this started, I believed I was eating correctly: I ate granola cookies, pasta, bread, pizzas, chocolates, rice, meat, yoghurt, cheese... everything. Only now do I understand that these foods -made with processed sugars and industrial flours- are of little nutritional value and can even damage the body through inflammation. This is a key concept: inflammation. As I know now, this is a natural process the organism uses to protect itself from alien substances, infections, or viruses. The bad news is that, sometimes, the immune system can activate inflammation even if the organism is not facing any external threat. Although, strictly speaking, it is facing one: It's withstanding the attack of a poor diet.

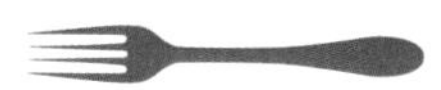

Dairy did its part as well: I was convinced that milk and other dairy products were a good source of calcium, because this is a worldwide belief. So, I drank milk and consumed dairy without knowing how they made my organism swell up. However, in 2013, the Harvard School of Public Health erased milk from its guide to healthy eating (Healthy Eating Plate) and replaced it, preferably, with water. This guide states, in between other things, that the chemical components found in most dairy products and which are used for their production, make them foods that should be avoided. The advice is to substitute dairy with spinach, cauliflower, broccoli, alfalfa sprouts, coca flour (the best source of calcium on the planet) and by different grains, to obtain calcium. Also, this guide clearly states that the consumption of milk increases the risk of ovarian and prostate cancer. Shocking.

Furthermore, milk is one of the hardest foods to digest, as casein, which represents 80% of milk's protein, accumulates and makes digestion difficult. In fact, casein is one of the ingredients used in glue sticks used by children, and this is also how it acts in the body: as glue that gets stuck to intestinal mucosa. Plus, according to the same source, more than two thirds of the population is considered to be lactose intolerant. Lactose is a type of sugar that is present in all mammal milk, and it's used as an ingredient in many manufactured foods. This intolerance means that we don't have enough of a specific enzyme (lactase) in the small intestine to decompose the ingested lactose. This, either partially or completely digested, will flow through the large intestine and will be decomposed there by its bacteria, leading to symptoms such as pain, abdominal swelling or diarrhea, among others. I would have never known this, obviously, if I hadn't suffered from cancer and, also, if I hadn't met **Iván Mimica.**

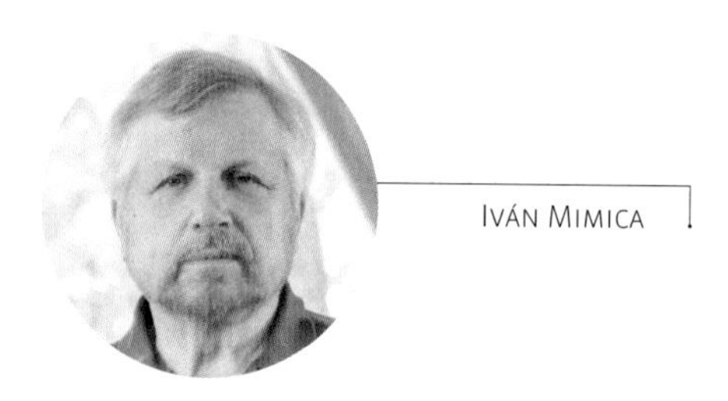
Iván Mimica

Iván was the first person to tell me about the consequences of a poor diet and the benefits of following a a specific and informed one. He suggested I visit naturopathic Doctor Mark Mincolla in the United States, the first important step to really taking care of my health and start changing the structure of my diet: ***Mincolla's motto is "Mind the body or the body minds".***

Mark Mincolla is an eminence in nutrition and health. He is a sociologist from Franklin Pierce University, has a Master's degree in nutrition from Goddard College, and a PhD in health and human services from Columbia Pacific University. He has more than 30 years of experience and combines Chinese energy techniques with nutritional science. He treats patients with many different types of diseases or conditions at the Santi Holistic Healing center, in Cohassett, Massachusetts. And he also hosts TV and radio shows, gives seminars and lectures, has a website (**MARKMINCOLLA.COM**) which includes information on his work and an active Twitter account: @markmincolla.

Dr. Mincolla has also published different books on his theory, including: *Maximum Healing* (1999), *Customized Healing: Blending the Best of Eastern and Western Medicine* (2012), and *Whole Health: A Holistic Approach to Healing for the 21st Century* (2014).

In the first chapter, *My Story*, I talk about my experience during the appointment I went to with my parents and from which we left convinced by the doctor's advice of becoming healthy by changing your diet. Mincolla addresses body and mind care through diet. We need to identify what we eat and the effects of that food on our organism. Chemically speaking, all that surrounds us has an alkaline and an acid part. Due to the fact that saliva's pH is less precise, a urine pH test is recommended as it is a direct indicator of pH the body's tissue. It is worth mentioning that the organism's pH has its own circadian rhythm: it has an acid pH from 3:00 a.m. to 3:00 p.m.; on the other hand, from 3:00 p.m. to 3:00 a.m. it has an alkaline rhythm. This is why you should test pH during the afternoon, when one should really avoid having an acid pH. The pH scale measures the media's acidic or alkaline values; in people, the ideal pH varies between 6.5 and 7. If a person's pH is 7, their blood is more alkaline than acid. If their pH is 10, it is too alkaline and it means there is a chemical imbalance. And vice versa. These two aspects are also present in food, as acid and alkaline values are related to food digestion. When the body reaction is acid, inflammation is produced.

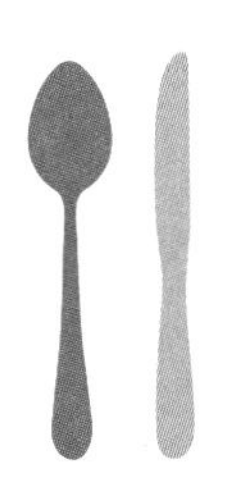

Mincolla suggests keeping a proportion of 4 to 1 in food: four alkaline parts for every acid part. But there is no universal recipe: "My mantra is personal, individualized healing. One size does not fit all", he often repeats.

Inflammatory foods

Alcohol	Artificial Additives	Wheat	Trans fat	Grain Fed Meats	Peanut oil	Egg yolk	Fried Foods
Dairy	Eggplant	Tomatoes	Carbonated Beverages	Vegetable oils	Sugars	Synthetic Sweeteners	Caffeine

Anti-inflammatory foods

Green Leafy Veggies	Ginger	Pumpkin and Pumpkin seeds	Sole Fish	Oregano	Bone Broth	Clove	Celery
Brussel sprouts	Salmon	Chia and Flax Seeds	Berries	Nuts	Turmeric	Coconut Oil	Cilantro and Parsley

Credit: Mark Mincolla, Ph. D., Ph. D. Suzanne E. Landry, MS, RD, LDN and María Paz Calvo.

I like the comparison Mincolla made between care provided to plants in a nursery and to humans. He says that each plant has a tag describing the care it has to receive; some need more water, others more sun than shade. Human beings also have an imaginary tag that we do not know about. For instance, *we do not know that for cancer to develop it needs an acid environment; i.e., a low pH, some chemistry that favors the spread of the disease.* Mine was 5.5.

Most significantly, I ate few fruits and vegetables, which are top basic foods, mainly green stems or leafy greens. Sugar, starch, red meat, some big fish such as tuna, and dairy are acid. Apart from food's pH, Mincolla also considers the inflammation these foods may cause. Dr. Mincolla estimates a high percentage of diseases are precisely due to organism inflammation; so, taking care of your body means protecting it against inflammation-causing food. It seems important to highlight that inflammation is not a negative process in itself, as it is the only way our body has to respond to any stress and finally repair damage. This is why balance is key. When you eat sugar, blood glucose levels explode and the body reacts: in order to be in equilibrium, the body produces insulin. When this process is repeated over and over again the system suffers a general imbalance and, to fix this, it is inflamed and produces fat. When inflammation is high, an indicator called Protein C shows up in the blood. This is one of the biological markers used for cancer detection and follow-up. If it is detected in a test, it may mean you have cancer. The following is one of the many things Mincolla told me:

–"The concept of inflammation is usually related to painful joints, but we now know it is a factor indicating the presence of eicosanoids, hormones that act as enzymes and express themselves through the production of certain fats or lipids".

According to Mincolla, there are six types of eicosanoids, hormones that work as mediators in the central nervous system, the immune response and inflammatory effects of the organism, although only one is inflammatory: arachidonic acid. Those foods that produce this acid in great amounts, such as peanuts, red meats, egg yolk, and dairy, present Cox-2 hormonal factors that are very inflammatory. Among the less inflammatory fats we can find oily fish, linseed, and chia, among others, because they all have omega 3 fatty acids. In fact, Doctor Stevens explained that linseed has interesting nutritional properties and potentially beneficial health effects due to its chemical composition. It has a great amount of dietary fiber, polyunsaturated and phytochemical fatty acids.

This sounds complicated, but I can explain it this way: chronic inflammation is not good for the organism, it affects the immune system, and is a risk factor to developing diseases.

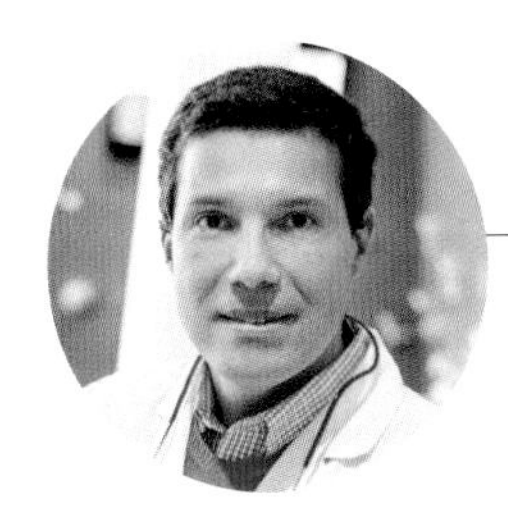

As a result, eating greater amounts of less inflammatory fats while rarely tasting foods with inflammatory fats is advisable.

Significant is that eicosanoids are involved in the immune response of the organism when facing inflammation. Mincolla explains that tumors, whatever their nature -cancer included- are inflammations. In fact, when you are subjected to a PET/CT exam to control the potential progress of cancer in your body, it detects inflammations, no matter how small or microscopic they are, and glucose concentrations. These indicate the eventual presence of tumors. What are the main differences between a normal and a cancerous cell? Normal cells have alkaline pH, consume oxygen, have a temperature of 37 degrees and are recognized by the immune system. Cancerous cells, on the other hand, live in acid media, consume sugar instead of oxygen, have low temperatures of 8-10 degrees and are not recognized by the immune system. According to Mincolla, if you reduce or eradicate sugar and keep a balanced pH, your body will no longer be a propitious environment for these inflammations.

Mincolla has carried out research on the power of some foods to improve the health in a person with cancer and discovered many good foods, such as beans (red and black), berries, spices such as turmeric or curcuma, green-leaf vegetables and green tea. This last infusion contains EGCG (epigallocatechin 3-gallate), a very powerful antioxidant when taken in moderation (max 2-3 cups per week). Also good are extra virgin olive oil, oregano oil, avocado oil, coconut oil (extra virgin as well), and black cumin seed oil, which is difficult to find in Chile, but easy to get in the United States (500 mg capsules). There are also other oils that are sold in capsules and have a great antioxidant effect, such as borage oil, evening primrose and blackcurrant seed, which change natural fats into omega 3. Hydrogenated corn and sunflower oils should be mostly avoided.

Mincolla recommends eating pumpkin seeds and nuts because they are dried fruits that produce anti-inflammatory fats, which is not the case of peanuts. Other good supplements for the body are alpha-lipoic acid, glutathione and n-acetylcysteine, the three most important antioxidants in the process of converting free radicals into good cells. I take a cocktail which includes these antioxidants; in fact, it is called Antioxidant Therapy and is prepared in Chile following Doctor **Mario Sandoval's** strict indications. According to the doctor, whether you have cancer or not, taking a basal level of an antioxidant is good and does not require much effort if one eats correctly and leads a well-balanced life. However as this isn't always that easy to achieve he suggests constantly providing the body with cofactors (zinc, selenium, magnesium, manganese) and ideally, with n-acetylcysteine (glutathione).

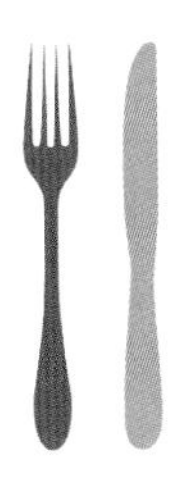

Other antioxidants, such as lycopene, vitamin E (mainly in women), berry extract or vitamin C are useful in specific moments, but do not make a difference in life, whether you have family history of cancer or not. I met Doctor Sandoval because he opened a center two and a half years ago, the *110 Sport & Health Center,* just across from my former office. I attended his center to rebuild muscles and found a doctor devoted to medicine, as redundant as that may sound, and who is a good person. In his opinion medicine has become so specialized that doctors rarely stray from their particular fields of expertise. Sandoval aims at an integrative medicine, focused on the patient and on improving their quality of life. When I told him everything I had gone through and my current condition, he suggested strengthening my antioxidant defense system with his cocktail. He recommends it to many cancer patients undergoing chemotherapy who arrive to his center looking for a way to feel better. As I did.

Doctor Sandoval explained that the Antioxidant Therapy has co-factors, for the body's enzymes to work when they have to, and direct antioxidants. These co-factors and n-acetyl-cysteine activate the glutathione peroxidase enzyme –our main defense mechanism– and superoxide dimutase and catalase enzymes. In fact, glutathione is one of the most important substances produced by the body to protect its cells. In a link Doctor Sandoval sent me, I read some information I reproduce here, as I found it very interesting: ***"Glutathione has three primary functions, detoxifying effects, immune system booster, and antioxidant (...)".*** On a daily basis the body is exposed to numerous factors that involve a reduction in glutathione reserves: stress, pollution, radiation, infections, drugs, poor diet, aging, sports, and injuries. Without adequate protection with glutathione, cells may end up damaged, and there might be some aging in them, as well, and in the long term, the development of diseases. Glutathione exhaustion interferes decisively in many illnesses. This is why keeping good reserves of this substance is crucial in complementary medicine. Until recently many scientists were convinced that glutathione could not be entirely absorbed and that the best way to increase its level in the organism was to use precursors, such as n-acetyl-cysteine and other substances like alpha-lipoic acid. Recently, though, it has been observed that glutathione can be correctly absorbed in considerable amounts, turning supplements into a justified and good option to stimulate its levels in cells. ***Glutathione is present in fresh fruits and vegetables, fish and meat; asparagus, avocado and nuts are also rich in this substance. Under normal conditions, the body produces it according to its needs.*** However, when one ages and has higher oxidative loads, one's own

This following suggestions in A and B boxes are given by Mark Mincolla to patients on their first visit to his practice.

Do not eat:

A. High fat processed foods

- **Sugar:** sucrose, dextrose, glucose, maltose, corn flavor, turbinate, honey, raisins, molasses and anything made with these.
- **Fried foods, white flour.**
- **Refined carbohydrates,** including white rice, muffins, donuts, pizza, crackers, chewing gum (with or without sugar), soft drinks (including diet drinks), cakes, cookies, sherbets or dairy ice creams (unless they are 100% made out of fruits, water and honey or maple syrup), pasta flour, flavored juices.
- **Condiments such as relish,** barbecue sauce, sugared jellies, sauces, jams, sour cream.
- **Excess fatty foods** as cream soups.
- **Alcoholic beverages and drinks with caffeine or derivatives.**

B. Fermented and highly acidic food

- **Yeast**
- **Wine and beer**
- **Bread with yeast**
- **Mushrooms**
- **Corn**
- **Vinegar**
- **Soy sauce**
- **All types of dairy**
- **Coffee and tea**
- **Dried fruits**
- **Aged foods,** such as blue cheese
- **Melons and watermelons**

Supplements:

Complements for my diet

- **Chlorophyll Extract** (to reduce acidity)
- **Maqui Berry extract , Gluthathione or N.A.C** (Powerful Antioxidants that at a cellular level prevent damages caused by free radicals)
- **Pau D'arco Pills** (Anti Microbial, Anti Fungal, fights Candida and Yeast infections.)
- **Probiotics** (Gluten and lactose free and never less than 20 Billion organisims per day. (To balance "good" and "bad" bacteria in the gut)
- **Vitamin D** (regulates cellular growth and DNA differentiation. Probably the most important vitamin if fighting/preventing cancer)

* It's terrible how used we are to eating great quantities of white flour and sugar. When they are taken away from us, it's as though we were going through cold turkey, withdrawal symptoms and all.

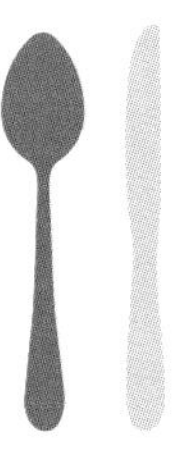

production cannot be enough. The body often has an important need for glutathione, which is quickly consumed in times of disease, stress, fatigue, and physical effort. Also, there are some factors that may exhaust the available amount, such as radiation (ionizing), stress, bacterial or viral infections, environmental toxins, tobacco, some drugs, high-level sports, chemical pollution, and heavy metals, excess iron, surgeries, burns, and glutathione precursor or cofactor insufficiencies. The body tries to reduce oxidized glutathione through antioxidant cascades and thus consumes other antioxidants, such as vitamin C, vitamin E and alpha-lipoic acid".

All of these should be studied in depth and Mario Sandoval and Iván Mimica helped me understand the importance of what we provide to our organism. It is also true that with so much information on antioxidants and free radicals, we can sometimes go too far and trigger chemical reactions that hinder the body from recovering, as they inflame it even more. Free radicals are key agents in the eradication of bacteria and viruses or tumor cells, but they can migrate to other places in the body and cause harm as they are like little bombs that destroy whatever they come across. As Doctor Sandoval explained: it's as though the kitchen of a house were on fire, and in an attempt to put out the flames the firemen were to flood the living room and dining room. The same happens with free radicals: we need them, but in the right proportions. The problem with free radicals only starts when the antioxidant mechanisms of the body are exceeded. In my case, as I need to protect my joints and muscles, glutathione and n-acetylcysteine also incite the natural production of hyaluronic acid which is like oil that lubricates joints.

Getting to know Mario Sandoval was a kind of re-affirmation. He approved the way I ate and reinforced my strict but not over-the-top attitude which allows for some occasional relapses. He said my attitude humanized my diet and, obviously, that encouraged me.

In view of the seriousness of my cancer – stage III A–, Mincolla gave me a very strict diet because my system was particularly inflamed. He gave me a comprehensive list of foods that I cannot eat and, since I follow it, always read the labels on food packaging.

Mark Mincolla explained that my inflammatory process was related to the presence of fungi which proliferate in my blood, because my immune system was depressed. Thus, he insisted on cutting mushrooms and yeast out of my diet.

It's terrible how used we are to eating huge amounts of white flour and sugar, and when they are taken away, it's as though we were enduring cold turkey, withdrawal symptoms and all.

On the day you decide to start the diet and completely change the way you eat, you react like an addict, you suffer from a sort of withdrawal syndrome. You feel sick because your body asks for what you have always provided and you feel physically tired and anxious. *At this point you immediately realize you were eating things that intoxicated you. No milk, sugar, wheat flour, white rice or processed foods: I had to leave all that out of my diet if I wanted to heal.* Assuming this new reality in relation to food was hard at the beginning, and it's still hard. I felt I was being deprived of everything and found this unfair. I didn't go to parties, meals and other social meetings because I didn't want to be tempted or have to walk around with a pot containing special food. It is already difficult to follow a diet when one is healthy, but it is even worse when you have recently been diagnosed with cancer and your head is spinning. Above all, you need to follow a strict diet, be rigorous and take care of your body, because nobody else will do it for you. And, although on the one hand this is a pain, on the other hand it is the best thing that can happen to you as it will help you heal. Wasn't following a diet better than facing the insecurity caused by treatment with Interferon? I had no other choice: I had ruled out Interferon –the only therapy for melanoma– due to its secondary effects and for it not being certified. Of course, the option I chose is not a universal formula, nor one that should be considered on your own: you need to talk about this with your family and the treating physician.

I chose to be responsible with my diet. And it's not easy; life keeps testing you, day in and day out. How to cope with stress? If you follow a diet like mine and for any reason you get anxious, you can no longer eat anything that used to calm you down. I ate chocolates or cookies, but now I couldn't and this made me even more anxious. Normally, if you have a bad day or you want to celebrate, what do you do? You call some friends and go out to drink *pisco* and coke, right? Your day improves, you relax and get distracted; or you go out and eat something tasty.

With this diet I couldn't go to restaurants because ordering ended up being long and tiresome: "What does this dish have? What are its ingredients? Does it have cream? Does it have butter?" You end up stressing waiters because they may not know exactly what each dish contains or they may simply make a mistake... "Does this have sugar? Has this been prepared with flour?" And so on with a lot of questions you need to ask.

If I forgot to ask or the waiter was wrong, I'd later come down with a stomach ache or diarrhea As I said before, I suffered from diarrhea long before I was diagnosed with a melanoma although, when I visited Mark Mincolla I understood that they were not isolated events: The reason I had chronic diarrhea was that my body was repeatedly rejecting certain foods

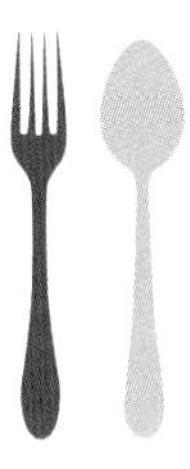

Food chart with color code

Alkaline foods   Neutral foods   Acid foods

Acid foods that turn into alkaline ones whenever there is a stable pH.

Animal protein

- Beef
- Chicken
- Clam
- Cod
- Crab
- Egg White
- Yolk
- Sea Bass
- Southern Ray's Bream
- Sole
- Ham
- Lamb
- Liver
- Lobster
- Pork
- Salmon
- Sardine
- Prawns
- Shrimp
- Octopus
- Tuna
- Turkey

Dairy and its substitutes

- Cheese
- Rice milk
- Rice cheese
- Cow milk
- Yoghurt
- Almond milk
- Soy milk
- Soy cheese
- Soy yoghurt

Legumes

- Beans
- Black beans +1
- White beans +1
- Soy sprouts / Tofu
- Lentils +1
- Chickpeas
- *Pinto* beans

Nuts and seeds

- Almonds
- Cashew nuts
- Macadamia nuts
- Peanuts
- Nuts
- Pistachio
- Sesame
- Pumpkin
- Sunflower

Fats

- Avocado
- Butter
- Coconut
- Cream
- Margarine
- Ghee
- Vegetable oil
- Olive oil

Vegetables with low starch content

- Arugula
- Asparagus
- Brussel sprouts
- Cabbage
- Khale
- Cucumber
- Cauliflower
- Celery
- Chinese cabbage
- Eggplant
- Endives
- Lettuce
- Iceberg lettuce
- Hydroponic lettuce
- Garlic
- Green beans
- Turnip
- Leek
- Mushrooms
- Onion
- Parsley
- Cilantro
- Basil
- Radish
- Chive
- Sprouts
- Chard
- Watercress
- Zucchini

Vegetables with high starch content

- Artichoke
- Beetroot
- Carrot
- Chestnuts
- Corn
- Lima beans
- Peas
- Potatoes
- Pumpkin
- Sweet potato

Grain produce

- Amaranth
- Barley
- Buckwheat
- Milet
- Quinoa
- Oats
- Rice
- Brown rice
- Rye
- Wheat
- Spelt

Sugars

- Barley malt
- Sugar
- Brown sugar
- Honey
- Maple syrup
- Rice syrup
- White bread
- Cane sugar
- Stevia
- Yeast

Acid fruits

- Grapefruit
- Kumquat
- Kiwi
- Lemon
- Lime
- Orange
- Pineapple
- Strawberry
- Tomato

Sub-acid fruit

- Apple
- Apricot
- Blackberry
- Blueberry
- Cherry
- Grape
- Mango
- Peach
- Nectarine
- Papaya
- Pear
- Plum
- Raspberry
- Mandarin

Sweet fruit

- Banana
- Pomegranate
- Figs
- Raisins

Melons

- Cantaloupe
- Honeydew
- Amarillo Oro melon
- Santa Claus melon
- Watermelon

* This is the table of acid and alkaline foods that Mincolla prescribed to me and that still guides my diet. The general guideline is very simple, for each gram of acid food you eat, you have to compensate it with four grams of alkaline food. Be aware that the recommendation is to avoid high doses of fructose present in all fruits. We should seek alkalinity mainly from the consumption of vegetables.

that I ate; food my body did not accept and, thus, caused diarrhea. My body was intoxicated and my immune system depressed. So in my body the entry barriers for cancer –or any other disease– were low.

When I changed the way I ate, I started going out less. At home, everybody changed their diet empathizing with me, because it is not easy being the only one at the table eating differently. After coming back from the U.S., we started eating salads, black beans and lentils. I won't deny it: during the first months I ordered meat or drank a glass of wine more than once, but it ended up being a bad idea as I immediately felt sick. In general, I have strictly followed the diet and it has helped me get better, I've got more energy, my moods are better and I feel more focused.

Before all of this happened I used to drink quite a lot. I won't deny that I still drink now and again, but much less than I used to. If I go to *Taringa* (a bar I own with other partners) during the week, I drink *Taringa* Water (a very tasty lemonade sweetened with stevia), although I also may drink one (or two) vodkas. I drink and don't feel guilty. So while this might be slightly irresponsible of me, it's hard to maintain an iron willpower, especially between December and March - the Chilean party season! I know a zero-alcohol policy would be the ideal, but my aim is to heal, not to be completely rigid about everything.

And in any case, every time I cheat the diet my body gives me a good kicking! Once I was in a meeting with a client and there was no water, so I drank a soft drink and, as I was fairly detoxified, my body reacted. Our bodies speak to us and we need to know how to listen.

I firmly believe that diet works. Yes, I've sometimes felt like a slave to it, but it has helped reduce my body's inflammation. My diet might not be the same as for someone else my age who receives the same diagnosis; there are many specific elements that make a difference depending on what your medical records show up.

Mincolla says it strongly depends on the organism and genetics, so it's important to be examined and to test the pH regularly - you can do this with pH strips available in the pharmacy.

One of the frustrating consequences of the diet was that I was forced to suspend my plans for independence. I lived with my parents, and my Mom used to say –as a joke, but with an element of truth–: "Don't move out Roberto." They sometimes suggested that if I left home I should go and live with friends, look for a big house with a garden so that I could live with my dogs, because my parents know they make me happy.

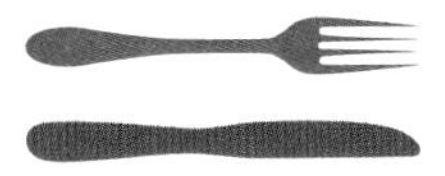

If I was looking for independence, it wasn't because I wasn't comfortable at home, but because I wanted to face new responsibilities in life and deal with them. But the diet made this difficult, as I needed special food which, while it's just healthy food, is a bit more complicated if you're living on your own. I didn't want to take the risk that I'd throw in the towel the moment things got difficult... Staying with my parents seemed like the sensible option. In any case I always had The House of Joy in Matanzas as a refuge, where I could hang out with friends, cook, and enjoy being by the sea.

Drago Gluscevic, with whom I spoke in depth to write this book, also follows a strict diet. Eight years ago, he suffered from Non Hodgkin lymphoma and as part of his recovery (which included chemotherapy) he changed his lifestyle and eating habits. He's convinced that human beings actually need much less food than we consume, and that diet is directly related to health:

"Today I'm healthy, I don't eat meat, but I do eat a lot of fish, fruits and vegetables. I've cut out sugar, although not completely. I love sweets, but if I used to eat five cakes, I now only have one, and not a complete one. This turned out to be one of the most difficult things for me." ■

Guillermo Acuña also provided many ideas during the conversations we had, and which are in the main part of this book. He had melanoma in one eye and considers that the most important fight is not against death, but in changing the way you eat:

"Melanoma is directly related to the skin and liver, because these are the places it is usually located and grows. So it was really clear that the way one eats has a connection with melanoma. Shortly after I was diagnosed with melanoma, I met Iván Mimica who showed me a world full of possibilities to recover my health through diet. And as I like cooking, it was fun." ■

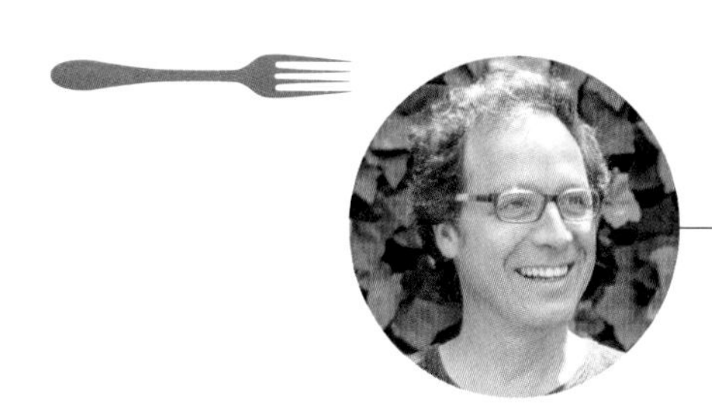

Iván is one of the best kept secrets in Santiago. He is a sociologist from the Catholic University and has doctoral studies in Harvard on cognitive sciences and artificial intelligence, but has been dedicated to studying holistic medicine and natural diets. He knows a lot about food toxicity, botanical drugs and the relation between emotions and health. Iván is a walking encyclopedia, always attending seminars and reading. *And I say he is a well-kept secret because he does not work as a doctor, but he is a generous man who shares his knowledge with people who are lucky enough to meet him, like me.*

Mimica, who is 73 and does not look it, started down this path in response to a particular situation.

In 1990 he lived in Boston and was CEO of a company of artificial intelligence applied to voice recognition. Suddenly, and without any warning signs, he started feeling sick, losing energy, although medical tests all came up clear. So he decided to start studying on his own and arrived at the conclusion he was intoxicated: "I thought it was arsenic, because I'm from Northern Chile, and everybody there is exposed to pollution. However, when studying the symptoms, I realized I was closer to mercury poisoning", he said. He had his hair and urine examined in Switzerland and was told, with the results in hand, that they did not understand how he was still alive. Then he chose natural medicine and homeopathy to slowly detoxify. He started a diet based on a great variety of vegetables, fishes, lentils, beans, algae (sulfur-rich food)... and no sugar.

IVÁN MIMICA SUPPORTS INTEGRATIVE MEDICINE, WHICH COMPLEMENTS ALLOPATHIC MEDICINE WITH NATURAL ORIGIN MEDICINE.

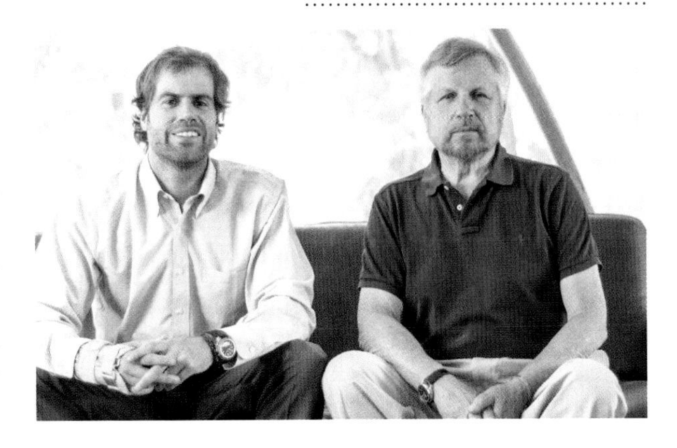

His mercury intoxication originated in his dental amalgam, which used to be 80% mercury. He recalled having his dental amalgams changed all at the same time and probably having inhaled mercury vapor in the process. It took him seven or eight years to get clean. Over this time he decided to study how the human body works. Iván attended seminars delivered by natural medicine specialists worldwide, such as Hanna Kroeger, who studies the cause of diseases derived from parasites, bacteria, viruses and fungi, and is the author of nearly twenty books.

Iván Mimica also researched the relation between supplements of vitamins and minerals, and studied areas related to allopathic drugs and their secondary effects. He reviewed in depth the principles established by the Japanese Doctor Hiromi Shinya, on the power of enzymes present in the body. In his book, *The Enzyme Factor* (volumes 1 and 2), Shinya suggests a diet to recover health which includes lots of interesting suggestions, such as eating 85-90% foods of plant origin and 10-15% of animal origin. He says –unprocessed– grains should be 50% of a diet, fruits and vegetables 35-40% and food of animal origin 10-15% (fish, chicken, turkey, duck, and eggs). He suggests avoiding milk and derivatives, eradicating margarine and chewing each bite between 40 to 70 times, as well as eating in small quantities.

Mimica also valued the ideas of Néstor Palmetti, a specialist in diet and natural nutrition (**ESPACIODEPURATIVO.COM.AR**) and creator of the purification process based on being aware of the hygienic and physiological needs of the body. In his center located in Córdoba, Argentina, one can learn about intestinal hygiene, hepatic cleansing, internal fluids depuration, treatments again internal parasites, rest of the digestive system, internal oxygenation, and how to change eating habits.

Mimica also focused on research carried out by neuropsychiatrist David Servan-Schreiber, cancer specialist and author of *Anticancer: A New Way of Life and The Instinct to Heal: Curing Depression, Anxiety and Stress without Drugs and Without Talk Therapy.* In both books, the French scientist states that the key to XXI century medicine is the bond between mind and body.

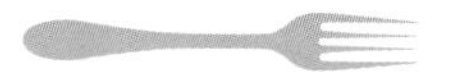

Then, Iván Mimica became a supporter of integrative medicine, which complements allopathic medicine with natural origin medicine. He considers that one needs to identify the cause of the disease first, then study the person, their story, genes, and family history, until reaching the emotional component of the disease. The book *The Healing Code,* written by Doctors Alex Loyd and Ben Johnson, expanded his point of view. In order to make the most accurate diagnosis, Mimica believes it is fundamental to determine if the person has been exposed to any toxicity levels through bacteria, fungi, parasites, viruses, or heavy metals. He knows, based on his experience, that these may contaminate our body and make us sick.

In 2011 I travelled to Boston for check-ups with all the information provided by Mincolla during the two times we met, and after profound conversations with Iván Mimica, *I can say my diet has helped me be healthy. As time went by, I noticed some transformations I would like to point out. For instance, my weight. I am 1.87 m [6.1 ft., approx.] high, and used to weigh 94 kilos [a little over 207 lb.]; now, my weight varies between 83 to 85 kilos [183 to 187 lb.]* Impressively, I lost those 10 kilos [22 lb.] in little over 2 months since I started my diet, and never gained that weight again. I did not lose more weight, either. Now my body temperature is always below 36° Celsius [96.8 Fahrenheit]. I stopped sweating like I used to. My back is free from the pimples I always had. My body is more... how can I put it?... at ease. The same physical exertion resulted in a lower pulse rate. I love this feeling.

"I stopped eating meat and drinking milk and almost completely eliminated sugar. In the mornings, my breakfast consists of 2 loafs of organic gluten and lactose free bread, topped with half an avocado each, non GMO organic turkey breast, some basil leafs and Himalayan pink salt. Also I prepare my own Chia Pudding with organic coconut milk mixed with half a cup of blue berries and cinnamon. Finally with my wife we prepare our own secret alkaline "solution" blending: a bunch of spinach, some ginger, the juice of one lemon, a couple of celery sticks, 1/8 of avocado, cucumber and water. We call it "the solution", because we not only have it as part of our breakfast but it is also a great shield against colds, canker sores, fatigue, headaches, sore throats and of course cancer."

On Mondays, Tuesdays and Wednesdays I measure my urine's pH and get an average. I need to keep it between 6.4 and 6.8. If my pH is under those values, my body is acid and I need to eat more alkaline foods. I take chlorophyll extract three times a day by dissolving a spoon in a glass of water every time. I buy the extract in Nature's Sunshine, Chile (**SUNSHINEANDINA.CL**). And Mark Mincolla suggests adding 1/4 of a spoon of sodium bicarbonate every night before bed.

In the mornings we also take a supplement called Delphinol, a powerfull extract of *Maqui*. This is a wild berry growing in the south of Chile that, according to research carried out by Universidad Austral de Chile, sponsored by the company producing Delphinol, stimulates the immune system. Furthermore, it has anti-inflammatory properties and all signs show that it is very effective in controlling blood sugar levels. It has more antioxidants that any other berry, including blueberries (**DELPHINOL.COM**).

To complement my diet, I went to **NUTRICIONINTELIGENTE.CL** and they told me to take Pau D'arco capsules, which are sold at Nature's Sunshine and prevent bacterial, fungal and viral diseases. And at the very beginning I also drank gold water –Colloidal gold– that fights infections. This was suggested by Mark Mincolla, but it is not sold in Chile: it is water containing gold particles; ancient kings and their courts, who drank in gold cups, were discovered to be healthier than other people. Mincolla said those microscopic gold particles helped to activate the immune system. I now drink ionized water, almost three liters per day. As soon as I get up, I drink two cups, just before breakfast. *This gives me energy, helps me to not feel sleepy, tired or fatigued.* It helps to reboot the operation of the organism that has been working during the night to drain the toxins that are then eliminated in the first pee in the morning.

Iván suggested I read *The Miraculous Properties of Ionized Water: The Definitive Guide to the World's Healthiest Substance*, written by Bob McCauley. Reading it I realized the incredible benefits of ionized water, which counteracts the effects of acid food in the body, among other things. So I bought an ionizer machine that can make water more alkaline, it's not cheap, but makes me feel good. The machine is sold at the **SHITIVEGOTCANCER.COM** site.

There are no strong scientific studies that prove the benefits of this "alkaline water", but I have personally seen that it fills me with energy, particularly, those two glasses of water I drink every morning while fasting, when I wake up. I start my day in a different way.

Another important aspect is that I now eat with the least amount of condiments and salt possible, trying to use sea salt. I no longer eat corn, as it ferments during digestion and contains a lot of sugar. I don't drink beer because yeast inflames my organism, but I do eat bread, although not much (it should be none). I used to eat only brown rice, but I now mix it with white rice (against Iván's recommendation to eat only brown). If I did not cut myself some slack, I would not resist this lifestyle that has benefitted me a lot.

It has really been worth it, I feel much better and my diarrhea has disappeared. This diet has helped me heal, feel better, and protect my body against future dangers. And the good news is that anyone can change the way they eat. You don't need to wait until your body sends an alarm. You can start right now!

8 *golden rules* for **health**

IVÁN MIMICA HAS SUMMARIZED HIS KNOWLEDGE IN EIGHT RULES, THAT MAY BE USEFUL FOR SICK OR HEALTHY PEOPLE. HERE THEY ARE; IN ORDER AND SUMMARIZED.

1. EVERY PERSON IS UNIQUE: THERE ISN'T ONLY ONE RULE FOR ALL. Each person has a different background which should be investigated. Their metabolism and physical make-up should be studied. A person whose system metabolizes sugar correctly does not produce high amounts of insulin or go through inflammation processes, *thus needs a very different diet in relation to someone who does not correctly process those sugars.*

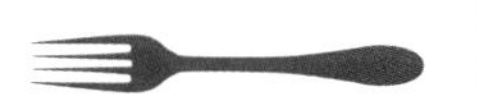

2. SUGAR MAY CAUSE INFLAMMATORY PROCESSES. At this point one needs to really pay attention, as we eat "disguised" sugar all the time: pasta, white rice, white flour. When talking about sugar, it is important to reduce foods composed mainly of carbohydrates particularly, those rich in starch. The fructose some foods naturally have may also be harmful to your health, although not all organisms react in the same way to sugar. Some metabolize it better than others.

3. HUMANS NEED TO HAVE A MAINLY ALKALINE DIET. Acidity may cause the death of a person and a body with low alkaline volume will try to get resources to be more alkaline from sources such as bones –from where it gets calcium, potassium or magnesium–. In books *Alkalize or die*, written by Dr. Theodore Baroody, and *The Reverse Aging*, written by Dr. Sang Wang, there is information for those who are interested in this topic. An especially **ALKALINE DIET** (70% alkaline and 30% acid) must include low glycemic index food, focused on fruits and vegetables, which should be complemented with fish, almonds, nuts, beans, lentils and chickpeas. Potatoes, rice, pasta, meat, milk and all proteins are acid.

4. MILK, IN GENERAL, IS DANGEROUS FOR YOUR HEALTH. As with all its derivatives, milk may cause the human being different allergies and internal inflammation, which make the immune system weaker, paving the way for various diseases. According to Hiromi Shinya, milk is a dead food that has been heated at high temperatures to kill bacteria. This process also kills the enzyme we need to digest it adequately. In his books, *The Enzyme Factor* (Volume 1, Aguilar 2008; volume 2, Aguilar 2014) and *The Rejuvenation Enzyme* (Aguilar, 2010), Shinya assures *that by enzymes and if we exhaust them, we will not have enough to repair cells and, therefore, in time we could develop some diseases.* **WHAT ABOUT BREAST MILK?** It is healthy and necessary during a stage in life, but adults do not need to eat dairy, not even as a source of calcium because calcium in milk is lost due to the phosphorus found in processed milk. It is much better to get calcium from vegetables, such as broccoli.

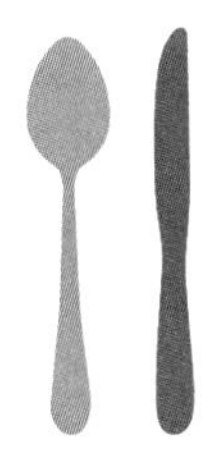

5. THE WAY WE DEAL WITH STRESS, EMOTIONS AND THOUGHTS IS IMPORTANT. When a person is under stress or has negative thoughts, their organism reacts with a dangerous rise in cortisol levels which lead to inflammation. According to Mark Mincolla in his disclosure articles, is one of the various functions of cortisol, regulating inflammation of the body is one, by providing instructions to the immune system to reduce or increase its work. During periods of stress, cortisol levels rise to increase the availability of "emergency" energy. Chronic stress reduces sensitivity of tissues to cortisol due to permanent exposure, and this affects the body's capacity to react when facing an infection. For instance, this takes place where inflammation plays the key role of transporting more white blood cells to damaged areas to improve immune defenses. The books *Biology of Transformation*, written by Dr. Bruce H. Lipton and Steve Bhaerman (Esfera, 2010), *The Healing Codes* by Jerry Graham, *Secrets of Your Cells* by Sondra Barrett and *Breaking the Habit of Being Yourself* by Joe Dispenza (Urano, 2012) include a lot of information on the topic.

6. Be aware of how toxic the food you eat is. Many foods have contain heavy metals and parasites. You should prefer fruits and vegetables from your own garden, one you know or an organic one. You may find more information on *Cure for all Diseases* by Dr. Huida Regehr Clark, and *The Parasite Menace* by Dr. Skye Weintraub.

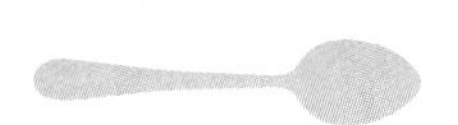

7. The importance of oils. Human beings need a healthy balance of fatty oils to survive. There are three types of these oils: omega 3, omega 6 and omega 9; the state of our health greatly depends on their correct combination. The healthier ones are omega 3, which can be found in blue fish, such as tuna, horse mackerel, sardines, bonefish, sole fish, anchovy, codfish, herring and salmon. All of these have more than 5 grams of fat for every 100 grams of edible meat (5%), compared to white fish that have a lower percentage. It can also be found in lobster, shrimp, crab, squid and octopus, egg yolk, rabbit meat, chia seeds, Brussel sprouts, pineapple, nuts, almonds, chickpeas, spinach, strawberries, lettuce, cucumber, parsley, cauliflower, soy, purslane and pumpkin. **Ideal balanced consumption of these oils:** three portions of omega 3 for every one of omega 6. Currently, it is common to have 12 portions of omega 6 for every one of omega 3, a combination that swells up the organism. In *Healthy Fats for Life*, Dr. Lorna Vanderhaeghe, and in *Fats that Heal, Fats That Kill*, by Dr. Udo Erasmus, one may study in depth the importance of the combination of oils we consume.

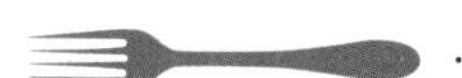

8. What and when is important. Raw foods have more active enzymes than cooked foods. Enzymes as well as nutrients found in fresh and raw foods are very sensitive to heat and may die at temperatures above 30°C. This is why frying food is one of the worst cooking methods.

Also, letting the body digest is important. It is highly recommended to respect a food schedule and for the last meal of the day to be three or four hours before going to bed.

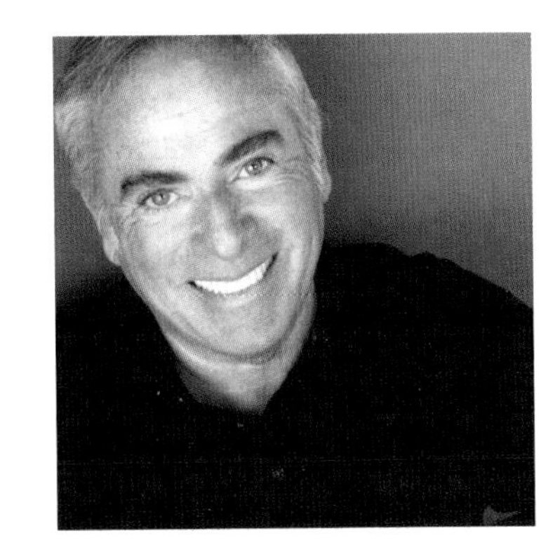

INTERVIEW WITH MARK MINCOLLA

"Mind and body are **inseparable**"

To better understand why I follow such a strict diet this interview Mark Mincolla gave me for the writing of this book, is enlightening. He spoke about his philosophy and the integral nutritional approach he advocates.

–What type of patients do you see?

–A wide variety. I see people that have been sent home to die from some disease, people that choose not to take drugs as a treatment and people that want to mitigate a condition without using certain drugs. I believe a disease is the result of a body expressing itself: symptoms are its language. When there are symptoms it means that the mind and body are not in balance. My aim is to understand where this unbalance takes place and how to approach it. People get stressed because they create stressful patterns of thought and this directly affects the organism. If you don't approach these problems directly, don't address the cause, you are disguising the issue. You are camouflaging.

–So your approach is not specifically to do with nutrition?

–Mind and body are one. There is a widely used expression in the world of natural medicine: *mind the body, or the body minds*. It is more appropriate to see things under this light. Mind and body as one, inseparable. But be careful, mind is not a synonym for brain. The brain is a local organ; the mind is not. The mind speaks to the brain, the brain speaks to the autonomic nervous system and this system speaks to the body. These are the connections and depend on the mental dialogue you have with yourself through the day (check the book *The Biology of Belief*, by Dr. Bruce H. Lipton).

–Do you work with patients who follow traditional medical treatments?

–Yes, this is called dual therapy and the patient has the option of following that path.

–What do you do in those cases?

–I support the patient in the same way, being conscious that there is another specialist working from other disciplines. Sometimes an oncologist asks us to stop using some vitamins or natural supplements because they don't coincide with the philosophy of chemotherapy of denigrating the cell, degrading it until cancer can no longer live in it. On other occasions, I am asked not to use certain vitamins or minerals, depending on the case, and we have to adapt: this is what dual therapy is about.

–How do you treat a person with genetic predisposition to develop his disease?

–We all have some genetic trends and I believe that genetic expressions want to be revealed. When one faces a trauma, strong stress or is exposed to poison or toxicity, negative expressions will tend to manifest.

I usually say that I can teach people habits, but they cannot change their genes.

–Which is the best test to determine the level of our pH?

–Blood tests are not very useful because human blood needs to be between 7.4 and 7.42, and this is a very small variation. Urine tests are much more precise. In the United States there are nitrazine strips which are very precise, calibrated up to .067. They measure tenths, between 5.5 and 8 pH. The correct way to use them is by measuring pH with the first morning urination using the strips. The aim is to keep pH between 6.4 and 6.8.

–What are the less acid foods?

–All green leafs, all vegetables that grow under the sun are alkaline, and fruits as well. On the contrary, sugar, starch, meat and fish are acid. Acids should not be completely removed; the key is to keep the proportion of 4 alkaline foods for each acid one.

–What is your professional opinion on milk?

–Many consider it neutral, but it is not, at least not for the human body because it is converted into a mainly acid food. It is usually considered that calcium is absorbed from dairy; however, there are many environmental estrogens in dairy products. If milk is not organic, it is almost certain that it has growth hormone and this increases the risk of IGF answer ("insulin-like growth factor"). And it has been proven that IGF increases the risk of cancer up to five times.

–Does this extend to all dairy products, such as yoghurt, cheese, etc.?

–Yes. Many of these foods, apart from being dairy products have sugar and are fermented, thus I prescribe patients to stop eating them as the main cause of cancer is sugar fermentation. The next step is eradicating inflammation-causing foods and, finally, conducting an individual test. If a person is intolerant to broccoli, they won't eat broccoli. There are three filters or exams: first fermentation and sugar; second, inflammation-causing foods, and third, individual reactions to foods.

–Which are fermented foods?

–Vinegar, marinades, beer, wine, champagne, soy sauce, miso, teriyaki sauce, peanut butter, foods with fungus –such as mushrooms–, breads with lots of yeast and melons.

–You talk about slowing down the growth of tumors through diet...

–We need to add by subtracting. I have a philosophy: *to solve a problem you cannot lift one layer after another, you need to discover the origin of the unbalance.* Is peanut butter causing your skin problem? Or is your allergy to dairy and eggs the cause? I had a patient in New York who was the most depressed person I'd ever met; she took six different antidepressants. Nothing was wrong with her, except for one thing: she was allergic to wheat. She suffered from reactive allergy which was sensitive around her head so I told her to try and avoid wheat and see what happened. She did this and has already returned to work, does not take drugs and is no longer depressed.

–In your opinion, taking into consideration all your patients, what percentage have illnesses caused by stress, or an underlying environmental or psychological reason?

–Most of them. The mind cannot be separated from the body. It is impossible. If someone is physically unbalanced, their mind is also unbalanced. ■

patient
EMPOWERMENT

Being a patient is hard because the fear is very real. There's constant uncertainty, you can't be sure of anything. That's what happened to me with cancer. The situation itself was very delicate and, at first, I was in shock; things happened and I wasn't able to assimilate them. Conversations with doctors which, at first, I assumed were only directed at Dad when, in fact, what happened was that I was not 'connected' with my melanoma. Facing cancer is like staring at the gates of hell, and with retrospect I can see that I just wasn't able to do that maturely. I threw tantrums, went into denial, and on top of everything I criticized Dad for the way he was handling things when he'd given himself over body and soul to finding solutions. Now, analyzing the trip I made with my family to Boston and Los Angeles, I understand that after writing the *No Tie* email where I told them I wanted to take the lead in my recovery, my family changed, because I started connecting with the emotional and practical aspects of my cancer, leaving aside the concerns which I now see as having been superficial. I guess that the family support I received as we toured from one doctor to the next in the US gave me the necessary confidence to do so.

I discovered that, in the US, doctors establish a very professional relationship with patients. They tell them everything directly, as harsh as it may be. They cover all possibilities and answer all their questions. I am not saying this does not happen in Chile, but in my case, as I was disconnected from my situation, the doctor-patient relation took a while to flow, so to speak. Only after realizing what was going on did I start asking all the questions I had. ***This is key: The first person that needs to understand the disease is the patient, as hard as it may be.***

I am not saying I never asked questions, but but perhaps I did so at the wrong moment, when I was too emotionally vulnerable: Just before my first surgery, for example. My parents and siblings were with me in the room in the hospital, and in the surrealism of the situation, I asked them to go out because I wanted to talk to Doctor Gustavo Vial *in private*. I needed him to in detail explain what was going to happen to me, because I still didn't know much about melanomas. I was not standing on firm ground at all. Despite my being puzzled by all of it, I was able to ask the doctor for that information, even though I was about to be wheeled into the operating room. And, naturally, he settled my concerns. A long time afterwards, and far away from that operating table, during

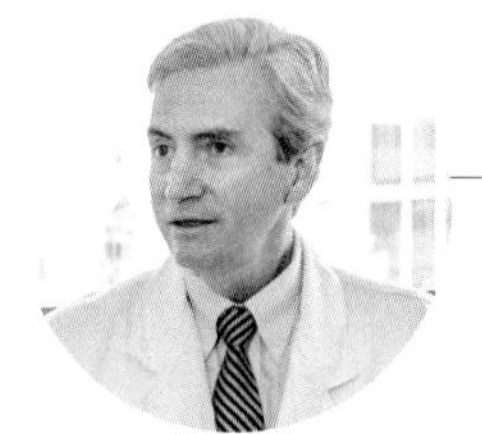

DR. GUSTAVO VIAL

one of our conversations for this book, Doctor **Gustavo Vial,** surgical oncologist of melanoma, sarcoma, head and neck, explained his perspective, which I found very interesting:

"Communicating with patients is never easy. It's hard to convey the whole idea of their illness or disease, with all its consequences. I believe the time we have to do this is never enough. I make an effort to be as precise as possible with the information I deliver and, of course, I never hide medical history. And, above all, I need to make sure the person understands the importance of their condition. Whether the patient decides to attend my office –or chooses another specialist– will depend entirely on the patient, but I need to make sure I provide all the necessary information for that person to make their decisions." ■

As Dad says, while the doctor has the duty to inform patients about the treatments and interventions he will perform, in order for the patient to analyze their situation with the doctor, it is his/her obligation to be interested, to learn about the disease. Until there are no further doubts. And patients must repeat questions as often as they feel like it, without being intimidated. I did what I could; I hope others have their doubts answered as soon as possible, as basic or strange as they may seem. ***"Study, analyze and talk, because listening makes you powerful. You need to be a good patient",*** Dad told me, thinking about the experience he went through trying to understand my cancer. He wasn't the one who was sick, but knowing him I can imagine that he'd much rather have been in my place...

One of the reasons for writing this book was to make patients (and to a certain extent their doctors) aware of how they need to empower themselves when they face this illness. Patients can and must be proactive and have a voice. It is a hugely important topic to discuss. Yes, patients can be afraid and therefore eager to blindly follow through the instructions they receive from the doctors, but it is vital to learn about and assess the potential, scope and consequences of treatments suggested, without shame. ***It is your duty to be informed and your right to demand an explanation on what you don't understand, and to be presented with all possibilities, with their positive and adverse effects.*** And also, for doctors to share with you the incidence of the disease and chances of survival. I decided to write this chapter after living a progressive empowerment process. One I feel like sharing. Everybody should know that, as a patient, you need to be as active and powerful as possible.

"Nobody sees what they don't know, this is a basic principle", said Doctor Bruno Nervi, oncologist from *Universidad Católica,*

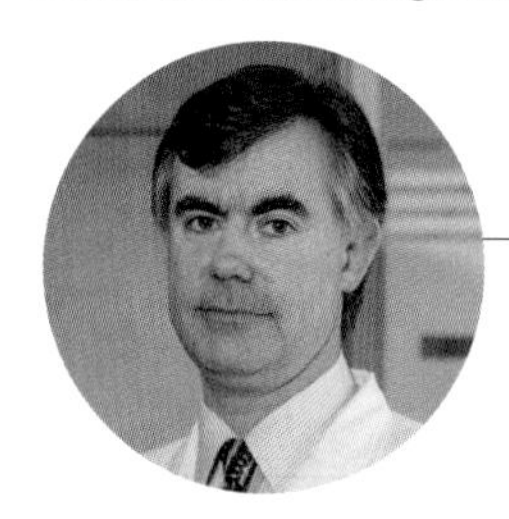

DR. BRUNO NERVI

when I interviewed him for this book. Doctor Nervi was one of the specialists my father consulted while he was doing his research and collecting information for his database. There's no question that having doubts about what one is going through increases anxiety, leads to possible misunderstandings and mistakes, and potentially wrong decisions taken about possible treatments. A patient also has the right (legally, as I will detail in the chapter *Questions on Cancer*) to ask for second and third medical opinions.

"If you don't acknowledge the disease, you don't acknowledge the problem. Then, you cannot solve the problem or be focused, you cannot be helped and we cannot help each other." ■

Doctor **Benjamín Paz** named this the *blindness of the disease:*

I went through that. I didn't know what a melanoma was and, therefore, didn't see the risk of the mole I had and which I found ugly but never deadly. You start seeing cancer once it has been diagnosed and it breaks into your life and stays there forever. You may think you can hide it, but it is there, sneaking up behind the door. If you don't know your disease, it's difficult to see it, and even more complicated to accept it. Doctor Paz is absolutely right.

In order to really see the cancer you've been diagnosed with, and which has left you in shock, it is crucial for the doctor to answer each and every one of your questions. And for the doc to support you when the struggle is uphill. Everyone needs to know where they stand and what their possibilities are. Doctor Nervi and Doctor Vial are convinced that, except if a person has a condition that hinders them from accepting information, or if the patient is a child, patients need to know exactly what their situation is. What statistics say about their disease, what the possible treatments are. Inversely, it is very important for doctors to know their patients. This is what Doctor **Bruno Nervi** thinks:

"We, oncologists, have to show perspectives to patients, what can happen. I like listening to patients and getting to know them, to see what their tools are; if their family supports them, if they have spiritual or economic support to face their future. It is key for me and the patient to determine where we stand from the very beginning." ■

Also, Doctor Vial explained he is more at ease with patients that act autonomously to make decisions regarding their health: ***"I need them to fully know what undergoing or stopping a treatment might mean. The consequences. The potential complications. And to be clear on the results. For instance, patients need to understand that if they don't treat their cancer aggressively, there is a chance the tumor may reappear, and they can face death. The more complete the idea a patient has of this disease, the better the decisions that person will be able to make. And this, for me as an oncologist, is also better."***

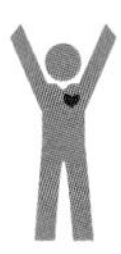

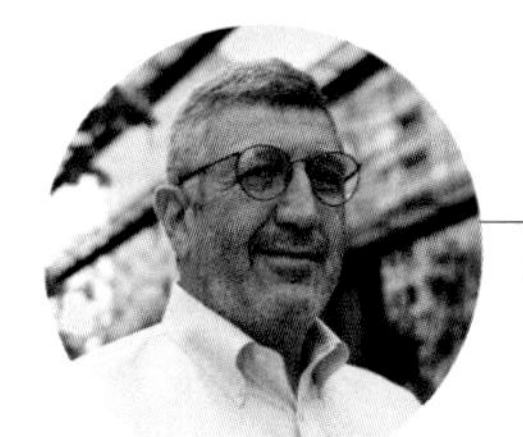

Dr. Benjamín Paz

It is also key to learn to find one's position within the cancer context, which is a new and difficult one. One of disease and weakness. In this sense, Doctor **Benjamín Paz** is convinced the specialist may help achieve this delicate situation:

"There are different ways in which one can lose autonomy, and this disease is only one of them. Our work is to help patients understand what it means to be vulnerable, and to show them they have always been vulnerable. I teach cancer patients to deal with the risk in a way that does not paralyze them. To go on with their lives." ■

I like the point of view proposed by Doctor Paz. Both Doctor Nervi and Doctor Vial believe the art of being an oncologist consists of informing patients, making them understand what they are going through, clarifying what their options are, and whether the treatment will cure or palliate. And most important: to respect their decisions. ***"Patients must completely understand what will happen if they choose one treatment or another, and what if they do nothing," Nervi says. "I show them what the most adequate treatment for their cancer offers and, also, how long they could live without doing anything."***

Here, I would like to make clear that, although doctors intend to share all the information patients need, sometimes circumstances make this impossible. I imagine they see so many cancer patients that the information ends up feeling repetitive. This is why I insist on being very proactive. Just in case your doctor is not. As Doctor Vial puts it, oncologists should not be feared, they should be seen as partners.

Once all medical history has been delivered to patients, they must make a decision within a reasonable time span. Most specialists mention this. Doctor Vial considers that patients cannot take a year to decide on one treatment or another. Nor can they wait months until they decide to undergo a prescribed surgery. If certain deadlines are not met, a diagnosis may worsen and projections regarding the initial situation may change, he explains. I underwent surgery really fast, only six days after I was diagnosed, while I still didn't completely understand why I was on that operating table or the possible consequences. If I had waited, I could have been under serious risk because, in the case of melanomas, from the time of the biopsy to the definite treatment there is quite a limited time frame during which prognosis remains the same. Doctor Vial told me that time is a month, as when one manipulates an injury, some growth factors may activate. My biopsy was from over three weeks earlier. The clock was ticking.

With other cancers, it may be good to wait for one or two weeks for the patient to internalize what's going on. And that doesn't endanger the patient's health, provided that doctor agrees, of course. Doctor **Mercedes López,** immunologist from *Universidad de Chile* confirmed this. She was the one who gave me the autoimmune vaccine, the only treatment I followed, apart from changing my diet and lifestyle. ***She told me that "Except for a medical emergency, you may always wait a little to clear your head. You could just do what your doctor tells you to do but it's better if you understand it, knowing you have the right to fully comprehend what you will be subjected to, and what may happen afterwards, such as secondary effects."***

Therefore, my advice is to ask EVERYTHING before surgery. Before the growing storm and uncertainty surround you. Take your time, be informed, and ask before taking the next step. Yes, wait, although obviously not too much, and always with your oncologist's knowing support.

In connection to everything that surrounds Patient Empowerment I had a profound conversation with **Amaro Gómez-Pablos.** His first wife died of colon cancer, and he was beside her from the moment she was diagnosed until she died. He dealt with lots of specialists, had experienced when information is not forthcoming, and found out doctors also have an unsuspected human side. Amaro said it is crucial for a treating physician to really know his patient: "I am a journalist who is always careful to find out the name and surname, and possibly also familiar circumstances of a person who is describing a dramatic situation, and I am not even interfering with their body. Therefore, from the beginning of the whole process, I find this vital."

His wife lived for five years with cancer. After that experience Amaro assures me that in his opinion oncology must be approached by a team of medical professionals: "I am interested in the exchange of opinions between professionals. I don't care about the momentary star of the clinic. The first question a patient must ask is not what doctor will treat him, but what medical team will give him the complete picture of his disease. Then, patients must demand not to be considered a liability at the hospital. Therefore, interpersonal relation with doctors is key. Finally, ***it is the patient's right to know all information right away. Doctors don't have to ration out information, please! They are not in charge of psychological therapies, which will be considered later. Patients have the right to be provided with all the information."***

I agree with Amaro here. I believe patients need to click with a whole medical team, not only with the oncologist.

On the doctor-patient relation, **Drago Gluscevic,** who suffered from non-Hodgkin lymphoma, had a good experience. He started on the wrong foot, because he didn't click with his first doctor, and was clever enough not to wait long before looking for a second opinion and,

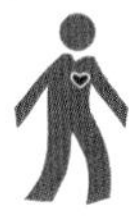

above all, establishing a relationship that suited him better: "It was really important for me to feel I was in good hands. And that meant dealing with a doctor who looked me in the eye when talking to me, who told me everything and did not engage in small talk that had nothing to do with cancer. I didn't make a mistake: my doctor –former doctor now– and I are friends. ***I always trusted him because I knew he made decisions with me, not on his own. He empowered me, gave me the tools I needed to have my own opinions."***

Medical records may, often, change decisions one might make as a patient. At first, when my family –and above all I– were blindly searching for a path to follow, I almost joined the Ipilimumab clinical trial, a clinical trial to test the drug, one of the treatments for melanoma. This drug has very strong secondary effects, one of them being the deterioration of the digestive system. I was willing to take part in one of the clinical trials in the U.S. until I told doctors in Los Angeles that I had had intermittent diarrhea for 3 years. I just happened to tell them, without giving it any importance and just as part of my clinical history. But when the doctors heard this they rejected my request to participate in the trial as one of the most common side effects of Ipilmumab is bad diarrhea. In fact, there are records showing some cancer patients have died from diarrhea and not from cancer.

I guess what I'm trying to explain here is that a patient with a different medical record could have participated in the trial, but I couldn't. Also, Ipilimumab is suggested for patients in cancer stage IV, and I was in stage III A. This shows how important it is to understand material that can look completely indecipherable before making a decision.

According to Doctor **Bruno Nervi,** an oncologist must, apart from making a good diagnosis and determining the exams that will enable choosing the most effective treatment, accompany patients at all times:

"One of the most painful things that can happen when you have cancer is not being able to choose your treating physician in the public system. It is really hard to be diagnosed by a specialist with whom you start establishing a very close relationship, due to the circumstances, and then being sent to see someone else. I assure my patients I will be by their side during the whole process, even though they are assigned other doctors. I like speaking to the doctor that will receive the patient and share with them our plan for the patient to live this transition in the best possible way." ■

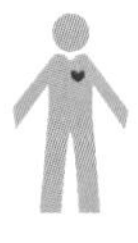

Doctor **Mercedes López** coincides:

"If you are an oncologist, you need to go along with your patient from the very beginning until the very end. You cannot leave them halfway through. You cannot allow other doctors that don't know them to be in charge of their process, because sometimes more medical procedures are undertaken than is necessary, and the patient and their family suffer without there being need for it." ■

Doctor **Elisa Herrera,** based on her experience as an oncologist in the public health system, states that every patient can understand a diagnosis: "The challenge a doctor faces is communicating it with the right words, taking into account that not everybody understands at the same pace. Some understand immediately; others, on the contrary, need a second interview." She suggests for patients to always go with someone to the doctor's office, as it is not the same receiving the news that you have cancer alone than with a relative that supports and embraces, hugs and cries with you. "In any case the medical specialist should be the first to give support when a diagnosis is given." She builds special relationships with her patients:

"I stay connected with the patient forever. If the patient wants to, they can call me 3 years after having been discharged, just to tell me they've got some new pain and are worried. Although the patient has healed, that person will always live with the idea and anguish that cancer may return. We oncologists need to be with our patients forever." ■

Doctor **Mercedes López** has seen lots of patients with serious conditions, some at a terminal stage, and she says that, above all, patients are grateful when they are given an honest and undramatic evaluation of the situation, when they are made aware of options and assured that they will be part of any decisions taken. The truth she mentions opened my eyes and made my world turn upside down: She was the first doctor to bluntly tell me that melanoma is the most aggressive cancer and that had I not seen that mole in time, I would have died. ***In this sense, the source of information chosen by the patient to answer their questions is very important. I remember what Doctor Vial told me about not looking for answers on the internet because most of what I read would make me assume and fear the worst-case scenario. Or it would just confuse me.*** And although I didn't do it, many may believe that surfing the web in search of answers is a great alternative. It's not. In my opinion the best path is to ask for many different opinions, to ask every imaginable question, and then to compare the answers. In the event you feel relieved by looking for information on

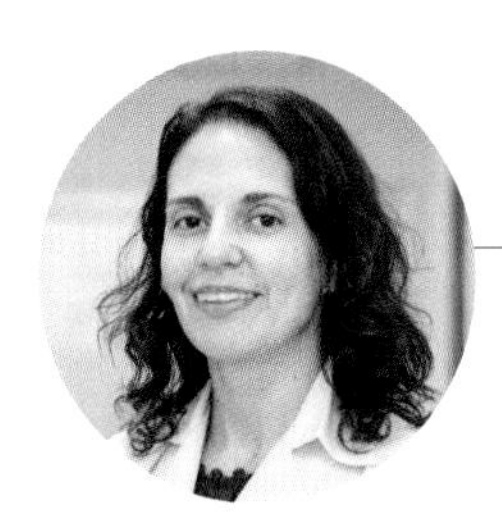

DRA. ELISA HERRERA

your own, it is better to ask doctors to mention reliable sources. As Doctor Vial said about this: "Patients can be scared by what they read on the web, because for a person without medical experience it's hard to filter and appraise information. But I do find it interesting for patients to arrive with questions based on the doubts they have after searching the web."

Doctor **Benjamín Paz** thinks that choosing that source of information is one of the most dangerous aspects of cancer. He calls this search the *new car syndrome* and describes it as follows: When you want to buy a car you ask others for opinions and, almost guaranteed, someone will tell you they just bought a spectacular car. And above all, they will contact you with their salesman, who will call you and try to sell you the same model. With cancer the risk is that the treatment that works for one person may not be the best for someone else:

> "We tend to validate our decisions based on what the rest of the world does. The source of information provides a social context, but it is not a source that enables taking a decision. The fact you know somebody else with cancer will allow you to understand the social context, but will not help you make a decision." ■

Doctor **Bruno Nervi** explains that one of the most important elements of the oncologist-patient relationship has to do with the assessment and proposal of the best treatment:

> "Treating a patient who suffers from a disease that cannot be cured and who can only receive palliative cure is very different to treating a patient that has a good chance of recovery. In the latter case, one can choose an aggressive treatment, despite its toxicity, as a good prognosis and the possibility of survival support that choice. If there is no treatment, I choose accompanying the patient in the process of their palliate cure, I don't suggest treatments that have a dead end." ■

Doctor Nervi says it's very important to make the toxicity of treatments known. Although most of the time results are optimal, there is always a chance things go wrong and the patient needs to know this.

And what if the patient refuses treatment as they intend to live their last days on their own terms? Doctor Paz believes nobody decides to die

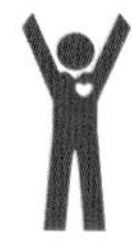

just for the sake of dying. But when a patient considers the circumstances, it's their choice whether to undergo a treatment or not. Facing this situation, he explains to the patient how long life can be prolonged with the treatment, and what the time frame is without any intervention.

Decisions as important as this one need to include the effect of the disease in the patient's environment. The impact the situation causes on their daily lives and, above all, the way others look at them. Cancer is almost never visible, others only see the effects of treatment, such as hair loss or extreme thinness, but they don't see the disease. In fact, when I say I had cancer people tend to believe I am lying, because they cannot tell. When the melanoma was first removed, I was left with scars from the surgery, but they were under my clothes and went unnoticed.

For Doctor Nervi the oncologist must accompany patients in their process when the stigma of being sick arises. In relation to this difficult issue, Doctor **Benjamín Paz** calls everyone to be very alert because there is a risk of a patient feeling isolated and cut off from their old world -the world of healthy people- either because they fear that they won't live long, or because they feel that their professional and social possibilities are reduced:

"The first thing I make my patients aware of is that when they go out of my office they will have already survived cancer, and I remind them of the importance of living, not surviving. I tell them that cancer is a moment or an accident, but in no way a punishment. It is an experience that needs to be used to change, to grow, to make decisions. Each day I focus on making my patients return to their daily lives, to their everyday routines and the stigma of cancer. And I do so by telling them: ***Tomorrow you will continue working.***" ■

One needs to be alert to avoid making a person with cancer feel sick. I was sick and worked, practiced kite, travelled and was in a relationship, because I didn't want to live as a patient. I acknowledge the endless support I received from my companions at work. Pepe Masihy, my partner, especially made this possible. Every time we faced stressful situations, he gave me space so that I wouldn't get stressed, to help me take care of my mind and body. In fact, keeping stress as low as possible was one of the suggestions made by doctors and this was and is well-known by the people who surround me.

In the end, the truth is that you will settle again into life and will continue doing the same, or similar, activities you used to do before, which is good, but you need to take an important fact into account: at some point, and without a specific reason, you will remember you have or had cancer. Doctor Paz explained this to me when I went to Los Angeles. He talked to me about cancer days and cancer moments, the days that the cancer peaks out from where you'd hidden it –because you have to see a doctor, or you catch a glimpse of your scar or someone mentions the word cancer– and suddenly you feel sick and scared. He told me I had to learn to deal with these cancer moments because they were now part of who I was. One needs to learn how to transmit this to family, friends, workmates, and even nurses and doctors you visit ***so that they know you don't take it personally and that the problem is not with them, but with yourself. They are part of the process you have to lead.***

Doctor Paz believes it is important to teach his patients how to live this experience in a good way, so that they can change negative into positive aspects.

Doctor Bruno Nervi, on his side, is convinced that an oncologist must be involved in another relevant process of any patient who has been given a complicated diagnosis: not leaving things pending. Doctors must help patients complete their grief and share information with them to help them deal with what they are living together with their families:

"The most painful deaths are the ones in which the person hadn't enough time to give closure to things. I had a patient who died. She was 40 and had a 9-year old daughter, and she didn't want the girl to know what happened. She was strict with this and the husband didn't want to intervene. The woman did well for several years, but from one moment to another she suffered from a complication and it all escalated. She thought she would recover as she had before, but she suddenly lost consciousness and could no longer talk to her daughter and explain what was going on. Neither could she say goodbye. The daughter learned her mother had cancer and that she was going to die when her mother could no longer speak with her." ■

According to **Amaro Gómez-Pablos,** apart from this, an oncologist must be delicate, close, alert and careful. In summary: sensitive. Ask how they're dealing with pain, smile and embrace. "When everybody already knows therapies are insufficient, oncologists must examine the quality of the palliative attention their patients will receive, confirm whether it is the best place to have it and establish a connection with doctors.

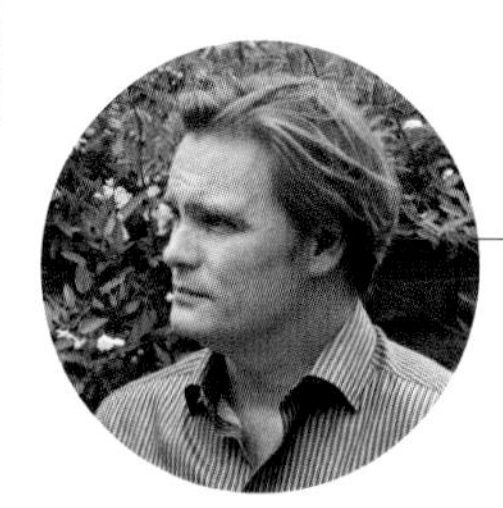
Amaro Gómez-Pablos

CONSTANZA LARRAÍN

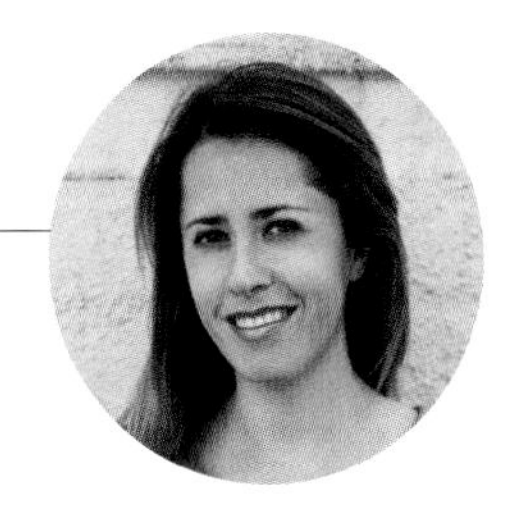

It would be unimaginable for a patient to be starting palliative care -so with the possibility of a near death very much on the horizon- and be unable to contact their doctor. A few days ago that same doctor was trying to save the patient's life. A few phone calls, the answers to some questions... It doesn't take much of the doctor's time, and if we don't do it out of sensitivity then at least out of politeness".

Within the scope followed by oncologists, there is not always space to complement chemotherapies, radiotherapies or other treatments with natural alternative medicine. This struck me, as I believe that it isn't useful to disqualify alternatives. Of course it is best to follow the advice of the treating physician, but sometimes doctors are unwilling to accept alternative therapies out of fear that they compromise the more orthodox treatments they themselves have prescribed. The only person who gave me a correct diagnosis on my constant diarrhea was Mark Mincolla, a natural therapist I visited in the United States (see chapter You Are What You Eat), although I had gone to prestigious doctors and clinics in Santiago. I believe it is best to research and collect information, and have a good discussion with your doctor on the subject. It is in this topics where Patient Empowerment becomes more difficult to attain because two opposite points of view can conflict. But I believe they can be complementary. I followed a natural treatment to recover after melanoma, by eating consciously and changing my lifestyle, and I used none of the drugs doctors in the United States offered me – with some resistance– as possible ways to get better. This decision ***also helped me face situations, such as telling a Medical PhD, with absolute conviction, that I would not get injected with the drug he was suggesting for me because I knew its diverse secondary effects and I was not willing to go through that. I made a bet to change my life.***

Coni Larraín clearly knows what I am talking about. We shared many conversations about this after her dad, the magician Fernando Larraín, was diagnosed with prostate cancer: "Dad took very strong medicine, he was even given morphine for pain, and taking so many drugs wore him down, he could barely walk and this demoralized him, discouraged him, his only thought was how much time he would have to use his wheelchair. Some drugs made him hallucinate and see aliens or think he was at a hotel and not recognize his house. At one point he mistook my mom for his nurse. As time went by everything got worst. Then, and although doctors found it useless, my mom and I suggested that he should follow some natural treatment or holistic medicine to counteract the effects of traditional drugs. We went to a very well-known iridologist in *Viña del Mar*, to a therapist who practiced reiki on him, to a shaman in *La Florida* –lots and lots of people were waiting for him–, and he had magnets applied. At first, Dad did not agree, especially because he didn't want to defend his decision in front of his doctors, but I was beside him through all this and he went from being sceptical to convinced, because he started feeling better."

During the long road I started on 27 April 2011, when I was diagnosed with malignant melanoma, as a patient I faced different specialists, natural therapies, holistic doctors, and with all this experience, created a personal list of tips for patients.

12 things a **patient** should do:

1. Get a clear and informed diagnosis.
2. Decide, if possible, who will be your **treating physician.**
3. *Ask to be **addressed directly,** in an honest and open way.*
4. **Know** the treatment **options** for your disease, the chances of success, secondary effects, and how much this will cost. And whether they will cure or palliate.
5. *Know the details of the disease: **what it is, how it works, what happens to those who suffer from it.***
6. Ask all the **questions** you need to and get **answers** for each one.
7. *Get for second, third and even fourth **opinions.***
8. **Change** doctors if you believe it is more convenient, without providing explanations nor feeling guilty.
9. Assess the possibility of **complementing** your treatment with relevant natural therapies.
10. ***Consider** the option of quitting and doing nothing.*
11. **Inform** your doctor about prior medical conditions, as well as any drugs you're taking.
12. Share your **lifestyle** with your doctor, for them to take this **into consideration.**

Also, I would like to share a relevant issue Doctor Vial brought to my attention, and it is that when I underwent surgery, Chilean Law 20,584, which sets forth people's rights and duties in connection to actions connected to health care, did not exist and was passed in April 2012, a year after my melanoma was discovered. This law is a summary of what I have been writing in this chapter: "Every person has the right to accept or deny being submitted to any procedure or treatment related to their health care, with the limits set forth under article 16. *This right must be exercised freely, voluntarily, expressly and in an informed manner and, therefore, the attending professional must provide the correct, sufficient and comprehensible information, in accordance to what is expressed under article 10.* Rejecting treatments will in no way aim at artificially accelerating death, the practice of euthanasia or providing assistance for suicide. As a general rule, this process will be carried out orally, but it should be stated in writing in the event of surgical procedures, diagnoses and invasive therapies and, in general, to follow procedures which carry a relevant and known risk for the health of the patient. *In these cases, the information and its provision, the acceptance or rejection, must be stated in writing in the patient's medical record and make reference, at least, to the content established in the first item of article 10.* The person is assumed to have received the relevant information to provide their consent when their signature is placed in the document that explains the procedure or treatment they needs to undergo." This is the same law that guarantees patient's access to a second professional opinion, as it is mentioned in the chapter *Questions on cancer*. The law is worth looking at and reading to be completely informed about current rights. ■

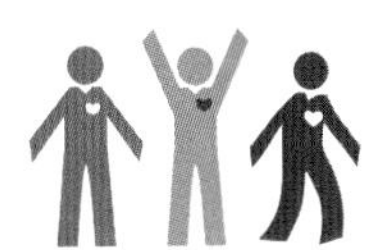

100 frequently ASKED QUESTIONS ABOUT CANCER

(WITH THE SIMPLEST, FOOLPROOF, ANSWERS)

* The information collected in the following pages has been obtained from Chilean website www.canceronline.cl, edited by biologist Flavio Salazar, current Vice President of Investigation at the University of Chile, Doctor Diego Reyes, urologist at the Clinical Hospital of Universidad de Chile and the National Cancer Institute.

I. *General* information

1. What is cancer?

It is a disease produced by the uncontrolled proliferation of abnormal cells, with the capacity of invading and destroying other tissues of the body. This causes a tumor, that may harm nearby tissues due to pressure or spread to other body parts. This is called metastasis. When this happens, the tumor is malignant and is diagnosed as cancer.

2. What is metastasis?

Metastasis takes place when cancerous cells can multiply in other organs. The immune system has mechanisms to stop and destroy them, but when they survive, they multiply and organs are harmed. Blood irrigation is key at this point, because cancerous cells are transported in blood or in the lymphatic system. Therefore, organs that receive more blood have more chances to have metastasis, such as the lungs and the liver, have a greater chance of having metastases.

3. Is melanoma, or any other cancer metastasis, a new cancer?

No. A melanoma metastasis in a lung, for instance, is caused in cells from skin melanoma that moved using the bloodstream or lymphatic system towards the lung. This is why it is called melanoma metastasis that has adhered to the lung, and not lung cancer.

4. Does displacement of malignant cells always imply a metastasis?

Technically, no. Displacement of malignant cells towards other body parts does not always mean metastases will develop. These malignant cells would have to adhere to tissue in the host organ and would then also have to have a supply of blood and nutrients in order to survive and multiply. If this does not take place, there will be no tumor from the same cancer.

5. What causes cancer?

The body is formed by millions of cells that, when grouped, form organs and tissues. These cells are constantly multiplying to replace those that are weak or die, so that organs can continue working: the cell doubles it components and then is divided into two equal parts, with the same structure and function. The body has control mechanisms that detect and correct mistakes that can take place during duplication to make sure the new cells are identical to the original one. When a mistake cannot be repaired, ***the defective cell is self-destroyed and the immune system rejects from the organism.*** However, if these control mechanisms fail, the abnormal cell is kept and its replicas continue multiplying in the body. This proliferation of defective cellular tissue is called tumor.

6. Are these tumors always malignant?
Not always. There are benign and malignant tumors. In both cases, the cells that compose them multiply uncontrollably, but those from a malignant tumor are capable of invading other body tissues, and this is called cancer.

7. So, benign tumors are not life-threatening?
Benign tumors cannot develop metastasis, but they can imply risk of death if they compress nearby vital organs as they increase their size. This is especially important in benign brain tumors, where the skull does not enable the movement of tissues and the risk of compression is higher.

8. How does cancer start?
Although the diverse types of cells in the organism have different functions, their internal structure is very similar. They all include a center, the nucleus, which holds DNA, the molecule containing all genes with all the information that controls cell functions. Genes determine what their function is, when they have to divide and when to die and be replaced. *The process through which normal cells are transformed into cancerous cells is called carcinogenesis, and it can last for years.* The first phase starts when agents external to the organism act on a cell and damage its genetic material. This affects the mechanism of error control and, with each new division, the process becomes more chaotic, until new cells finally lose their specific function and acquire the ability to spread across the organism and infiltrate nearby tissues.

9. How does cancer disseminate?
Defective cells are very different to normal cells: they reproduce quicker, the result of the duplication is not the same as the original one, the specific function disappears and they may lose the capacity to attach to similar cells. This is why cancer spreads in the body: apart from invading and destroying nearby tissues, malignant tumor cells may move towards tissues located far away through the bloodstream or lymphatic system.

10. Is it contagious?
There is no scientific evidence that shows a healthy person may get cancer by directly touching or breathing the same air as somebody that suffers from the disease. Cancerous cells don't survive in another body as they are recognized as alien by the immune system and are destroyed.

11. Does it have symptoms?
Cancer is a group of diseases that may cause almost any type of symptoms, depending on where the cancer is located, the size of the tumor and how it is affecting organs and tissues. If a cancer disseminates ("makes metastases"), symptoms may arise in different parts of the body. However, sometimes cancer develops in places where no symptoms will arise until reaching advanced stages of the disease.

12. How many types of cancer are there?
There are more than 200 types of cancers identified, each one with different symptoms and treatment methods.

13. What are the main types of cancer in existence?

Medicine separates them into carcinomas, sarcomas, leukemias, lymphomas and myelomas, according to the type of tissue where the cancer has developed.

Carcinoma: It is the tumor which is developed in epithelial cells, which cover almost all external and internal surfaces of the body (cavities, hollow organs, body ducts, skin, mucosa and glands). Therefore, it is the most frequent cancer (85% of diagnosed cases). The usual ones are breast, prostate, colon, rectal, lung and skin cancer. Melanoma is a malignant carcinoma and is one of the most invasive cancers because it is easy for it to make metastasis.

Sarcoma: They are tumors formed by muscles, cartilage, bones and adipose tissue (fat). Sarcomas represent 1% of cancer cases in the world.

Leukemia: It is cancer of the cells of the bone marrow, the tissue located inside bones that produces blood cells. It usually manifests itself by uncontrollably increasing the production of white blood cells or leukocyte. If these get into the bloodstream, they can cause imbalance and weaken the organism's defenses. Leukemia is the most common type of childhood cancer.

Lymphoma: They appear in the cells of the immune system and are located in lymphatic nodes, which are part of the circulatory system. There are two categories: Hodgkin lymphoma and non- Hodgkin lymphoma. Both are tumors are characterized by their origins in lymphocytes, a cell from the immune system which turns into a tumoral cell and multiplies. Within tumor cells, Hodgkin lymphoma has a very particular one called Reed-Sternberg, which can be observed in biopsies. Non-Hodgkin lymphoma, a much more frequent type of cancer, includes a large number of different lymphoma which do not show Reed-Sternberg cells.

Myelomas: This is a type of cancer that starts in white blood cells, produced by the bone marrow. It is also called Kahler disease, multiple myeloma, plasma cell myeloma and myelomatosis. It is the second most common blood cancer in the United States, which represents 1% of the total cancer cases. There are no figures in Chile reflecting its incidence. Other body tissues may also cause malignant tumors, such as the brain, but they are rare.

14. How is the level of advance or cancer dissemination classified?

"Staging", using exams and tests, is a process used to indicate the degree of advance of the cancer one the diagnosis has been established.

Generally, cancer is classified in categories that range from I to IV, the first one relating to a localized tumor and the last one to a tumor that has spread to distant organs. Between the tests performed during staging there are computerized tomographies, blood tumor markers, magnetic resonance, PETCT and some typical biopsies, among others.

15. Which are the most aggressive cancers? And the deadliest ones?
Cancer is a worldwide public health problem. According to the World Health Organization, more than 14 million cases of cancer are detected every year. Three-quarters of cancer deaths are registered in countries with low and medium income, such as Chile, where cancer is the second cause of death (20-25%) following cardiovascular diseases. Cancers with the highest mortality rates in the world include, lung, liver, stomach, colon, breast and prostate cancers. The most aggressive ones are melanoma, pancreatic, lung, liver, esophagus, leukemia and breast cancer. In Chile, the main cause of death due to cancer in men and women is stomach cancer.

16. What cancers have methods or exams for early diagnosis?
Depending on the age and gender, it is possible to carry out exams to detect breast, colorectal, cervical, lung, prostate, thyroid, oral cavity, skin, lymphatic node, testicular and ovarian cancers.

17. What is a PET and what a PET CT?
PET (for its acronym in English) means Positron Emission Tomography. It is an exploratory exam of nuclear medicine ***that shows images from the inside the body based on its chemical structure, as opposed to its physical structure, which is shown by radiographies.*** PET is used to detect cancer and assess its response to treatment, using chemical substances called radionuclides, which release small amounts of radiation to the patient's body to identify tumor inflammation. Combined with a computed tomography (CT), PET CT provides detailed information on any increase of cellular activity, which helps locating new tumors. However, it also exposes patients to higher radiation levels.

18. What is a biopsy?
It is a surgical procedure whereby a doctor removes a sample from an organ's tissue to exam it in detail using a microscope.

19. What is a magnetic resonance?
It is an exam that allows to be obtained images based on the movement of the human body's molecules after being submitted to a magnetic field in internal organs without using radiation. It is especially useful to detect and locate certain types of cancer, such as brain tumors. It is also used to track signs of metastasis.

20. What is a medical oncologist?
Medical oncology is the subspecialty of internal medicine that focuses on diagnosis and treatment of neoplastic diseases. It is mainly dedicated to the systemic cancer therapy, the most common of which is chemotherapy.

21. What is a surgical oncologist?
A specialist surgeon who treats cancer with surgeries. They are usually specialized on an organ or specific system.

22. What is an oncology nurse?
Oncology nursing is a specialty related to early diagnosis, multidisciplinary handling and coordination of therapies for cancer patients. Oncology nursing work includes, among others, administrative, promotion and prevention tasks.

23. What is terminal cancer?

Cancer is considered to be at a terminal stage when there are no more cure therapies that may extend the time of survival for a patient. At this stage, the disease evolves naturally towards death and palliative care is crucial.

24. What is survival?

Survival is a term used in oncology to define *a period of time between cancer diagnosis or therapy and its consequent evolution.* For instance, there is general survival, which is the time between diagnosis or treatment and the death of the patient, notwithstanding the cause of death (accident or other disease). In turn, specific cancer survival is referred to the time between diagnosis or treatment and the death of the patient, only in relation to the cancer they develop. Progression-free or sickness-free survival is also usually measured, which relates to the period from the moment the patient underwent treatment and has no evidence of cancer until it reappears.

25. How do doctors estimate survival in a metastatic cancer?

Doctors may provide close information on a cancer patient's survival based on statistical data from clinical trials of a group of patients, and a survival average is estimated under similar conditions.

26. What is palliative care?

Care provided to people who suffer from a disease and have no cure. They It aims, as far as possible, to accompany the patient, and provide comfort and pain relief. Palliative care is not in favor of euthanasia but nor does it endorse the prolonging of life through any and all media that may actually increase suffering. This is about accepting death as inevitable, but taking care of the patient until the last moment, ensuring the best quality of life possible, even taking physical, psychological, social and spiritual needs into account, in relation to the patient as well as their family. The World Health Organization defines it as the active and global care of the patient and their family, provided by a multidisciplinary team when the patient's disease is considered not to be subject to cure therapy.

27. What symptoms are treated in palliative care?

Although pain is the symptom most frequently related to cancer, there are other symptoms that affect patients' quality of life, such as poor appetite, anxiety, weight loss, constipation, nausea, vomiting, and suffocation. Someone with cancer may suffer from around 10 symptoms simultaneously.

28. Do all cancers produce pain?

Pain is the most important symptom for cancer patients and its presence affects people in all areas (physical, spiritual and psychological). Almost 30% of cancer patients feel pain, and this percentage raises to 80% in cases of patients with advanced cancer.

29. **How can one handle pain?**
Oncological pain is, generally, treated according to the Analgesic Ladder established by the World Health Organization. This scale divides pain into mild, moderate and severe, and suggests drugs to be used. For instance, for mild pain non-opioid anti-inflammatories and analgesics such as paracetamol or metamizole (dipyrone) are suggested; for moderate pain mild opioids are used, such as tramadol or codeine; and for severe pain strong opioids, such as morphine, fentanyl or methadone are used.

30. **What are the alternatives besides analgesics?**
Besides analgesics, contributing drugs may be used to relieve pain, as they improve the efficacy of analgesics. The use of physical and kinetic therapies is also important, and in some selected cases, surgery and radiotherapy may contribute to handling painful injuries.

II. *Therapies*

Chemotherapy

31. **What is chemotherapy?**
Chemotherapy is the main therapy used by modern medicine in tumors that have spread, this is that have metastasized. The word literally means therapy with drugs. It is a systemic cancer therapy, which means it has an effect on the whole body, and not only on specific areas. It is based in the use of certain drugs whose aim is to kill tumor cells.

32. **What types of chemotherapy exist?**
Chemotherapy may be used to cure some specific tumors, as well as to stop or control the growth of an advanced tumor that cannot be completely eliminated, in order to extend a patient's survival time, reduce the size of a tumor before conducting local therapy (such as surgery or radiotherapy), or reduce the risk of cancer recurrence. Finally, chemotherapy can also be used in palliative care to improve patients' quality of life, reducing symptoms.

33. **What does chemotherapy contain? Why is it so aggressive?**
Due to it being a systemic therapy distributed in the entire body, chemotherapy drugs also damage cells from healthy tissue, mainly those with quick cell multiplication. This causes undesirable secondary effects, such as partial or total hair loss, poor appetite, nausea and insomnia. Some secondary effects can be reduced with the use of drugs.

34. **How does chemotherapy work in the body?**
Drugs used act on all body cells so that malignant cells are not able to survive and then die. Due to quick multiplication, tumor cells have greater chances of being affected by drugs than normal cells. An important characteristic of tumor cells is their high resistance to environmental adverse conditions; therefore, many chemotherapy treatments combine different drugs to avoid this resistance.

35. How is chemotherapy administered?

In general, chemotherapies are administered in cycles: *There is an intensive period of treatment, followed by a recovery period so that the body gets prepared to tolerate the next one.* Treatment schema may include one or more cycles, depending on the drugs used, the type of cancer, its degree of advancement and the obtained results. The way drugs are administered depends on each drug and their possible combination. Some may be taken as pills, orally, although most of the time they are administered intravenously. In some cases, chemotherapy cycles are provided on an outpatient basis: the patient goes to the oncology center where they receive treatment for some hours and then goes back home. Other cases need strict medical supervision, thus the patient needs to stay hospitalized.

36. Why does chemotherapy have secondary effects? Why does it cause hair loss? Can this be avoided?

When they are healthy, some body tissues such as the skin, mucosa covering the digestive tract, hair follicle (hair root) and bone marrow work based on a quick cell replacement. These tissues are the ones chemotherapy drugs affect the most, which explain their secondary effects. This cannot be avoided, although each person has a specific tolerance to the toxicity of the therapy.

37. How will I feel with chemotherapy?

Fatigue is unavoidable during or after each chemotherapy cycle, because it is an intensive therapy which consumes great amounts of body energy. Poor appetite is also frequent, thus it is very important for patients to eat many times a day so that their bodies don't become even weaker due to the lack of nutrients. Secondary effects on bone marrow affect the production of blood cells and platelets in blood, which also leads to generalized weakness. On the other hand, bowel transit is usually affected by uneasiness, such as constipation and diarrhea, patients feel nausea or vomit, and they sometimes temporarily lose their sense of taste. However, the appearance of these effects depends on each patient and varies according to different drug schemas.
When one is going to undergo chemotherapy, it is advisable to consult the oncologist which are the possible symptoms related to the treatment.

38. Do chemotherapies have determined protocols or do they depend on the oncologist's experience?

Protocols of use *aim at maximizing the elimination of cancerous cells and minimizing negative effects on healthy cells. Advances in the development of successful chemotherapies have allowed be related to many types of cancer to specific and efficient protocols.* However, much remains to be done and the oncologist's experience continues to be an important factor in the choice of protocol.

39. Is there a limited amount of cycles of chemotherapy which a patient may undergo?
There are no absolute certainties. The duration, frequency and number of chemotherapy cycles will depend on factors, such as the type of cancer, its extension, administered drugs, toxicity levels and the necessary time to recover from each cycle, as well as the patient's general condition. A weak patient may not be able to deal with toxicity derived from chemotherapy and thus not be administered this type of therapy.

40. Will chemotherapy make me infertile? Should I freeze sperms or eggs before undergoing one?
This may be advisable. In some young patients, chemotherapy drugs may affect fertility in both men and women, so this is an important issue to take into account before starting a treatment.

Radiotherapy

41. What is radiotherapy?
It is a method to treat cancer that uses radiation to destroy cancerous cells, blocking their capacity to multiply. It destroys all tumor cells without compromising, at first, healthy surrounding tissue. It is a therapy used in most patients who have been diagnosed with some types of cancer (more than 50% receive radiotherapy at some point) and it can be used as the only therapy or applied combined with surgery and/or chemotherapy, in a specific order, depending on the diagnosis.

42. Is radiotherapy stronger or weaker than chemotherapy?
The most important difference between them is that ***radiotherapy is a local treatment, while chemotherapy is systemic. Radiotherapy only affects the area where it is applied,*** while chemotherapy, as with any other drug, reaches all of the organism's corners. Therefore, there is a wide range of adverse effects of chemotherapy, and these vary from patient to patient, according to the administered drug and the treatment stage the patient is in.

43. How does radiotherapy work?
It consists of irradiating cancerous cells to eliminate them from the organism. The necessary doses depends on the tumor's volume and its location, as some tumors are very sensitive and others are more resistant to radiotherapy. It is important to determine a dose that eliminates the tumor without transgressing the critical tolerance threshold of nearby healthy tissue. Therefore, prior simulations are performed to confine the area that will be irradiated. Diagnosis and the stage of the disease will determine how the treatment will be carried out: Usually, it is provided on an outpatient basis, as sessions are short and secondary effects relatively minor.

44. What are those secondary effects?
Although, at first, they do not affect healthy tissue, sometimes they do have secondary effects. Skin may be pigmented or remain sensitive and hair may be lost in the radiated area. Radiotherapy may also reduce blood cell replacement and so patients may suffer from anemia and, less frequently, from a reduction of cells of the immune system. Usually, these are mild effects and disappear once the treatment ends.

45. How will I feel with radiotherapy?
Apart from secondary effects, whose occurrence or intensity depend on the type of tumor and where it is placed, the majority of patients feel tired and weaker due to treatment.

46. Is there a maximum of radiation sessions a patient can be submitted to?
The administered doses includes a security margin which is lower than what tissues and organs of the treated area are able to support. The radiation remains absorbed by the organism for many years. This is the reason why, in most cases, radiotherapy can be applied only once to the same body area, notwithstanding a different area may be irradiated, in case of metastasis. Radiotherapy doses are measured in Gray (Gy) and the radiotherapist indicates the total dosage and its daily amount, which determines the treatment's duration. The usual treatment protocol is 10 Gy per week divided into 5 daily sessions of 2 Gy, although the total dosage varies according to diagnosis.

Surgery

47. When do I need to undergo surgery?

Oncological surgery is a fundamental therapeutic resource as 60% of tumors are only healed with surgery.

However, surgical oncology procedures have different objectives: identifying the disease (biopsy), determining the grade of tumor advance (exploratory surgery), removing the tumor (resection) or improving symptoms in a patient (palliative surgery).

48. Can all tumors be operated on?
Although some types of cancer are statistically more common to operate, each tumor has its own specific conditions which determine their resection options. But medicine advances quickly and many cancer patients with tumors which where once considered not treatable through surgery, today have available technologies that may achieve what was considered impossible a few years ago.

49. If a tumor is removed, can it reappear?
The reappearance of a removed tumor is called recurrence and may be produced by the proliferation of residual tumor cells, because they were not completely removed by the therapy. Recurrence may happen in the organ where the tumor first developed or in an area of previously treated metastasis.

50. Can I wait before operating the tumor or must it be removed immediately?
The answer to this question is provided by the type of tumor. If it is a benign tumor, it has no capacity to spread and multiply on other organs, which offers a broader waiting margin. If it is a malignant tumor, the quick proliferation of cancerous cells and the possibility of a metastasis make the idea of undergoing surgery soon advisable.

51. Can a benign tumor turn into a malignant tumor if it is not removed?
Some cancers start as a benign disease or tumor which during their development acquire a "pre-malignant" condition and end up becoming cancer. However, most cancers start and show as a malignant tumor.

Bone Marrow Transplant

52. When is a bone marrow transplant necessary?
Bone marrow is the soft fatty tissue inside bones and includes stem cells which give origin to three types of blood cells: Leucocytes (white blood cells), erythrocytes (red blood cells) and platelets. A bone marrow transplant restores marrow that is not correctly working or which has been damaged.

53. Why are marrow transplants carried out to treat cancer?
In certain types of cancer such as leukemia, lymphoma and multiple myeloma, the bone marrow transplant is performed to restore stem cells destroyed during the use of radiotherapy or chemotherapy. The aim is to normalize the production of blood cells, mainly of white blood cells, in order to restitute the immune system and contribute to the destruction of remaining cancerous cells in the recipient organism.

54. Where is bone marrow obtained for a transplant?
In order to use bone marrow in a transplant it is usually aspirated from the iliac bone, which is part of the pelvis and offers ideal conditions because it is a spongy and flat bone.

55. Why do patients that undergo marrow transplants need to be isolated?
In the first six weeks after the transplant, while the new bone marrow starts producing new white blood cells normally, *the patients is susceptible to infections which would not represent any risk for a healthy organism.* This explains why recently transplanted persons are isolated.

56. When can autotransplantation be carried out? When is a donor necessary?
Autotransplantation consists of extracting stem cells from the patient's bone marrow before they undergo treatment for cancer which may destroy them. Stem cells are collected from the patient's own bone marrow or blood, and are then frozen. This is more effective in relation to rejection possibilities or risk of infection, but less effective as to achieving the desired effect against cancer. Transplants received from compatible donors, almost always a patient's brother or sister, have the advantage that the donor's stem cells tend to be more effective in supporting the elimination of the remaining cancerous cells after the treatment provided with high doses of radiotherapy or chemotherapy. *This is the most frequent type of transplant in cancer cases, although some risks of rejection or infection are higher than in cases of autotransplantation, mainly when the donor has no consanguineous relationship with the receptor.*

57. Who is compatible as a donor?
A donor's compatibility is shown by the similarity between tissues from their bone marrow and that of the receptor. Many factors influence the way the recipient organism will react to the transplant, but the most important one is related to the compatibility between the correspondent human leukocyte antigens, proteins that can be found in the surface of almost all cells of tissues. These antigens distinguishes own substances from alien ones in our organisms and start alerts that activate the immune system to defend ourselves against infections. For two people to be compatible, antigens in bone marrow must be identical or have certain coincidences, which are previously detected with a blood test.

58. What are the risks in a marrow transplant?
The main risk in this type of procedure is the same as in any other transplant: organic rejection due to unforeseen incompatibility. This takes place when the body rejects new stem cells and they do not engraft in the bone marrow nor multiply as they should. An important risk is the spread of eventual infections during engraftment. Other possible complications may be the effects of necessary drugs after transplant, damage to other

organs that have no cancer, abnormal lymphatic tissue growth, hormonal changes, infertility and cataracts. The extent of these risks is always related to each patient's particular conditions.

59. What cancers admit transplants as treatment?
Transplants are mainly used for certain types of leukemias, lymphomas and multiple myelomas.

Other treatments

60. What is interferon therapy?
Interferons are some proteins produced by cells, mainly by those of the immune system. Their main function is acting against viral infections, but there is evidence they also have an antitumoral role. Also, some types of interferons can activate immune system cells to boost their function. In a melanoma, interferon alfa showed, besides its antitumoral activity, the capacity to stimulate NK cells and T-lymphocytes to kill tumor cells. Interferon alfa-2beta (IFNa- 2b) was used as treatment for patients with advanced malignant melanoma. It was one of the first to achieve improvements in survival. However, high toxicity at the beginning of the therapy and the appearance of new treatments have lead to it not being used as standard treatment.

61. What is radioactive iodine treatment?
Radiopharmaceuticals are drugs that include radioactive elements. They are intravenously injected and accumulate in some specific tissues from where they produce radiation that eliminates cancerous cells. Radioactive iodine is also considered a radiopharmaceutical, although it is not concentrated in bony areas, but in tissue from thyroid nodules. It is used to treat thyroid cancer when it has spread.

62. What is immunotherapy?
Controlled manipulation of the immune system is the principle of immunotherapy. It is a systemic cancer therapy based on active molecules named immunomodulators that are injected to stimulate said system for it to act with more or less specificity on cancerous cells. It sometimes uses synthetic versions of certain proteins from the immune system to eliminate cancerous cells. There are many types of immunotherapies, depending on the type of molecule used, thus the variety of names used: Biological therapy, biotherapy or biological response modifier therapy.

63. What is hormonal therapy?
Hormones in the body may contribute to the progression of some cancers, such as breast and endometrial cancers (uterus inner layer) in women, or prostate cancer in men. This is why one of the available treatments to stop the disease consists of avoiding specific hormones that stimulate the multiplication of cancerous cells. Reduction of hormone levels can be achieved with procedures that range from the provision of drugs that inhibit hormone release to surgical removal of the organs that produce them. Another method consists of blocking hormone action in cancerous cells. All these options have some secondary effects.

64. What is the current role of supplementary and holistic medicine?
There are a great number of products, practices and treatments suggested to help relieve symptoms and improve quality of life during treatments against cancer. Modern medicine calls them "supplementary" treatments as they are used in parallel to conventional medical attention. Other times, when methods claim to prevent, diagnose or treat cancer, medicine calls them "alternative" because they tend to replace conventional medical attention. Many hospitals have already adopted them, some of which are as simple as a change in diet and lifestyle (exercise, sleeping hours, avoiding stress).

III. *Relationship with* treating the physician

65. How do I choose my oncologist? What do I need to pay attention to?
Most testimonials collected during the creation of this book highlight the importance of establishing the most honest and close relationship with the oncologist, as the chemistry or human factor may also be very important for treating a cancer. Unfortunately, Chilean health coverage (AUGE/GES) usually do not allow choosing a treating physician.

66. Can I choose another oncologist at any time?
It is paramount for all cancer patients to feel safe with their medical teams, which includes the human capacity to understand and answer the large number of questions and doubts the patient and their family may have. If the event a patient dos not feel comfortable they are completely free to choose an alternative that best fits their requirements.

67. What should I ask my doctor?
There is no suggested specific questionnaire, it is important to ask everything you think is pertinent to understand the situation better, including the prognosis.

68. After having a first diagnosis, can I legally search for a second, and even third opinion before starting a treatment?
Second opinions are set forth under the Chilean Health Guarantee General Regime included in the Chilean AUGE Act No. 19966 and they are a RIGHT (not an obligation) patients have since February 2013, understanding patients as those subscribed under the National Health Trust (*Fonasa* for its acronym in Spanish). This guarantee can also be used when the diagnosis has not been provided by a doctor from the public system: "This right will also be enjoyed by beneficiaries who have been diagnosed with a health problem by a professional who is not part of the Providers Network, in the event this diagnosis has not been confirmed by the relevant Network professional." Thus, the law establishes that both *Fonasa* and private health insurance companies in Chile (*Isapre* for its acronym in Spanish) must contemplate a mechanism for patients to exercise this right.

69. What do other institutions say about second medical opinions after a cancer diagnosis?
It is considered usual for patients to ask for a second opinion after a diagnosis, as this can allay doubts, answer questions, and empower the patient as they face treatment options for their illness. The American Cancer Society provides suggestions on their website (**CANCER.ORG**) on how to face this change of course, as many patients may be afraid or feel ashamed to let their treating physicians know about this concern. It can be read on their website that "You may discover you want to talk to another specialist to review your exam results and who will maybe give you a different

point of view." To this end, and for patients' peace of mind, it is highlighted that most doctors are used to this type of request. In fact, there are some insurance companies -also in Chile- that demand a second opinion to approve a treatment. It is very important for patients to have their original medical records at hand before consulting a new doctor.
Mayo Clinic, an excellent and not-for-profit US organization which provides medical assistance to patients worldwide, has the same idea: "Cancer can be complicated to diagnose and manage. Getting a second opinion helps you feel more confident about your diagnosis and treatment plan," is what they state on their website (**MAYOCLINIC.ORG**). A person may be motivated to look for a second opinion for various reasons,

but whatever these may be, getting a second opinion may clarify ideas on new treatment options. Sometimes it is the treating physician who can suggest where to access a second opinion. However, in the event this does not take place, the patient is recommended to contact State entities or well-known centers –such as the National Cancer Institute (**CANCER.GOV**)– to look for orientation. They are also advized to talk to their insurance company to verify coverage in the event of attending a new treating physician.

70. What can be expected from a second opinion?

The Breast Cancer Organization mentions, on their bilingual website (**BREASTCANCER.ORG)**, what can go on during this process: "A second opinion may confirm your original doctor's diagnosis and treatment plan, provide more details about the type and stage of breast cancer, raise additional treatment options you hadn't considered, or recommend a different course of action." This organization believes that a good doctor will not feel offended for such a request, but –on the contrary– will offer their help to find another specialist that will provide an opinion on the case. And warns: "If your doctor gets angry or defensive, stand your ground -and if he or she continues to react in this way, it may be a sign that you're better off finding a new doctor anyway."

71. Do all cancer patients receive the same treatment?

No. Clinical protocols consist of designing, after all supplementary tests have been carried out, a planned treatment that adjusts to the type of cancer, the stage of the disease, the age of the patient and all variables the oncologist, their patient and network consider relevant.
It is increasingly more frequent for cases to be discussed by an oncology committee, where different specialists get together (medical oncologists, radiation oncologists and surgeons) to jointly agree the best treatment for each patient.

72. If I am diagnosed with cancer, can I choose not to receive any medical treatment?

All oncological treatments, whether medical or surgical, require authorization by the patient, by signing a document named Informed Consent. Some people have no doubts, about undergoing all medical procedures available, while others don't feel comfortable with options offered by modern medicine and give up that type of treatment for supplementary therapies or palliative care. Other factors involved on the decision of not following a medical treatment are the fear of secondary effects, the lack of economic resources, doubts as to the real benefit compared to expectations and, even, religious beliefs. Patients have the right to choose, notwithstanding being able to later reconsider their decision.

73. Should I start a treatment as soon as I get a diagnosis or can I wait?
It is usually recommended for patients to promptly act and plan the commencement of their medical treatment with the oncologist as soon as possible. In most cases, two or three weeks is a reasonable time. However, sometimes the type of tumor and the stage of the disease offer a wider margin to take decisions.

74. What do statistics refer to exactly?
Incidence and mortality are basic terms to understand cancer's impact on the population's health. Incidence is the number of new cases of a specific pathology in a year. Mortality refers to the number of deaths caused by a pathology in a year. Both terms are expressed in number of cases over a total universe ("for every 100 thousand inhabitants"), which make comparisons easier, for example, between two countries.

75. Can I also use other therapies?
Supplementary or alternative therapies are increasingly being suggested by oncological medicine to treat secondary effects and offer palliative care during cancer treatments. The list of options is almost infinite and very dynamic, as each patient may react in a different way to a specific type of supplementary therapy.

IV. *Recovery*

76. Does one get better after cancer? When am I free from cancer?
Completely recovering from cancer means a treatment achieved eradicating all symptoms and signs of cancer and that the tumor will not reappear. "Remission" means that symptoms and signs of cancer in a person have partially or totally reduced. ***If a patient is under complete remission for five or more years, they may be considered cured. However, being well does not guarantee that the person is safe from developing the same or other type of cancer in the future.***
The body may host cancerous cells for years, even for decades, without them being detected. These cells may cause a recurrence (or "relapse"), although in most cancers this happens during the five years following the initial diagnosis. Less frequently there is also late recurrence, thus almost no doctor states a patient has definitely recovered. Possibility of recurrence, which of course statistically varies according to the type of cancer and the specific case of each patient, make doctors keep controlling their patients for years, looking for signs of recurrence or late adverse effects caused by received treatments. Very rarely will a doctor give a definite discharge.

77. Do diets have an effect on cancer?
The bond between diet and cancer is complex and not easy to determine with certainty, mainly because our diet includes very varied products. However, scientifically-validated researches have determined a relation between the type of food we eat and cancer development.
In 1984, the U.S. National Cancer Institute determined that 35% of malignant tumors are

originated or related to food factors, making a comparison to the risk of cancer produced by tobacco. Therefore, experts include diet as one of the most important risk factors within the group of environmental factors that can be prevented. A change in diet is estimated to reduce global cancer incidence between 30 and 40%, which equals between 3 and 4 million cases in the world.

78. What are antioxidants? How do they work?

The term "antioxidant" is generally used to name a group of natural substances that are part of the diet and whose action may offset the effect of reactive oxygen species (ROS), byproducts formed during cell metabolism whose accumulation may cause cell damage that lead to the development of various diseases, such as cancer. Antioxidants include vitamins A, C and E, and other substances such as polyphenols (resveratrol and flavonoids, found, for example, in cacao in the form of dark chocolate, green tea or red wine), carotenoids (such as lycopene and beta-Carotene, found in fruits, vegetables and yellow, red or orange cereals), glutathione and melanin (see chapter You Are What You Eat page 170). In laboratory tests these substances have shown antioxidant, antiproliferative, antitumoral and antiangiogenic properties –they block the formation of new blood vessels–, and their presence in diets has been related with a reduced possibility of developing certain types of cancer.

79. Does sleep help recovery?

Yes. Research has increasingly related sleep patterns with the proper function of the immune system. Cells in our organism regenerate faster when we sleep than during the day.

80. If I healed from cancer, may I have the disease again?

As already stated, a recurrence is always possible, even a late one, or also the development of another type of cancer. This is why it is so important to change habits during the development of the disease and keep them even when cancer has been medically eradicated from the organism. Cancer carries a very important transformation in a person's life: healthy habits adopted during treatment must be followed during one's entire life.

81. What symptoms should I be alert for to avoid cancer recurrence?

Follow-up is very important after a cancer treatment -more than tracking signs and symbols- which includes the periodic suggested check-up carried out by the treating physician.

82. What is the most important research carried out the world in relation to cancer?

The most important research conducted in the world about cancer aims to identify its cause and to develop prevention, diagnosis, treatment and recovery strategies. It encompasses epidemiology (distribution in a population) and biomolecular structure of cancer, to compared effectiveness of clinical trials performed in different countries around the world. From the nineties onwards, the most advanced research has been focused mainly towards the development of therapies based on progress in nanotechnology.

V. *Psychological* process

This group of questions was answered by psycho-oncologist Jennifer Middleton.

83. How can a psychologist help during the process of cancer?

Psycho-oncology provides support to cancer patients during treatments and surgery. It accompanies the patient and his family, and provides help during anguish and depressive states that usually appear with the disease, without necessarily working with preceding processes. In our line of work, which I call proactive psycho-oncology, we also help patients actively in their recovery process, with the premise that the disease may be the result of a person's self-abuse. This tends to be confused with guilt, but it is never the case: It is simply about assuming responsibility. If I used to smoke two boxes of cigars every day and I have lung cancer, first I need to understand why I did so and how can I be a healthier person now, despite cancer, and maybe reverse the disease. We approach all areas of life. We ask cancer patients to change their diets, to meditate and, hopefully, practice yoga and physical exercise; also, to make a deep revision of their relation with stress and their lifestyle. We aim at achieving persons to participate in their recovery and, also, help prevent the disease's recurrence by leading a healthy lifestyle.

84. Does one cause its own cancer?

We are responsible for our health, but it is difficult to exactly define such responsibility because when cancer arises many uncontrollable factors are involved, such as, the unnoticed exposure to heavy metals, environmental contamination, or hereditary genetic factors. Multiple factors form part of cancer, but people may become part of their own recovery with certain factors that may be decisive, such as lifestyle and vital priorities.

85. Is it convenient to treat the whole family?

Each member of a family will have an influence on the recovery -or not- of a patient. ***This is the reason why it is very important for the family to understand this process and to be willing to tolerate some changes, which are not always pleasant. Having a cancer patient in the family is not only critical for the person suffering it, but also for the family.*** Roles are changed, there are economic, social and working consequences. In this context, it is important for the family to express and make their sadness, rage and inquiries known in a therapeutic space, and to get psychological support or orientation. Taking care of a person with cancer is a very long and demanding process, this is why the invitation is extended to the family to take care and enjoy some free time, share the care of the patient, ask for help and get distracted.

86. Does introspection make sense for people facing this process when they are searching for the origins of their disease?

From my point of view, patients need to change their vital priorities and find themselves at deeper levels. This process is basically about being in connection with one's emotions and expressing them, assuming the responsibility of the disease and one's health, learning to love life again, committing to living each day and having a good time. It is about using one's intelligence in relation to emotions and their biology. Also, about stopping to think "what is happening to me? Why am I so tense? Why am I scared?" and assessing the alternatives to face the threat in a different way. Many issues come across and some patients find something more useful than others. But I am sure that by making use of all of these, cancer can be reversed. However, much work needs to be done every day during the entire day.

VI. *Incidence* in the U.S.

Source: *The American Cancer Society

87. In 2016, an estimated 1,685,210 new cases of cancer were diagnosed in the United States and 595,690 people will die from the disease.

The most common cancers in 2016 are projected to be breast cancer, lung and bronchus cancer, prostate cancer, colon and rectum cancer, bladder cancer, melanoma of the skin, non-Hodgkin lymphoma, thyroid cancer, kidney and renal pelvis cancer, leukemia, endometrial cancer, and pancreatic cancer.

88. The number of new cases of cancer (cancer incidence) is 454.8 per 100,000 men and women per year (based on 2008-2012 cases).

The number of cancer deaths (cancer mortality) is 171.2 per 100,000 men and women per year (based on 2008-2012 deaths).

89. Cancer mortality is higher among men than women (207.9 per 100,000 men and 145.4 per 100,000 women). It is highest in African American men (261.5 per 100,000) and lowest in Asian/Pacific Islander women (91.2 per 100,000). (Based on 2008-2012 deaths.)

90. The number of people living beyond a cancer diagnosis reached nearly 14.5 million in 2014 and is expected to rise to almost 19 million by 2024.

Approximately 39.6 percent of men and women will be diagnosed with cancer at some point during their lifetimes (based on 2010-2012 data).

In 2014, an estimated 15,780 children and adolescents ages 0 to 19 were diagnosed with cancer and 1,960 died of the disease.

91. Incidence Worldwide

- Cancer is among the leading causes of death worldwide. In 2012, there were 14 million new cases and 8.2 million cancer-related deaths worldwide.

- The number of new cancer cases will rise to 22 million within the next two decades.

- More than 60 percent of the world's new cancer cases occur in Africa, Asia, and Central and South America; 70 percent of the world's cancer deaths also occur in these regions.

The World Health Organization's website has more information about cancer statistics across the world– **WWW.WHO.INT**

VII. *Financial* support

Source: *cancercare.org

The Cancer Financial Assistance Coalition (CFAC)– The Cancer Financial Assistance Coalition (CFAC) is a group of financial assistance organizations, including CancerCare, that have joined forces to help cancer patients experience better health and well-being by limiting financial challenges. The coalition's website, www.cancerfac.org, includes a searchable database of local and national organizations that provide financial assistance to people with cancer and their families. The site allows you to search for resources by diagnosis or by the type of financial assistance you need.

Nonprofit Programs For Co-Pay Relief

A number of nonprofit organizations provide help for expenses such as drug co-payments, deductibles, and other medical costs. these programs have their own eligibility rules and may cover only certain cancers. contact each organization to learn more.

- **92.** CancerCare Co-Payment Assistance Foundation
866-55-COPAY
www.cancercarecopay.org

- **93.** Good Days
877-968-7233
www.mygooddays.org

- **94.** HealthWell Foundation
800-675-8416
www.healthwellfoundation.org

- **95.** The Leukemia & Lymphoma Society's Co-Pay Assistance Program
877-557-2672
www.lls.org/copay

- **96.** National Organization for Rare Disorders
800-999-6673 (Voice mail only)
203-744-0100
www.rarediseases.org

- **97.** Patient Access Network Foundation
866-316-7263
www.panfoundation.org

- **98.** Patient Advocate Foundation Co-Pay Relief Program
866-512-3861
www.copays.org

- **99.** Patient Services Incorporated
800-366-7741
www.patientservicesinc.org

National Collegiate Cancer Foundation

The National Collegiate Cancer Foundation's mission is to provide services and support to young adults who have been diagnosed with cancer. Our goal is to help these survivors and their families establish a "Will Win" attitude in their fight.
NCCF is committed to providing need-based financial support to young adult survivors who are pursuing higher education throughout their treatment and beyond. Furthermore, the Foundation promotes awareness and prevention of cancer within the young adult community.NCCF is one of the only national organizations to provide direct financial assistance to young adults with cancer.

VIII. *Community* support *Fighter* resources

Outdoor adventure

• **Send It Foundation:** Senditfoundation.org
The mission of the Send It Foundation is to inspire positivity, courage and gratitude in young adult cancer fighters through the gift of outdoor adventure and community.

• **First Descents: FIRSTDESCENTS.ORG**
First Descents provides life-changing outdoor adventures for adults 18-36 impacted by cancer through free surfing, kayaking and climbing programs and regional adventure communities nationwide.

• **Outdoor Mindset: OUTDOORMINDSET.ORG**
Outdoor Mindset unites and empowers people affected by neurological challenges through a common passion for the outdoors

• **Live By Living: LIVEBYLIVING.ORG**
Live By Living provides transformative outdoor experiences for cancer survivors and their caregivers.

• **True North Treks: TRUENORTHTREKS.ORG**
True North Treks is a national 501(c)3 nonprofit organization whose mission is to empower teens and young adults with cancer through outdoor adventure

Other resources

• **The Breast Cancer Fundraiser:**
The BCF helps to preserve the dignity of breast cancer patients and their loved ones by supporting their unmet needs through funding value added services such as massage therapy, acupuncture, fitness classes, beauty consulting, etc.
HTTP://WWW.THEBREASTCANCERFUNDRAISER.ORG/

• **ADC SCholarships:** AGC is nonprofit group committed to providing both advocacy and scholarships for those struggling with infertility in the United States.
HTTP://WWW.AGCSCHOLARSHIPS.ORG/

• **The Ulman Cancer Fund For Young Adults:**
We enhance lives by supporting, educating, and connecting young adults and their loved ones affected by cancer.
ULMANFUND.ORG

• **Livestrong Foundation:** We find new ways to raise awareness, increase outreach and facilitate collaboration in an effort to improve the cancer experience. Dozens of navigators are available by phone to assist patients with questions and support. **LIVESTRONG.COM**

• **The American Cancer Society:** Your American Cancer Society is in your corner around the clock to help you stay well and get well, to find cures, and to fight back. There is also a 24/7 lifeline to support cancer patients with questions. **WWW.CANCER.ORG**

• **Cancer Hawk Foundation:**
At the Cancer Hawk Foundation, our mission is to make the services, products and expertise needed to fight cancer sharply visible to patients and caregivers. Online navigator services direct patients to the right info quickly. **CANCERHAWK.COM**

• **Ihadcancer.org:** Get peer-to-peer cancer support from a community of survivors, fighters and caregivers by connecting with people with firsthand experience on life before, during

• **Caring Bridge:** Caring Bridge is an online space where you can connect, share news, and receive support. It's your very own health social network, coming together on your personalized website. And thanks to those who donate, we are available 24/7 to anyone, anywhere, at no cost.
CARINGBRIDGE.ORG

• **Cancer Care:** Cancer Care provides telephone, online and face-to-face counseling, support groups, education, publications and financial and co-payment assistance. **CANCERCARE.ORG**

• **Mylifeline.org:** is a 501(c)(3) nonprofit organization that encourages cancer patients and caregivers to create free, customized websites to keep their networks up to date on their health and lives. **MYLIFELINE.ORG**

• **Imerman Angels:** Imerman Angels carefully matches a person touched by cancer with someone who has fought and survived the same type of cancer (a Mentor Angel). **IMERMANANGELS.ORG**

• **Stupid Cancer:** Stupid Cancer is a non-profit organization that empowers young adults affected by cancer through innovative and award-winning programs and services. **STUPIDCANCER.ORG**

• **Testicular Cancer Foundation:** TCF provides education and support to young men to raise awareness about testicular cancer, the #1 cancer among men ages 15 – 35.
TESTICULARCANCERFOUNDATION.ORG

• **Cancer + Careers:**
Cancer and Careers empowers and educates people with cancer to thrive in their workplace by providing expert advice, interactive tools and educational events. **CANCERANDCAREERS.ORG**

• **Leukemia & Lymphoma Society:**
LLS exists to find cures and ensure access to treatments for blood cancer patients. We are the voice for all blood cancer patients and we work to ensure access to treatments for all blood cancer patients.
LLS.ORG ■

MORE THAN

600 TIPS

MORE THAN

90 PEOPLE

testimonies

TECHNIQUES | *tricks*

information | SECRETS

natural drugs

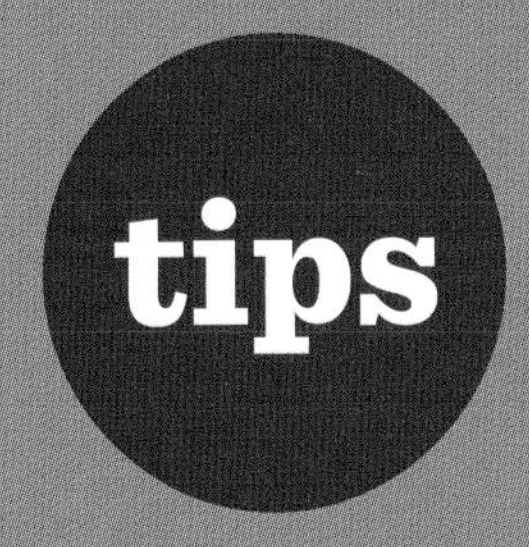

Very generously, more than ninety people accepted sharing, in this book, an important part of what they learned from the moment their cancer diagnosis changed their lives: among them are patients, friends or relatives of people affected with cancer, and therapy specialists. They all immediately understood the aim of sharing their experiences for a very simple reason: they would all have preferred to have known in advance what they had to discover on their own.

MORE THAN **600**
TIPS
MORE THAN **90**
PEOPLE

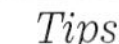

introduction

I say this based on my own experience: Cancer not only impacts on the lives of patients who have been diagnosed. It also affects their families and those around them in social and professional environments.

After the initial shock, I experienced the unavoidable sensation of uncertainty, emptiness, pain, as well as some –many unknown– emotions which were mixed with the obligation to think, evaluate and act firmly in dealing with the disease.

Within this whirlpool, I found out the importance of having initial guidance information, which helps the patient as well as their family and close friends face the new situation from a realistic and, above all, empathetic point of view.

With this in mind, throughout the four years I took to write this book, together with the team of journalists I worked with, we collected testimonials, tips and suggestions from hundreds of people who, in some way or other, know or knew what it is to live in the shadow of this disease.

Some of these people were also cancer patients and, unfortunately, were not able to see this work finished. However, they shared their experiences knowing that with their testimonials they could help others lead a better life with cancer.

I share a close relationship with about twenty of the people who were interviewed for this book and who knew my story before this book's existence. I got to know others during my treatment and, today, I feel closer to them. I also share here my own tips. Although they are spread throughout the book, they are repeated here.

Everyone who contributed to this book is confident that the advice given here could be useful for someone facing cancer.

To all those who are closely living the process of the disease and have this book in their hands, apart from giving you all my support, I hope this book is useful as a good starting point.

Roberto.

TABLE OF CONTENTS

patients

family

specialists

therapists

friends

In the following pages, white background color states that this is a testimony of a breast cancer patient. Light blue background, in turn, indicates that people have some relationship with the disease, as specialists, doctors, therapists, family or friends of patients. Each type of cancer is identified with a different color.

Melanoma *Skin Cancer*

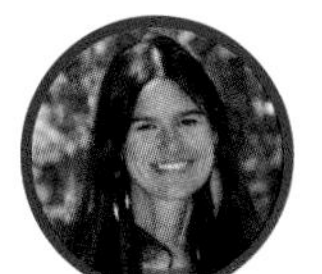
Loreto Agurto
PATIENT
p. ***236***

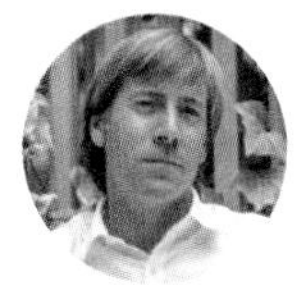
Gonzalo Tagle
FAMILY
p. ***238***

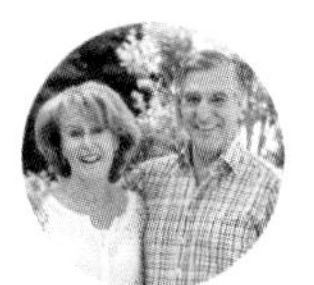
Familia Ibáñez Atkinson
FAMILY
p. ***240***

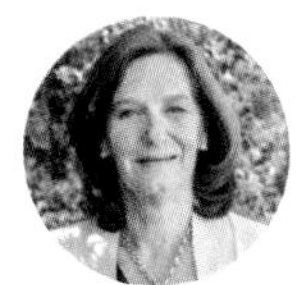
Loreto Fuentes
FAMILY
p. ***244***

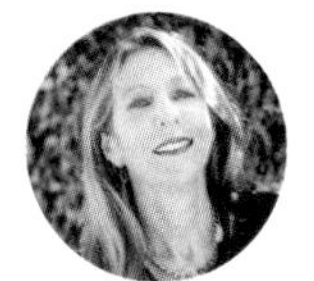
María Isabel Orpinas
PATIENT
p. ***246***

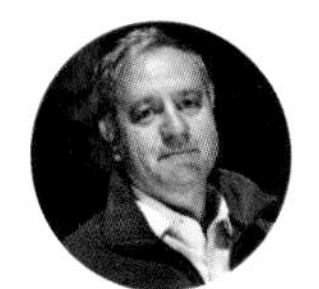
Mario Valdivia
FRIEND
p. ***248***

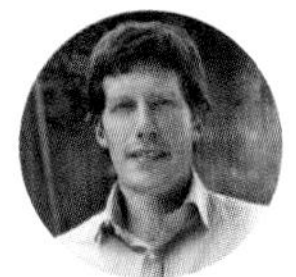
Christian Verteneul
PATIENT
p. ***250***

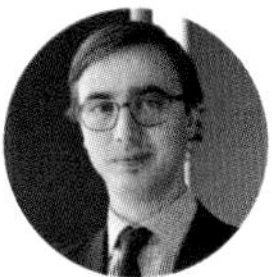
José Coz
FRIEND
p. ***252***

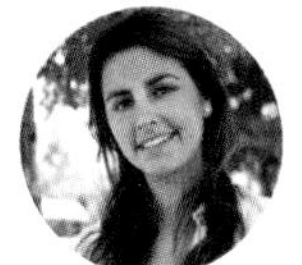
Florencia Uslar
FRIEND
p. ***254***

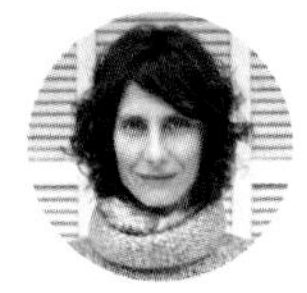
Diana Strauss
PATIENT
p. ***258***

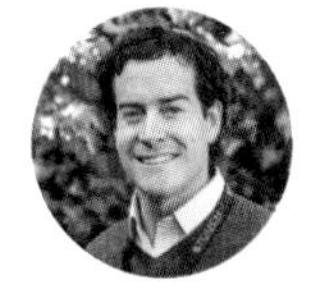
Antonio Monckeberg
FRIEND
p. ***260***

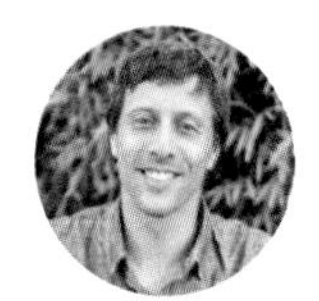
Eduardo Pérez de Castro
FRIEND
p. ***262***

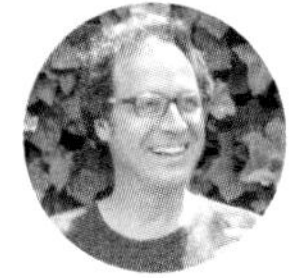
Guillermo Acuña
PATIENT
p. ***264***

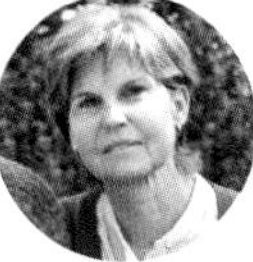
Quequi Mingo
PATIENT
p. ***266***

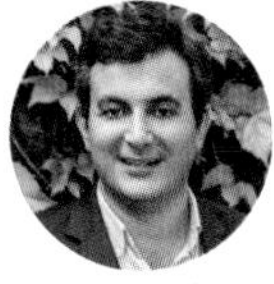
José Masihy
FRIEND
p. ***268***

Breast cancer

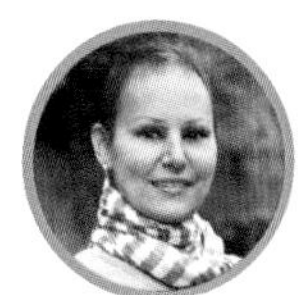
Marcela Lorenzini
PATIENT
p. ***272***

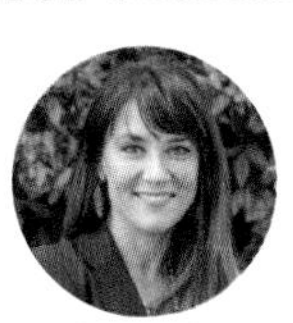
María Paz Aldunate
PATIENT
p. ***276***

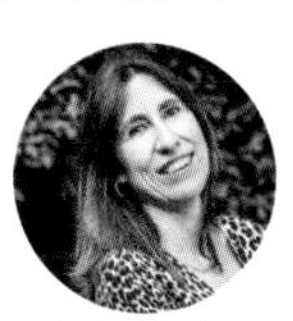
Paula Warnken
PATIENT
p. ***278***

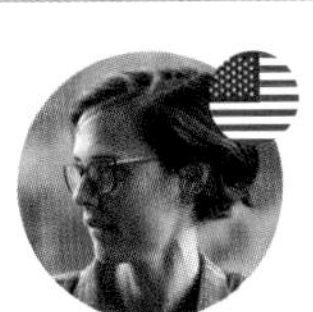
Natalie Conforti
PATIENT
p. ***280***

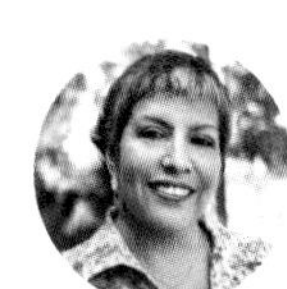
Flora Molina
PATIENT
p. ***284***

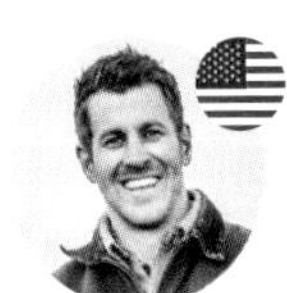
Brad Ludden
FAMILY
p. ***288***

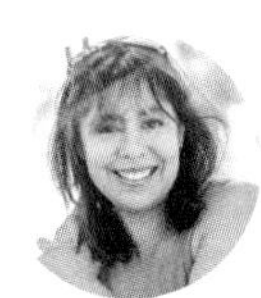
Claudia Palomino
PATIENT
p. ***290***

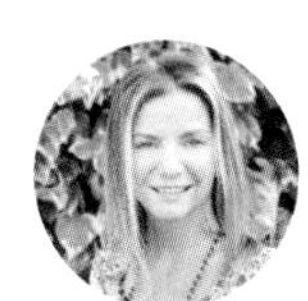
Bernardita Swinburn
PATIENT
p. ***294***

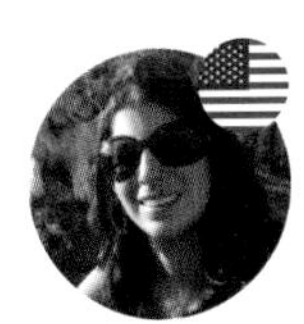
Nadia T
PATIENT
p. ***296***

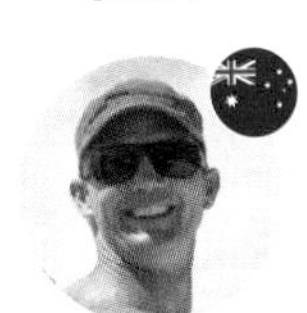
Paul Viney
PATIENT
p. ***298***

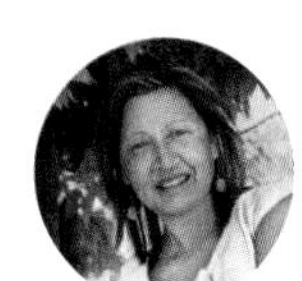
Aurora Opazo
PATIENT
p. ***300***

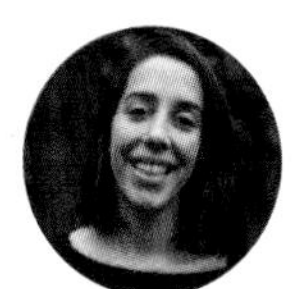
Karla Amaro
PATIENT
p. ***302***

Non-Hodgkin's Lymphoma

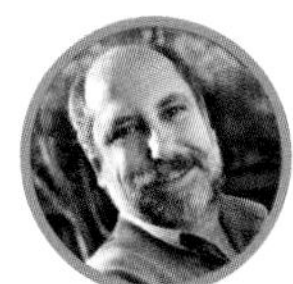
Ricardo Larraín
PATIENT
p. ***304***

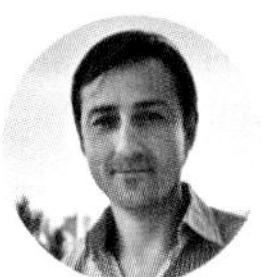
Pablo Hernández
PATIENT
p. ***308***

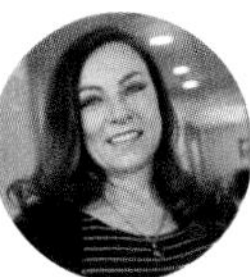
Isabel Infante
FAMILY
p. ***312***

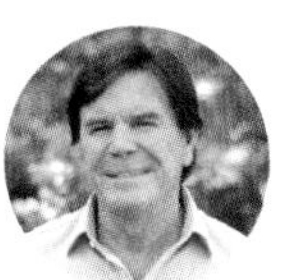
Drago Gluscevic
PATIENT
p. ***314***

Hodgkin's Lymphoma

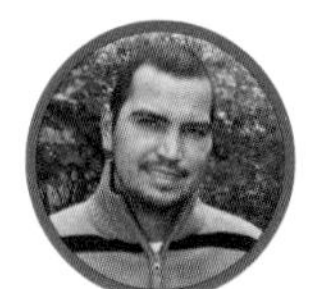
Luis Silva
PATIENT
p. ***318***

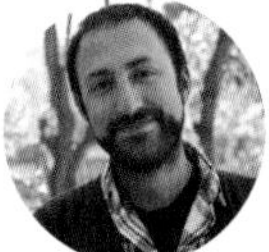
Nicolás Stutzin
PATIENT
p. ***320***

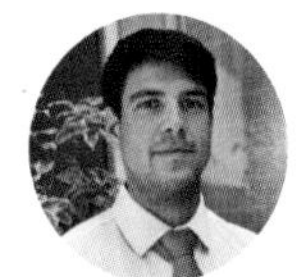
Max Valdés
PATIENT
p. ***324***

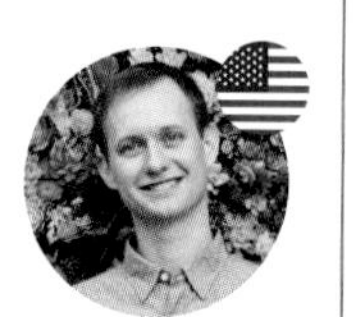
Peter Moore
PATIENT
p. ***326***

Brain Tumor

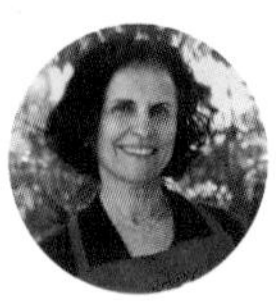
Marcela Zubieta
FAMILY
p. ***330***

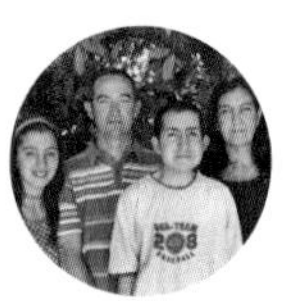
Familia Gross Sarrazin
FAMILY
p. ***334***

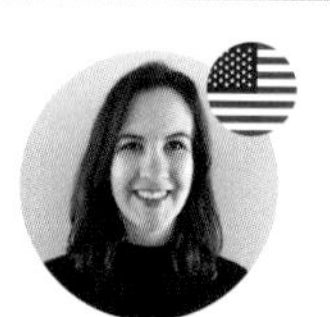
Sabine Schwab
PATIENT
p. ***338***

Leukemia

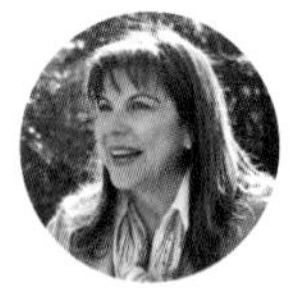
Patricia Marchesse
FAMILY
p. ***342***

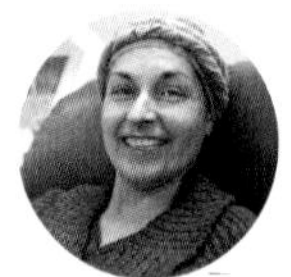
Aldrida Matamala
PATIENT
p. ***346***

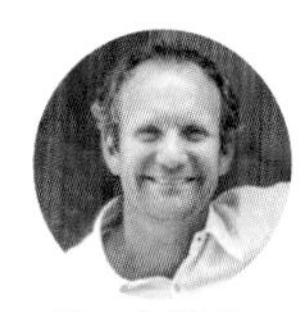
Gonzalo Muñoz
FAMILY
p. ***348***

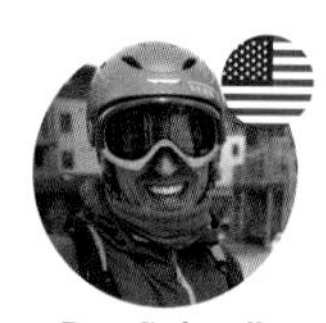
Dave Carbonell
PATIENT
p. ***352***

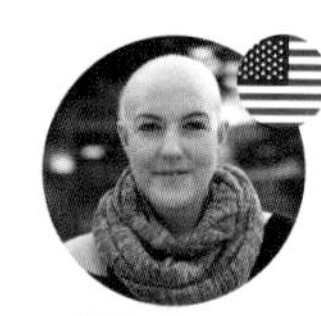
Abbie Alterman
PATIENT
p. ***354***

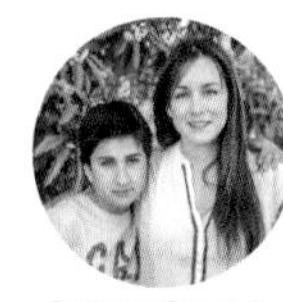
Javiera Chinchón
FAMILY
p. ***356***

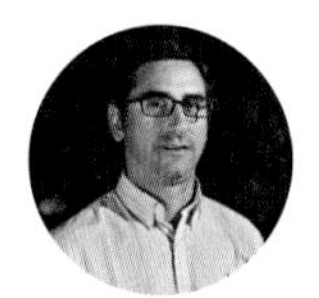
Juan Andrés Lira
FAMILY
p. ***358***

Ovarian Cancer

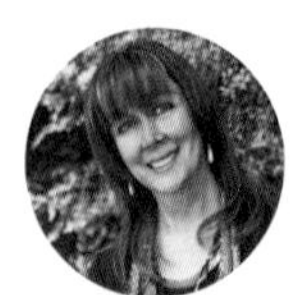
Leonor Gacitúa
PATIENT
p. ***360***

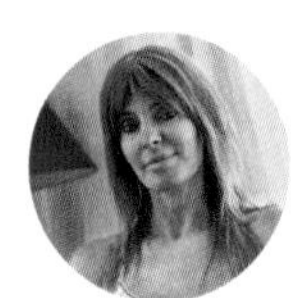
Isabel Mahou
PATIENT
p. ***362***

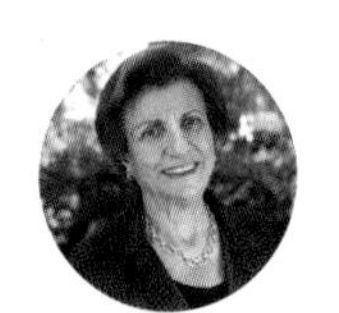
Jaennett Cattan Cattan
FAMILY
p. ***364***

Thyroid cancer

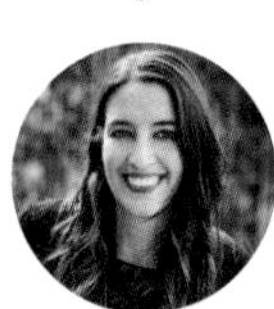
Daniela Rozental
PATIENT
p. ***366***

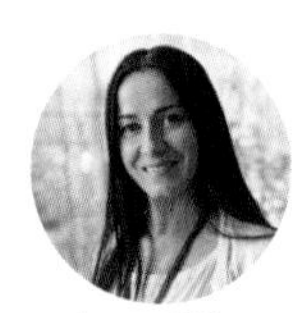
Loreto Wahr
PATIENT
p. ***368***

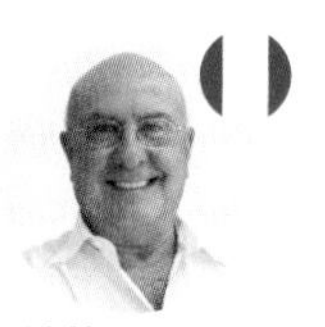
Adolfo Dammert
PATIENT
p. ***370***

Sarcoma

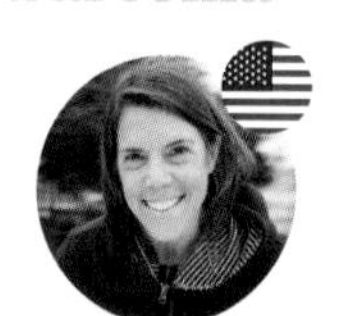
Katie Schou
FAMILY
p. ***372***

Oral cancer

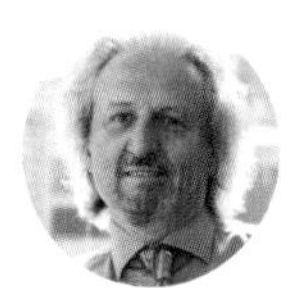
Francisco Javier Ibáñez
PATIENT
p. ***374***

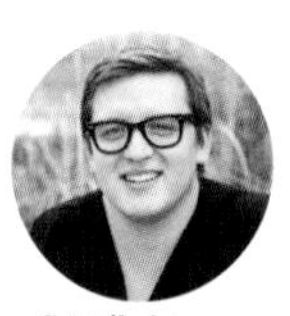
Cristóbal Araya
DENTAL SURGEON
p. ***376***

Pancreatic cancer

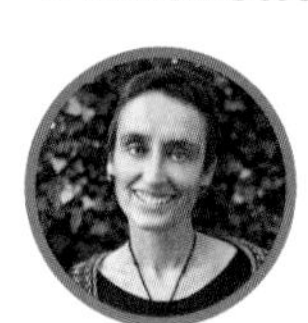
Carla Vidal
PATIENT
p. ***380***

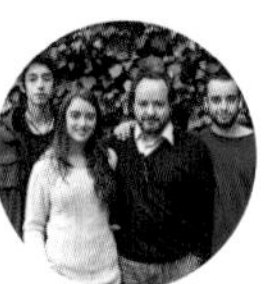
Familia Aguiló Vidal
FAMILY
p. ***384***

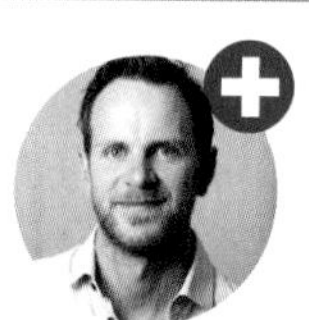
Martin Inderbitzin
PATIENT
p. ***388***

Uterine and cervical cancer

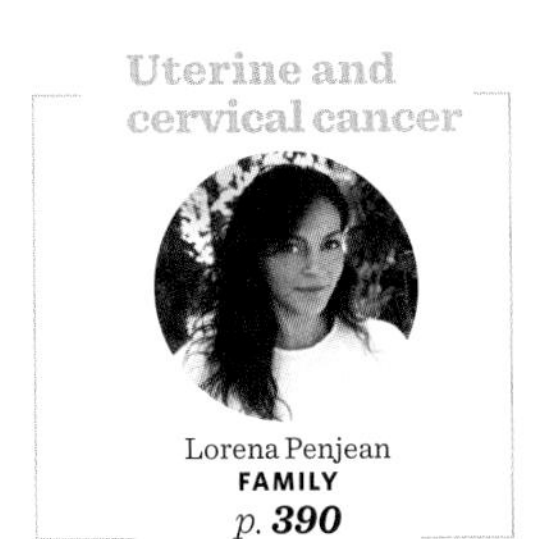

Lorena Penjean
FAMILY
p. ***390***

Osteosarcoma

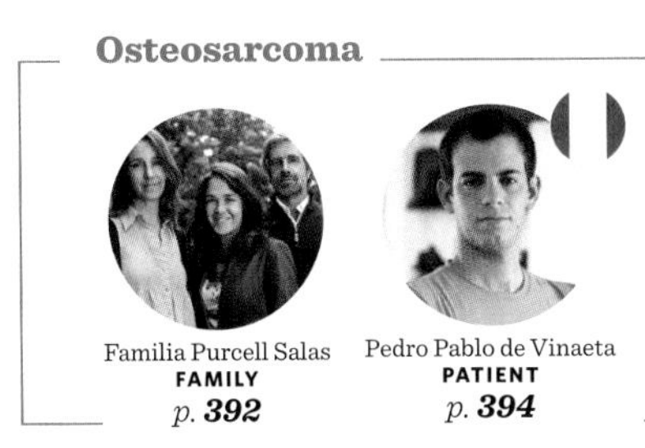

Familia Purcell Salas
FAMILY
p. ***392***

Pedro Pablo de Vinaeta
PATIENT
p. ***394***

Colon cancer

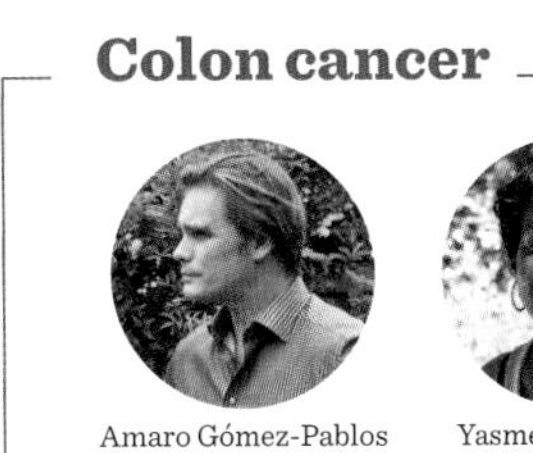

Amaro Gómez-Pablos
FAMILY
p. ***398***

Yasmeem Watson
PATIENT
p. ***402***

Lung cancer

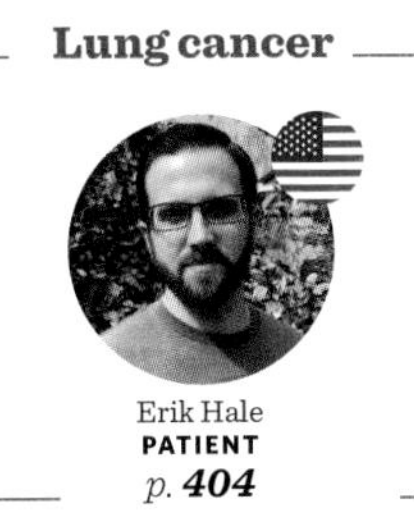

Erik Hale
PATIENT
p. ***404***

Testicular Cancer

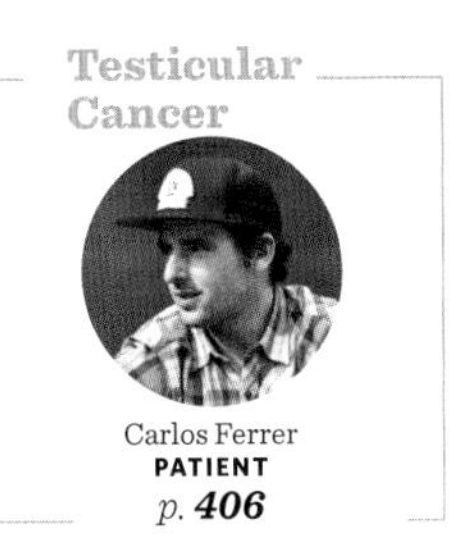

Carlos Ferrer
PATIENT
p. ***406***

Ewing Sarcoma

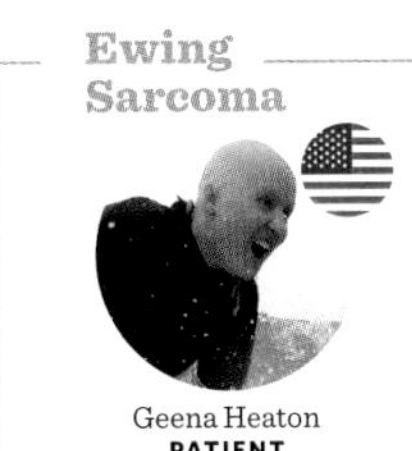

Geena Heaton
PATIENT
p. ***408***

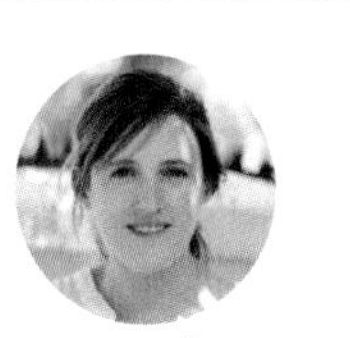

Carmen Hodgson
PATIENT
p. ***410***

Prostate cancer

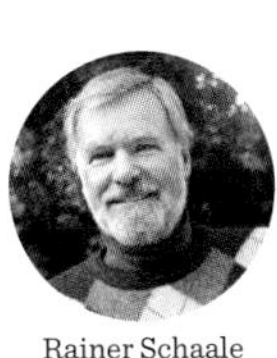

Rainer Schaale
THERAPIST
p. ***414***

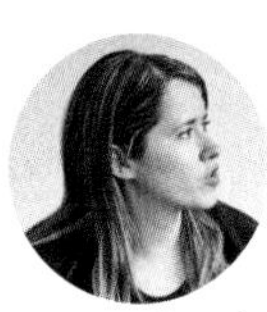

Constanza Larraín
FAMILY
p. ***416***

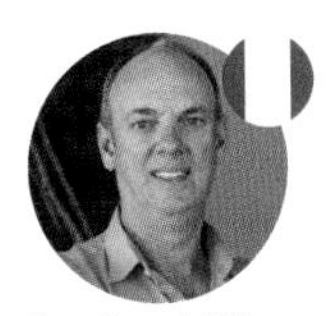

Juan Antonio Dibos
PATIENT
p. ***420***

Clear-cell cancer

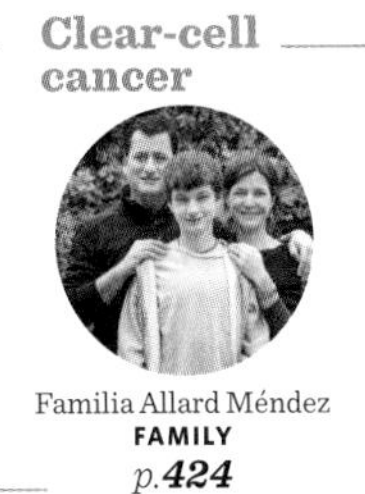

Familia Allard Méndez
FAMILY
*p.****424***

Specialists

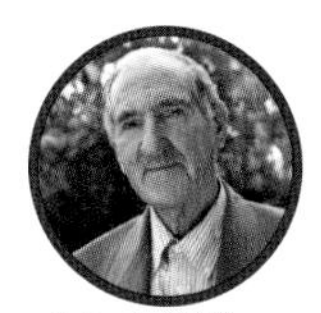

Roberto Williams
NATURAL THERAPIST
p. ***428***

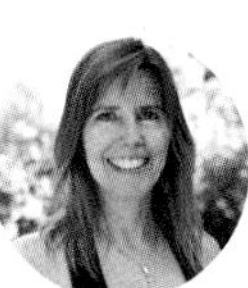

Patricia Eing
THERAPIST
p. ***430***

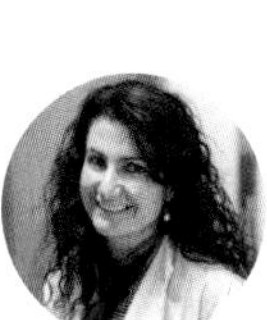

Pamela Salman
ONCOLOGIST
p. ***434***

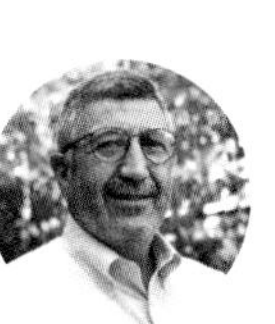

Benjamín Paz
ONCOLOGIST
p. ***436***

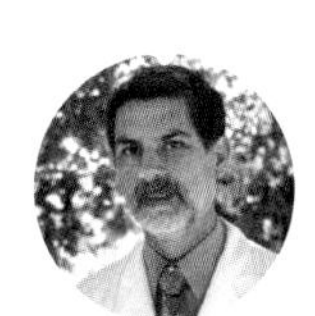

Robinson Guerrero
DERMATHOLOGIST
p. ***438***

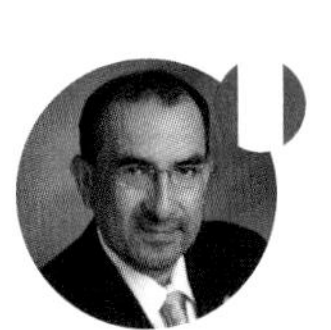

Elmer Huerta
ONCOLOGIST
p. ***440***

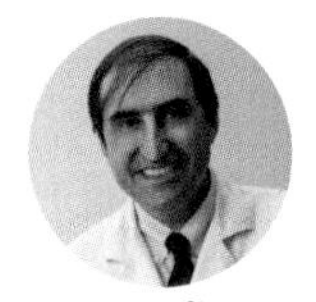

Francis Palisson
FRIEND AND DERMATHOLOGIST
p. ***444***

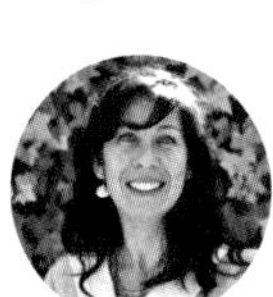

Isabel González
SOCIAL WORKER
p. ***446***

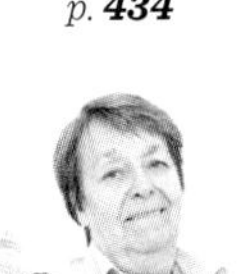

Jennifer Middleton
PSYCHOLOGIST
p. ***450***

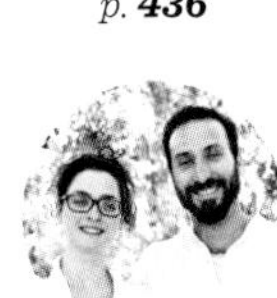

Scott & Rojo
PSYCHOLOGISTS
p. ***454***

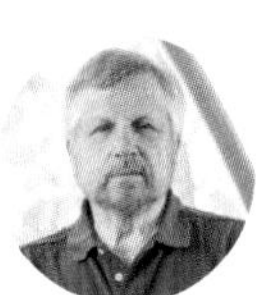

Iván Mimica
FRIEND AND PSYCHOLOGIST
p. ***458***

Author

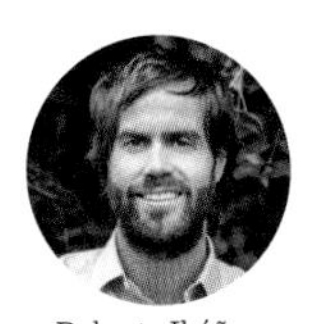

Roberto Ibáñez
PATIENT
p. ***462***

ILLUSTRATIONS: WWW.FREEPIK.COM

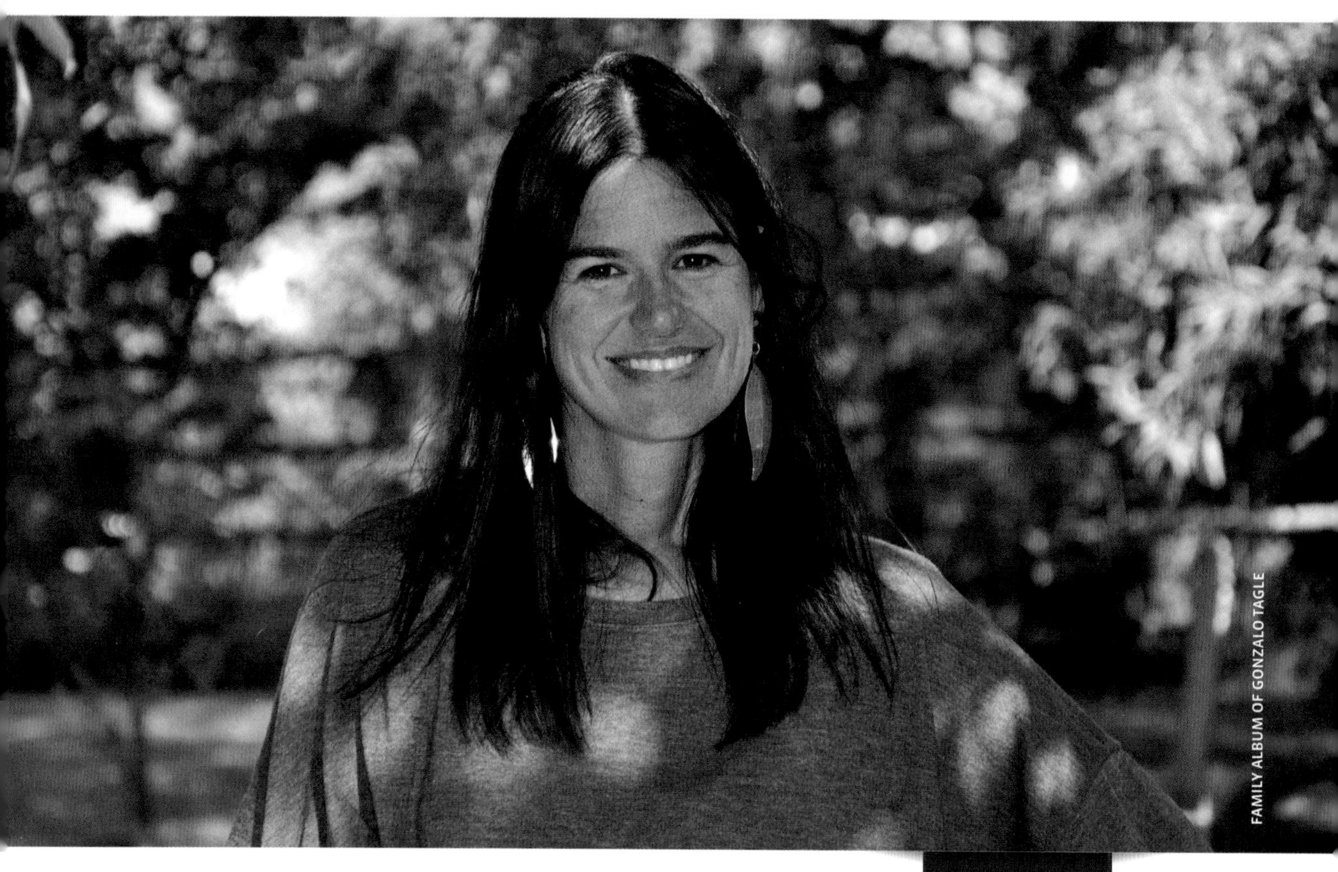

FAMILY ALBUM OF GONZALO TAGLE

Loreto Agurto

melanoma
PATIENT

AGE: *37*

OCCUPATION: *Agricultural engineer who worked 12 years in Iansa.*

DIAGNOSIS: *Melanoma.*

WHEN: *2006*

CONTEXT: *Loreto, who discovered she had melanoma on her right thigh during one of the usual check-ups with the dermatologist, is the woman who inspired and motivated Roberto Ibáñez to write his story. She was the first person who gave tips to him, by email, when he told her he would gather together the contributions of people who were living or lived with the same cancer she was dealing with, to share those tips in a book. Loreto died in 2012 after another melanoma developed in her scalp, which metastasized in the lungs and brain. Here you will find all her suggestions as she wrote them in 2011.*

1.

"Surround yourself with positive people and keep away from those who are negative."

2.

Doctor Mercedes López. She injected me the autoimmune vaccine against melanoma. (oncobiomed.cl)."

3.

"Stop worrying about nonsense."

4.

"Vitamines Ritestart 4life (4liferitestart.com). They are sold in the United States and need a prescription.

5.

"Take into account the treatment the patient wants to undergo. I preferred surgery over a drug treatment."

6.

"Conduct tests rigorously every three months."

7.

"Surgeon Gustavo Vial from Las Condes Clinic."

8.

"Have a spiritual and an earthly guide to pour your heart out to."

9.

"Oncologist Arturo Madrid from the *Clínica Alemana*."

10.

"Don't leave pending issues with anybody."

11.

"Live each day at a time, without egos."

12.

"Dermatologist Robinson Guerrero."

13.

"Do whatever you want to do and say no to what you don't want to do." ■

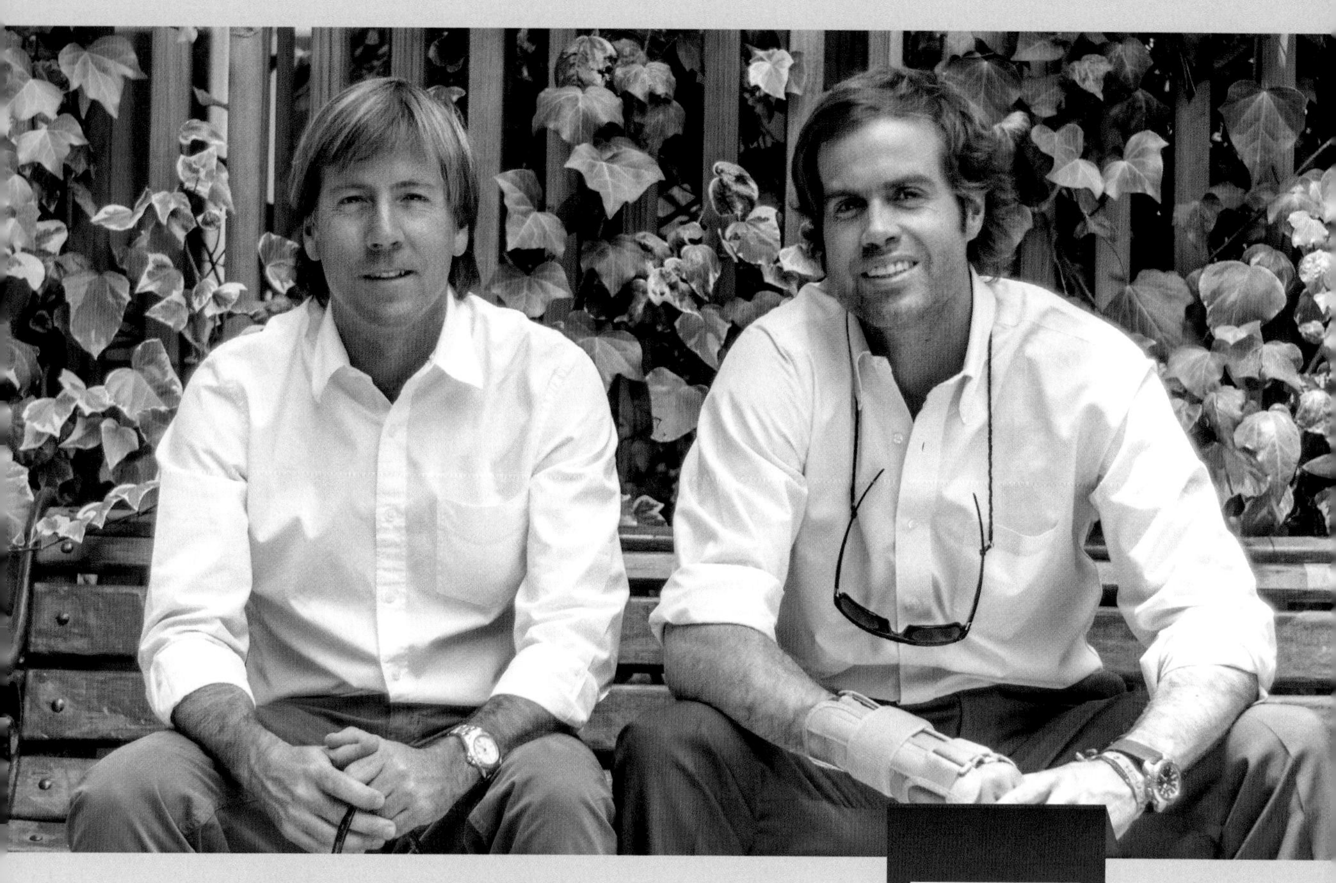

Gonzalo Tagle

Husband *of* **melanoma patient**

AGE: *42*

OCCUPATION: *Businessman*

RELATIONSHIP: *His wife had different melanomas*

WHEN: *2012*

CONTEXT: *Gonzalo is Loreto Agurto's widower, the woman who inspired this book. They were together for 17 years and had three kids. Gonzalo highlights here how his wife faced cancer and the lessons he learned from her before she passed.*

1.

LIFE IS NOT THE SAME: "I believe cancer helped Loreto live her life with much more intensity. We should all lead our lives as she did, although we don't have cancer. At least, that's what I try to do."

2.

KEEP MOVING FORWARD AS A FAMILY: "All this is filled with good experiences, stories, contributions, and that's what we have left from Loreto. Pain and suffering will always exist, but the good things are so many that it is useful to live and move forward as a family. We have such a strong connection that my children and I try to do things as she would have liked us to."

"**Life** is meant to be *enjoyed*. We are born to be ***happy,*** and to make *others* happy."

3.

MAKE HAPPY TO BE HAPPY: "We are born to be happy and make others happy in a transparent and ego-free way. This is what Loreto taught me and was of great help for us as a couple. We are devoted to life, not death. She didn't like people to know she was sick, because she didn't feel that way. It wasn't denial: it was her positive way of facing the disease."

4.

FEEL DIFFERENTLY: *"A sick person does not feel the same as a healthy one, in the same way I don't feel the same as someone who has not gone through the death of his wife. I feel differently, because I went through a different experience. This difference allows me to reconsider the way I lead my life. This, finally, is a privilege."* ■

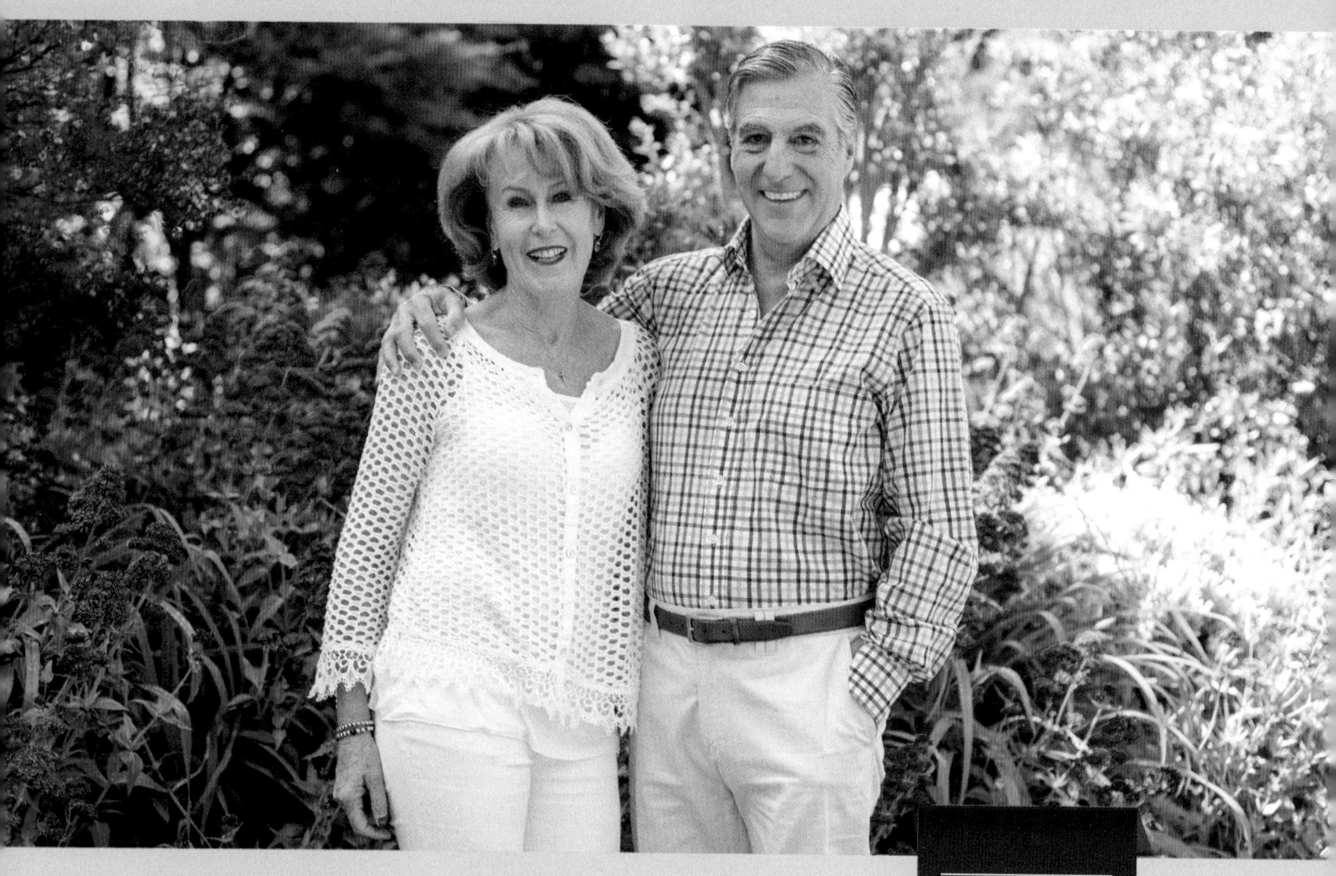

Ibáñez Atkinson Family

Family *of a* **melanoma patient**

Felipe Ibáñez
AGE: *61*
OCCUPATION: *BA in Business Administration and businessma*

Heather Atkinson
AGE: *62*
OCCUPATION: *Historian and social entrepreneur*

CONTEXT: *Overnight, the routine of the Ibáñez Atkinson family changed when the dermatologist called Roberto to tell him the biopsy showed the existence of melanoma. Each one, from a different front, devoted their lives to support, take care and protect him, researching on melanoma and recovery possibilities 24/7. This strike changed all family members forever -not just Roberto- and, currently, none of them regret this experience. These are tips from one family to another.*

1.

AFTER THE INITIAL IMPACT:
"The first three days were emotionally hard for the entire family, as we were trying to understand that this was our reality now. That's approximately how long we took to decide we had to get ready to act. We didn't see death was close, but we felt the need to get well organized to prevent it. We gathered strength, accepted the situation and started getting organized and coordinated to face it."

2.

FIRST GET INFORMED: "We found out everything, consulted other doctors and worked non-stop. The diversity of opinions is impressive, that's why at the beginning you feel a huge uncertainty which needs to be separated into three main questions: What is the illness being suffered? What can we do? What is the timing in this situation? We finally arrived at the conclusion that surgery was necessary, that it could be very well performed in Chile and, also, that it was urgent. But we needed to understand the scenario in full in order to make the best decisions in connection to an unknown subject."

"You have to have a certain degree of *confidence* that things may be done the way **you want** them to be done."

3.

REALITY AND EXPECTATIONS: "You need to be optimistic, but you also you have to be clear what chances are and keep your feet on the ground. It's useless to dream everything will turn out great, although you don't need to get stuck thinking on what can go wrong. Reality needs to be explained with optimism, but without making omissions or creating false expectations."

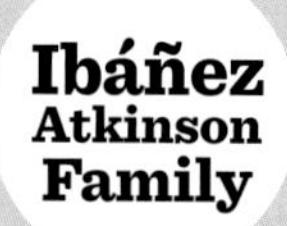

4.

CONTINUE WITH YOUR LIFE: *"We couldn't avoid talking about the subject, but we also tried doing other things, clearing our minds, going out for walks, talking about something else. Because in this shocking situation you tend to stop doing things, but you need to keep going, you can't stop moving."*

5.

CREATE A SUPPORT NETWORK: "Not only the family should be aware of what's going on; also friends should know about the situation, in order for the patient to feel support from all the aspects of their life. People tend to react immediately and the patient receives warmth, closeness and special consideration of their family, friends and even workmates."

6.

AUTONOMY IN DECISION-TAKING:
"You receive advice from doctors, but the problem is that they, as expert as they may be, sometimes have different opinions. Then, you need to make decisions after considering all aspects of the patient's medical history and situation. You need to study all possibilities and make a conscious decision."

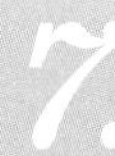

PATIENT HAS THE FINAL DECISION:
"In the end, all visits and inquiries have the purpose that the patient has enough information so as to make their own decisions. It is very important that, independently of advice and disagreements or agreements with the opinions of the patient's environment, nobody takes decisions, but the patient."

8.

FIGHT: "Being pessimistic and waiting for death is the worst you can do. And if you're part of a family, it is a very bad sign, because you can make others feel the same. You need to hold your head up high, support others, be organized and methodical, but always being optimistic at the –not small– possibility that everything may go well."

9.

LOOK FOR POSITIVE TESTIMONIALS: "Learn from others: through acquaintances we met people who had had melanoma and recovered, and this was very reassuring at the beginning, when you don't understand anything, everything makes you angry and news confuses you."

"Reality needs to be explained with **optimism,** but without making **omissions** or creating false *expectations.*"

10.

BE A GOOD PATIENT: "The sick person needs to form their own opinion on subjects they don't know in depth and this can only be done if such subjects are discussed with experts. We had the opportunity to travel to the United States to talk to many melanoma specialists. We heard their answers and understood the consequences of this cancer, and its contraindications. You need to do homework and understand what doctors talk about. Studying, analyzing, talking and listening make patients powerful."

11.

LOOK FOR CONVERSATION MOMENTS: "When a family member has cancer, it is very important for the family to have moments in which they talk about the disease. This could be once a month, or once a week, depending on the family. The whirlpool of formalities, information and medical history is so overwhelming that sharing some calm moments helps reduce anxiety and bring the family together."

12.

WALK THE ROAD OF THE HEALTHY, NOT THE ROAD OF THE SICK: "A phrase that pushed us forward from the beginning and kept our spirits high at all times." ■

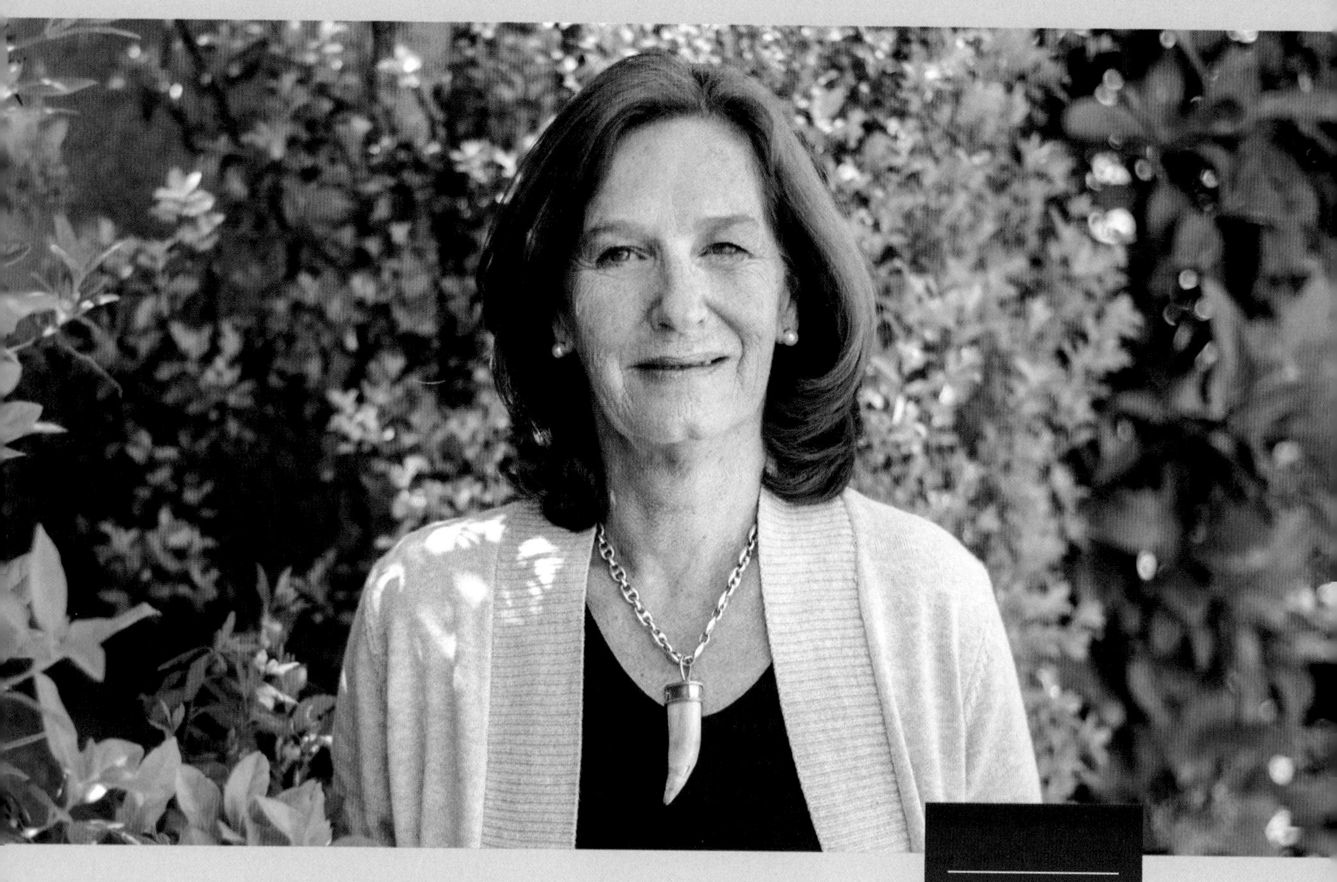

Loreto Fuentes

Mother *of* **melanoma patient**

AGE: *63*

OCCUPATION: *Decorator*

RELATIONSHIP: *Her daughter had several melanomas*

WHEN: *2008*

CONTEXT: *Loreto Fuentes is Loreto Agurto's, La Negra's, mother, the woman who suggested Roberto Ibáñez leave egos aside and simply be happy. After her daughter died in March 2012, Loreto suggests enjoying your children as much as you can, until they are grownups.*

1.

TALK ABOUT EVERYTHING YOU CAN WHEN IT IS STILL POSSIBLE: "It's not that I feel I owe her something or anything like that, but I would've loved to speak more with her!"

2.

SIMPLICITY: *"Share simple things of life, which are wonderful."*

3.

RUN AWAY FROM PESSIMISM: "Don't make the patient feel sick or limited."

4.

CHILDREN ARE FOREVER: "Enjoy every minute with your children. Even when they're grown ups. They're your children, no matter how old they are. My parents are alive. They loved *La Negra*. She gave us strength, we miss her, but that will help us move forward."

5.

A NICE FAREWELL: "I continue living outside the city. In Santiago there's no time to share, to enjoy the simple things of life. For instance, we had a beautiful farewell for my mother-in-law. We took a a beautiful picture of the whole family together just fifteen days before she passed away."

6.

ENJOY EVERY SECOND OF THE TIME YOU HAVE TOGETHER: "Don't let days go by. Call. See each other. In this life. Being together." ■

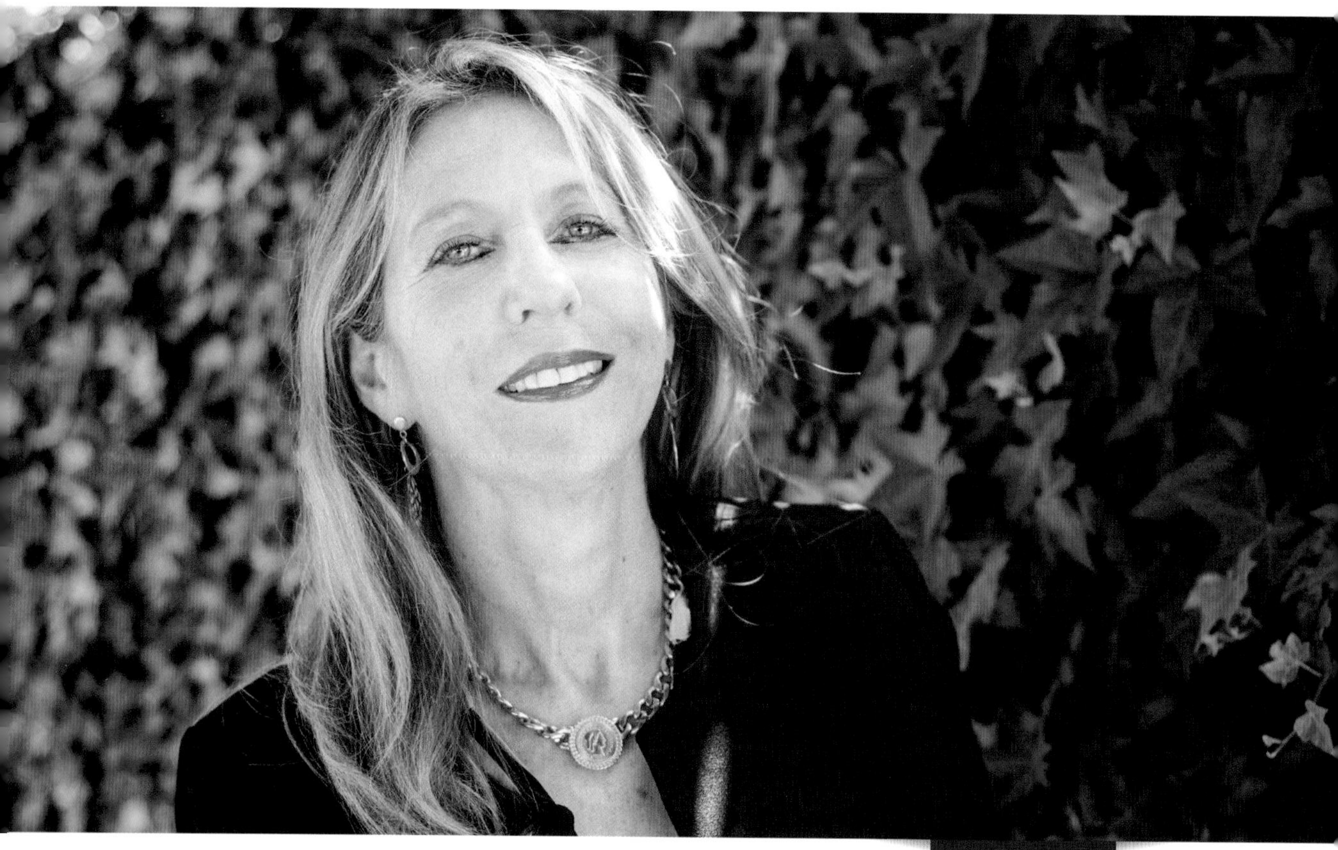

María Isabel Orpinas

melanoma
PATIENT

AGE: *56*
OCCUPATION: *Business woman*
DIAGNOSIS: *Melanoma*
WHEN: *2000*
CONTEXT: *Sixteen years ago, an abrupt melanoma marked the start of María Isabel's experience with skin cancer. She was 42 years old, and six months before her father passed away from lung cancer. In 2015 was the 15th anniversary of her surgery and she now considers herself to be completely healthy.*

1.

A CHANGE IN PERSPECTIVE: "It didn't turn my life upside down, because after surgery I did not undergo invasive treatments related to cancer, but I started looking at life from a different perspective. I'm a neurotic workaholic; I'm working on everything and try resolving it all. From then on, I realized that no one is safe from this disease. The world may stop turning but through all of it, I try to stay calm."

2.

USEFUL ACTIVITIES: *"I was told to practice yoga and practiced it for a while in a meditation center. I also started painting and spent an entire day each week in a workshop in Buin, in the countryside. Deep down, these are things one does to avoid thinking about cancer all the time and to be relaxed."*

"From then on, I realized that no one **is safe** from this disease. The world may **stop** turning but through all of it, I try to stay *calm.*"

3.

ATTITUDE IS EVERYTHING: "You need to have a lot of faith and try moving forward. I never thought these would be my last days. I continued living my life, although more frightened than before. When cancer is discovered on time, there are always some possibilities. The most important thing was that I never felt I was sick. I thought *this couldn't be happening to me.* I continued living my life as if nothing happened; I had 8-year old twins and thought *God, you need to help me, I can't leave them alone yet.* And I have continued each day of my life thanking Him." ■

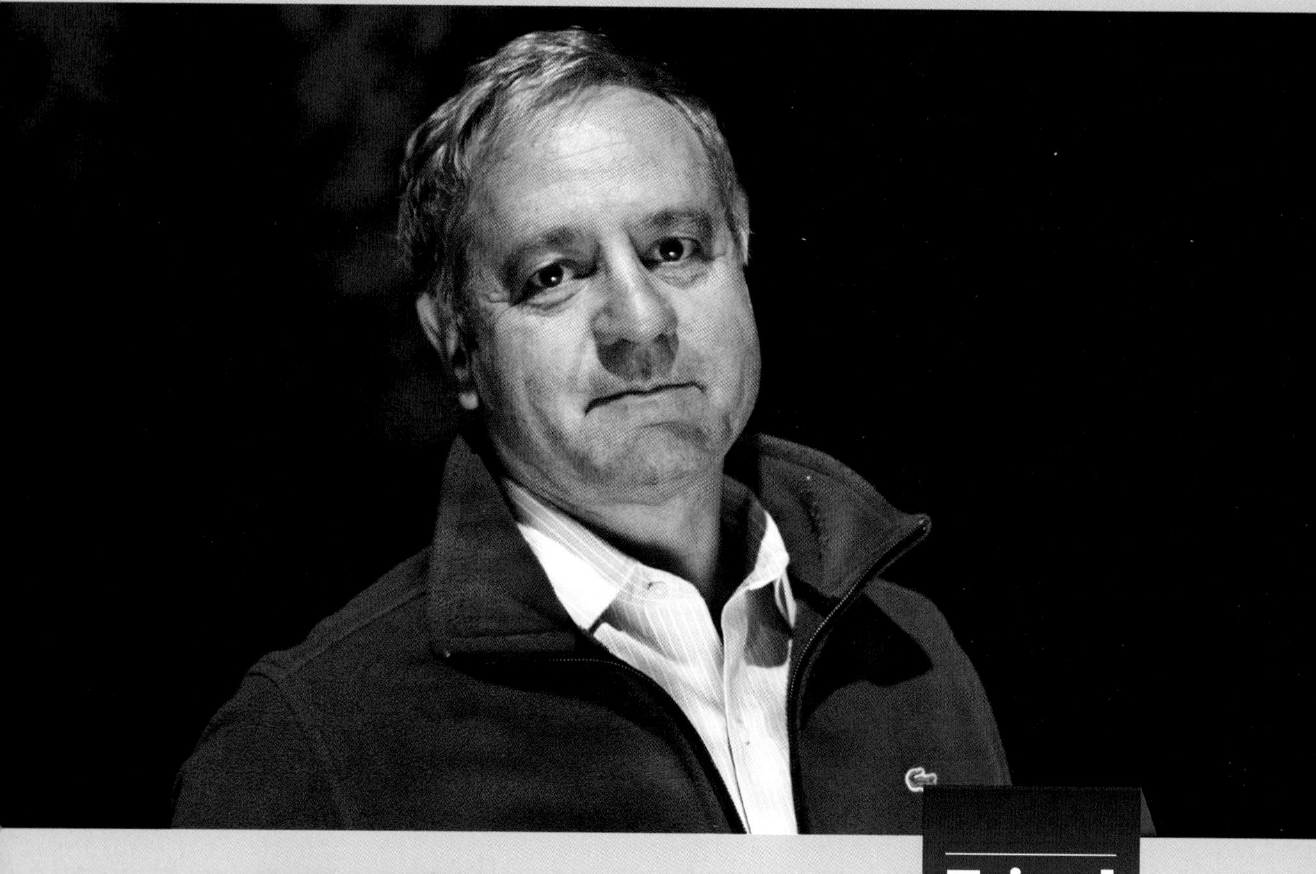

Mario Valdivia

Friend *of* melanoma patient

AGE: *56*

OCCUPATION: *Business man*

RELATIONSHIP: *Friend of melanoma patient*

WHEN: *2011*

CONTEXT: *Business man and advisor of Roberto Ibáñez's father. He was close to the family in the initial stage of the diagnosis and during the trip to the United States looking for answers to the doubts and questions.*

1.

MY WAY OR...: "When the patient is an adult, one must never forget that all decisions must be made by them and by nobody else. This, naturally, is especially difficult for parents, but it's a rule that must be followed."

2.

COMPARE OPINIONS: "Most cases in medicine are not black or white, there's always some hope. You need to receive good counseling related to medical decisions and this means it's worth comparing opinions."

3.

YOUR SUFFERING IS DIFFERENT, BUT YOU DO SUFFER TOO: "When news of a diagnosis which implies serious life risk is given, all members of the family suffer. But each member has a different reaction: some accept reality before others, others evade it for a long time and others magnify it. You need to know how to respect and accompany each member of the patient's family in the process."

4.

CONSCIOUSNESS AND LEARNING: *"Only God gives and takes lives. These processes let us realize our fragility as humans and, many times, they get us close to what's transcendent."*

5.

ALTERNATIVE MEDICINE: "A valid choice." ■

"When the patient is an adult, one must ***never forget*** that all decisions must be made by them."

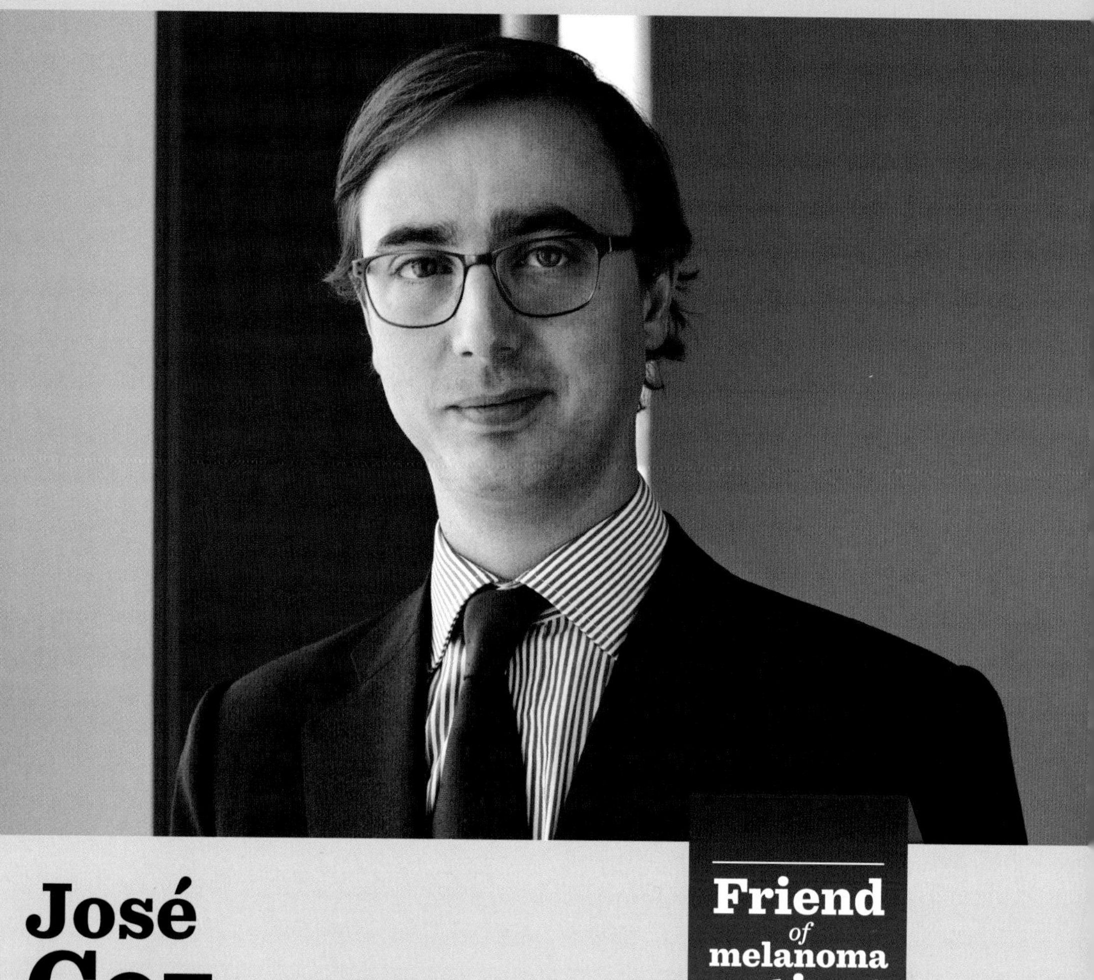

José Coz

Friend *of* **melanoma patient**

AGE: *31*

OCCUPATION: *Lawyer*

RELATIONSHIP: *Friend of melanoma patient*

WHEN: *2011*

CONTEXT: *Schoolmate and friends ever since, lawyer José Coz closely followed Roberto Ibáñez's process from the very beginning. He shared the initial anguish, was beside him during treatment, but –above all– he always made Roberto feel he could be completely honest with his emotions in connection to what he was living.*

1.

THE FIRST REACTION: "A friend of my mom had died of melanoma not long ago, so I knew it was not a joke. As a friend, you try to avoid the subject and reduce the problem to avoid giving the impression you're frightened. At first, when he was just diagnosed, as friends we decided to focus only on facts. We knew he had a mole, which was going to be removed, that the mole was dangerous, that it was not sure it had spread and that there was a treatment. Therefore, we had to be prepared and get hold of cancer in advance."

2.

THE TWO SIDEWALKS: "There's a phrase my dad, who is a doctor, told me once: in cancer situations you can walk on two different paths, that of the sick and that of the healthy. Walking on the path of the healthy means understanding that, above all, you have a life which goes beyond cancer. And if you have to face cancer in this life, well, that's what the tests and the treatment you're following are for; but, the main axis in your life should not be *I have cancer....*"

3.

DON'T LOSE TRACK: "I believed it was important to be updated on Roberto's health all the time, not allowing days to suddenly go by without me knowing about him and see him again in very bad conditions. I made sure not to let a long period of time go by without finding out personally how things were with him."

4.

HOW TO SUPPORT FRIENDS: "I believe that in supporting Roberto, it's more important for him to know he can count on me and that if he is scared he doesn't have to act like a tough guy. Providing support by saying don't worry, everything is going to be fine is not useful between friends, they should create the possibility of relief, of talking about the real experience." ■

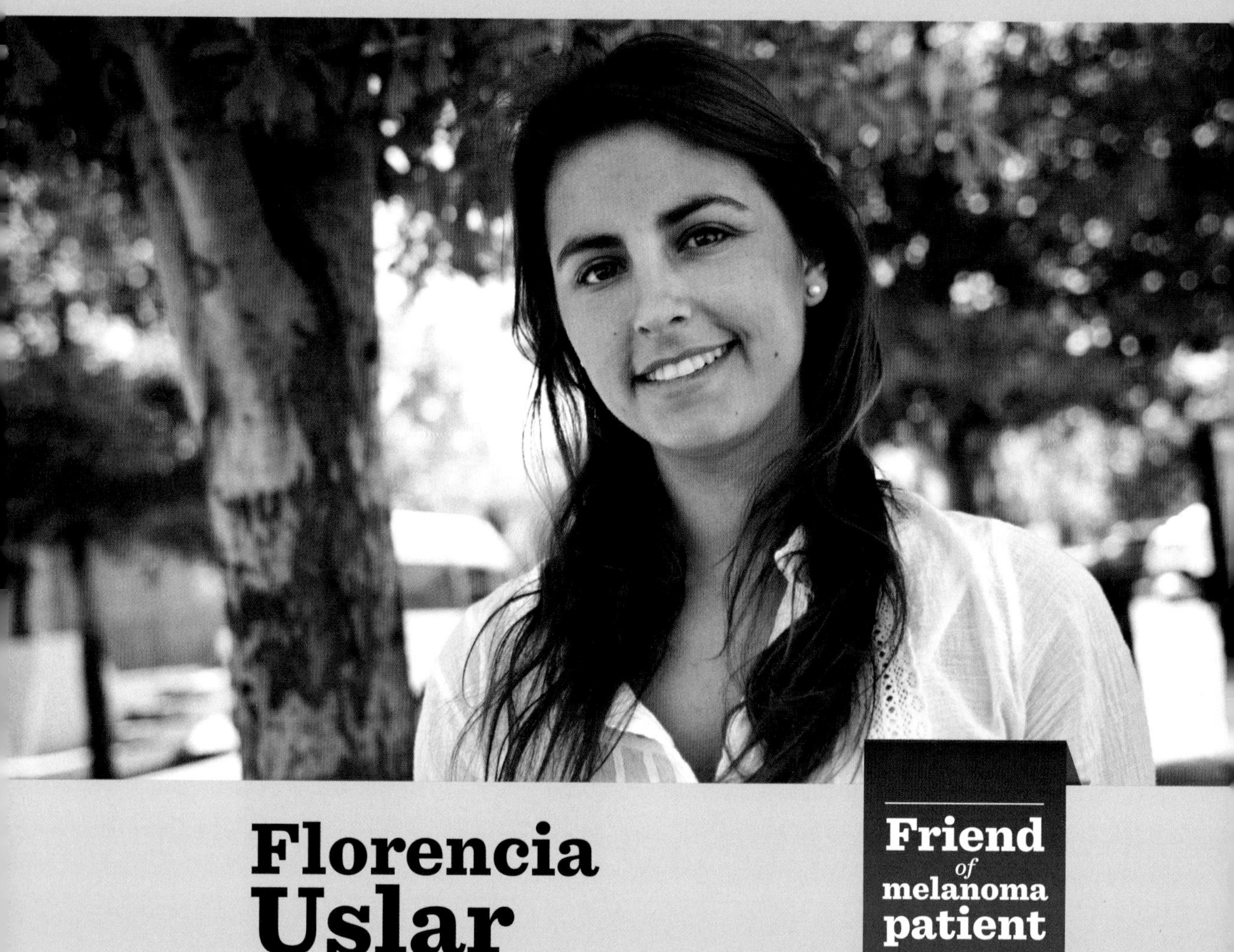

Florencia Uslar

Friend *of* **melanoma patient**

AGE: *27*

OCCUPATION: *BA in Business Administration*

RELATIONSHIP: *Friend of a melanoma patient*

WHEN: *2011*

CONTEXT: *When the bond is friendship, embracing and supporting a cancer patient has its own techniques. A person who is really aware of this is Florencia Uslar, to whom fate brought Roberto Ibañez just as he was starting to understand the diagnosis.*

1.

SPEAK ABOUT CANCER?: "Yes, because it's always an issue. Many of the things he was going through at the moment were because of or somehow related to cancer, because he was at a very vulnerable stage and everything was hitting him three times harder than normal. Besides, when you know your life is at risk and you live waiting for test results that, to some extent, defines your future possibilities of success with a treatment, you reconsider many things which are always worth talking about."

2.

HELP ASSIMILATING THE NEWS: "At the beginning, the best you can do is listen. There are people, like Roberto, whose minds get clearer while they speak. Therefore, when listening with attention and patience, you enable them to create soothing thoughts. On the day of the second diagnosis I hugged him and told him *be calm, that it meant nothing and there are more options left, not everything is said, the next test would also be important.*"

3.

THE ROLE OF A FRIEND: "I met Roberto before he was diagnosed and he was *El Cholo*: good for partying and going out. It hadn't occurred to me sitting beside him to talk about more profound subjects. After this happened, he really changed. He now sees things in a new light and appreciates them more. That's my role as his friend: listen to him venting emotions and being beside him during the process."

4.

ROLE INVERSION: "When my cousin was diagnosed with cancer, it was a strong experience for me, because he had just gotten married and had a whole life in front of him. As soon as I found out, the first person I called was Roberto. Who could better understand what all this was about? He helped me a lot then and it was strange to hear him giving me suggestions on the role I had to take in my family."

5.

GENERAL GUIDELINES: "Having shared a lot of time with people I cherish and who were cancer patients, I believe the best way to face the disease is with lucidity, without letting the idea that you may die gain control. Have positive thoughts, good vibes and live the happiness of each moment, making them feel heard and supported." ■

Loreto Besa

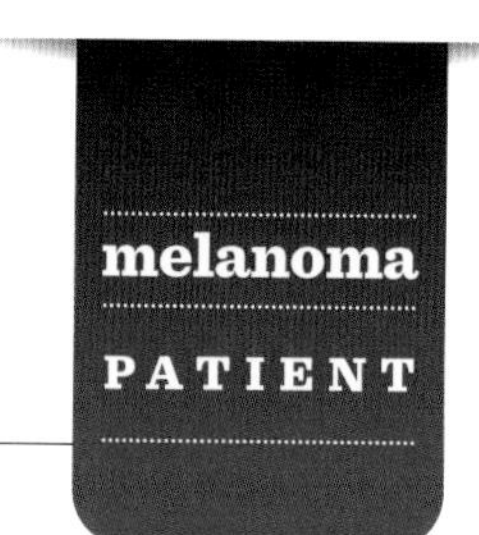

AGE: *50*
OCCUPATION: *hotelier and sales manager*
DIAGNOSIS: *melanoma*
WHEN: *2005*
CONTEXT: *In 2005, Loreto was told to sit before she could hear the results of the biopsy she had undergone ten days before. She had melanoma, a skin cancer which spread very quickly when it is not detected on time. Loreto was lucky. That's why now, after four surgeries and with her disease under control, she doesn't stop highlighting the importance of its prevention by periodic check-ups.*

1.

IMPORTANT MOLES: "I always had lots of moles and with pregnancies more appeared. I had an especially ugly one on my back which I never gave importance to, I didn't imagine the consequences it could have. One day I bent over enough for it to be visible under my dress. A friend was able to see it and told me: 'Loreto, you have a mole there that you should get checked.' Luckily, I followed her advice because it was the right time: If I hadn't had it removed, I wouldn't be telling my story. I now know which moles are risky if they increase sizes. I've had four moles removed since I carefully check them up."

2.

THE STRENGTH IS WITHIN YOU: "When I thought about the pain I could cause others, I found a special strength. At first, I felt almost beaten down because I had cancer, but then I started feeling that this wouldn't defeat me, how would I cause them such pain? That worry, that sadness of not wanting to cause such pain to my loved ones, is where I took my strength from."

3.

YOU CAN MAKE YOUR OWN DIAGNOSIS: "I now know my body and look at my moles. The doctor who conducted my surgery taught me that those which grow, have irregular borders and different colors may be melanomas. Therefore, I make my own diagnosis. Self-care and control. If you do this on time, you are saved."

4.

APPREHENSION VS. OPTIMISM: "When you're too apprehensive you trigger worry and excess pain. You need to be moderate, because you don't win anything by being desperate and crying thinking the world is over. You need to take it easy and commit the necessary time to it, and then forget about everything, except your check-ups."

"No, it is not going to *win*, *How* could I cause them such pain?"

5.

MESSAGES FROM CANCER: *"I believe life needs to suddenly shake you for you to understand what the most important thing is. Working in excess, postponing children, lifestyles. In my case, melanoma was a warning.* ■

Diana Strauss

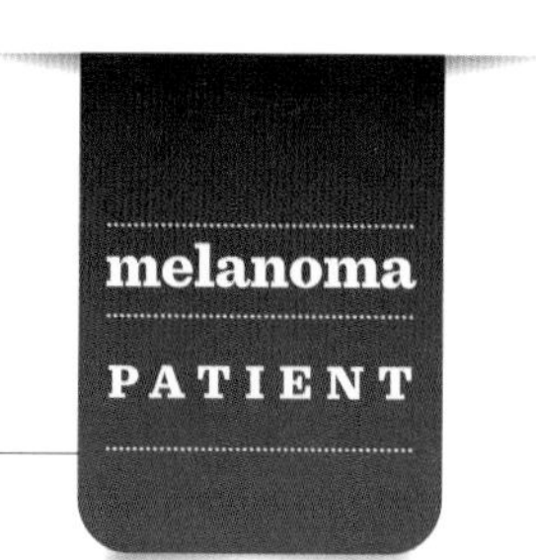

AGE: *40*
OCCUPATION: *Self-educated student on health and diets*
DIAGNOSIS: *Melanoma*
WHEN: *1999*
CONTEXT: *At the age of 24, Diana found a very small blue mole in her thigh which itched a lot. It was an encapsulated stage II melanoma; but the strong experience she lived triggered questions and opened former wounds that had never been closed.*

1.

SEEKING FOR REASONS: "One of the reasons I thought I had developed cancer was because I had gone through difficult episodes, where fear was a constant emotion. When I was diagnosed with melanoma, after being paranoid at first, I reached a stage in which I asked: *what is really going on here?* I told myself: *I have an injury in my skin which is located there because my body and immune system are not working correctly; they couldn't defend me properly.* And so I faced this situation and freed myself."

2.

PROVIDE A MEANING: *"I assigned cancer a sense of opportunity to learn to build my individuality in a more empowered way."*

3.

CANCER AS THE DRIVING FORCE FOR CHANGE: "Every situation you live is saved in the body and generates emotional stages which work in their way and lead to a change in you. Cells work differently when you're happy than when you're depressed; therefore, a constant state of depression will alter your molecular formation and will help the development of some health situations. Melanoma was that: a hard landing which forced me to undergo constant check-ups. I now live each situation searching how to change negative emotions into positive ones."

"I assigned cancer a sense of ***opportunity,*** to learn to *build* my individuality".

4.

TRANSFORM FEAR: "When you have cancer, what you feel the most is fear. The first thing you think is you're going to die and this is why processing fear turns into a crucial task: you have to do it or, otherwise, you get sick."

5.

HOW I UNDERSTOOD THIS: "Cancer is a deep wound in your heart, in your life. It's something that harmed you a lot, or harmed you for a long time. Cancer is also the possibility of opening your eyes to life and being more conscious, of waking up." ■

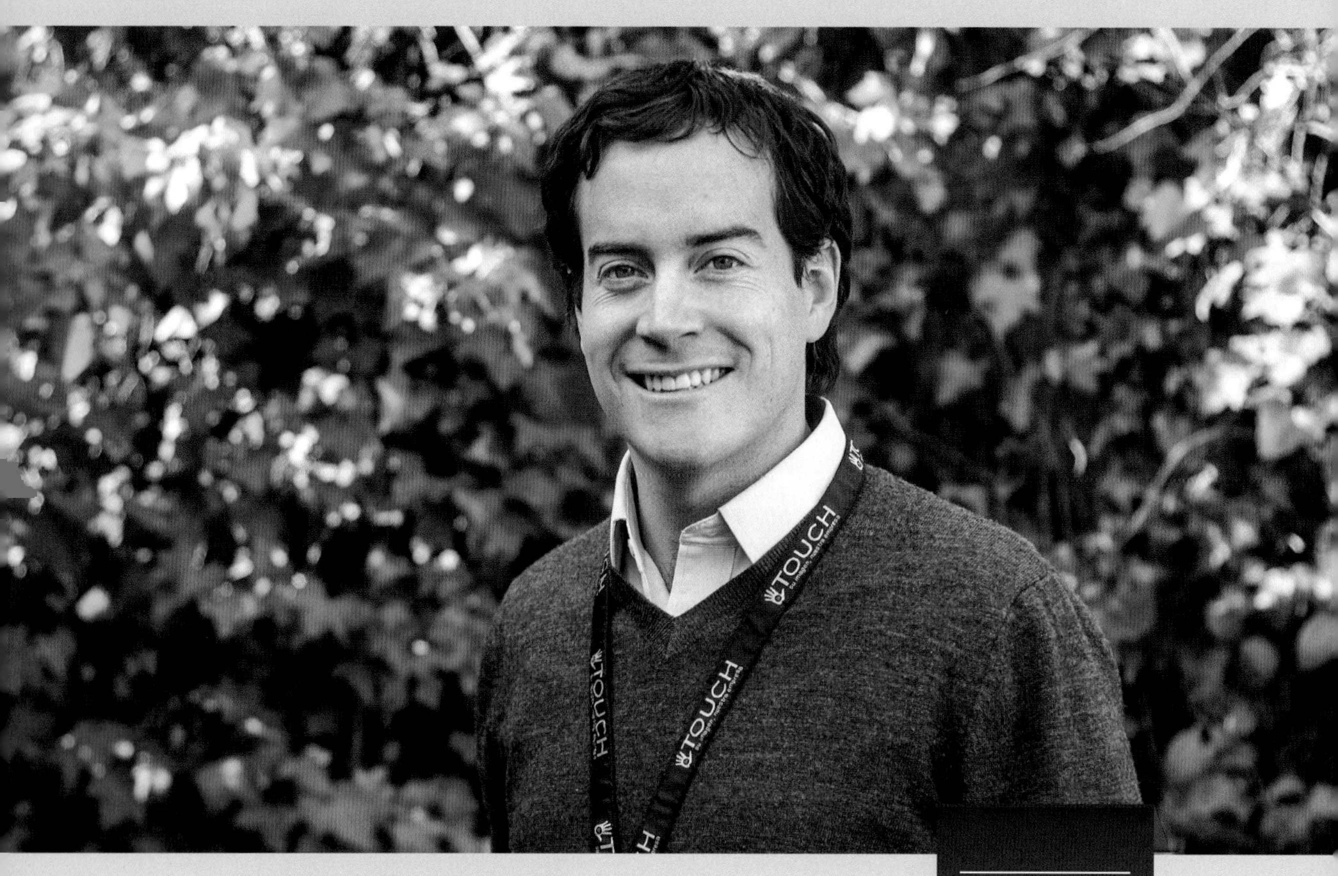

Antonio Monckeberg

Friend *of* **melanoma patient**

AGE: *31*

OCCUPATION: *BA in Business Administration*

RELATIONSHIP: *Workmate of a melanoma patient*

WHEN: *2011*

CONTEXT: *Antonio is a partner and the commercial manager for Touch, the company that he founded with Roberto Ibanez and what he ran while he allowed Roberto to focus on his treatment.*

1.

HOW TO SUPPORT A WORKMATE: "I aimed at making him understand he was indispensable. I wanted him to know that, beyond the uncertainty and urgency of his situation, he was necessary at Touch. Then, when the disease decreased and he was feeling better, I asked him to help me with concrete duties, in which he is an expert, and indispensable for Touch.

2.

NOT TO ALWAYS TALK ABOUT IT: At first we often asked Roberto about the situation but later we tried to steer conversations away from the subject. If he was already spending 99% of his time thinking about it what was the point of us asking him questions that would bring it back to the forefront of his mind?"

"I **propose** to make him understand he was *indispensable*. He was ***necessary*** in Touch."

3.

TAKE HIM AWAY FROM SELF-ABSORPTION: "When someone faces serious problems, they become self-absorbed. If I saw Roberto like that, I asked for his help for a project and included him in the relevant team, because at Touch people rejoice when he is part of a project. I believe it made him feel always important, and although he had less time on his hands, key to the team."

4.

OFFICE MANNERS: "My recommendation is try to see a workmate with cancer as the person they have always been, not as someone different. They're just going through a different process. There was no pity in Touch. Roberto is a valuable asset to the team and the attitude at Touch was that if he was going to be less in the office then we just had to make better use of the time he could spend with us."

5.

NO DRAMA AT THE OFFICE: "In Touch we chose not to dramatize the disease, although we assumed it was going to take time and we couldn't know how long Roberto's absence would last." ■

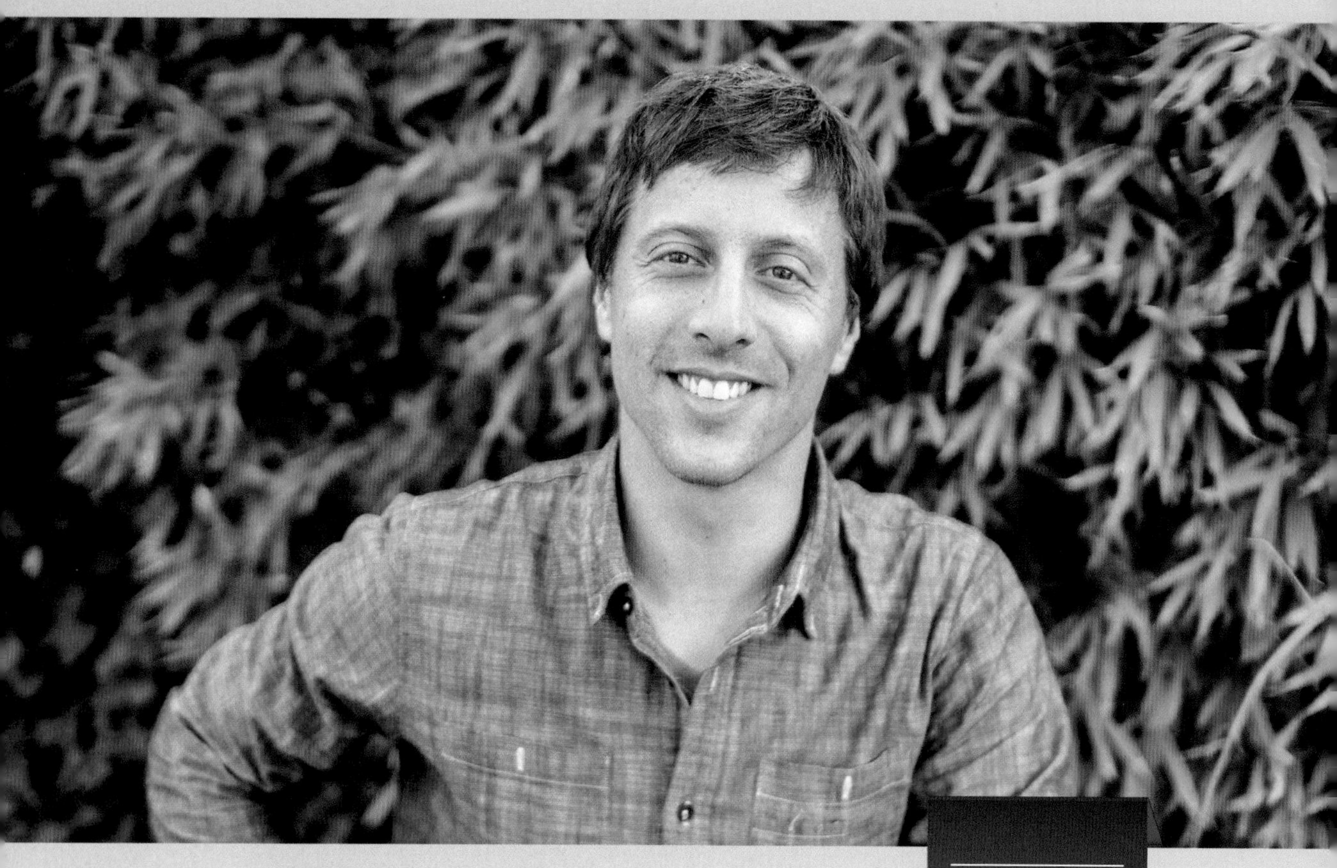

Eduardo Pérez de Castro

Friend *of* melanoma patient

AGE: *39*

OCCUPATION: *Industrial Civil Engineer*

RELATIONSHIP: *Friend of a melanoma patient*

WHEN: *2011*

CONTEXT: *From several years, Eduardo has been a friend of Roberto Ibáñez through the sports they both practice, especially kite. Eduardo knew about the fragility that lies below the armor of youth and gave Roberto all his support.*

1.

THE MYTH OF THE INVINCIBLE: "Youth gives you a feeling that you're invincible; you never feel fragile. You never expect cancer, these problems are always far-off, so when it happens to a friend the shock is huge, especially if they're younger than you (Roberto is eight years younger than me)."

2.

HOW TO APPROACH THE ISSUE: "In order to speak with the patient you need to be delicate, but don't use euphemisms, because it is crucial to have an open conversation, without *hiding in the bushes*. This kind of news makes you understand your time may be limited, because –although nobody wants to say it– it's a possibility."

3.

THE FAMILY SHIELD: "I believe that, in these complicated situations, what fills you with energy to get by is feeling the love, tenderness and energy of those who are close to you. It's incredible how close I felt Roberto's family was. The way they organized and assumed tasks and responsibilities was really nice."

4.

SPORTS THERAPY: *"I can feel it. When I go through very stressful periods, in work and all, my great escape is going to the beach, taking my kite or surf board and diving into the sea. I have an amazing job that brings serious consequences for my actions and any mistakes I might make. The moment I dive into the water I can switch off and be somewhere else in my head."* ■

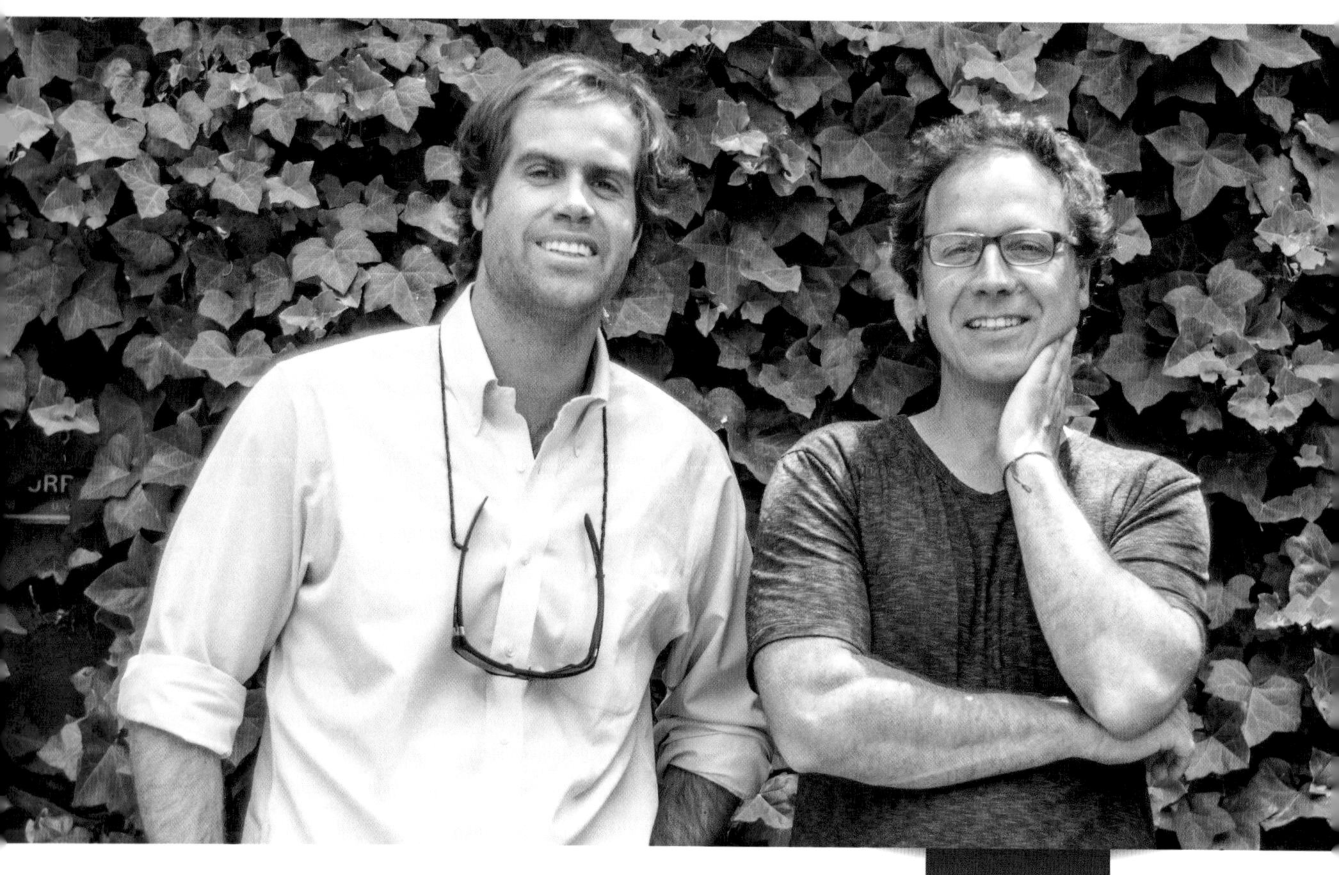

Guillermo Acuña

melanoma

PATIENT

AGE: *51*

OCCUPATION: *Architect*

DIAGNOSIS: *Melanoma*

WHEN: *2012*

CONTEXT: *After having eye surgery, Guillermo learned to live with his disease, rejecting conventional therapies which are invasive and massively destroy cells. He is a living testimony that, sometimes, the most effective treatments start from an inner awakening.*

1.

DO IT YOURSELF: "Try understanding what you have, don't make others responsible for it. Understand what the problem is, how it developed, at what stage you are and how you think you can be saved."

2.

TELL ME WHAT YOU EAT: "Melanoma is a symptom that an organ is not working properly in your body. If my melanoma is related to my liver and skin, I believe it's reasonable to think that diets played an important role in their appearance and –after having overcome the disease– in it not spreading. It's all about chemistry, that's why I believe eating healthy foods helps prevent the disease proliferating and to support the body."

3.

THE DANGER OF EXPECTATIONS: "Invasive treatments place you in the dilemma of the survival expectancy, its percentages and probabilities. On the contrary, when you live one day at the time, the variable of expectations is eliminated."

4.

IT'S A MATTER OF DISCIPLINE: "I do certain activities, such as going once a month to get balance and alignment massages. Music therapy has also helped. Both therapies help reorganizing corporal energy channels and feeling balanced. They help remembering that, from time to time, you need to establish new limits and for this you require discipline and conviction."

5.

HELP YOUR BODY: "Your body completely regenerates every seven years and you become a whole new person in terms of your cells. Our organism gets intoxicated through air and food, two things that access our body and may cause diseases. I now try to eat well, but we all continue breathing a horrible air. This needs to be compensated to some extent."

6.

PERSONAL STRATEGY: "I have chosen to avoid being surrounded by people with cancer. I know this sounds selfish, but it's because I suffered when those close to me die, so I don't get near them anymore." ■

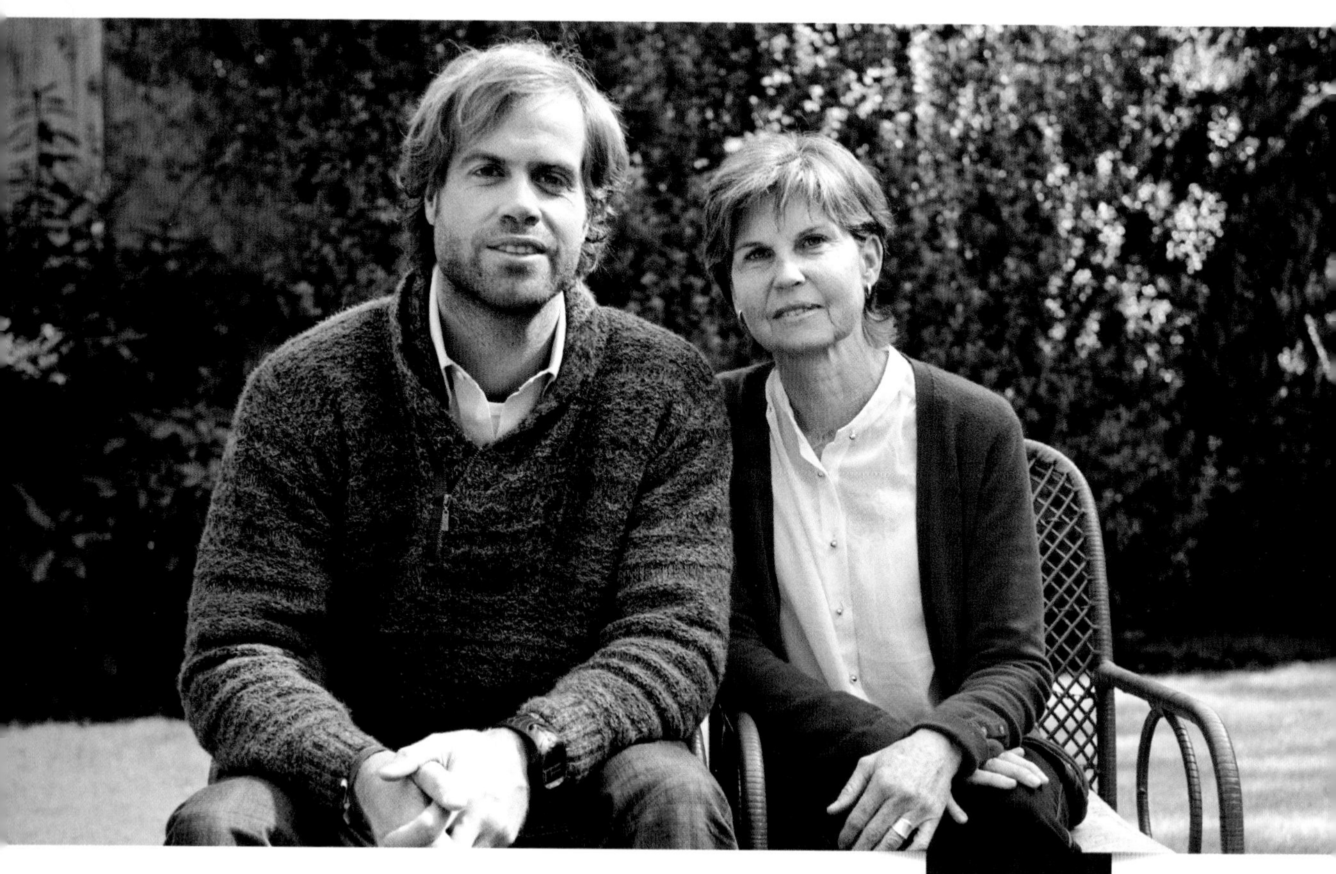

Quequi Mingo

skin cancer

PATIENT

AGE: *60*

OCCUPATION: *Tapestry artist*

DIAGNOSIS: *Skin cancer*

WHEN: *2005*

CONTEXT: *Her four children were still young when she learned that she needed an urgent lung and kidney transplant. It was hard, but a donor was found. After surgery she discovered that the strong drugs prescribed to avoid organ rejection gave her a carcinoma, and then at 50 her life again took on a dramatic twist.*

1.

YOU START THE FIGHT: "Attitude is key. I always knew my transplant and its consequences would not defeat me, because there was no way I would leave my four children. This made me stand firm and prepare to get by."

2.

TO AVOID FIGHTING WITH THE CATHETER: "In order to hide the catheter, I used t-shirts and buttoned sweaters. I used the catheter underneath and attached the tubes on the back in a backpack I used all the time. It was funny because when somebody came to see me and I opened the door, they would ask me if I was going out... I never remembered I was wearing it, except during night and morning treatments.

3.

WITH YOUR CHILDREN, PUT ON YOUR BEST FACE: "I minimized my pain in front of my children and I do this even now. I don't need to tell my children I feel sick if I know something is not serious. If they were worried, they did badly at school, didn't go out to play and felt sad. My children have always seen a mom with energy to move forward."

4.

TAKING CARE OF YOURSELF IS A MUST: *"Your life belongs to you, and there is no one who can take better care of yourself than you. Neither your mom, children nor closest friend will take better care of you, because you know what you're going through and know your body, when it's working correctly and when it's not."* ■

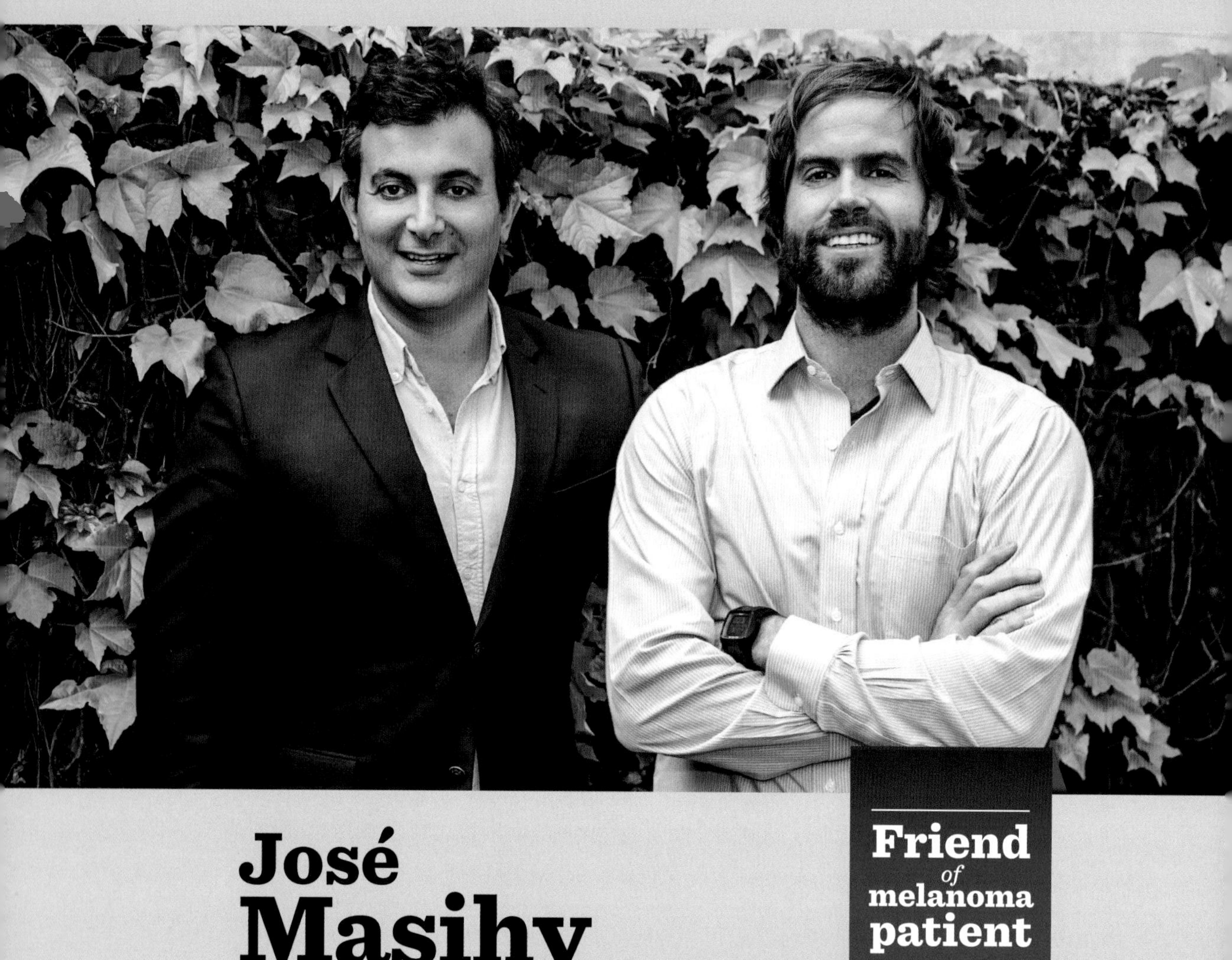

José Masihy

Friend *of* **melanoma patient**

AGE: *32*

OCCUPATION: *Founding partner at Touch*

RELATIONSHIP: *Friend of a melanoma patient*

WHEN: *2011*

CONTEXT: *José is a friend of Roberto Ibáñez since university and together they founded Touch when they were on their twenties. Since then they have walked a solid professional path together. José was the first one to arrive to the clinic when Roberto went into surgery. He has provided his unconditional support throughout Roberto's recovery.*

1.

PREVENTION FROM THE HEAD: "I truly believe all these diseases come from emotions. In my family there are many cases of skin cancer and I have seen this. One of the important things my mom taught me was not holding on to material or physical things, and being a good manager of my life. A good manager knows that the good and bad things that happen, most of the time, depend on and are the responsibility of every person, so you need to face challenges in the best possible way, handling the freedom that has been given correctly, without affecting other people's freedom."

2.

RESPECT LIMITS: "Everybody is different. Some need more affection and require you to be closer. Others need their own space; therefore, you can't be always be pushing and talking about the disease because, in the end, they will get tired and this won't help the patient or the people around them. You have to have sufficient tact to address the matter at the right time."

3.

PROVIDE THE NECESSARY SUPPORT: "People with cancer, at the beginning, don't know what is happening to them and it's hard for them to understand. Doctors don't find this easy to explain either, so, as a friend, you need to offer support and say we'll find out. It's important not making cancer a tragedy, but a phase in life that needs to be overcome to move forward. And that you'll be there to provide support."

4.

KNOW HOW TO READ EMOTIONS: "A person with cancer jumps from one emotion to another, and as a friend you learn how to interpret and approach the issue properly. If you intervene too much, you may make the other person feel anxious. You need to provide calmness and, above all, commitment, love, space and unconditional support."

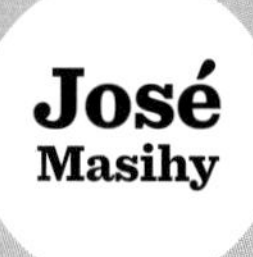

5.

SUPPORT A FRIEND: "You need to hug them and tell them that you're there for them, that they'll overcome the problem. You don't want them to feel down, because that just makes everything worse. Let them know you're always there. Find a way to cheer them up. Always be full of energy and strength when you're around them. Crying and being upset around them really doesn't help."

6.

WORKMATE ATTITUDE: "My advice to any workmate of a cancer patient is to take them out of their medical environment to help make them feel better. If you're close, listen to them when they need someone to pour their heart out to. If they want to come to the office, make it possible."

"I truly **believe** all these diseases come from *emotions*."

7.

GROW POSITIVE EMOTIONS: "I know we're all going to die, but cancer is such a strong disease, it can take you before your time and I will do all I humanly can for this not to happen to anyone. That's why I'm such a pain in the ass in relation to emotions: you need to have a good time, within the margins of the disease, and not spin around thoughts and ideas that can cause even more stress."

8.

HEART LYSATE: "My mom's sister was given two months to live due to cancer. She finally lived 12 more years thanks to a drug she found in Uruguay. The drug was heart Lysate, now sold as Bio Vital, which raises your defenses when you go through chemotherapy. This natural drug, a healthy diet and mud poultice made my aunt better."

9.

AVOID PROBLEMS IN LIFE: "Considering other people's problems as your own is never a good idea. A person needs to understand that they first need to lead their own lives, enjoy what they have done and share it with their families. Be calm and avoid making too much trouble about things that happen. Assuming problems is one thing, but being problematic all the time is another."

10.

OPEN UP TO FREEDOM: "Problems come from your mind and emotions. Then, if you don't talk about your stuff, if you don't feel capable of sharing your fears and uncertainties, you cannot feel calm. Deep inside, you cannot be free."

"It's important *not to make* cancer into a tragedy, but understanding that it's a phase in life that needs to be overcome and **surpassed.**"

11.

BE CLEAR WITH THE PATIENT: *"In my experience, any cancer patient would like for everybody to be as honest as possible with with them, starting with their own doctors and their responsibility to make good explanations of issues, risks, procedures and probabilities. Finally, ambiguity isn't helpful because a cancer patient needs a clear head to be able to feel in control of the situation. It's frustrating to feel they can't take control of their destiny."* ■

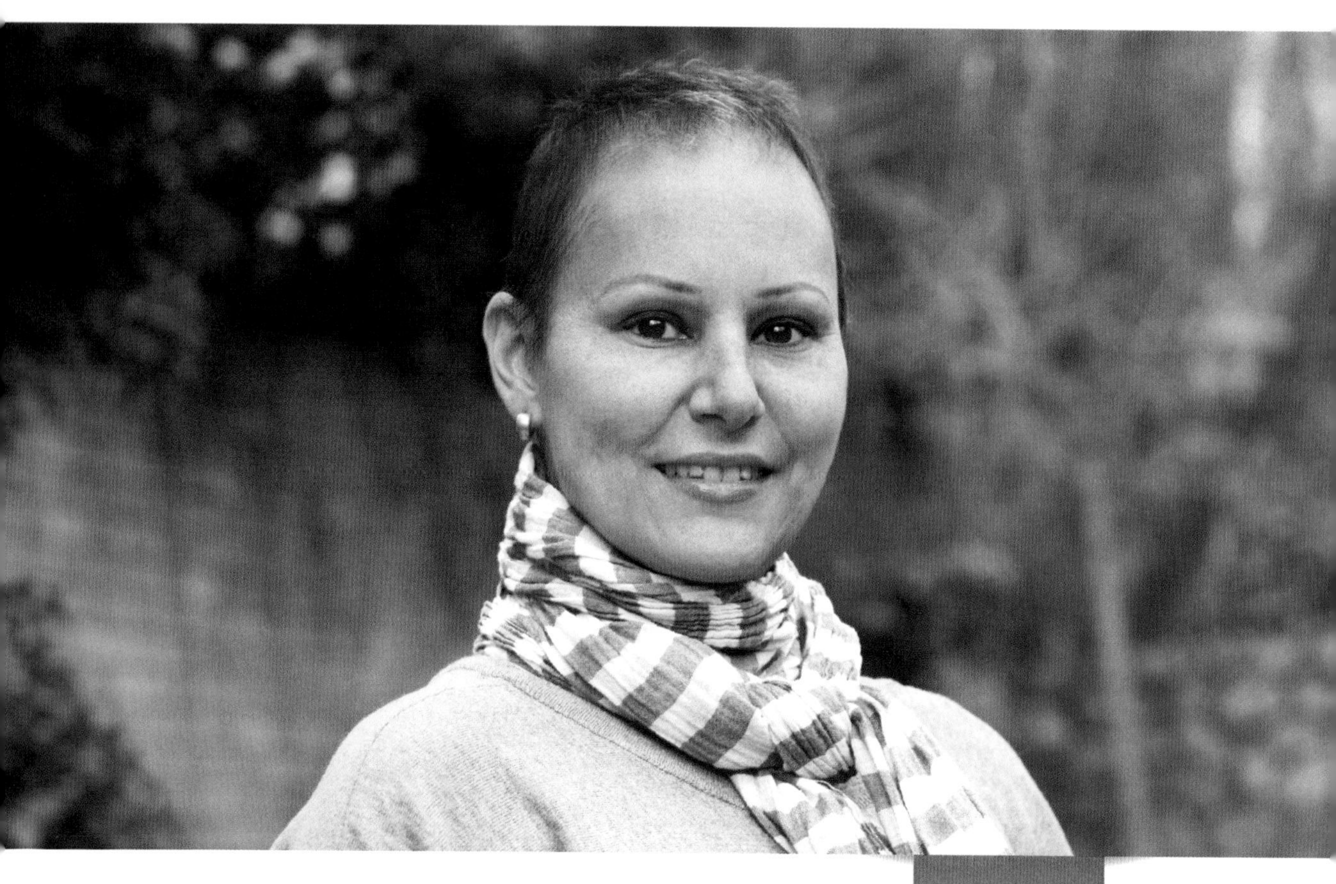

Marcela Lorenzini

breast cancer

PATIENT

AGE: *43*

OCCUPATION: *Special education teacher*

DIAGNOSIS: *Breast cancer*

WHEN: *2005*

CONTEXT: *Marcela was diagnosed with breast cancer with metastases in the nodes and the liver, which is very complicated to treat. She wanted to give her son Alberto a brother, but a lump she detected on her body made her visit a doctor first. She had all tests conducted in three days and a special treatment protocol was followed, because her metastasis was really aggressive. She never lost the desire to live and resisted firmly for nine years, until she passed away on Wednesday, May 21st 2014. Here you will find her testimony, which now is a legacy.*

1.

LIVE WITH IT, NOT FOR IT: "From the minute I was diagnosed with cancer I told myself I wouldn't live for cancer, I would live with it. This has become my slogan and gives me strength to live enjoying each day. I have a normal routine, I go out and go on vacations. I believe it's important to spread your love to the family and remember how wonderful it is to share, talk and pamper each other, always living in the moment."

2.

NORMALITY: "My son Alberto, who is now ten years old, has gone with me to some chemotherapies. He lies in bed, watches TV, and does his homework and plays. The first time my chemotherapy sessions were interrupted, I took him to a psychologist to be examined. I am pleased to say the psychologist told me he was doing fine, because I tried for the situation to be as normal as possible."

3.

TAKE IT NATURALLY: "I never wore a wig. When I lost my hair, it turned out that I had a nice head so the issue didn't bother me or my husband. My son was younger than two years old, thus we decided to face the situation so as naturally as possible. He now remembers his mom without hair, but I show him pictures of me with hair and he understands his mom has a bug and that's the reason she goes to the clinic."

4.

ADJUST PROJECTS: "When facing this disease, it is key for you to review your life plan. Before this, we wanted to have another son, travel, study abroad, but we can't do all these things anymore. Creating a new life plan helps a lot and allows us to enjoy each day we are given. Despite the diagnosis related to death, we are not dead: we have the chance of doing things, expressing love and enjoying everything that surrounds us."

5.

TREATMENT IS TO LIVE, NOT TO KILL CANCER: "When I went to have chemotherapy, I liked staying at a room that had a window which looked directly to a tree. I felt the tree represented life and I was there to live, not to kill cancer."

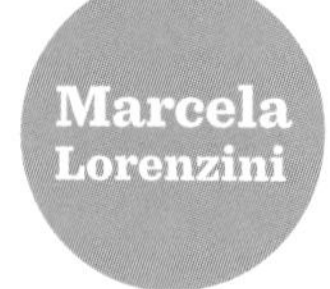

6.

PAIN WITH A PURPOSE: "From the first day I learned to offer my pain to God and to those who suffer, and this helped me assign a meaning to the situation and strengthen my spirit. I now avoid focusing on pain, on the treatment's consequences, and instead I focus on the meaning of my existence."

"When I go to chemotherapy I use something **white** to represent light and divine *love*."

7.

CHOOSE THE NURSE: *"If I'm going to undergo chemotherapy, the first thing I do is check the nurses present at the clinic. I like for long-established nurses to inject me and if a new one arrives, I ask for a nurse I already know. I understand they may not like it, but they inject you and continue with their lives; in turn, if I get a badly placed injection, it is me who is going to be carrying that my whole life."*

8.

WARM RELATIONSHIPS: "Without looking for it, you start being friends with nurses and assistant nurses, it's something special. That's why I don't think I am going to have chemotherapy, but that I'm going to meet people who care about me and so I don't wake up in a bad mood that day. I undergo chemotherapies on Mondays so that I'm rested at the weekends."

9.

WEAR WHITE: "Every time I go to chemotherapy I use something white to represent light and divine love."

10.

LIVE TO REMEMBER: "The three of us usually go everywhere together. It's very important for me to be with Luis and Alberto, because we bond and create memories. I have started to understand that memories give you life, because they make you feel you're with people."

"You need to think about *new projects* that make you **as happy** as the ones you had before the disease."

11.

FEEL BLESSED: "In spite of having cancer, I am thankful for receiving treatment at a good place, my doctor is really warm and professional, and nurses and assistant nurses have been very warm. My parents have been beside me with their care and love, and a good friend has always been by my side; her dedication, patience and help with transportation were key during the first period. Family, friends and acquaintances express their love in different ways that nurture you with their time and mood."■

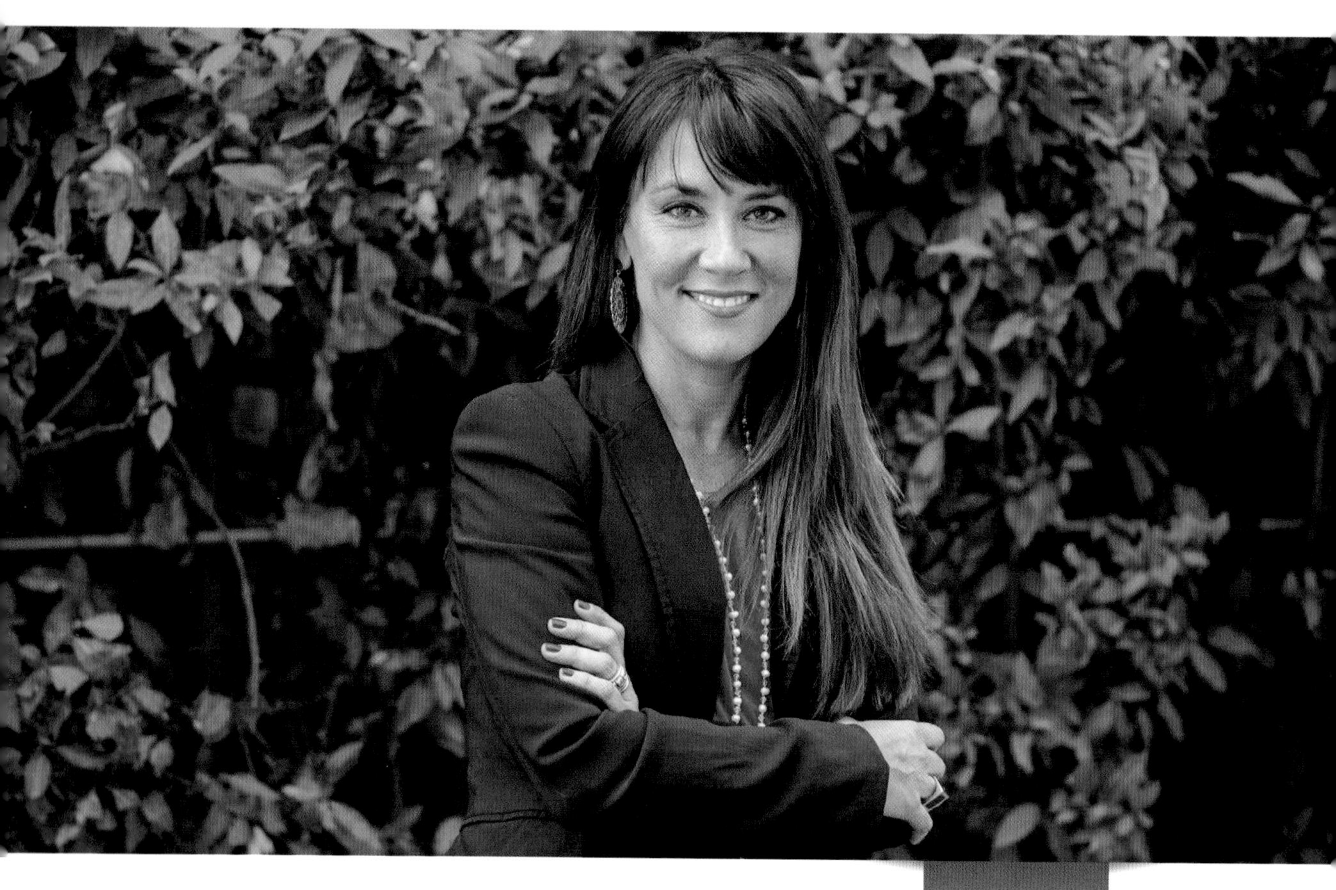

María Paz Aldunate

breast cancer

PATIENT

AGE: *42*

OCCUPATION: *Lawyer*

DIAGNOSIS: *Breast cancer*

WHEN: *2008*

CONTEXT: *María Paz was 35, and had two daughters of 4 and 2 years old when she was diagnosed with extended ductal carcinoma in situ on her right breast. She had a mastectomy with immediate reconstruction. María Paz was willing to have a double mastectomy at the time, but doctors asked her to assess the true risk of having cancer on the other breast before deciding. A year later, and with medical approval, she had a mastectomy of her left breast and a subsequent reconstruction. "I knew I would live more calmly" she explains.*

1.

THINKING ON THE FUTURE: "Not being able to breastfeed again is one of the things I considered before I had the mastectomy. But I thought: it is what it is and that's it. I need to get by and win this war. It was an option which allowed me to have a better prognosis and be calmer, and I believed it was key to do all I could to be with my little girls and husband. That's why I never regretted the decision and I still believe it was the best one."

2.

AFTER TOTAL MASTECTOMY: "The scars I now have are war injures which are part of my story and make me remember having lived and, I hope, overcome the disease. Anyways, time is on your side and the appearance of those scars start to mitigate. Using dermatological scar creams, among other things, such as lassar's paste and silicone sheets, which are sold in drugstores, helped me a lot."

"The scars I now have are **war injures.** They are part of my *story* and may be concealed if I need it."

3.

GOODBYE TO UNDERWIRE BRAS: "I now use seamless sport bras because I don't need to use wires anymore, they bother me. Apart from being comfortable, you need to see the bright side. For instance, having silicones allows me to do some things, such as running and being more comfortable, or wearing strapless dresses that many of my friends can't wear."

4.

SELF-ESTEEM: "I spent one year with only one breast that had been operated on and they ended up looking really different. This is quite important. Implants made out of silicone are much harder, but you finally get used to it. I used inserts to make them even; they looked quite symmetrical. In summer I used strapless bikinis because they hid imperfections and scars better. I have now assumed and been reconciled with that part of my body, and thanks to my husband's support, I feel a stronger woman in all aspects." ■

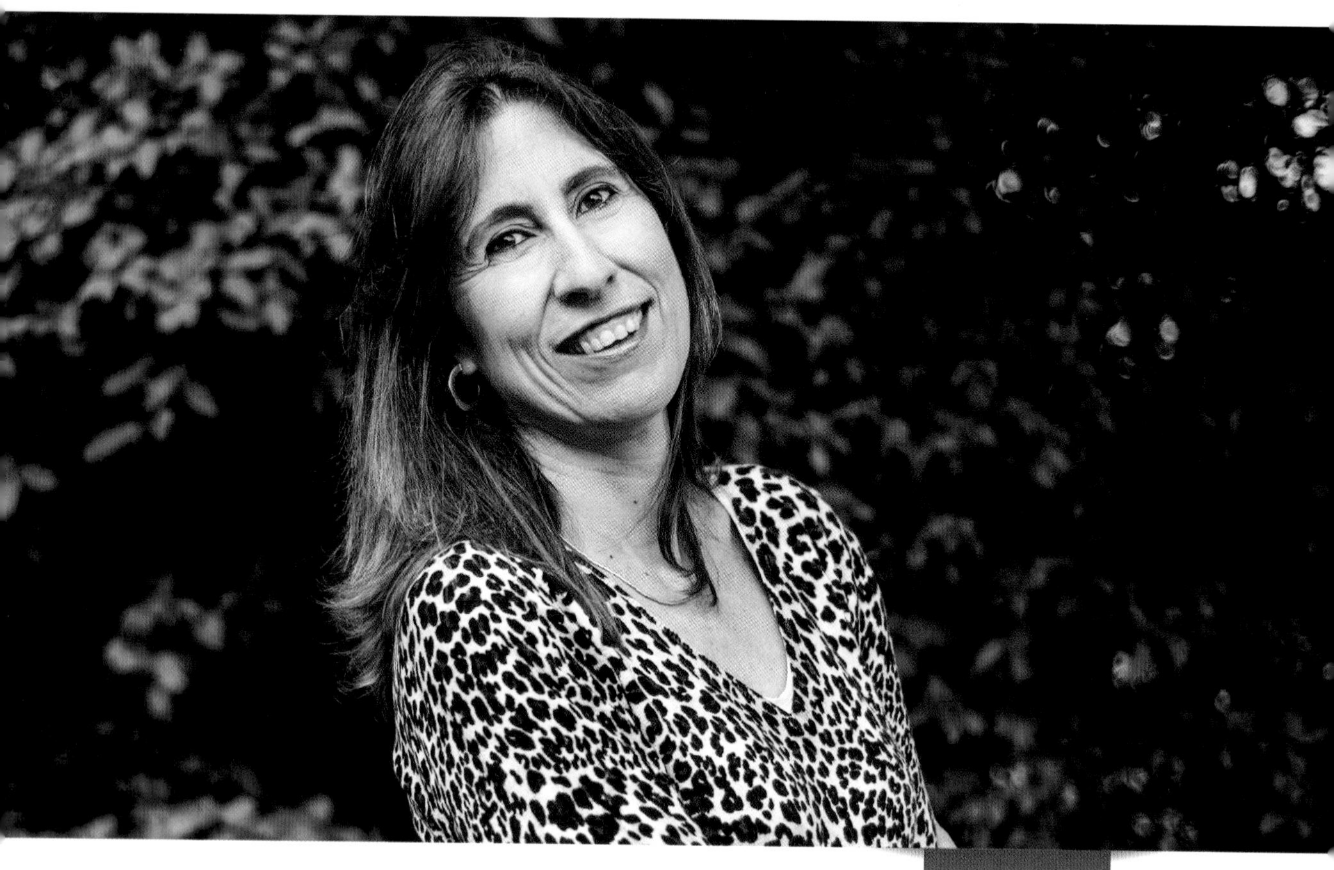

Paula Warnken

breast cancer
PATIENT

AGE: *52*

OCCUPATION: *Protocol assistant*

DIAGNOSIS: *Breast cancer with bone metastasis*

WHEN: *1999*

CONTEXT: *without any apparent reason, just because she felt she had to, Paula had a mammogram at the age of 35, before she went to live to the United States. "A bean showed up. It was the first voluntary medical test I had in my life and I "won the prize" she recalls. It was quickly removed and she had radiotherapy. However, five years later a metastasis from her breast cancer was discovered in her humerus. This time she had chemotherapy and radiotherapy, as well as having her ovaries removed.*

1.

POSITIVE THINKING: "Even what you read and the people with whom you make relationships with must be full of light. When I finally travelled to the US, after receiving my second treatment, doctors told me that between two patients with the same diagnosis, the one with the most positive spirit has better possibilities of recovery."

2.

FILTER: *"Everyone has their bit of advice, but your head gets saturated. It's good to read and chat, but you need to learn to use a filter. Aloe Vera is not useful for all of us; taking meat out of your diet won't save everyone."*

"*Feeling* **loved** makes you feel fantastic, because you think 'I'm needed in this earth, ***I can't*** die now'."

3.

EXPELLING SORROW IS A BASIC: "If you have been diagnosed with cancer, being afraid or feeling rage is normal. You need to cry, expel the sorrow, because having cancer is that: a great sorrow. Writing was useful to me. My psycho-oncologist Jennifer Middleton, who wrote a book called *I (don't) want to have cancer*, encouraged me to write and it was very therapeutic. I wrote some long notebooks for each my two sons and they still ask to read it."

4.

SEARCHING FOR BALANCE: "Everyone knows what their own equilibrium is: family, friends, diets, exercise. You learn to recognize when something makes you feel good and when it does not. Although it's impossible to ignore everything that makes you feel bad, you need to make an effort to listen to your body."

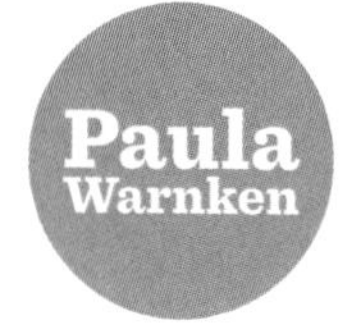

5.

OPEN UP TO SUPPORT NETWORKS: “Feeling you are loved makes you feel fantastic, because you think you’re needed in this earth and you can’t die now. Feeling love is always great, we all like to be told *I love you.*”

6.

GIVE CHEMOTHERAPY A NEW POINT OF VIEW: “The idea of chemotherapy may be scary, but when I was in the clinic, with the drug going into my veins, I looked at it and said: *you’re not my enemy, you’re my ally, you will heal me, and you’re welcome.*”

7.

HELP YOURSELF WITH SUPPLEMENTARY THERAPIES: “I had magnets applied and reiki. I also practiced yoga at the Mukti center in Vitacura [Santiago, Chile]. I took Bach flowers, did relaxation exercises and meditated. It is key to find what you feel more comfortable with and not doing alternative therapies if you don’t believe in them, because that makes no sense.”

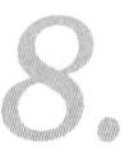

TALK AND LISTEN: “It is really good to be with people who have experienced what you have and have recovered. Before undergoing the first chemotherapy I was terrified, but I spoke to a woman who had had brain cancer and our conversation was essential. I now talk to every person, because I learned the importance of knowing someone with the same disease and who is now doing well.”

9.

THINK ABOUT YOU: "One of my everyday tasks at night was to stop and think what I have done for me during that day, what I have liked, what was the minute I spent for me. In essence, it was about spending time each day on me and not always on others. For instance, I tried to play tennis when I felt well because it really calmed me down."

"Aloe Vera is not useful *for all* of us; stopping eating meat won't save everyone. In some way you learn to recognize when something makes you ***feel good*** and when it does not."

10.

RESTRICT SELF-INFORMATION: *"You don't only need to be surrounded by optimism, but it is also important to be exposed to positive information. A friend's husband was diagnosed with pancreatic cancer and the first thing I told him was not to surf the Internet, because there you only find misfortunes which provide little help to keep your mood positive."* ■

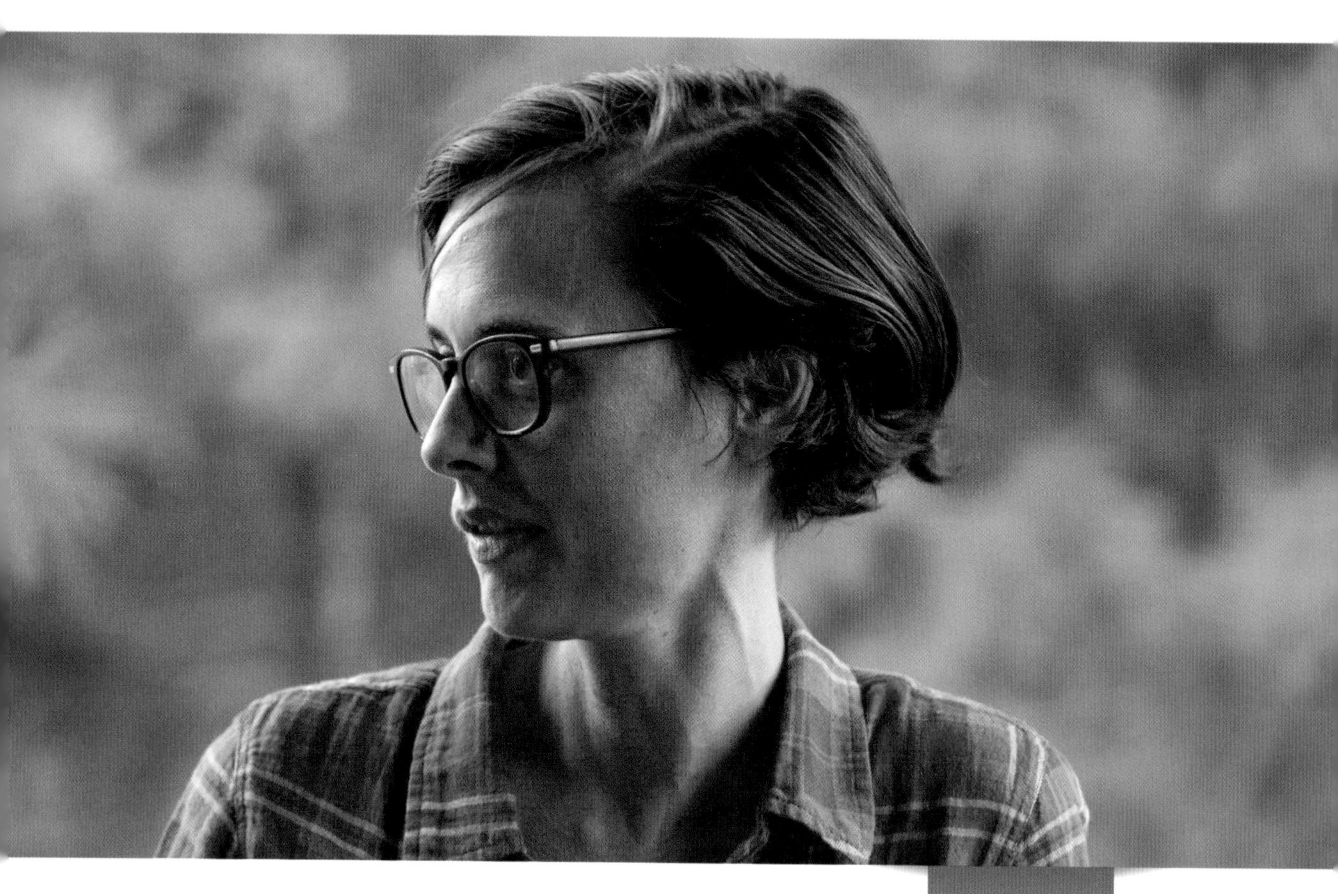

Natalie Conforti

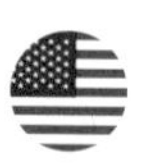

breast cancer PATIENT

AGE: *14, 25, 28*
OCCUPATION: *Designer*
DIAGNOSIS: *non-Hodgkin's T-cell lymphoma, parotid tumor, breast cancer*
WHEN: *Diagnosed in 1994 at age 14, then 2004 at age 25 then again in 2007 at age 28*
CONTEXT: *I've had cancer three times. As a teen, I faced the worst of it and went through a full year of radiation and chemotherapy treatments. The second time, I had started an industrial design program, and could not face having to delay my studies for illness so the parotid tumor was treated as I began my program. By the third, I was aware of the young adult cancer community and it was much easier meet others thanks to groups like Stupid Cancer and First Descents.*

1.

BE CLEAR WITH YOURSELF AND OTHERS: "Including family, supportive friends, and medical professionals what it is that you need from each of them every step of the way. It'll be much easier on you if you are able to do this from the start. People want to help, they often don't know how or what to say in order to do so."

2.

EDUCATE YOURSELF: "Get as much information as you can possible handle before making any decisions regarding your treatments. Doctors will often push for a quick decision, but unless they demand it you can research using the information they offer to come to your own conclusion using the time you need. If your doctor won't allow a second opinion, or treats your medical decisions as though they are inconsequential find another doctor."

"Do your best to *listen* without being **judgmental.** You will be able to hear ***much more*** that way."

3.

THERE IS SOMEONE WITHIN THE MEDICAL SYSTEM YOU HAVE ACCESS TO: "Be it a doctor, a nurse, an acupuncturist, etc. who you trust. Let that person guide you through some of the medical insanity. It's a long, rough ride, someone who knows the system can help to guide you through it, or at least make your time within it more bearable. A good friend, or a nurse who becomes your friend along the way who knows the ropes can often help beyond belief."

4.

WORK ON TELLING YOUR DANCE STORY WHILE YOU ARE LIVING IT:

"Organizations such as Send It, Esperity, First Descents, mAss Kickers, A Fresh Chapter, etc. will give you the time away from your everyday life to reflect and listen to others who not only have been where you are, but are doing amazing things as a result. They will inspire you as you inspire them to continue on in a positive manner."

5.

FIND A DIET THAT WORKS WELL FOR YOUR BODY AND STICK WITH IT:

"I find it easiest to maintain a diet when I do all of my own cooking, but eating out is part of socializing. Try not to be too hard on yourself if you don't always stick with a diet. I love cooking soups, stews, salads, and roasts because they're simple and can be filled with the freshest ingredients."

6.

BUILD EXERCISE INTO YOUR DAILY ROUTINE:

"I try to build it into my commute by commuting to a local job, but others do so by taking public transportation and getting off at a stop a mile or two before they have to. Join a sport club if you have a history of playing that sport, or have a standing date with a friend to keep the workout on your schedule regularly. Find a friend and get outside to enjoy the beauty."

7.

MAKE FRIENDS WITH ANYONE WHO SEEMS TO BE WILLING TO LISTEN: "Most people know someone who has dealt with cancer, bend people's ears until you find their connection. Then converse with them about what your experience is like. They will be interested to know your experience if you are willing to share."

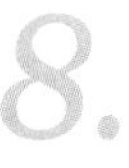

TAKE ADVANTAGE OF EVERY SERVICE YOU ARE OFFERED: "You never know how long it'll be around, and the people offering it want you to take advantage of their experience. There are so many good people to meet who run, and volunteer for these organizations. You can pay it forward one day by becoming a volunteer, or starting an organization of your own."

"*Find a friend* and get outside to enjoy the **beauty.**"

9.

IF YOU ARE TRYING TO SUPPORT A LOVED ONE THROUGH ILLNESS: *"Do your best to listen without being judgmental. You will be able to hear much more that way, and your friend will be relieved to have somebody around who will support them in every way."* ■

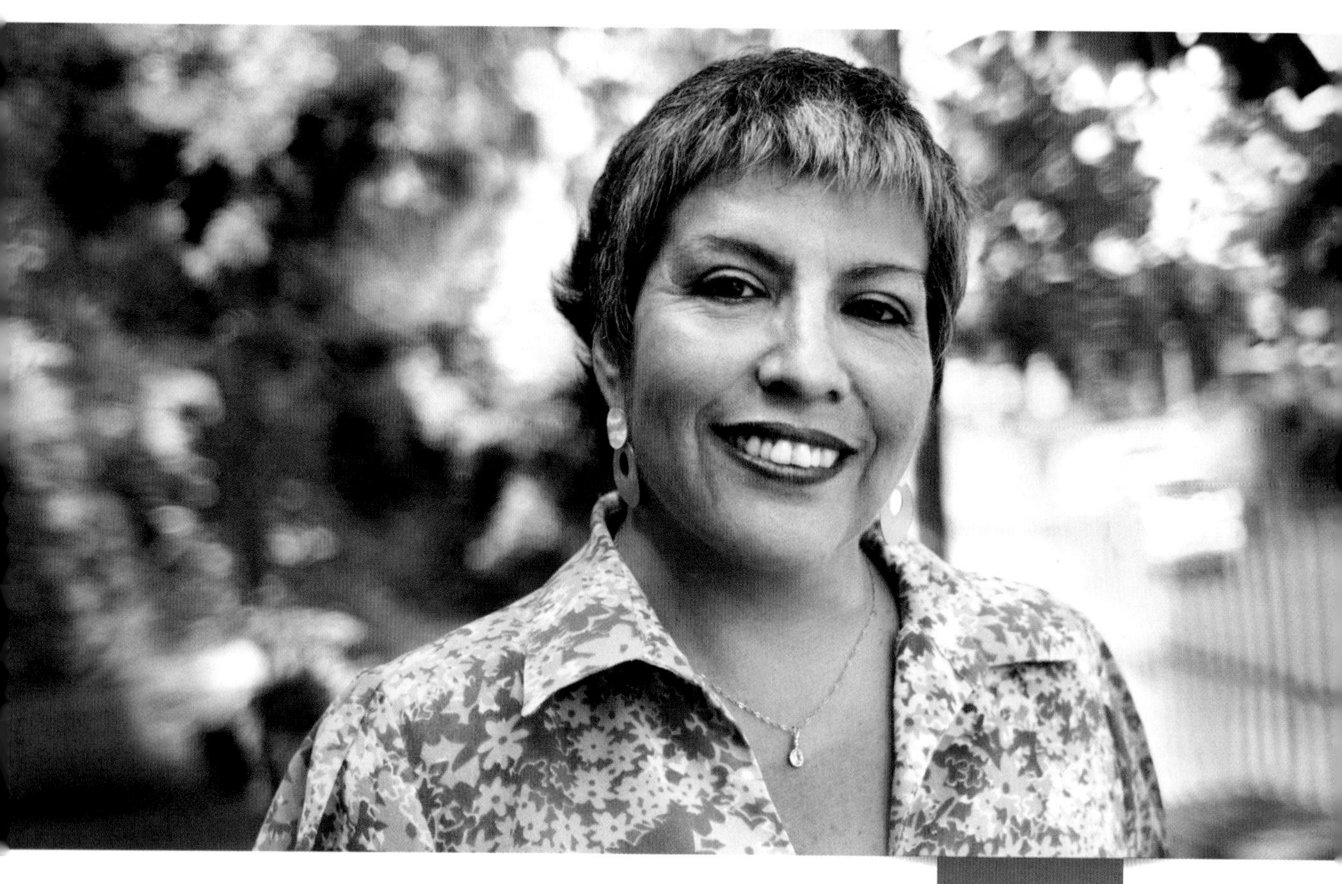

Flora Molina

breast cancer
PATIENT

AGE: *55*
OCCUPATION: *Secretary*
DIAGNOSIS: *Breast cancer*
WHEN: *2011*
CONTEXT: *Flora had annual check-ups, but in 2010 she skipped them due to lack of time. The next year she was diagnosed with breast cancer. It is the first case of cancer in her family. When she started recovering, she received some news: her husband, David Piña, had a 12-centimeter tumor between his rectum and colon. "The first thing I felt is that life is very unfair, but then I understood everything happens for a reason. Our love became stronger in an incredible way." David died in 2012.*

1.

HAVE CHECK-UPS: "Have annual check-ups and also echotomographies. There are tumors hidden on the back of mammary glands which are so small they aren't detected by mammograms."

2.

FILL YOUR DAY WITH ACTIVITIES: "I took a lot of work home to be updated with computer programs. I created many databases and also read a lot. Thanks to the book *Mother in Heaven*, written by Pablo Simonetti, I understood not all of us see diseases in the same way and there are some people who really suffer.

3.

NATURAL DRUGS: "There was a time I was fed up of drugs and chose to fight the pain with natural medicine. They act slower, but they are as effective. Rinsing with *Matico* water and bicarbonate, or fresh plantain water is useful for teeth, mouth and gums pain caused by chemotherapy. Water with ice and lemon was a balm for nausea. Lemon balm and rosemary, lemon verbena and *Oro del Inca* teas are useful to relax or fall asleep. These are all sold in the Chinese mall, downtown Santiago. The last chemotherapy was terrible and the lemon balm drops I drank helped a lot. During radiotherapy I took graviola and noni –which I also bought at the Chinese mall– and ginkgo biloba pills from Knop drugstores. Thanks to that I had no stomach problems."

4.

WORRY ABOUT OTHERS: "I spoke to many people. When I went to have chemotherapy or radiotherapy, I worried about how my roommates were doing and asked them how they felt. When you're starting it's useful to know."

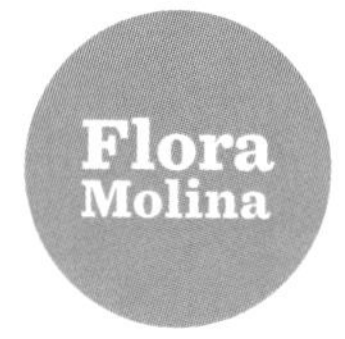

5.

LOOKING PRETTY: "I never stop wearing makeup. I wore earrings, took care of how I looked, I never lost that. When people told me I looked pretty that kept me moving forward. When I looked in the mirror and saw myself looking sick. I painted my nails, because chemos leave them black. I cleaned my skin with good quality creams, I lined my eyes, painted my lips."

6.

KEEP THE FAITH AND THE WILLINGNESS TO LIVE: "I believe in God and after receiving my diagnosis I had prayed a lot, so I felt spiritually strong. On my bad days I'd pray to be the Flora Molina I'd been before. I thought: *I have to be brave, I am coming out of this, I love life, I love my husband, my children, my grandsons, I have a wonderful life ahead of me, full of effort and work, but is the life I love.* All of that gave me of strength on a daily basis."

"I never stop wearing makeup. I wore earrings, I took care of how I looked, *I never* lost that. When people told me I looked pretty that kept me moving ***forward.***"

7.

YES TO LOVE, NO TO PITY: "A family doesn't need to overprotect you and be on top of you the whole time. The chemo process is clear and specific: on the days I felt bad I preferred to stay at home and I asked people if I needed anything. Actually on those days I really needed to be alone. The important thing is to feel love, not pity or overprotection."

8.

SCAR CREAMS: "Radiotherapy burns you. Besides the drug the doctor prescribed for me, called Platsul-A, I wore Aloe Vera. I placed the gel as is, squeezing it from the plant and it helped the skin. Calendula soap, sold in artisan fairs helped eliminating the stains. Pomegranate oil from Weleda improved my skin in an impressive way."

9.

JUST THE TWO OF US: "My husband was a fundamental support during my treatment. He was always with me cheering me up and telling me beautiful things, as that I looked hot without hair. When he got ill, I thought, *how unfair life is.* We that were like soulmates, that we deeply loved each other, we have to endure this. Now I see how it helped us as a couple: we could show each other all the love that we felt."

10.

ACCEPTING HELP: "All we had with my husband we used it to pay our medical expenses. Luckily I am very organized and we had some savings. My workmates were wonderful, deposited money in my account, gathered funds, organized collections. I thanked it with my soul, but it was hard. Is so good to help others, but being at the other side of the river, sometimes made me feel small."

11.

SCARFS VS WIGS: "When my hair was falling out I wore a scarf. I invented many ways of using them, practicing in front of the mirror. I was really creative. One day I discovered that, if besides the scarf I wore a nice hat, it looked even better. I never wanted to wear a wig as I didn't want to feel that I was hiding what I was going through."

"The chemo process is clear and specific: on the days I felt bad, I preferred to ***stay*** at home and people asked if I needed anything. Actually on those days I really needed to be *alone.*"

12.

MENTAL HEALTH: *"I used my head doing some domestic chores, I entertained myself with my grandson and my children. To maintain mental sanity was really important to count with my husband and the closeness of my family."* ■

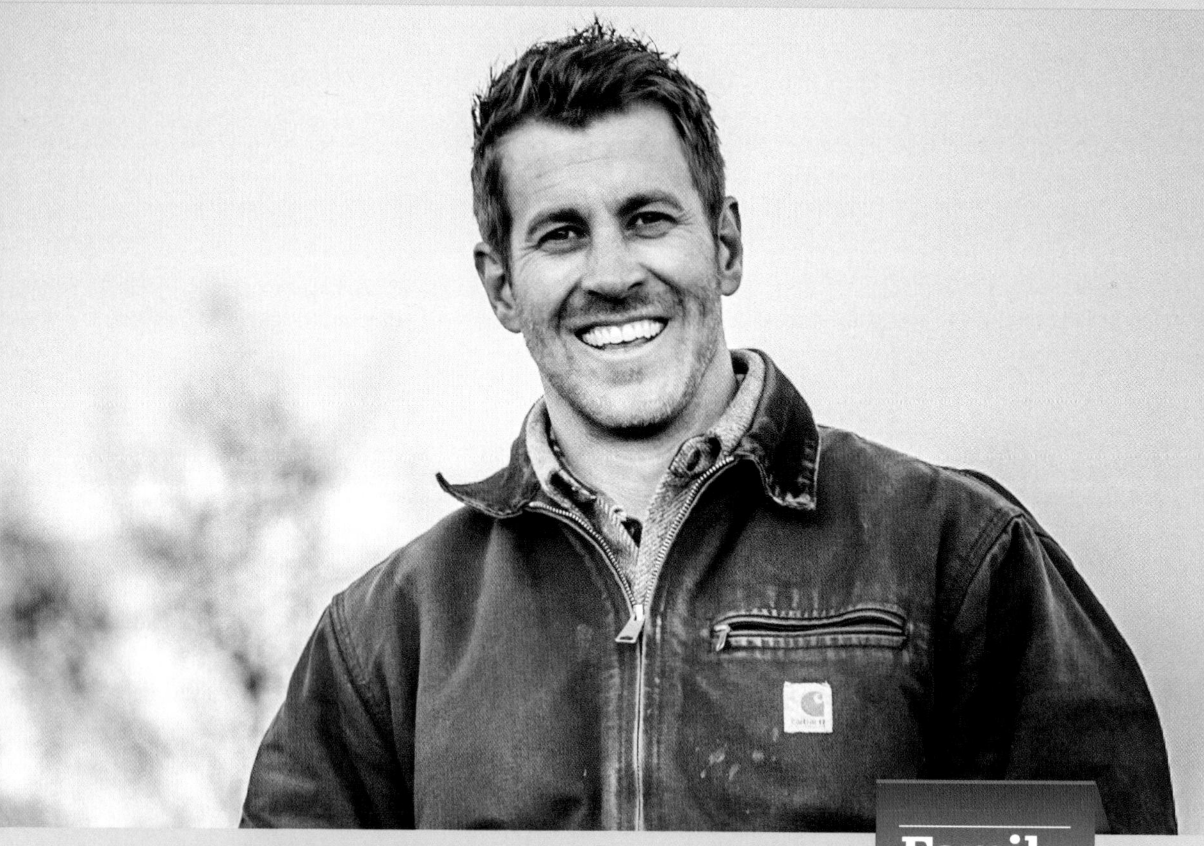

Brad Ludden

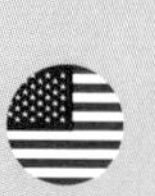

Family of breast cancer patient

AGE: *35*

OCCUPATION: *Founder of First Descents*

RELATIONSHIP: *Nephew of breast cancer patient*

WHEN: *1993, when Brad was 12*

CONTEXT: *When Brad's aunt was diagnosed with cancer, he realized the need for support, connection and healthy outlets in the young adult community. When they would kayak together, he noticed a change in her attitude towards the disease and her own capability and decided the outdoors could play an integral part in the lives of other young adults with this disease. He founded First Descents in 2001 to provide outdoor adventures to young adults age 18-39 impacted by cancer. His aunt fought the disease and is still alive today.*

1.

GO OUTSIDE: "Nature is the perfect place to remind us that we're alive today. She has a way of putting things in perspective and showing us our place in all of it. Fresh air, beautiful views, sunrises and sunsets, clean water, vast oceans and mountain peaks all gently bring us back to the present and help the events of yesterday and the worries of tomorrow evaporate in the beauty of the now".

2.

GIVE: "This might be the most important one. It can be all too easy to focus on our own hardships, shortcomings, and inabilities, but by being alive in this moment, we all have something to lend to someone or something in need. There is always someone or something in need of *you*. Just that simple recognition and the act of giving yourself to something else puts you in a place of power, gives and gets gratitude and lends a valuable perspective that we all need often."

3.

FIND YOUR TRIBE: "Too many of the young adults I've met have talked about feeling isolated and alone in their diagnosis. This doesn't have to be! There are countless others out there living your reality and waiting to share in your experiences, form close friendships and become a part of your new tribe. This process of connecting, learning and laughing heals, and from my experience, is the most important thing you can do in your life after cancer."

4.

LAUGH: "I've seen it happen all too often, the grimness of cancer can put out the flame of laughter. I've also seen so much health and healing come from that flame when it's ignited. Surround yourself with people who make you laugh. Be quick to laugh at those around you and yourself in the most loving of ways. Go to funny movies and comedy clubs. Buy a bulldog or wear a goofy costume to a dinner with friends. Make a point to belly laugh once a day."

5.

CRY: "As important as laughing is, crying is equally important. In today's society, especially with men, crying can be seen as a point of weakness. I believe the opposite. Crying is the release of important emotions that shouldn't stay in the body. It's honoring your state of being, the hardships your facing and the loss of the life you once knew. It's also honoring the beautiful things in your world, yourself included, and the new life on which you're embarking. Cry freely, amongst friends or in the quiet of the night. Just don't forget to cry."

6.

FORGIVE: "One of the greatest challenges I've faced in my life is having the ability to forgive. I've seen cancer create a lot of anger, resentment and frustration in people's lives, which makes it all the more important to focus on forgiveness. In doing so, you're freeing yourself and claiming another victory of cancer."

7.

MEDITATE: "When facing something as overwhelming as cancer, the mind tends to run, and often into dark places, so it's important to train the mind to be present. This is as much a skill as playing an instrument, and requires as much attention and energy as working out, socializing, our job and important relationships. The app called HEADSPACE is a great introduction to meditation." ■

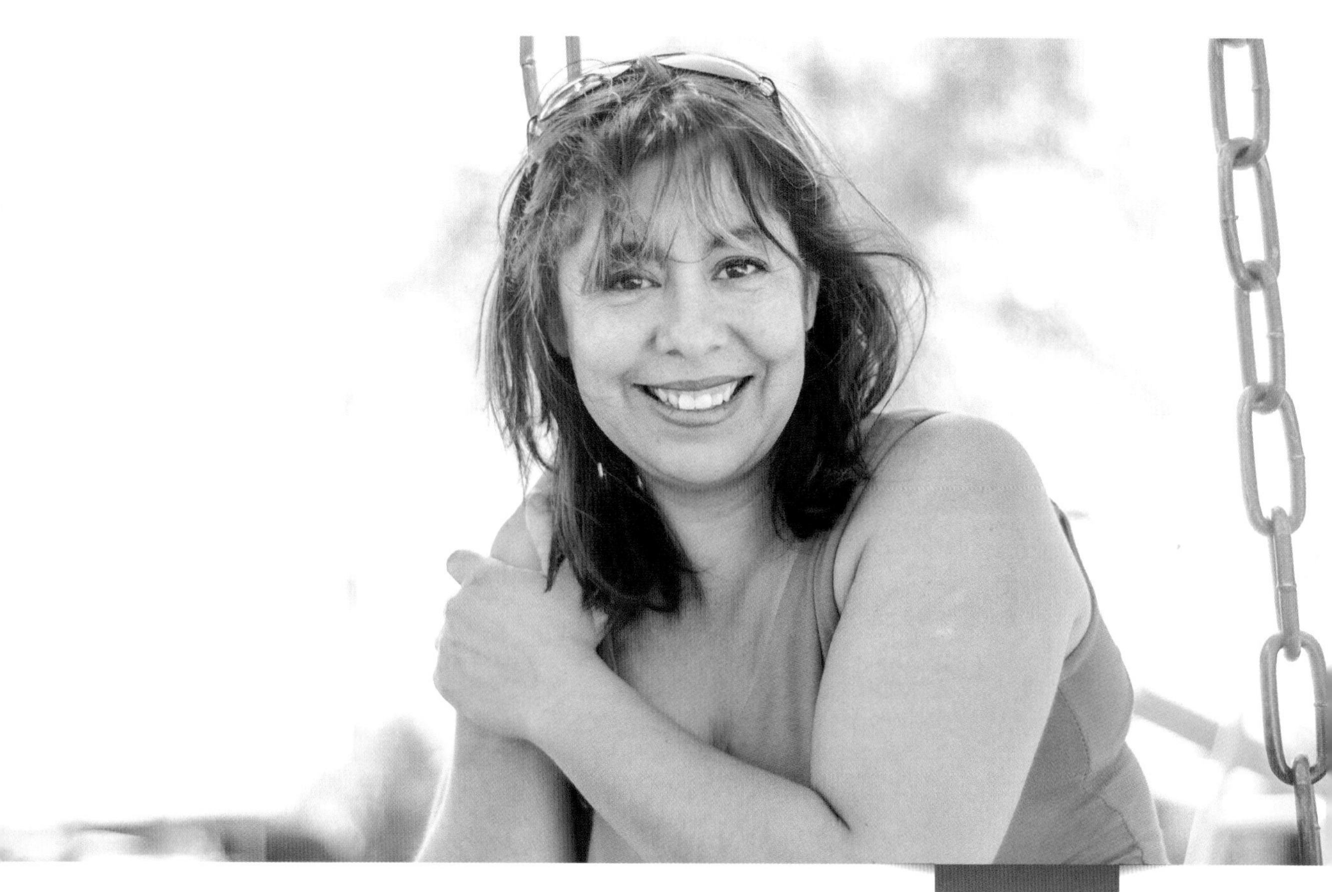

Claudia Palomino

breast cancer

PATIENT

AGE: *41*

OCCUPATION: *School transportation and sales*

DIAGNOSIS: *Breast cancer with metastasis in nodes and throat*

WHEN: *2006*

CONTEXT: *At the age of 32, Claudia had her left breast removed. After receiving chemotherapy she recovered, but tumors developed on her throat. She didn't give up and requested a treatment with Herceptin, a new drug. She collected 24 million Chilean pesos in bingos and raffles. Claudia recovered, but in 2012 a spot appeared in her thorax. She waited and some months later it had disappeared. There no new appearances and she underwent surgery once again to close the cycle with a desired breast reconstruction. "I was told I was going to die; I now know I, God and people's good energy have the last word. There's a reason I'm still here."*

1.

KNOCK ON ALL DOORS: "Nobody else knocked all the doors I knocked on. When I was diagnosed with cancer, my husband and I earned US 1,538.46 a month, we had no savings and I had never been admitted to a public institution. I went to ministries, got together with cancer experts, queued at the municipality to get funds and made *Roche* lab give me the third dose of Herceptin that I needed. You don't have to wait until things happen."

2.

ALIGN WORK AND LIFE: "I commuted two hours to work and used to think only about how I could afford things, until I realized that having things made no sense if I didn't have the health to enjoy them. I reduced my expenses and quit my job. I now sell homemade food, transport children and sell make up via catalogue. I do everything at my rhythm and I am happy this way."

3.

CREATE SUPPORT NETWORKS: "Treatments are really expensive and I have paid for many with my own money. But I was lucky: my workmates gave 20% of their salaries to help me and my boss cooperated with half of the first drug doses and gave me the breast prosthesis as a gift. My family helped me organize bingos, raffles, and fundraising parties. My brother told my story, opened a bank account and created a support system using social media. We didn't collect much money, but people expressed words of encouragement. I will never forget that."

4.

DO WHAT YOU HAVE ALWAYS WANTED TO DO: "When this happened to me I said: *I won't limit myself.* If I'm going to die, first of all I'll do the things I've always wanted to do. I had always wanted to learn to play guitar and so I did. I now play the guitar and sing folk music. When Madonna came to Chile I was receiving chemotherapy, but I said: *I was not going to die without seeing Madonna.* I fulfilled my dream."

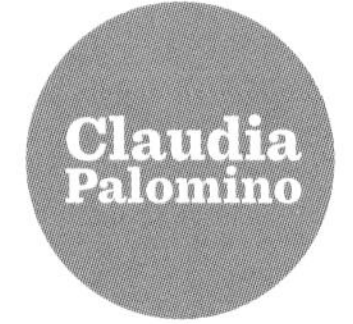

5.

STATE OF MIND: "State of mind is key. I am optimistic and joyful, I feel no pity for myself. Nothing would have worked if I'd been depressed, thinking I wouldn't recover."

"Now I know ***time*** is to enjoy, to ***live***"

6.

PREPARE THE ROAD: *"When I was given no more hope, my husband started crying uncontrollably and asked what he was going to do without me. I calmed down, calmed him down and told him he couldn't afford to break down, because he had two children to take care of."*

7.

ENJOY LIFE: "After cancer, I started enjoying life as never before. I don't give importance to silly things. I sometimes fought with my husband over silly things, but we now know time is to be enjoyed, to be lived. I know I will live with this disease for the rest of my life, but I will lead it as best as possible; I won't die a minute earlier."

8.

PAVE THE WAY: "One day I decided to keep a photographic record of all we did as a family and write down what my children said, wanted and needed... even how they liked their food! It was a way to start paving the way for the moment I would no longer be with them and it made me feel calmer facing the future."

"*Nothing* would have worked if I'd been ***depressed*** thinking I would not get better."

9.

KNOW WHERE THE SHOE PINCHES: "I practiced Yoga for a while. It helped, but I then started exercising on my own. I visited a psychologist also, but cried a lot during sessions and wondered whether it caused me more pain than relief. I started realizing I was not so sick, so I stopped going. Exercise, on the contrary, helped me release tensions. My husband and I go out biking; I run with my children... sports relax me." ■

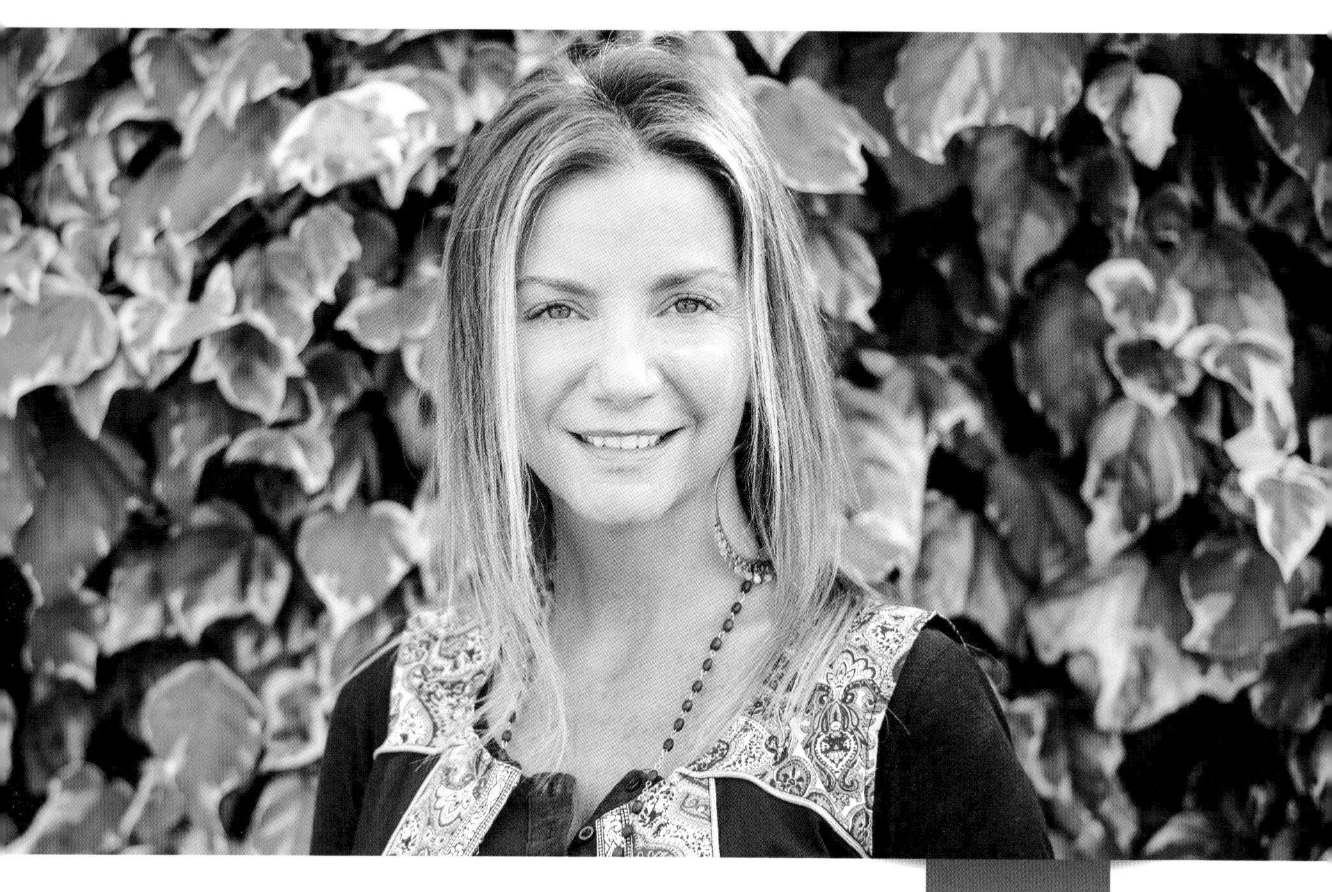

Bernardita Swinburn

breast cancer

PATIENT

AGE: *40*

OCCUPATION: *PRs professional and businesswoman*

DIAGNOSIS: *Breast cancer*

WHEN: *2009*

CONTEXT: *After her sister and mother were diagnosed with breast cancer, Bernardita also had the tests done. The result was the same. She never asked "why me", she was convinced the origin of the disease was in some way genetic and in another way emotional: "My mother, my sister and I had felt great sadness at the death of my father." Today, they're all one hundred percent recovered.*

1.

LIFE AS NORMAL AS POSSIBLE: "Avoid staying in bed and worrying about leading a normal life, because it's easier to become depressed or frightened. As soon as I could, I dressed up, put on heels and went out."

2.

COMPLEMENT TREATMENT WITH NATURAL THERAPIES: "I ate chia, which has high levels of Omega-3; I drank cranberry concentrate and also had plasma injected in *Physis* center, in Santiago, to strengthen my immune system. You have blood extracted and with that plasma, plus an antigen, a special vaccine is prepared and applied for three months to strengthen defenses."

3.

FILTER PEOPLE YOU'RE WITH: "I suggest giving priority to people who transmit good energy and make you feel well, and avoiding those who feel pity for your disease."

4.

USE THE DISEASE TO BETTER UNDERSTAND YOUR OWN LIFE: "I thought I had accepted my father's death, but it was not true. While I was treating cancer I went to a psychologist, did family consultations and discovered I held a lot of anger. I now feel more relieved."

5.

GIVE YOURSELF THE CHANCE TO DO WHATEVER YOU WANT: "Before my cancer, I felt I always had to look happy, be in a good mood and posture. I now know I have the right to be sad and respond however I feel like it if I get angry." ■

"I suggest giving *priority* to people who transmit **good** energy and avoiding those **who** feel pity for your disease."

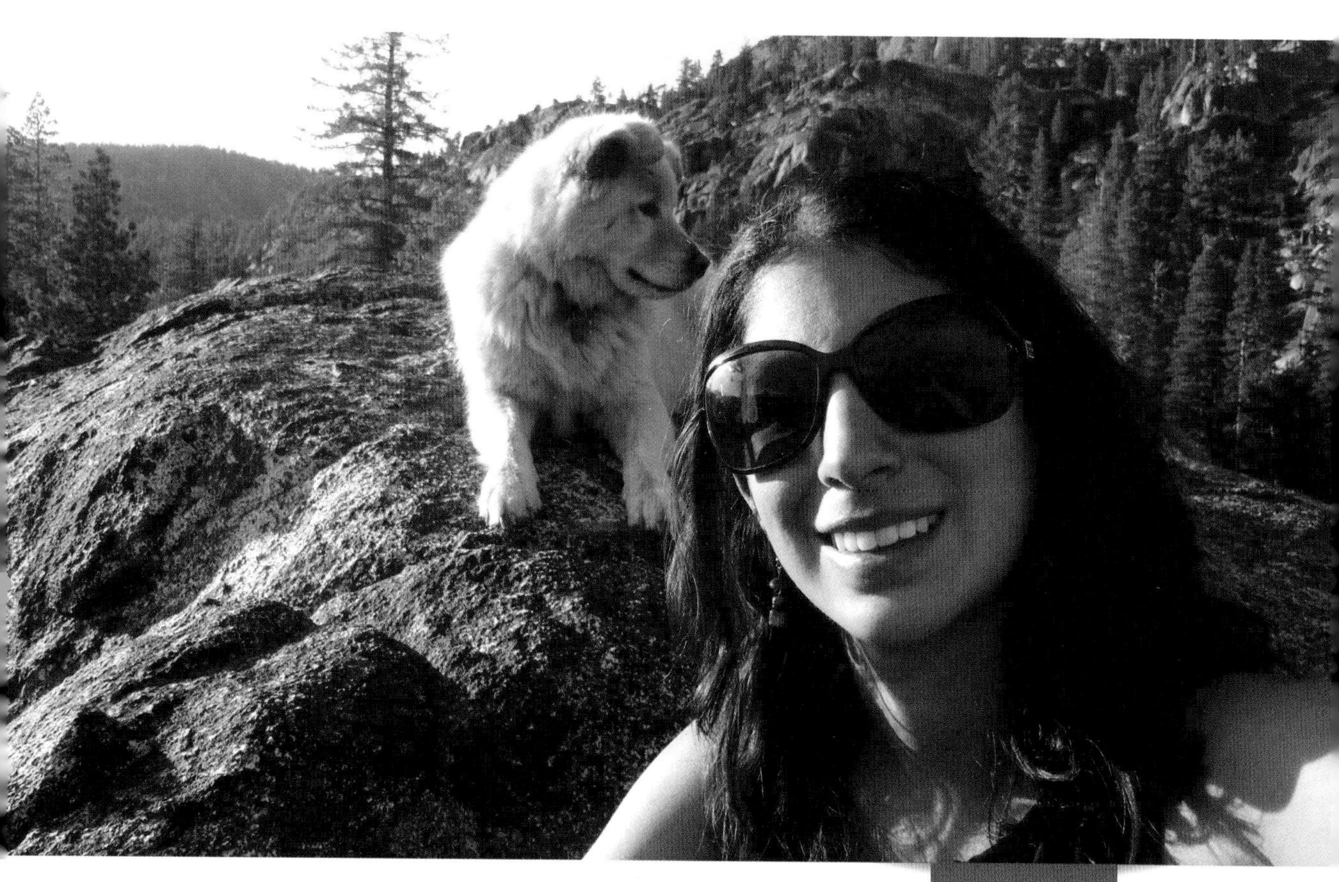

Nadia T

breast cancer

PATIENT

AGE: *31 at diagnosis, 34 now*

OCCUPATION: *Forester*

DIAGNOSIS: *Stage 3 Breast Cancer*

WHEN: *2014*

CONTEXT: *In late 2013, I found a small lump in my left breast. I was 31 years old and had no family history of breast cancer. At the time, my husband and I were trying to start a family, so cancer was definitely not on our radar. I waited 2 months to get checked out and it took a few more weeks to get a mammogram and ultrasound. After a double mastectomy, we found that I had cancer throughout my left breast and in my lymph nodes. I had months of chemo, radiation, immunotherapy, and hormone therapy. Three years later, I am doing well and even did a 200-mile bike ride last fall!*

1.

YOU KNOW YOUR BODY BEST. "If you think something is wrong, fight for yourself. Don't let doctors brush you off because you're "too young.""

2.

CONSIDER ALTERNATIVE TREATMENTS: "Acupuncture, massage, and reiki to complement traditional treatments. My care team was amazing and these other modalities helped me deal with treatment side effects and stay strong."

3.

FERTILITY: "Make sure you talk to your doctor about fertility if that's a concern. Many cancer treatments can affect it, for both men and women. Doctor's don't always bring it up because they think you should get started on treatments right away and that you should just be happy to be alive. That's pretty harsh and not their choice to make."

4.

DON'T BE AFRAID TO SEE A THERAPIST: "A cancer diagnosis and treatments are terrifying and it's hard to talk to your caregivers because you don't want to worry or upset them, so you end up keeping a lot in. It helps to talk to a professional to help you process what's happening or help you if you have anxiety or become depressed."

5.

TRUST YOUR DECISIONS: "Don't second-guess yourself. Have faith in your treatment plan."

6.

GIVE PEOPLE THE BENEFIT OF THE DOUBT: "People might say weird things to you because they don't know what else to say or how to be helpful. Like, that at least you got the "good cancer." Try not to take offense and give them the benefit of the doubt."

7.

SOME PEOPLE YOU EXPECT to be there for you will drop off the planet, and others will come out of the woodwork and surprise you with support you never knew existed. You're loved ones might be super upset about your diagnosis and unable to face you - just remember that they love you and in the meantime if there is someone else that is showing up with warm meals at your door, lean on them for that daily support instead.

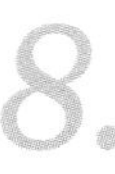

ADVICE ON HOW TO LIVE CANCER-FREE: "Can be overwhelming and sometimes unhelpful. Make the changes that work for you and don't stress about the rest. Some books that were helpful to me in learning about healthier lifestyle and nutrition choices were: "Crazy, Sexy, Cancer" by Kris Carr, and "Anti-Cancer: A new way of life" by David Servan-Schreiber." ■

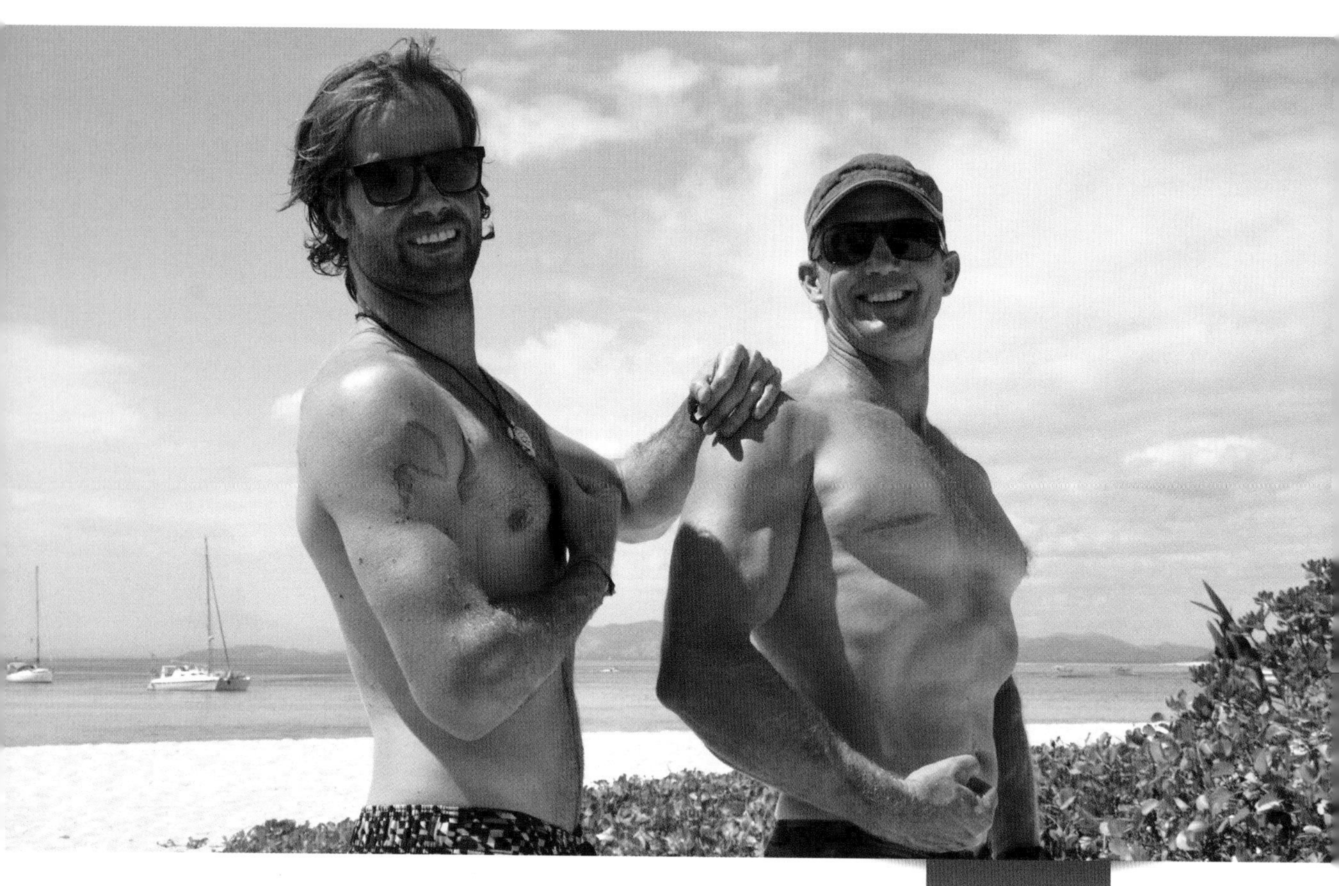

Paul Viney

breast cancer

PATIENT

AGE: *48*

OCCUPATION: *Owner of an oyster breeding center and a fishing company in the northern Tasmania coast, Australia*

DIAGNOSIS: *Breast cancer*

WHEN: *2007*

CONTEXT: *One day, when he was drying himself with a towel, Paul discovered a small bump above his right nipple. A few days later, he consulted a doctor and then a specialist. The diagnosis after the biopsy was unequivocal: he had breast cancer and needed to have a mastectomy, something most men believe could never happen to them.*

1.

KNOW YOUR BODY: "If you know it well enough you'll notice the changes. If you find something different, such as a lump, go straight to the doctor. Early detection is key to survive cancer."

2.

SCARS AS BADGES: "Today, I tend not to get worried because I lack one nipple on the right side. It's true, I don't need it. I could get one tattooed –it's sometimes done–, but I'd rather carry my scar as a badge of honor from a cancer survivor."

"Know your body **well** enough to notice *changes* in it".

3.

YOU'RE NOT THE ONLY ONE: "Suffering from cancer is a very emotional journey, a drastic roller coaster full of ups and downs. From time to time, I wasn't ready to feel so overwhelmed and thought I was going crazy. My oncologist calmed me down saying this happens to many cancer patients."

4.

VIRTUAL AND REAL SUPPORT NETWORKS: "Make sure you're surrounded by family and friends, because you'll need their love and support. There are many support groups for cancer patients, some local and others online. They may help you understand you're not the only one living this. It was hard for me as support groups for breast cancer are focused on women."

5.

AXILLARY WEB: "The AWS (Axillary Web Syndrome) may be a common condition among patients who had their lymphatic nodules removed or had a mastectomy. In my case, this syndrome left me with limited mobility in my right arm and the recommended exercises didn't seem to help much. However, when I started swimming every day, the situation improved immediately. I kept swimming until my arm could move without feeling any pain."

6.

SLOW BUT SAFE RECOVERY: "When my treatment ended, I took some months to recover. I followed a healthy diet, didn't drink alcohol and started exercising. I started slowly and increased the intensity each week. First, I took long walks, then jogged and finally ran, until my physical condition completely improved." ■

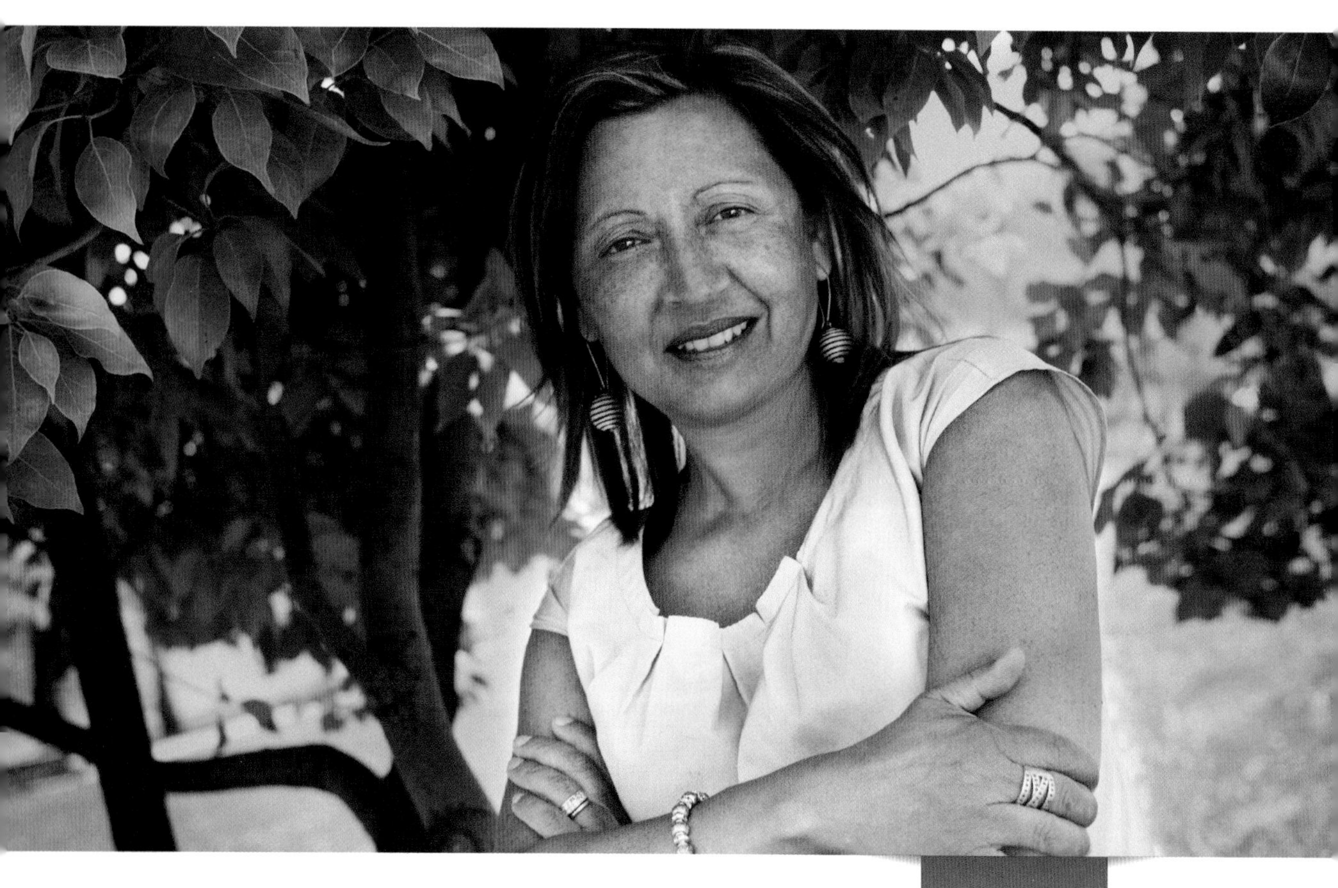

Aurora Opazo

breast cancer

PATIENT

AGE: *53*

OCCUPATION: *Businesswoman*

DIAGNOSIS: *Breast cancer*

WHEN: *2002*

CONTEXT: *Married with four children; in 2002 Aurora was diagnosed with breast cancer. After a year of chemotherapy and radiotherapy, doctors stated she was officially healthy. Thirteen years have gone by without her having any relapse.*

1.

DON'T TURN A DEAF EAR ALTHOUGH IT'S OBVIOUS: "The first advice is the most obvious one and, maybe for that, the less considered one: have regular check-ups. There are still many women who think that cancer will affect others and not them."

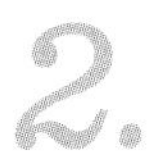

THE FIGHT: "You mustn't think that the initial diagnosis is a death sentence: You can't start convinced you're going to die. You must fight back and enjoy the good aspects of this experience, such as becoming closer to your family. I did so with my children and brothers."

"*I wrote* for a while each day and soon it became a kind of **meditation.**"

3.

TRIAL AND ERROR: "Take many herbs until you identify those that make you feel good. They cleanse the organism, eliminate toxins and all the dirt left inside due to the disease and its treatment."

4.

YES TO WORK: "Apart from thinking positively, you need to try to lead as normal a life as possible. I never stopped working and this made me stronger to face the most difficult moments."

5.

LISTENING AND SHARING: "It is important to talk and share experiences with people who have defeated cancer. That helped me."

6.

WRITE: "I wrote thoughts, anecdotes and information about my cancer in a notebook. I wrote for a while each day and soon it became a kind of meditation."

7.

CLASSES TO DRAW EYEBROWS: "I started taking makeup classes, where I learned to draw my eyebrows. And I went every week to the hairdresser to have my wig styled." ■

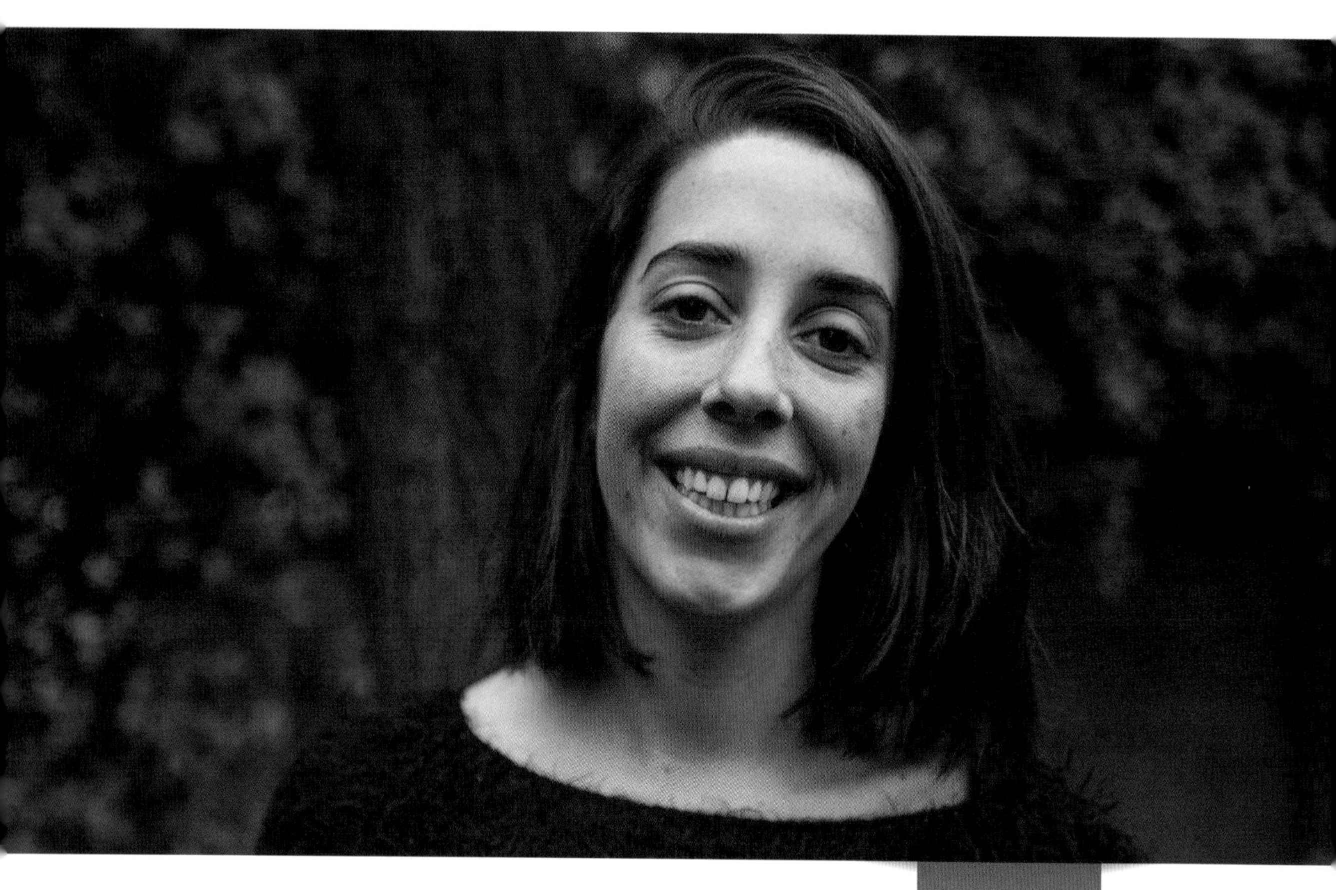

Karla Amaro

breast cancer

PATIENT

AGE: *28*

OCCUPATION: *Cook*

DIAGNOSIS: *Breast cancer*

WHEN: *2007*

CONTEXT: *The gynecologist found a little bean on her breast. She was about to turn 21 years old with a cancer which, luckily, was encapsulated and didn't develop. Karla currently submits to bi-yearly check-ups and enjoys a life she rediscovered based on self-knowledge she gained from that experience.*

1.

HEAL FROM A *GHOST* CANCER: "I didn't have to have radiotherapies, chemotherapies, or any other therapy. I lived my true healing process later. A year later I saw a psychologist and understood that cancer can be caused by locking your emotions away. I was very undemonstrative, I never used to talk about what was going on with me, I'd keep it all to myself. I changed this."

2.

HANDLE FEARS: "I became very scared. I'd never been afraid of nosebleeds but now they made me sick with fear. Fear of blood is fear of death. I slowly managed to control my fear, knowing that there was something very concrete that could cause my death. I went to workshops with other cancer patients and felt like such a coward as my tumor had been taken out and others were going through this with a cancer that was still developing."

"Diseases are signs and I discovered something was not going well in my ***life*** and I had to *change it.*"

3.

AN INDIVIDUAL PROCESS: "I suggest living the cancer process on your own, because it's not something that can be shared. You live surrounded by people who support you, but the true process is personal and you need to take the time to experience it in order to avoid the risk of making it endless."

4.

FAMILY TENDS TO BE OVERPROTECTIVE: "My family became very apprehensive and overprotective, they filled me with information: *Karla you can't eat that because you will develop cancer again, don't eat sugar because it can cause some disease,* that's just how they dealt with it. I now understand they wanted to prevent any relapses, but it ended up being too much for me to handle."

5.

KNOW YOURSELF THROUGH CANCER: "I live in *Puerto Varas* [Chilean southern city] and I'm happy. I feel calmer; I don't know if I'm totally complete because cancer is a process which is hard to give closure to. I now look back at it as an incredible period which helped me get to know myself in a way I would never have been able to before. I now live life to the fullest, I laugh and cry. I didn't let myself before, and that's what gave me cancer. Let yourself enjoy life: life is the here and now." ■

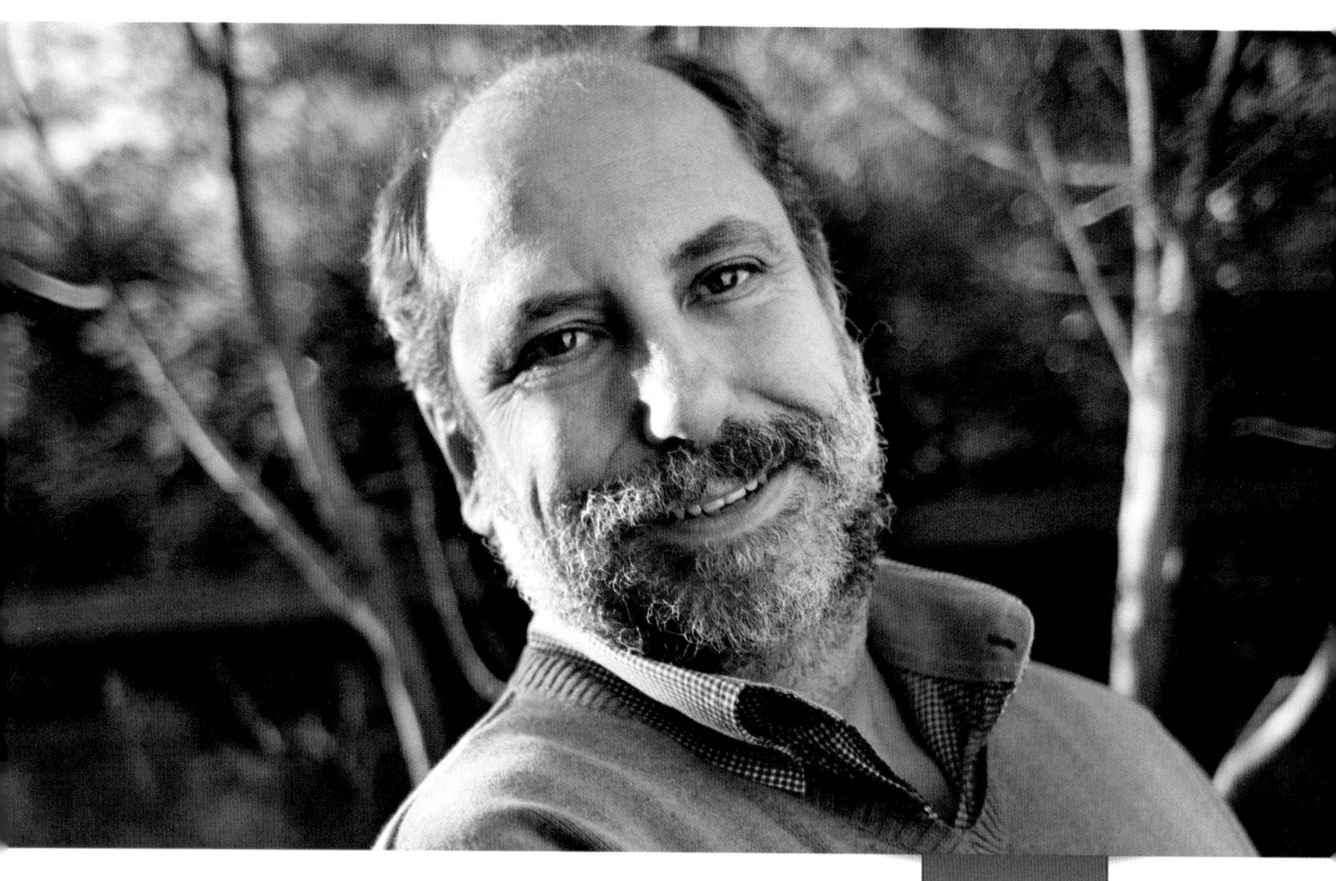

Ricardo Larraín

non-Hodgkin's lymphoma

PATIENT

AGE: *58*

OCCUPATION: *Filmmaker*

DIAGNOSIS: *Non Hodgkin's lymphoma*

WHEN: *2006*

CONTEXT: *Ricardo Larraín didn't have any symptoms anticipating cancer, but a routine examination confirmed he had Non Hodgkin's lymphoma. He never collapsed, so much so that while he was undergoing treatment he learned how to meditate, which he had wanted to do for years. And his life didn't stop. He didn't postpone any project, not even when he had a relapse. In fact, during the period -between "cancer 1 and cancer 2"- he studied and graduated as a psychologist. "I opened a door and don't know where it will lead me, but I'm happy I did." Ricardo's cancer is currently a chronic disease that he will have to look after periodically.*

1.

TRUST IN YOUR POSSIBILITIES: "The disease was never made visible, it didn't stop me from working, except when I was in the hospital. The most I had to do was slow down the pace. Non Hodgkin's lymphoma has an 85% chance of recovery. Supposedly, with the second treatment the possibility of cancer returning reduces a lot, but it does not disappear. If it develops once again, so be it; luckily, it's a cancer that can be treated. A friend tells me I'm a robust Basque..."

2.

SAY NO TO CLICHÉS: "There's a saying that people with cancer have, to a certain extent, caused their own cancer. I never accepted the idea I was killing myself; it's simply part of the vital process that I live through. I always rejected the idea of feeling guilty."

3.

DRINK A LOT OF LIQUID: "This is a valid suggestion for everybody, but from my cancer experience, I believe drinking a lot of liquid helped me. The doctor suggested this to me and it made sense, because of the amount of drugs being injected into your body; liquid helps to cleanse. I drank everything: waters, tea and homemade infusions of mint, ginger and basil, among others, because pure water started making me sick."

4.

OMMMMM...: "Before cancer I had been flirting with meditation for a while, that's why after my diagnosis I went to visit a friend who meditates and she suggested me going to the *Shambalha* center, where I started meditating and incorporating this practice in my everyday life. I assumed that if there is a thing that helps cancer develop, it's the alteration of moods, such as sadness and bitterness. I rigorously meditated for a long time. I now do it less regularly, but I learned it can be done at any time and in any place. Even during the morning's traffic jam. Stress is cancerous."

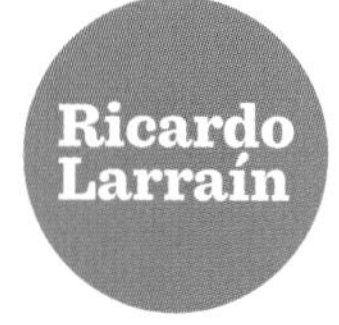

"When you are sick you *feel* the **love** of the people in a very **INTENSE** way. People you cannot imagine reappear and ***everybody*** gives you a very *caring* vibe, it is very enriching."

5.

LIFE AS A JOURNEY: "We only have one life and it is ongoing. We tend to see the disease as a setback without understanding it is part of that ongoing mode, of the life we have to live. It's not a parenthesis. I tell my daughters that I now see life as a journey that takes us through different places and, in the end, everything is an experience. When we fight against the disease, it's as if we are trying to deny something that just happens. If it hurts or prevents me from doing something it's not good, but it's part of the journey, such as when you drive along the road and think *'I'm starving'* but there's no place to stop and eat a sandwich. It's not good, but it's part of the journey. The disease is a great teacher who teaches you that life is a journey."

6.

POSITIVE FOOTPRINTS OF THE DISEASE: "When you are sick, you feel the affection of people in a very intense way. People you cannot imagine reappear and everybody give you a very caring vibe, very enriching. They are experiences that leave a footprint. Life is changing all the time and all experiences transform you, including the disease of course, which modifies you, sculping you and is an event leaving very positive footprints I think."

7.

TOLERATE CHEMOTHERAPY BETTER: *"After receiving suggestions from some relatives she treats, I visited* Socorro Cordeiro, *an anthroposophical Brazilian doctor who designed a parallel treatment to my chemotherapy in order to strengthen my resistance. It was about vaccines, capsules and drops; some sort of cocktail. I think it helped me bear the conventional therapies I had to undergo."*

8.

PATERNAL STRATEGY: "I'm father of four daughters who felt somehow overwhelmed with the news of my diagnosis. Therefore, I became very serious and told them: *'Darlings, nothing is wrong. I'm going to get better and if not, we have plenty of time to say goodbye, to fix everything'.* I felt that was acting as a father rather than as a sick person, and this helped me face the disease with a huge amount of serenity." ■

"If there is something that helps cancer develop, it's the **alteration of moods,** the sadness and bitterness. That is why I incorporated *meditation* as practice in my everyday life."

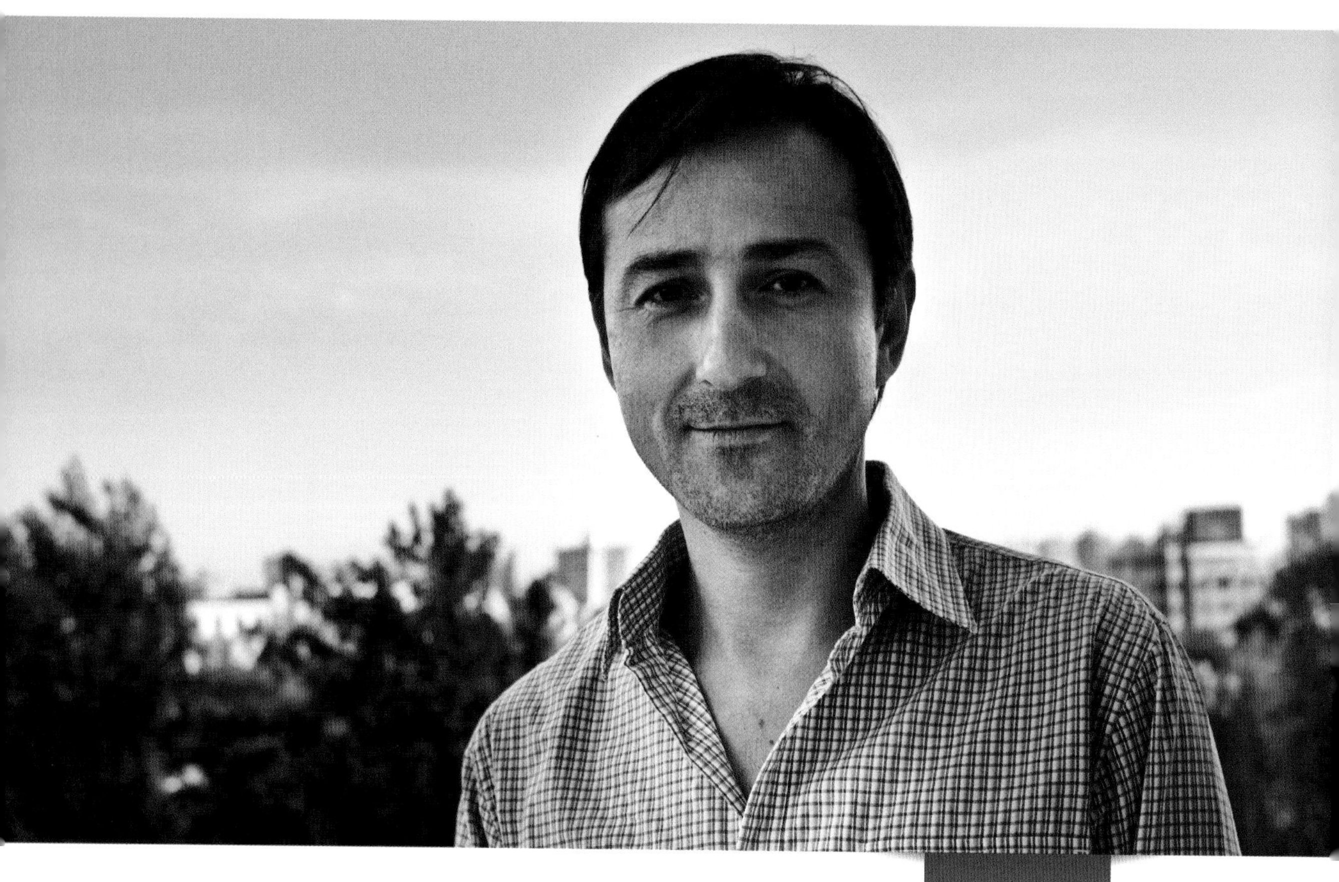

Pablo Hernández

non-Hodgkin's lymphoma

PATIENT

AGE: *48*

OCCUPATION: *Journalist*

DIAGNOSIS: *Non-Hodgkin's Lymphoma*

WHEN: *2001*

CONTEXT: *Finding a bump under the chin was the first alarm something was happening. Pablo was 34 years old; he allowed time to go by and only when the protuberance became visible at plain sight did he go to the doctor. He was found to have many other bump and the one on his neck ended up not being the biggest. He had a biopsy and obtained the results on the same day of his birthday: he had Non Hodgkin's lymphoma. 14 years after that diagnosis, Pablo has not suffered from any relapse.*

1.

PAY IT FORWARD: "Talking to someone who had gone through the same thing I was going through was the first relieving experience. Something really special happens, a "pay it forward" experience that enables you to learn about other cases, meet people and build a support network which is very important."

2.

ALLOW YOURSELF TO BE TAKEN CARE OF: "At first it's not easy to allow yourself to be taken care of because it's hard to lose independence. But it's essential to your recovery. I will always be thankful to my family and friends for having been beside me during that time."

3.

RESPECT YOUR SPACE: "If you don't feel like talking, don't; if you don't want to meet with someone, don't. Something really strange happens: usually, it's the patient that has to provide support to others and it ends up being exhausting. You need to respect those spaces and moments in which you want to be alone or with some specific people only."

4.

ALLOW YOURSELF TO BE SICK: "I would suggest you stop working, if possible. This worked for me, although I had to go against a system that pushes you to work in order to feel successful. When you don't work, you lose your role in society, especially if you're sick, but I refused that idea and worried about something much more important than professional success: my life."

5.

BE PATIENT": "As a doctor once told me: 'You need to be patient, as the word itself says'. I learned to take one step at a time, because the idea of spending six months in treatment, with its collateral effects, may sound overwhelming. If you're patient, in the sense of providing some time to see how your body reacts, time does go by and anguish diminishes."

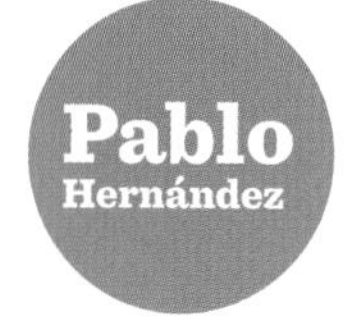

6.

CHANGE YOUR ATTITUDE: "I decided to leave sorrows aside and adopt a new proactive attitude after reading the book *Illness as Metaphor*, written by Susan Sontag, an essay where the author states cancer is a very heavy social term, full of negative connotations."

7.

KEEP ORDER: "I found keeping files and saving every classified and with a date written on it helped very much. The swarm of formalities you get surrounded by can be very stressful. I scanned everything: drug prescriptions, dated checks, drugstore invoices, and medical programs. In this way I had a backup for everything and didn't lose time searching for papers."

"If you don't feel like **talking,** *don't;* if you don't want to meet with someone, don't."

8.

LET YOURSELF GO FOR DISCOVERIES: "Cancer helped me discover new aspects in people. For instance, a person who didn't know me offered me two free reiki sessions a week. My mother held praying chains and, although I am not a believer, I could feel that energy. During that period my relationships became more loving, more human, and accumulated in a sort of love bank account."

9.

CLEAR CONVERSATIONS: "On the one hand, I knew I had to be really careful about being over informed in connection to my disease, but I was clear I had to confront this disease and accept it. Sometimes people find it to talk and deal with the doctor; being a journalist, I knew how to own up to that."

"I scanned everything: drug prescriptions, dated checks, drugstore invoices, and medical programs. In this way I had a **backup** for everything and *didn't lose time* searching for papers."

10.

BETTER RELATIONSHIPS: *"Apart from having a terrible physical time, you make valuable discoveries, such as relating with people in another way. Your bonds somehow change; my relationship with others became more loving, affectionate and human... I recall going through six months of physical discomfort and emotional pain, but also of huge support from people around me."* ■

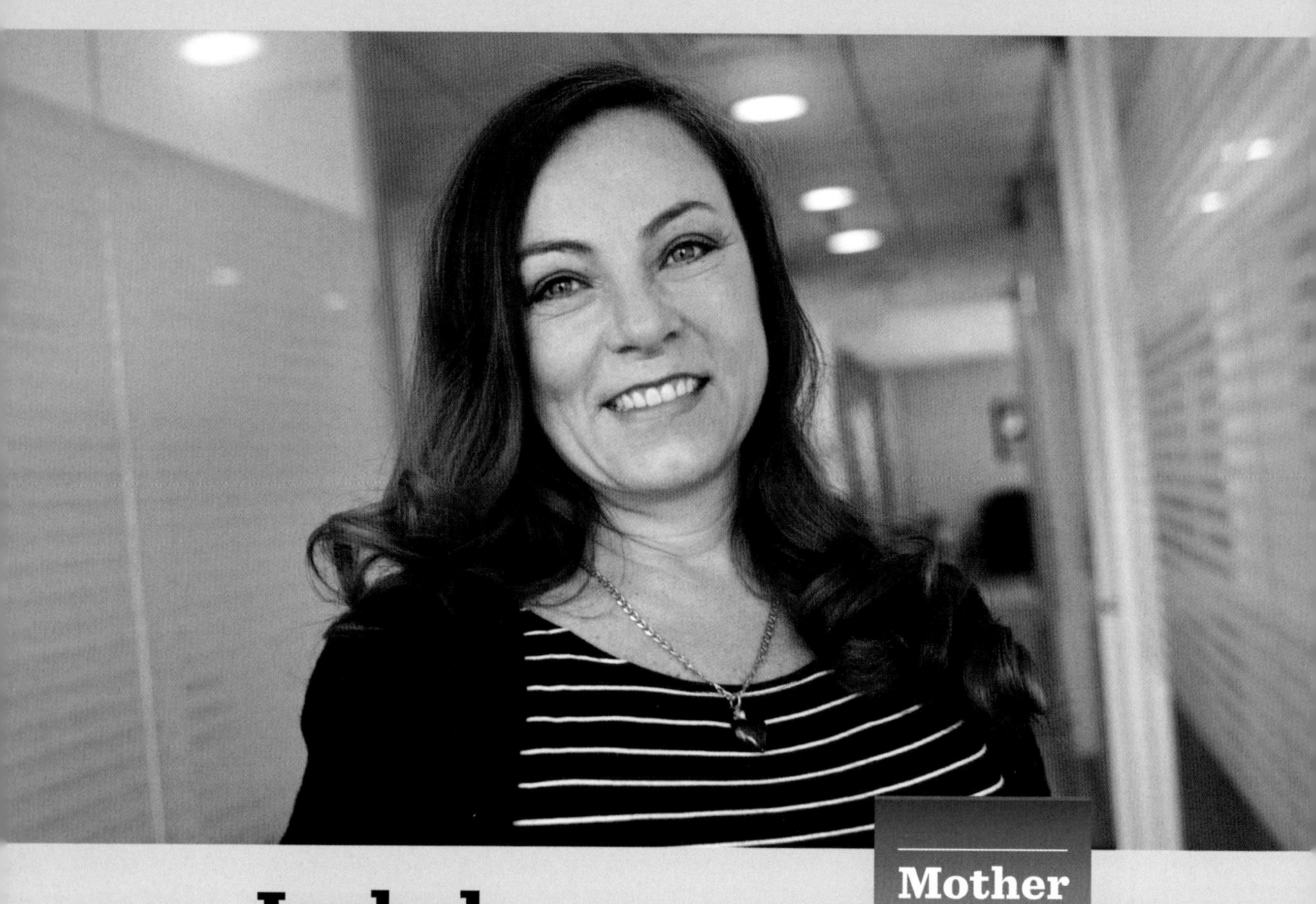

Mother
of
non-Hodgkin's
lymphoma
patient

Isabel Infante

AGE: *53*

OCCUPATION: *Wealth Manager*

RELATIONSHIP: *Mother of non-Hodgkin's Lymphoma patient*

WHEN: *2005*

CONTEXT: *Her son, Santiago, was fourteen years old when doctors detected a stage 3 Non Hodgkin's Lymphoma. It was an unthinkable scenario that changed Isabel's life forever; she faced the situation with some kind of pragmatism she now considers essential when the patient is a teenager. Santiago is now 24 years old and his mother remembers how she overcame the challenge: "My son would never need me so much as in that moment and the greatest test of my love was not giving up."*

1.

MANAGE VISITING HOURS: "It's paramount to filter visits made to the patient and to do so without the fear of defying formalities, because everything needs to be at the patient's service. I have a big family and at the peak of my son's disease they started visiting the clinic in turns. On the third day I hung up a sign on the door of the room: Santiago has cancer, but we're not interested in hearing your stories about other people's sicknesses. It was shocking for visitors, but when you go to visit a sick person, you need to take happiness, good energy and empathy."

2.

THE FAMILY FRONT: "Each one of the family members had a specific function. I told them we were all soldiers fighting a battle and the speech was that here there is no space for self-compassion or for anybody being depressed; let alone the two sisters lowering their grades. It was a very important life experience we had to seize positively, holding our heads high. This was what I asked of the family, and they all accepted."

3.

BE CLEAR WITHOUT TRANSMITTING INSECURITIES: "You need to stay strong for the children, to provide support. It's not about hiding emotions, but you need to make an effort to transmit assurance and strength."

4.

HERD OF ELEPHANTS: "I gave my daughters the example of a herd of elephants: When one of them gets sick, the rest of the herd places it in the middle, because they make it steady. We would keep Santiago standing all together. We needed all of us to succeed."

5.

***MATICO* TEA:** "Although every case is different, sometimes it is complicated to give a child weird or bad-tasting things. I gave Santiago *Matico* tea, a natural healer." ■

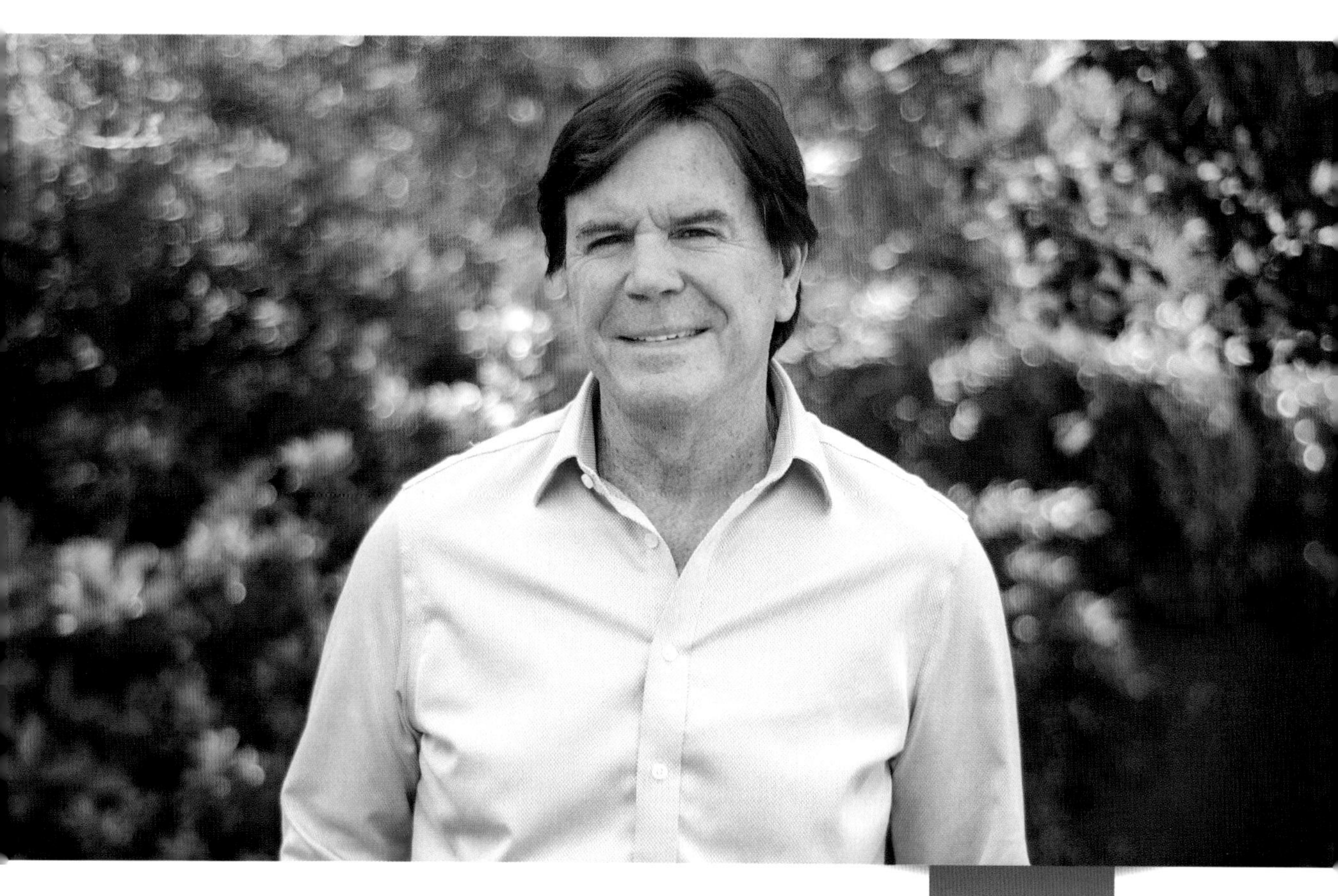

Drago Gluscevic

non-Hodgkin's lymphoma

PATIENT

AGE: *62*

OCCUPATION: *Businessman*

DIAGNOSIS: *Non Hodgkin's Lymphoma*

WHEN: *2007*

CONTEXT: *six months after his tumor was detected and in the middle of his own treatment, his battle against the disease took an unexpected turn when his wife was also diagnosed with cancer; breast cancer on her case. Drago then faced an improbable scenario which not only put him to a test in, but also tested the relationship with his wife and the whole family.*

1.

END POINT: "Now that I'm healthy, I decided to leave cancer in the past and eradicated it from home. My children see me now exercising every day, leading the same life I led before the disease –but much more relaxed–, spending more time at home. We celebrated the last chemotherapy all together in the clinic, with some *pisco sour*. That was the end of the story."

SECRET RECIPES: "A friend told me that to strengthen the stomach, one of the areas most affected by chemotherapy, he prepares a mix of an extract of Aloe Vera leaves, with honey and a little bit of rum, whisky or cognac, that are vasodilators. Before every meal I took a spoon-full of the mixture, and I never had pain in my stomach. Another habit I adopted was to take what is known as a transference factor, a compound invented by the Russians helping avoid infections. The formula is sold as pills, and during my treatment I took 10 pills a day."

"I don't want ***unnecessary*** fears or sorrows in my life."

3.

FIND THE ZEN SPOT: "I did everything possible to fight against the disease and feel better. If I was told to practice yoga, I did; to meditate every day, I meditated. From all the things I did, I regret none. I believe each one helped in some way. Just as there are many factors that converge to make you sick, the same logic applies to find the cure. It's not just the chemotherapy."

4.

EAT HEALTHY AND ONLY WHAT'S NECESSARY: "Before my disease, I was one of those people that ate a whole ice cream cake by himself. Now, I eat a portion. After I healed, I began to eat properly. I cut out sugar, exchanged meat for fish, increased the vegetables and fruit, and now only eat in reasonable quantities."

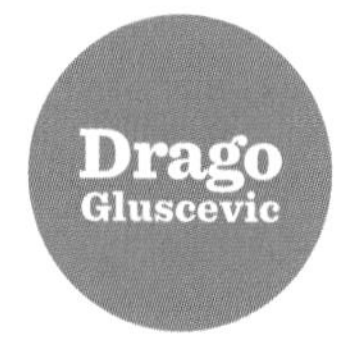

5.

BYE-BYE TO EMOTIONAL LOAD: "I no longer want unnecessary fears or sorrows in my life. I no longer tolerate those who irradiate bad energy. Nowadays, I do what I want. Before, I obliged myself to act thinking too much on what others wanted, I absorbed all their problems and the one that ended up sick was me, and they're all healthy. I decided I'm nobody's psychologist."

6.

PASS ON YOUR STORY: "After being recently diagnosed, an acquaintance called me to tell me he had suffered from the same and he gave me some details on what I would go through. He was doing really well and told me not to be worried, and that I could call him anytime. That conversation was like an interview with the best doctor in the world. This is why it is important to share your story."

"We **celebrated** the last chemotherapy all together in the clinic, with some *pisco sour*. That was the *end* of the story."

7.

IN THE HARD TIMES, WORRY ABOUT THOSE WHO SURROUND YOU: "Six months after I was diagnosed with cancer, my wife developed breast cancer and, for a while, we both were having treatments in the clinic. This really affected the kids; it's something you can't imagine. If breast cancer in women is not detected on time, it gets more complicated. I was finishing chemotherapy and it was my wife's turn. The doctor told me *you have to worry about your wife and yourself.*"

8.

THE HEAD COMMANDS: "It all depends on the way you confront the disease; this is why I say the head is so important. Apart from my family, I didn't get help from psychologists, psychiatrists or drugs. What I did was get a lot of support from spirituality and meditation, vibrational therapies, Reiki and that type of activity. You need to improve your self-esteem, your chakra, because you have to have your own energy balanced in order to face this kind of disease."

Just as there are **many** factors that converge to make you sick, the **same** logic applies to find *the cure."*

9.

YOUR OWN PATH: "I read books written by Brian Weiss, an American psychiatrist who writes regression stories and has a very good CD to meditate. I followed him. It was my starting point to explore about energies, sounds and vibrations; this took me to a person who has made me feel quite well and with whom I continue meeting twice a week."

10.

ABOUT FRIENDS: "There are friends that give you support and others that disappear. There are friends that you'd like to see more of, but who get scared; it's as if they believe these diseases are contagious. But we need to understand them: they get scared, don't want to interrupt the intimacy you have with your family when you're sick. Everything is understandable. You understand we are all different. Some more than others, they all show their love and deep down are worried. Some people never saw you when sick and then see you are well and start crying." ■

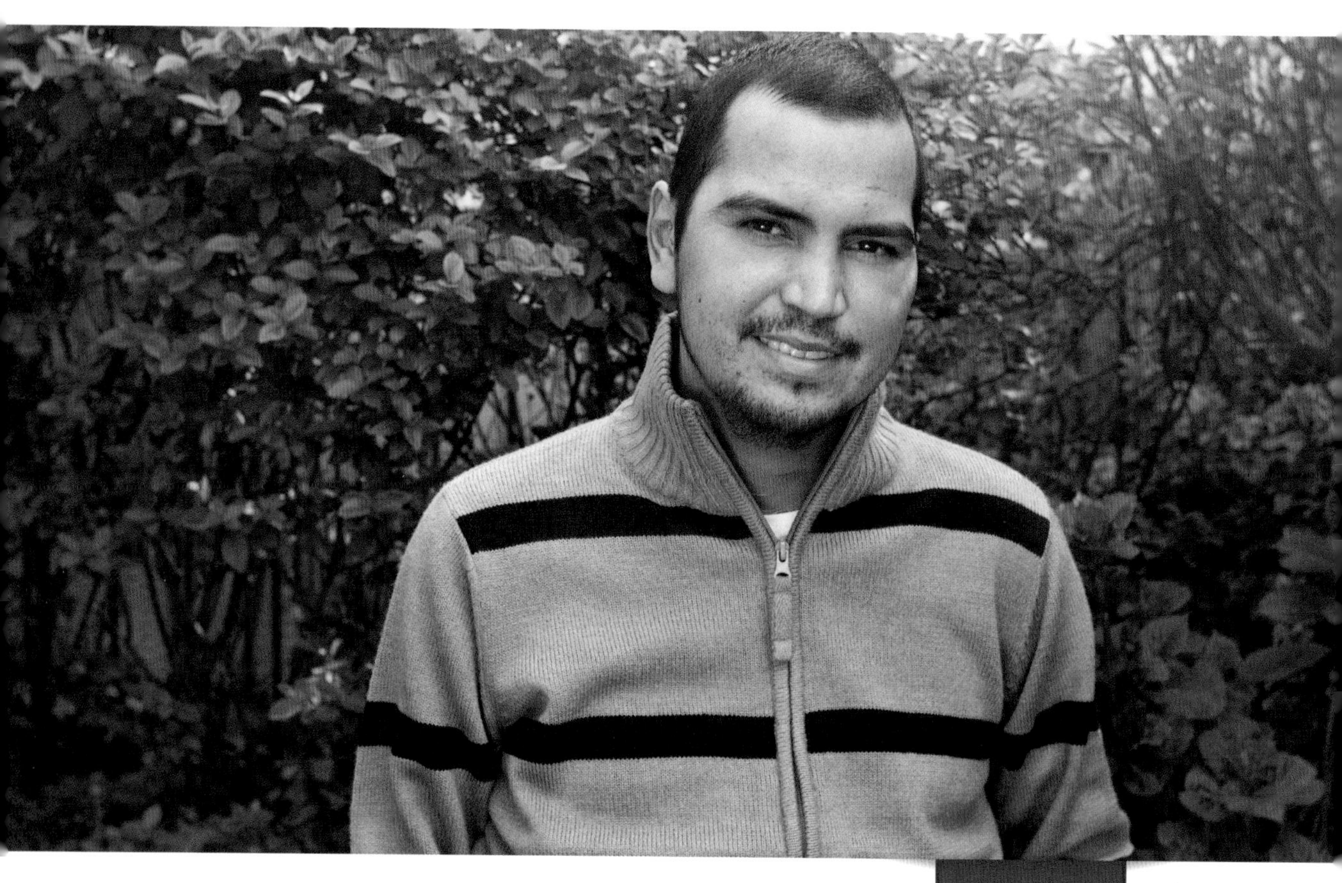

Luis Silva Piñones

Hodgkin's lymphoma

PATIENT

AGE: *26*

OCCUPATION: *Unemployed*

DIAGNOSIS: *Hodgkin's lymphoma and lung cancer with metastasis in the hip*

WHEN: *2008*

CONTEXT: *Five years ago, Luis detected a small ball in his neck. He was examined, but doctors couldn't explain the reason for his inflamed node. He spent one year being tested in private clinics. He was told it could be caused by a cold, lupus, the cat scratch disease... "My neck was increasingly swollen. When we ran out of money and patience, we turned to the public system, where I was diagnosed. Never before had I thought I could have cancer, but I had to face it. 'I'm young, I can hold on', I thought." Unfortunately, Luis passed away on 5 July 2014, and his testimonial becomes even more valuable.*

1.

DON'T STOP FIGHTING: "There are two options, either you fight or stand still, and my choice is to continue fighting. I have faith my disease will end someday, I will be able to resume my life, practice sports I used to practice and accomplish my plans."

2.

VALUE THE PUBLIC HEALTH SYSTEM: "We first visited private clinics because we had the economic resources and they are supposed to be quicker: there are consultations in hospitals which take months. However, doctors from the private clinics were never able to establish my diagnosis, they didn't know my symptoms. I learned that doctors from public hospitals have more experience than doctors of the private sector."

3.

CREATIVE FINANCING: "Plan *Auge* [public health plan in Chile covering some disease treatments] covered my chemotherapies from 2008 up to the end of 2009. I applied to all available state funds, but my condition needed to be worse for me to be eligible, so my family paid for everything. To finance chemotherapy treatment we ran raffles, bingos and parties to raise funds; we also took out loans. In 2010 I had to undergo another procedure that cost 6 million Chilean pesos. We applied for licenses from the municipality to hold fundraising events, the neighbors donated prizes, there were artists, a local musician, the municipality donated the use of the chairs and tables and the kitchens. We raised 500 thousand pesos in less than three hours."

4.

BEING INFORMED: "Many people told me that surfing the Internet was a bad idea because besides suffering from the disease, the surfeit of information can be stressful. Nevertheless, I did it and, thanks to this, I learned about all types and stages of seriousness of my cancer. This depends on you."

5.

ALTERNATIVE TREATMENTS: "I took scorpion poison for a year. It helped my cancer reduce, but I had to stop taking it because it became really expensive and we couldn't afford it." ■

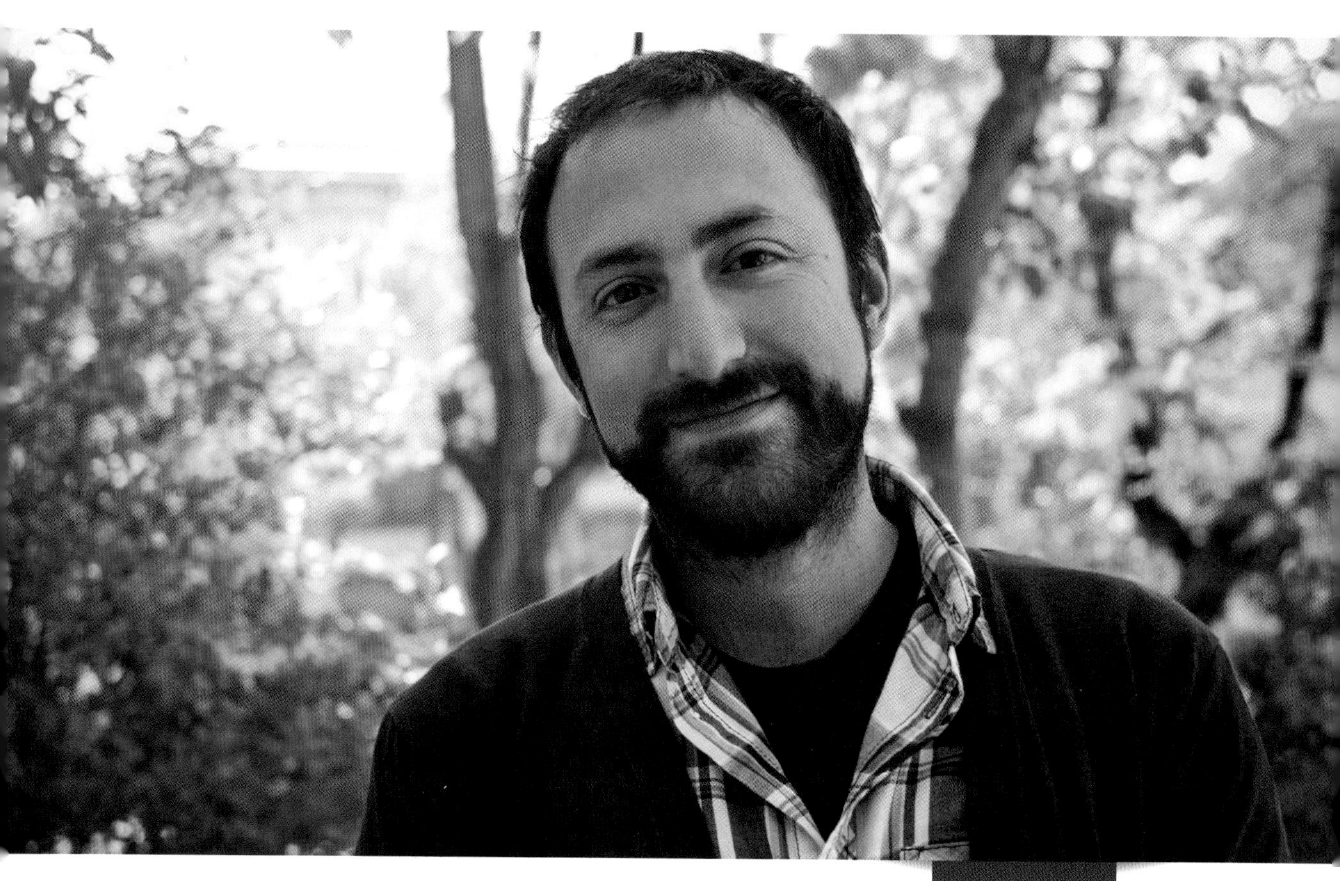

Nicolás Stutzin

Hodgkin's lymphoma

PATIENT

AGE: *32*

OCCUPATION: *Architect*

DIAGNOSIS: *Hodgkin's Lymphoma*

WHEN: *2012*

CONTEXT: *Nicolás felt sick frequently, got tired really quick and had a suspicious cough. He went to see a bronchopulmonary specialist and was hospitalized that same afternoon. A 13-centimeter tumoral mass was compressing his vena cava, trachea and bronchi. He was told he had lymphatic (Hodgkin's) cancer and that the journey was just beginning.*

1.

THE GLASS HALF FULL: "There are two types of lymphatic cancer, Hodgkin's and non Hodgkin's. According to doctors, the first one has a better prognosis and I had that one. Therefore, although I had cancer and it looked complicated, the balance was tilted towards the best side. Seeing it in this way was of great psychological help. It was bad, but it was the least bad option. It's a type of cancer from which people usually recover, but the process is difficult and the cost of getting better is exhausting."

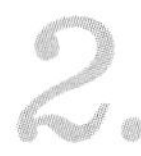

TRUST THE TREATING PHYSICIAN: "I thought about trying alternative therapies, such as vaccines of anthroposophical medicine. But my doctor is very methodical and told me not to do anything that could affect my treatment or the indicators he followed to measure my advances. I was willing to import vaccines from Germany, but preferred creating a more transparent bond with my oncologist, the person who was theoretically going to save my life."

3.

ALWAYS BE AWARE OF BODY WARNINGS: "It took months for my body to adapt to this cancer. I had blood vessels working inversely to compensate areas of irrigation. Until it couldn't resist anymore and I started feeling sick. I coughed because I had shortness of breath and tachycardia because my heart had a small space. It was a fragile balance. In the period prior to diagnosis, my body was compensating for what I was going through and I was sick without knowing it for around six months. This means I have a good physical resistance, but a bad capacity to acknowledge what happens to me."

4.

STRENGTHEN YOUR BODY FOR CHEMOTHERAPY: "After the disease I followed a treatment of anthroposophical medicine to strengthen my body's resistance to chemotherapy. It consists of a mix of drops, powders and lotions. The ingredients depend on who the patient is. Deep down I faced cancer and, at the same time, got informed on what was within me that could explain this disease. I didn't follow an alternative therapy against cancer, but tried to understand what happened before cancer and to prevent undesired effects of the treatment."

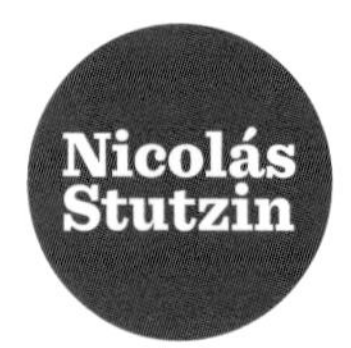

5.

SCIENTIFIC REASON AND ALTERNATIVE VISION: "I'm rational and scientific to understand the things that happen to me. In this sense, I know there is a medical reason which explains cancer, but it has been fundamental for me to acknowledge how I've led my life and what I do to achieve what's important to me, even things I've put off. Mainly considering lymphatic cancer affects the immune system, which acts as a 'police' informant in our organism. Its correct functioning depends on how you take care of yourself: how much you sleep, how you sleep, what you eat... And I was quite irregular and not systematic in relation to taking care of myself."

6.

KEEP UPDATED: "I kept taking classes at University and it was very important to know I could continue working. I know some people find it impossible, but it helped me very much, because I could leave aside the idea of being sick and having to heal. Also, because I proved to myself I could although I was sick. It is key to find moments of little satisfactions."

"It was very *important* to know I could continue **working.** I know some people find it impossible, but it helped me very much, because I could leave aside the idea of *being sick.*"

7.

RELAXATION PRACTICES: "During my chemotherapy treatment, I did reiki and reflexology every week to be relaxed and have a quiet moment. I want to be systematic in my aim of being aware of what is happening to me."

8.

REASONABLE LIMITS: *"With cancer, some sort of community is created where everybody speaks in plural: we're fine, as if they were all sick. On the one hand it's very nice, but on the other it can be invasive. How to do it will depend on each patient, but I believe you need to learn to establish limits for the benefit of the patient, their family and friends, because they sometimes believe you're worse than what you really are and get more worried."*

9.

DON'T OVERBURDEN YOURSELF: "Knowing how to delegate what you can no longer do without neglecting your disease is key: you may count on your family, wife and friends. You realize everybody accepts it willingly; knowing you have that kind of support is very valuable and helps you to face the challenges in a more efficient way."

"I know there are medical ***reasons*** which explain cancer, but it has been fundamental for me to acknowledge how I've led **my life** and what I do ***to achieve*** what's important to me."

10.

NO AMBIGUITIES: "It is paramount to be clear about what you want and do not want and when, which includes learning to say *please come another day, today I don't feel too good.* The best thing you can do is be clear and assertive." ■

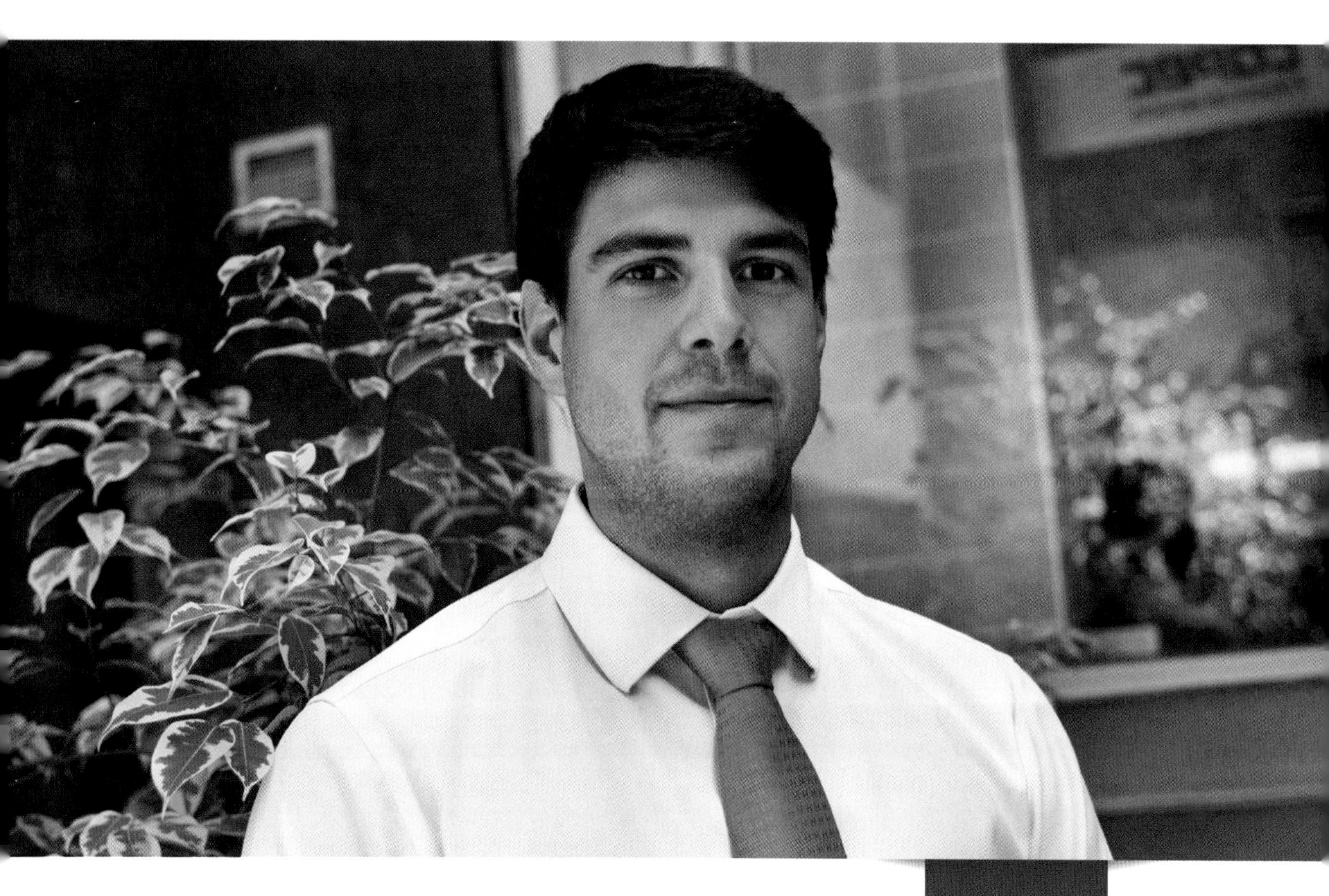

Max Valdés

Hodgkin's lymphoma

PATIENT

AGE: *30*

OCCUPATION: *BA in business administration and MBA*

DIAGNOSIS: *Hodgkin's Lymphoma*

WHEN: *2004*

CONTEXT: *At the beginning of the last decade, in his first year of college, from one day to another Max discovered a bump of the size of a tennis ball in the neck. Five months later, he finished chemotherapy and traveled to Boston to receive radiation and finally eradicate the cancer.*

1.

LISTEN TO THE BAD NEWS IN THE COMPANY OF YOUR FAMILY: "When the doctors got together to tell me the bad news, they sat me down and told me everything. They explained each procedure they were going to carry out, how I was going to feel and the effects they would have on me; all in the presence of my parents and my brother. It's good to have family around when you're given explanations so you don't need to repeat things or speak about things you don't want to repeat. When the doctor left, we stayed there all together and it was quite strange. We had been explained all, but didn't know where to start reacting."

2.

DIVORCED PARENTS SUPPORTING A SON TOGETHER: "My parents were divorced and didn't get in contact that much before my disease, but they faced the issue together. They even came together with me to Boston. My brother and sister were also with me there. It was strange having lunch all together again, but I enjoyed it. They also made an effort not to fight during the entire process and I thank them for that."

3.

THE CHEMOTHERAPY CYCLE: "Chemotherapy process, which had eight cycles distributed over five months, is usually scary. The good thing is you have plenty time to think, value what you have and try and be positive. Recently, my father's sister was diagnosed with leukemia and I spoke with her. I told her she needed to be well, that she knew her body better than others and that, in the end, it all depended on her. No matter how much others talk to you, no matter how much support you have, you need to learn to live with these new thoughts."

4.

MORE WARMTH IN CHILE: "I had the chance of doing part of my treatment in the United States. It's true they had all the equipment and state-of-the-art technology, but they are very distant people. Therefore, if somebody wants to have chemotherapy, I wouldn't recommend it. In Chile it's very different: nurses are very warm and doctors really embrace you and take care of you. The treatment patients receive is very different here than in the United States." ■

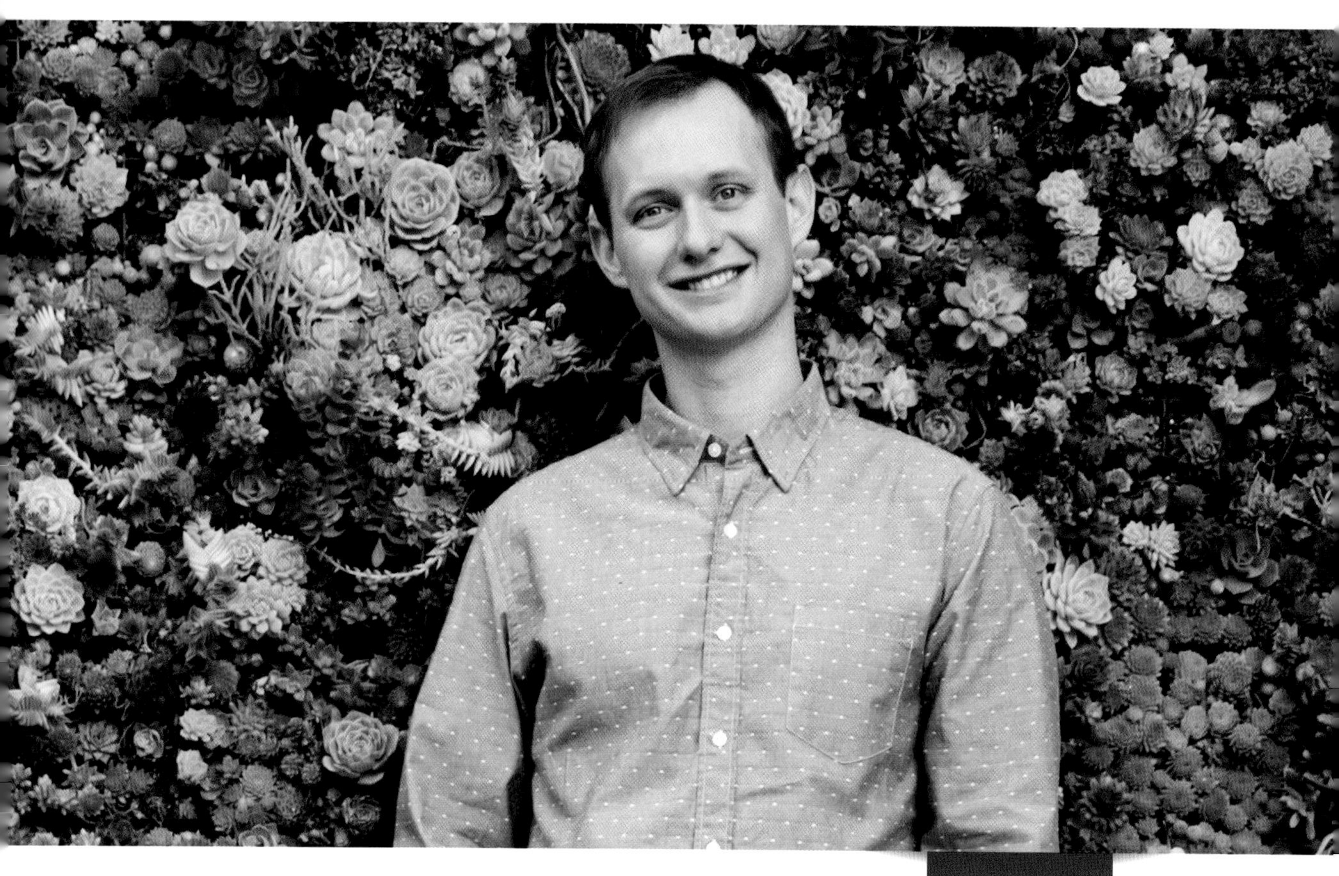

Peter Moore

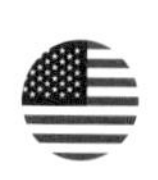

Hodgkin's lymphoma

PATIENT

AGE: *24*

OCCUPATION: *Internal Medicine Physician*

DIAGNOSIS: *Hodgkin's lymphoma*

WHEN: *2008*

CONTEXT: *At the time of my diagnosis I was a first year medical student, and had recently finished working for one year as a lymphoma researcher. I had noticed a lump in the right side of my neck that persisted for one year. After many laboratory tests, attempted treatment with empiric antibiotics, and several imaging studies, a surgical biopsy led to my diagnosis. Two years later I relapsed and have since been in remission. At the time of diagnosis I had just started a new relationship (had been dating approximately 2 weeks- we are now married).*

1.

BE EASY ON YOURSELF: "Cancer is exhausting, both physically and emotionally. It is normal to be scared, feel tired, and to not be in the mood to do things you usually love. Do not be hard on yourself. If you aren't in the mood for something one day, forgive yourself and try again tomorrow."

2.

FORGIVE YOUR FAMILY AND FRIENDS: "It is important to recognize the emotional distress that accompanies cancer is not limited to the patient, but is also experienced by family members and close friends. Just as every person with cancer has a different response to the diagnosis, those close to them will also experience a spectrum of emotions, including anger, anxiety, and depression. Remind yourself that they are going through a rough time also, cannot possibly understand how you feel at that particular moment, and (usually) mean the best!"

"**Don't let** cancer get the best of you. You need to *keep being you!*"

3.

DELEGATE A FRIEND OR FAMILY MEMBER TO BE A POINT OF CONTACT: "It may be easier to have a close friend send updates to your loved ones to take the burden off of you. This can allow those who care about you to understand what is going on and feel connected, without overwhelming you."

4.

BRING UP FERTILITY PRESERVATION EARLY: *"If you are planning on having children in the future, be sure to bring up fertility preservation with your oncologist."*

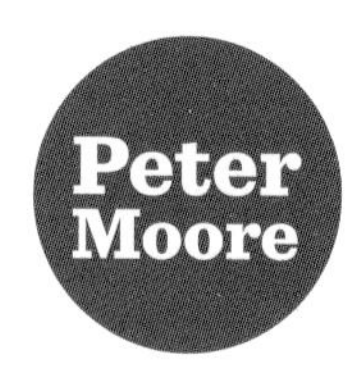

5.

TAKE CONTROL OF SOMETHING IN YOUR LIFE: "Getting diagnosed with cancer is the ultimate loss of control. I started a non-profit to raise money for lymphoma research during my radiation treatment, which made me feel like I was doing something to fight the disease. Many people make changes to their diets or start an exercise routine. All of these things allow you to take back some control, which will make you feel less powerless."

6.

FIND A HOBBY: "There is a ton of downtime during cancer treatment. I learned to crochet hats, and made over 50 of them during my chemotherapy to give to friends and to auction off for charity. You could become a Sudoku, crossword, or jigsaw puzzle master by the end of treatment!"

7.

SCHEDULE YOUR SURVEILLANCE APPOINTMENTS: "Once your therapy is over make sure to keep up with your doctor and radiology appointments. I made the mistake of prioritizing work and school and my recurrence was diagnosed on a scan that was 3 months overdue."

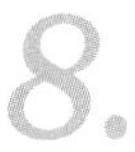

8.

MAKE A FOLDER FOR MEDICAL EXPENSE RECEIPTS: "Make sure to have a system for filing these, and keeping track of which bills have been paid. This will be handy when there is an inevitable dispute with your insurance company. Also, don't pay for hospital expenses not covered by insurance until you talk with the insurance company directly. These costs will often be covered be insurance when disputed."

Do not be *hard* on yourself. If you aren't in the **mood** for something one day, *forgive* yourself and ***try again*** tomorrow."

9.

KEEP DOING THE THINGS THAT YOU ENJOY: *"Don't let cancer get the best of you. You need to keep being you! I skied between chemotherapy cycles, even when I could manage one or two runs between breaks due to fatigue."* ■

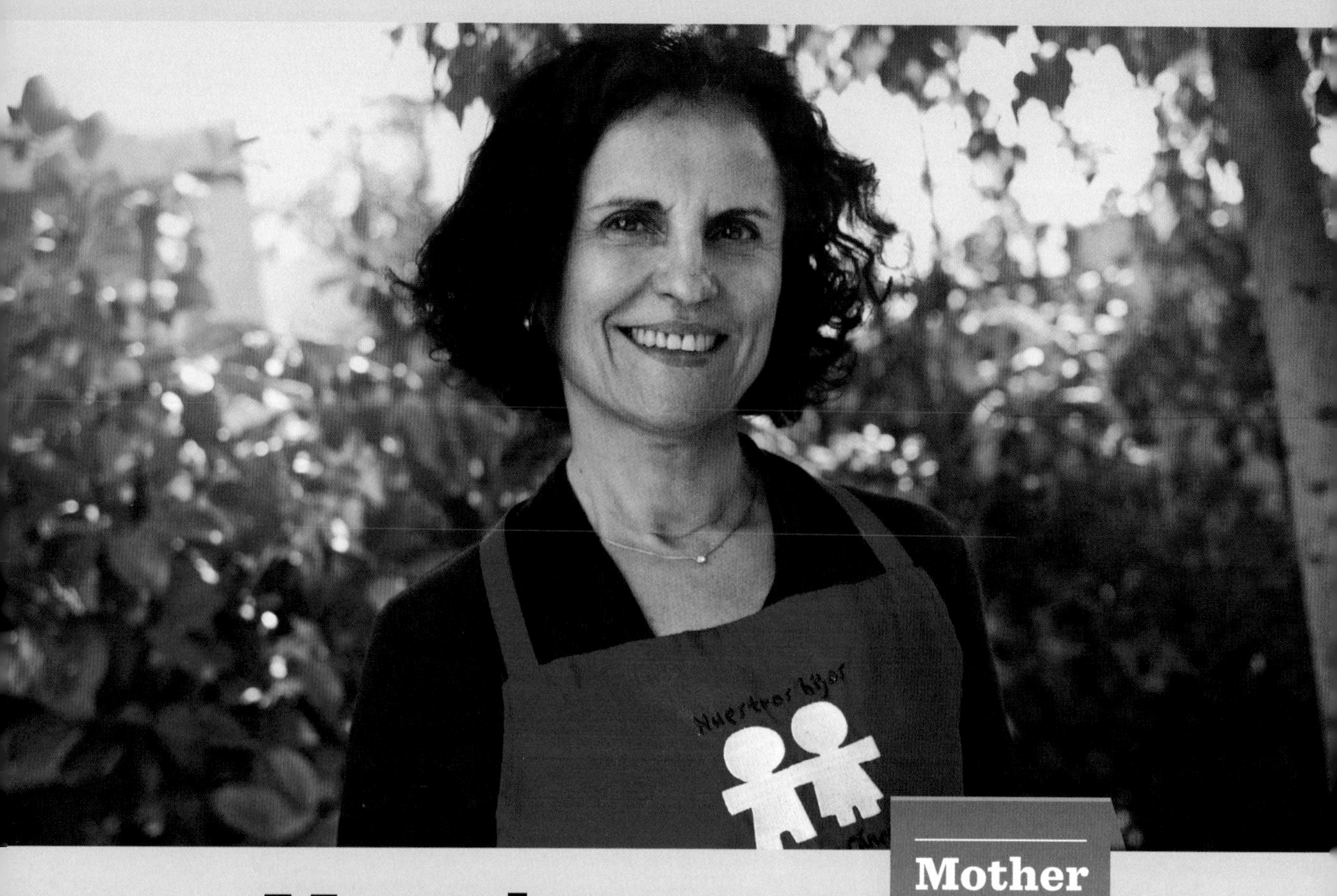

Marcela Zubieta

Mother *of* brain tumor patient

AGE: *60*

OCCUPATION: *Pediatrician*

RELATIONSHIP: *Mother of Brain Tumor Patient*

WHEN: *1988*

CONTEXT: *Her one and a half year old daughter's disease changed her life 180 degrees. Claudita Besomi's brain tumor couldn't be treated in Chile and they found hope in St. Jude Hospital in Memphis, a world premier pediatric oncology research hospital and the only one which had a research protocol at the time for her type of cancer. They fought a two-year battle in the United States, which finally Claudita could not resist. After such an experience, Marcela –together with other parents– created the organization* Nuestros Hijos *(Our Children), which today provides assistance to children from low-income families who have cancer.*

1.

THE BEST DOCTOR IS NOT AT THE MOST EXPENSIVE CLINIC: "In the rarest cancer cases, such as the one my daughter had, the best doctor is not always found at the most expensive clinic. We ended up taking her to the doctor with the most experience in pediatric brain tumors who operated on her in the Neurosurgical Institute in Chile. 80% of children with cancer are treated in the public system, and doctors from the Institute were those with the most experience."

2.

LEARN THE MESSAGE: "I wanted to be a general infectology specialist and I'm now trained as an infectology specialist for cancer patients. I totally refocused my professional life on children with cancer from the point of view of infectology and the creation of the foundation."

3.

ACCEPT THE INVITATION: "I felt I didn't need to be worried about why this had happened to me, but what for. Life is a puzzle. I believe in God, and believe He makes invitations you can either accept or reject; I felt this was an invitation for me to do something. I realized Claudita's passage through this world had had a purpose and I was willing to assume it."

4.

THINGS HAPPEN FOR A REASON: "A nurse at the hospital once told me *I bless the moment your daughter got sick, because you changed the life of thousands of children.* Of course, it has a strong side, but it's also good that it's recognized. The path I've followed has been so productive that I also feel all this has been, maybe not a blessing, but a very beautiful life. I believe I had a privileged life. Some people live for a hundred years and have a terrible time and others live for three and are happy. At the end of the road you decide if *everything had a meaning*. I'm completely at peace."

5.

FROM THINKING TO ACTION: "When my daughter got worse, we returned to Chile and she spent a month in a coma in Santiago before she died. At the funeral we started inviting our friends to become part of the *Fundación Nuestros Hijos* (Our Children Foundation). On the day following her death, I started working on it. We quickly formed a group of volunteers whose first mission was going to be making children cancer patients and their families have a better quality of life. That's how the story starts."

Marcela Zubieta

6.

QUALITY PUBLIC HEALTH SERVICE: "Many times you need to ask for two or three opinions, if the first two don't coincide. And know how to choose carefully where you're going to treat your children, which depends on your socioeconomic situation. There are some people who only want to go to a private clinic and end up mortgaging everything, when public health services currently have great units and, sometimes, get the same or better results than private clinics. Clinics and hospitals are working in collaboration and, the former are in line with international protocols."

7.

NO HERO-MOMS: "The person at the front row who accompanies the child patient is almost always the mother, and she must take care of herself. She doesn't need to act as a heroine and quit sleeping or eating correctly. In this mom-child duo, the small child looks to her to know if everything is okay because they don't understand about survival percentages."

8.

KNOW TO CHOOSE BETWEEN PRIVATE AND PUBLIC HEALTH SYSTEMS: "You need to be well-informed on cancer to take good decisions. For instance, cancer in adults is totally different from children's cancer, because although the disease advances more slowly, they respond less to treatment and have worst prognoses. Children have a 77% survival rate of 5 years, but time and periods are much shorter; so you need to act quickly. In order to have access to *Auge* (health coverage) you have a certain period of time to inform whether you're going to be treated with *Fonasa* (Chilean public health system) or *Isapre* (Chilean private health system). After that you can't change your decision. *Fonasa*, for certain types of cancers, may be a great option because you have access to public health treatment centers. If you're in an *Isapre*, you can't receive attention in public centers."

9.

NOT EVERYBODY HAS THE NECESSARY RESOURCES: "You need to activate the support networks and explore what institutions can provide help. I say this because I work in the public system and 80% of the people receiving treatment in hospitals have limited resources and have no local support networks, because people are focused on their own lives, just getting by. Therefore, who will give them money for their transportation, help them get a bed to avoid their child sleeping with his brothers because risks increase, or fix their bathroom, buy special milk or drugs? Only institutional support networks."

10.

FOCUS EFFORTS: "I believe that more than worrying, you need to *take care* of doing things well. This means that when you're diagnosed and, if you have enough resources, you need to look for the specialist you consider most prepared to treat you. Not the most famous one, but the one who knows more."

11.

CHILDHOOD CANCER PREVENTION: *"Before, it was considered that children's cancer couldn't be prevented, but there are increasingly reports stating there are factors that favor cancer development in children; not just the sun, for example. Pesticides the father had contact with before conceiving or the mother had contact with during pregnancy may cause leukemia; These factors have to be studied further to rule out that they are risk factors."* ■

Cancer in adults is very **different** from children's cancer, because despite the slower advance of the disease, they respond less to treatments and have worst prognoses. Children *survive* 5 years in 77 percent of the cases, but time and periods are much **shorter."**

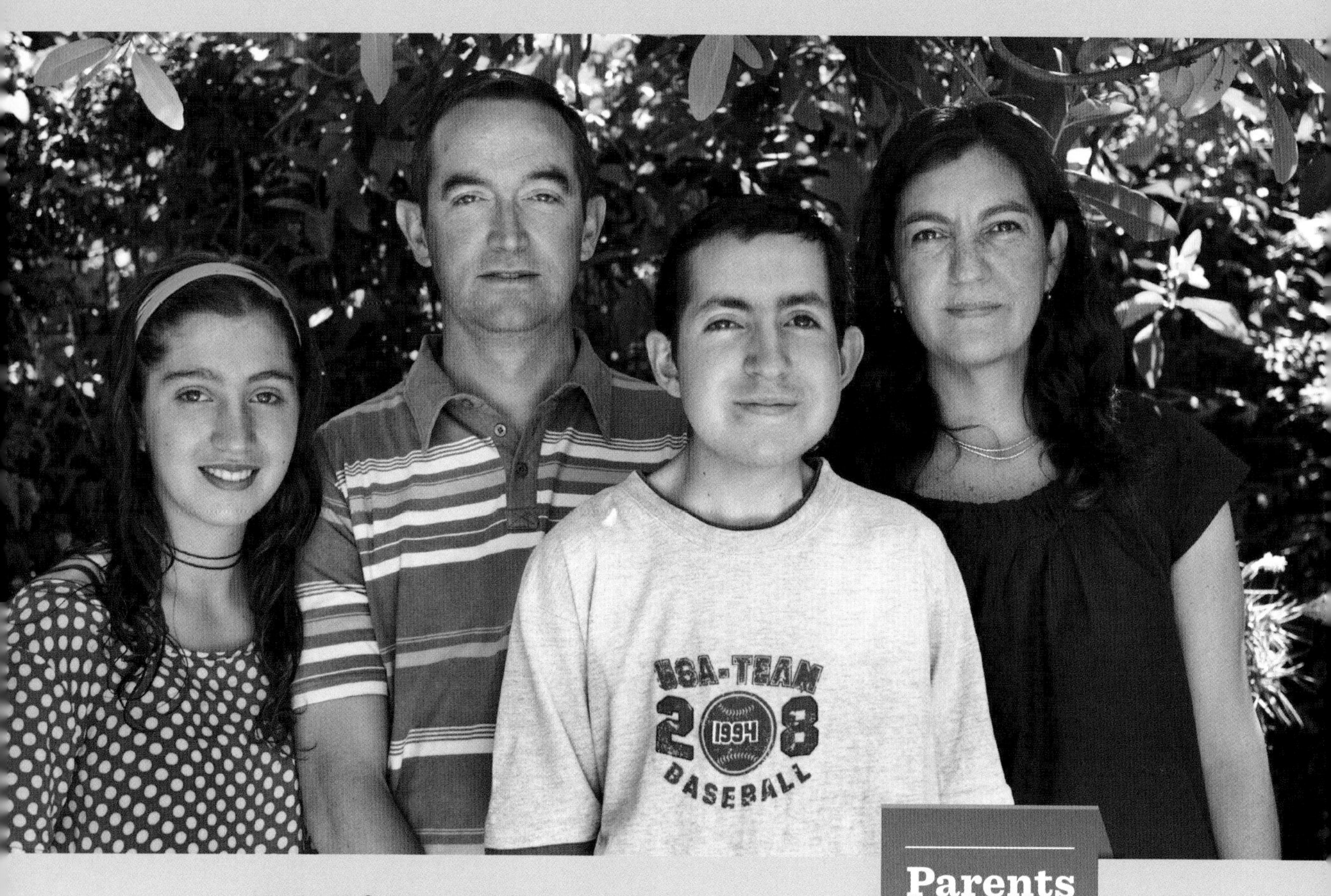

Parents *of* brain tumor patient

Felipe Gross & Claudia Sarrazin

DIEGO'S PARENTS

EDADES: *45 and 44, respectively*

OCCUPATION: *BA in business administration and clinical psychologist*

RELATIONSHIP: *Parents of a brain tumor patient*

WHEN: *2003*

CONTEXT: *Two weeks went by between when Claudia and Felipe noticed the first symptoms and the day in which they heard the word which, abruptly, took away the family's calmness: medulloblastoma. Their five-year old son, Diego, had been just diagnosed with a very aggressive tumor located on the back of his head, very close to the encephalic trunk. He had to undergo emergency surgery that same night and doctors warned that what was coming was going to be tough. They weren't wrong.*

1.

LEARNING THE HARD WAY: "You learn many things, such as what is a true problem and the true value of things. We value life over anything else, even over the conditions in which that life is developed. When we were told: *look, compare radiation plus chemotherapy possibilities versus only radiation or only chemotherapy...* the option with more survival possibilities was radiotherapy plus chemotherapy, but it had too many consequences, a cognitive impairment being one. Facing this, we placed the value of life over any other consideration."

2.

THE EXTREME QUESTIONS: "In the worst moments, bonding and being in contact with others helped us. At first, we were closely accompanied by a Jesuit priest, who asked us the hardest questions. He joined us on the night of the diagnosis; we were still in shock and couldn't stop crying. He faced us and asked us the main questions, those people who love you don't ask due to a misunderstood respect of your intimacy.

3.

RISING FROM THE ASHES: *"What is the worst that can happen?* was his question. We answered without addressing the issue; *well, Diego will go home anyway*; until we mentioned death and shook from head to toe. Only then did we realize what we were dealing with, but we could quickly start with the reconstruction."

4.

THE MEANING OF THINGS: "The meaning of Diego's disease is that of valuing life, the present, of enjoying more, of walking with a lighter weight in life seeking and deep happiness. It's really weird for people to understand, but that's how it has been. Either on the deepest pain or in the most spectacular happiness, one always finds God."

5.

PROVIDENTIAL CHARACTERS: "Diego's defenses lowered a lot after each chemotherapy and we had to give him a special drug for ten days. A nurse from the clinic came to our house every month to administer the drug, in order for Diego to avoid going to the clinic. Providential characters start appearing, people who gave us cakes, children who gave him their toys."

Gross Sarrazin Family

6.

PROMISES MUST BE KEPT: "When we were at the clinic, Diego met *Ogú* and *Mampato*: the film was just released and then he read the books. He told us he wanted to go to Easter Island; he knew all of *Ogú's* speeches. And there in the clinic we made a commitment with him: he was five and a half years old and we told him when you turn fifteen, we will go to Easter Island. And when he turned fifteen he did not forget. We fulfilled our promise in August, a month after his birthday."

7.

A TEST FOR THE COUPLE: "This experience is hard on the relationship. Going through something like this can break a marriage or make it stronger. When Diego's condition stabilized each of us had moments when we'd crumble and the other would hold us up."

"This is not a **parenthesis,** it's a new status. It's neither better nor worse, but it's hard getting *used* to it."

8.

OFFICIAL *PRESS RELEASE*: "We had great help from a friend taking over what we could call the *press release* for friends about Diego's condition. This way the story was spread and we didn't have to tell it twenty times."

10.

LEAN ON EXPERIENCE: "It is important to let yourself be supported by someone that has gone through the process. We did not have it, and that is why we like to be present for other families. At the beginning you think everthing starts and ends with surgery."

9.

NEW NORMALITY: "This is not a parenthesis in life, it's a new status. It's neither better nor worse, but another life, that in some cases can be very tough getting used to it. Is filled with very nice things, but it's hard and it always will be."

11.

PAIN AS OIL: "As a friend told us: pain is like oil. Oil is fossilized waste and it keeps being that as long as you keep it where it is, but if you extract it you can change it into something useful. The same happens with pain; you can remain crying and sad, but you can also take advantage of the situation personal growth and development within the relationship."

12.

OTHER EXPECTATIONS: "You may sometimes feel you belong to a group of chosen people, because you're living a unique experience. That's the most difficult thing to transmit, because when you're in the middle of the process, everything seems hideous: I could have hit anyone at the time who told me the disease would be for the better. Now, after time has passed, I have a different point of view; honestly it was good for us. We are a better family today, we changed our priorities and the way in which we fulfill our expectations in life."

13.

SMALL RESIGNATIONS FOR PARENTS: "Diego is deaf, meaning he hears very badly, and misses some high-pitched sounds in words. Cognitively, everything is more difficult for him than for others, mainly certain levels of abstraction, but he is very concrete and ordered and his organizational capacity enables him to advance. The social aspect is the hardest, not because he has difficulties to socialize, but because children his age see him differently. We haven't heard about him being mocked, but he is not included much. Adolescence is a complicated time for children and even more for Diego. We chose to send him to a small school, not very demanding, where he wouldn't stand out much. It was a great decision, but in order to take such a decision we had to forget some dreams, such as sending Diego to a well-known school, in a nice place, surrounded by our friend's children... His school is not like that, but it has a strong and clear aim for children's wellbeing, their healthy development and happiness. This, in our opinion, makes it a great school."

14.

SUGGESTED READING: "It was suggest that we read a book that was very beneficial to us which was very good for us. It's called *Yo Superé el Cáncer* ("I Overcame Cancer") and is written by doctors. The editor is Annette Becker and it includes testimonials from children – now grownups– and adult patients who defeated cancer. It includes phrases which make a lot of sense to those going through a similar experience." ■

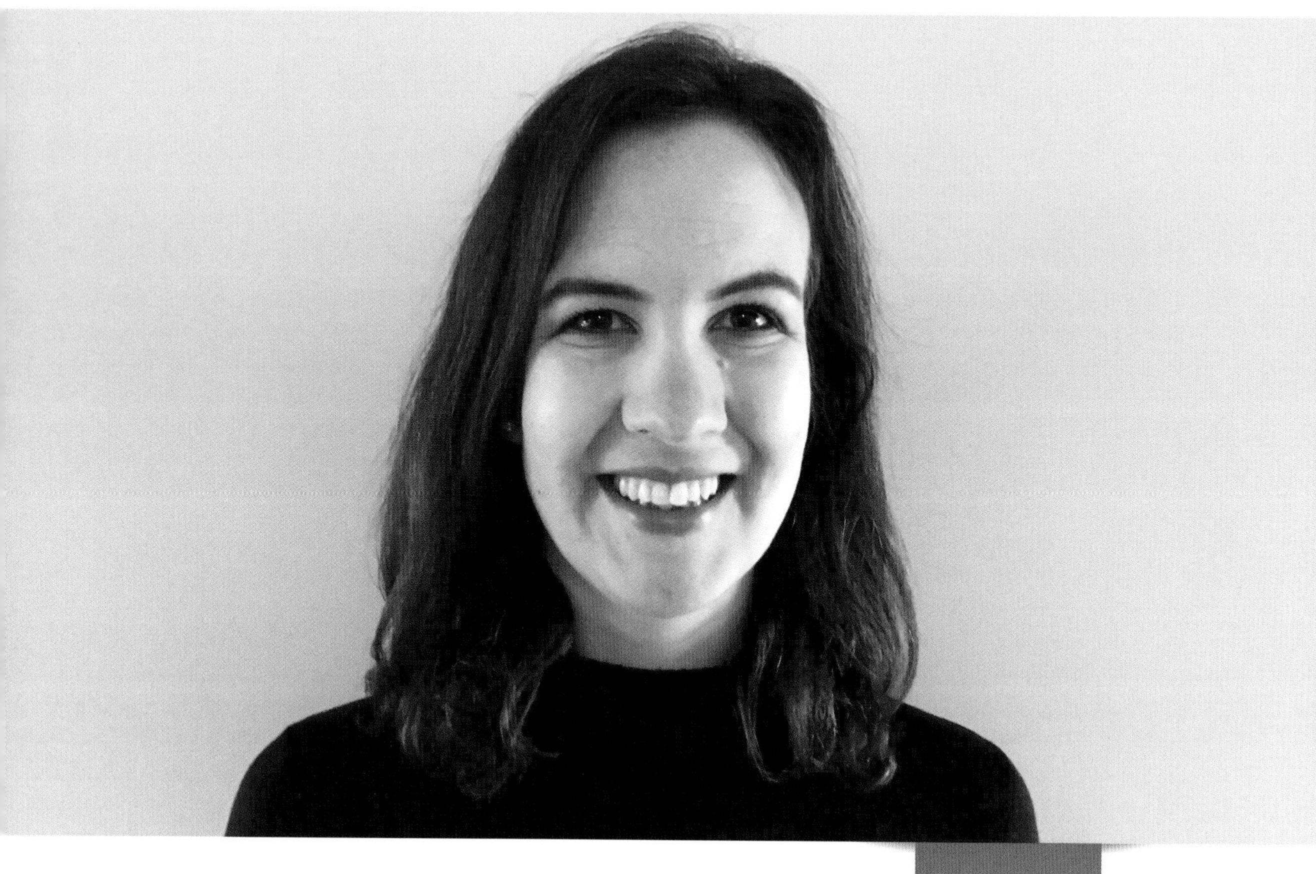

Sabine Schwab

brain tumor PATIENT

AGE: *35*

OCCUPATION: *ABTA volunteer and stay at home mom*

DIAGNOSIS: *Anaplastic Astrocytoma (grade 3 primary brain cancer)*

WHEN: *2014*

CONTEXT: *In 2014, I was living an amazing life with my husband and brand new baby girl. That spring, out of the blue, I had a seizure in the middle of the night and was rushed to the emergency room. They soon discovered a mass in my brain and I had to have emergency brain surgery. I was only 32 years old and diagnosed with primary brain cancer. Three years out, I am still facing some cognitive challenges, but I am happy and trying to live life to its fullest despite the negative outlook I am facing.*

1.

IT IS TOTALLY OK TO CRY!: *"A very important piece of coping with cancer is the recognition of emotions and feelings. While positivity plays a big role, you may feel pressured into keeping a good attitude at all times. In my opinion, it is not only acceptable to cry, it is healthy as well. Don't put your smiley-face on for others if you don't feel like it. Find that person you can cry with!"*

2.

START A DIARY OR BLOG: "You may ask why? Well, there are several reasons:
a) Writing is a powerful and excellent tool for the soul and self-healing process.
b) Chemo brain is real. In case you want to remember anything, put it in writing.
c) You will get tired of telling the same story or answer the same questions over and over again. By creating a blog or caring bridge page, you can update all your loved ones, family, friends, neighbors at the same time.
d) It serves as a source for inspiration in difficult times. You can see what you overcame and how badass you really are."

Eating the **right** kinds of foods helped me feel better and stay stronger."

3.

ACCEPT THE GIFT OF HELP! BE SPECIFIC WITH WHAT YOU NEED: "I am such a do-it-myself person. It took some time to accept help from others. Most likely, people will offer making meals. If you don't want to find your freezer stocked with soups until next year's winter, be specific about what help you need.. Have them do your laundry, run errands, walk the dog, pick up medication, watch a movie with you, rub your feet, etc."

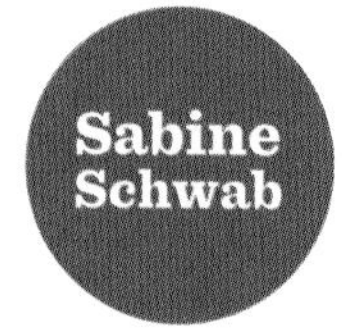

4.

PRE- AND POST-PREPARATION OF DOCTORS' VISITS: "Whenever you have a question concerning your diagnosis, treatment or side effects, make a note of it. Before each doctor visit, compile the list and sort by nurse/doctor questions.. Always bring a second person with you when seeing your doctor. Record your visits on your phone or a voice recorder. Always collect all your medical records including scans, blood work, reports, etc."

5.

FIND ONLINE SUPPORT GROUPS: "We live in a time of social media - make use of it! I am pretty sure there is a support group on Facebook for almost every kind of cancer. Also, you'll get support 24/7 and you don't need to wait for your spouse or friend to wake up. You can share your story and ask questions, pray and laugh and cry together. The knowledge within these groups is huge!"

6.

TRY INTEGRATIVE MEDICINE: "I am a true believer in combining eastern and western medicine. Mediation and breathing techniques have helped me to reduce my scanxiety. Daily Yoga gave me back my strength and keeps me active."

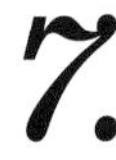

SLEEP! AND SLEEP SOME MORE: "Especially for primary brain cancer patients, like me, sleep is an important factor in the healing process. Sleep is the only time the brain heals from its trauma; it is when cells repair the damage and restore tissue."

8.

DON'T EAT C.R.A.P.: "C = carbonated beverages, R = refined carbs and sugars, A = artificial sweeteners, flavors, and colors, P = processed foods. Good nutrition is important for good health. Eating the right kinds of foods helped me feel better and stay stronger."

9.

#SENDIT #OUTLIVINGIT: "Cancer sucks, big time. But there are amazing organizations, willing to help you feel alive! Don't underestimate the power of nature and togetherness. Surround yourself with people who get it! My favorite quote: "When 'I' is replaced by 'WE', 'Illness' becomes 'Wellness'."

"A very *important* piece of coping with cancer is the recognition of ***emotions*** and **feelings.**"

10.

MAKE SURE YOU HAVE AN ADVANCE DIRECTIVE AND LIVING WILL: *"With a medical power of attorney, you can appoint a person to make healthcare decisions for you. A living will is an advance directive that guides your family and provider through the medical treatment you wish to receive. Both are important documents to have in case you are unable to communicate your wishes."* ■

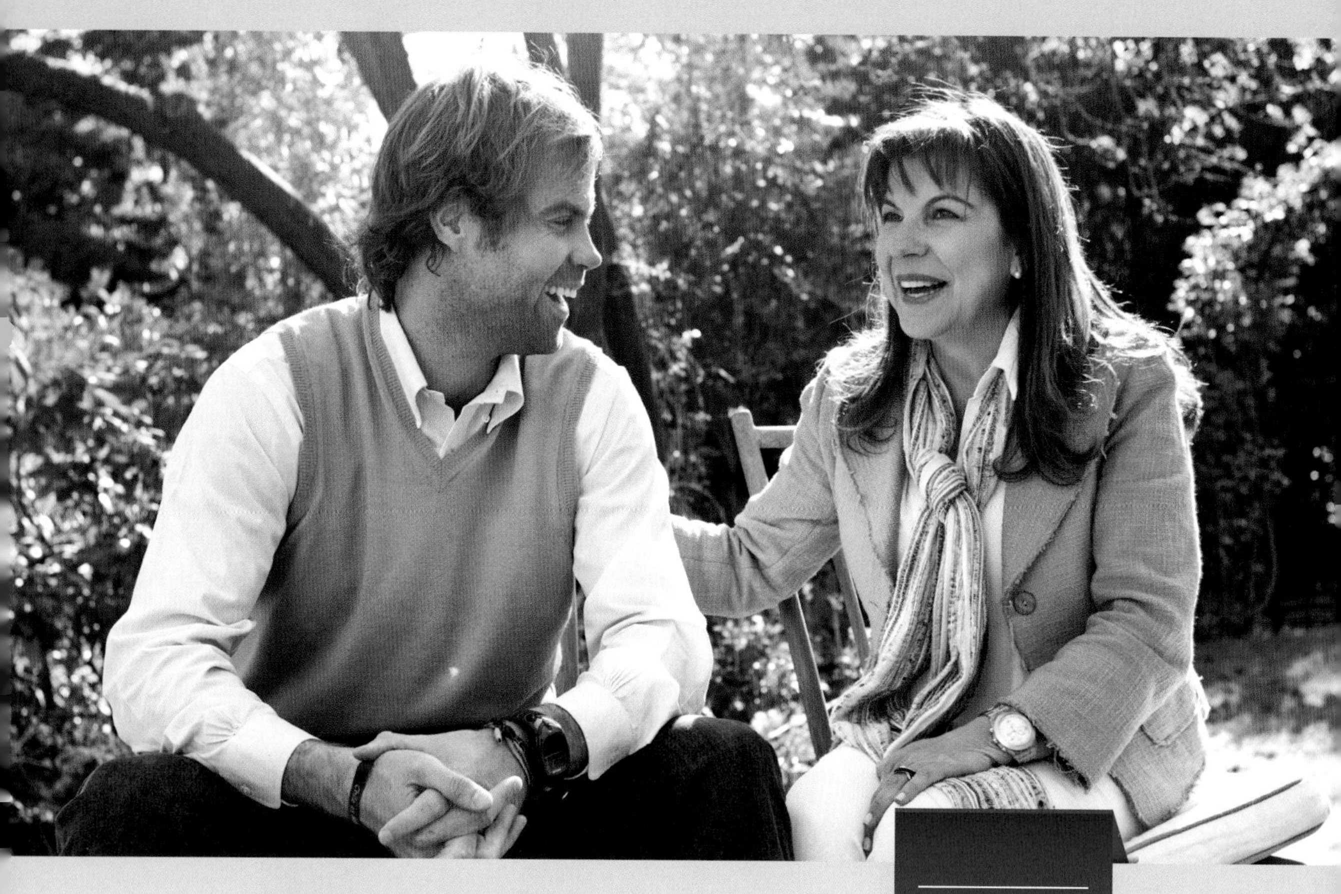

Patricia Marchesse

Mother *of* leukemia patient

AGE: *55*

OCCUPATION: *BA in business administration*

RELATIONSHIP: *Mother of a Leukemia patient*

WHEN: *1994*

CONTEXT: *They say there is no greater pain than losing a child, and Patricia experienced it first-hand. For seven years she fought the lymphoblastic leukemia of Tomás, her son, until nothing more could be done. The experience would leave its mark on Patricia and the rest of her family.*

1.

DON'T STAY WITH THE DOUBT: "Before we learned about Tomás' disease, the pediatrician examined him and found his nodes inflamed. The problem is that nodes get inflamed due to a cold, an infection or for many other reasons. However, my husband, an engineer, told her: I don't understand anything and I'm worried, why don't we get a scan? The doctor agreed and also asked for a hemogram. This is a job that starts with the parents in collaboration with the doctor. No one has the final word; the work is performed jointly."

"Mom, *I want to live!*, **Tomás** answered."

2.

AT FIRST IT CAN BE A GAME: "With the beginning of the treatment comes the hardest part: Seeing your child suffer. Despite everything that happens, you need to learn to switch and prepare to fight. Tomás was 4 years old when he was diagnosed with a lymphoblastic leukemia and we started talking to him about the 'little bugs' he had and how we were going to kill them. We even made some songs up about them. Therefore, at first it was all a kind of game for him. During a crisis in which he refused to be injected, my husband suggested a deal: If he agreed to the injection, he'd get a motorbike. They shook hands and the deal was fulfilled. The motorbike would be his great ally in the following years."

3.

SOMETIMES, PRIORITIZING IS MANDATORY: "One day my daughter Daniela, who was three years old at the time, was found inside a closet crying because her parents were never with her. I acknowledge all my time was for Tomás and the doctor told me something that, at first, I found very cold: 'Patricia, Tomás needs you now, the burden will be fixed later.' Of course my daughters weren't a burden, but deep down he was right. The risk that Tomás could die at any moment was high and if I didn't spend time with him I would regret it. Later I caught up with my two little girls and we are now very close friends."

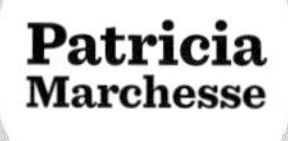

4.

TALKING TO A CHILD ABOUT DEATH: "Tomás once asked me if people could die of cancer. I answered that some did and that was why he needed to follow the treatment. The next day, the hemogram showed a bad result. I talked to him and said: 'My love, we won't do anything you don't want to do, but if we do nothing you'll die.' 'Mom, I want to live!' he answered; so I told him that he would have to resume the treatment. He was the one who decided to live."

5.

HOW CAN I TELL HIS SISTERS?: "You need to get support from people who know. The psychiatrist underscored that cycles need to be closed. It was important for his sisters to see him and be beside him in the room when their brother passed away. One of them realized that Tomás was no longer breathing. So I told her he was now in heaven."

6.

UNDERSTAND THE INEXPLICABLE: "The death of a son is something huge that causes an enormous pain, but it's another step. I miss my son very much, but I know he doesn't suffer anymore and I feel he's at peace, wherever he is. This is what I try to transmit to people: Sometimes you need to know how to let your loved ones go."

7.

TALKING ABOUT HIM: "I always speak about Tomás, so much so that people sometimes get confused. To be honest he is a part of me. I have another type of communication with him, sometimes I feel he cuddles me and is with me. At first I organized masses in his memory, but then I understood the grief was mine and I didn't have to make others accompany me to the cemetery. I sometimes ask if someone wants to join me, other times I say nothing. I tried not passing my feeling of grief to my little girls from the beginning. They already had theirs."

8.

LOSE A SON, WIN OTHERS: "It's a complete environment that supports you. His school mates knew him, went to the clinic, and wore masks and gloves because Tomás had no defenses after the chemotherapy. It was a very nice process, full of love. His circle grew as he did. It happened to us, but everyone prayed for him, supported him and, as I already said, during the process I gained true sons among Tomás' school mates."

9.

SPECIAL PEOPLE: "He wanted to live; if we had to take down a star from heaven for him to touch, we had to do it. The strength, bravery and courage this bald precious little person had was admirable. I believe the people who go through this are chosen; I say this with honesty, because they're special people who pass leaving marks in other people."

"What ***I try*** to transmit to people is that sometimes you need to know how to let your *loved ones go.*"

10.

THE FAREWELL: "He always fought and fought, but in that minute I felt he could not fight anymore, he was tired. Then I told him: '*Pelao*, I'm proud of your fight, because my God you've been brave! I love you, cherish you... but follow the light. I will take care of your father and sisters, I swear; no matter what I will always be there.' And his heartbeat started decreasing. Roberto, his dad, also told him very beautiful things: that he had been the most important thing in his life and that, although all children would like to be like their parents, in this case it was the other way around: he dreamed about being like his son." ■

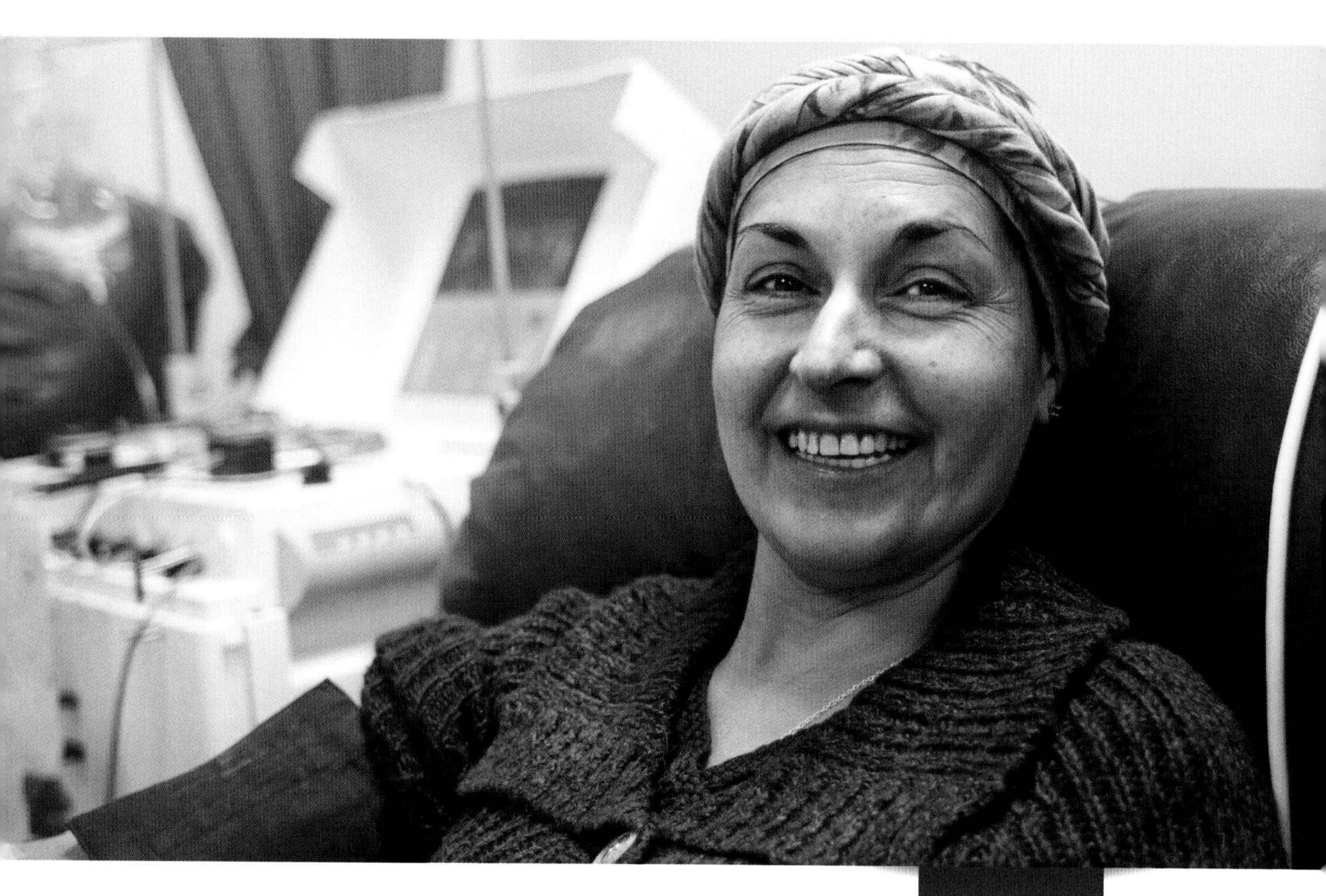

Aldrida Matamala

leukemia

PATIENT

AGE: *45*

OCCUPATION: *Housewife*

DIAGNOSIS: *Plasma cell leukemia*

WHEN: *2012*

CONTEXT: *After a series of post-surgical complications related to an anemia, Aldrida received a diagnosis that would change her life: plasma cell leukemia, the same cancer which had taken maternal grandmother. Thanks to the treatment, Aldrida is currently healthy.*

1.

RECEIVE THE UNEXPECTED ADVICE: "I never felt people looked at me with pity. One time I was approached by a lady who asked me if I wore the scarf for aesthetic reasons or for. When I answered, she told me 'you need to have courage, because I went through the same and look at me now.' We talked for a little while and, before leaving, she insisted on me having faith and courage, which would help me understand that this was not the end of the world."

2.

CONTAINED TRUTH: "My husband was told I was going to die, but he didn't tell me. Although I wanted to know everything and not be protected from information, I now understand it was for the best, because I would have probably felt even worst."

"I never felt people *looked* at me with pity."

3.

HELP OTHERS: "One of my mom's brothers who is 60 years old has stomach cancer. Thank God he is now doing fine. When I visit him I tell him the most important thing is not giving up. And I ask him to be encouraged and say it's common to feel terrible with the treatment. He told me he was scared and I asked him not to think that way: Only God knows when cancer will take you."

4.

WILL TO LIVE: "The state of mind is key after a cancer diagnosis. With will to live, strength and faith in God everything is easier."

5.

DOING WHAT YOU LIKE: "I live in *Villarrica* (southern Chilean city) and love the countryside. I enjoy working in the vegetable garden with my husband and keeping a nice garden; I love plants! Working in the garden relaxes and entertains me."

6.

VALUE WHAT REALLY MATTERS: "Before, I thought about working, owning things. That no longer worries me because I know that what's important is having health and being fine." ■

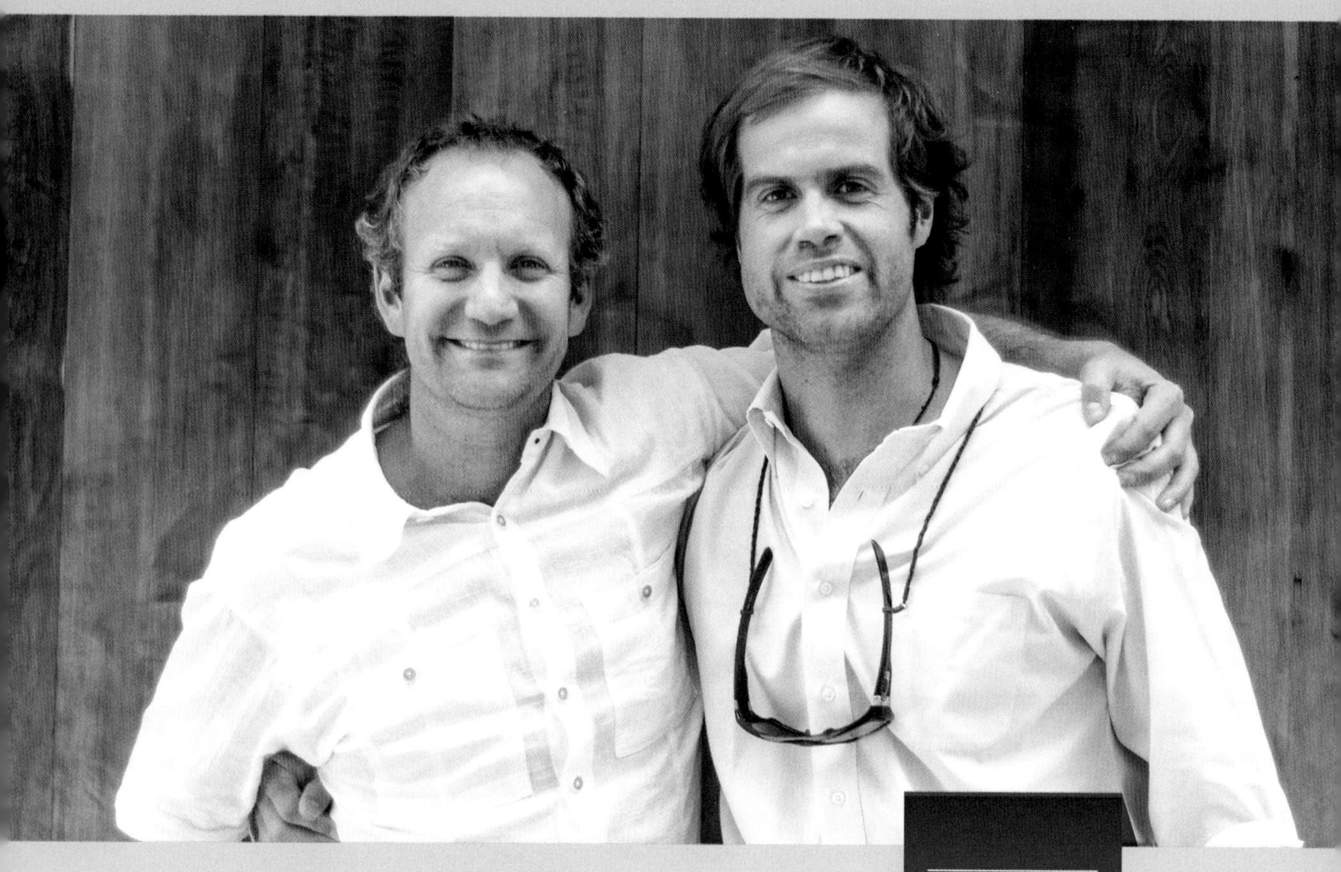

Gonzalo Muñoz

Father *of* **leukemia patient**

AGE: *42*

OCCUPATION: *Businessman and cofounder of* Triciclos

RELATIONSHIP: *Father of a leukemia patient*

WHEN: *2005*

CONTEXT: *When his daughter Rosario was 3 years old some spots appeared on her skin. And she lived with a cough that couldn't be stopped. She went from one doctor to another until she was diagnosed with leukemia. With conventional chemotherapy Rosario's life expectancy was 20%. Gonzalo and his wife visited foreign specialists and increased the intensity of the treatment. It was a long and risky process, but Rosario is now 13 years old, out of danger and there's a book on her story:* La Pequeña Trapecista.

1.

STRICT HYGIENE: "Anyone coming into the house would get totally disinfected. We built a channel: A space between the exterior and the house's entrance where you got disinfected, changed shoes, washed your hands and used Lysoform. Rosario didn't catch a disease, not even during chemotherapy sessions which really lowered her defenses."

2.

KEEP A RECORD: "Life was putting my family in danger and the way I faced that eventual danger was by writing. We started recording everything in two giant notebooks. We kept the drawings of the three little girls, took lots of pictures. I sent an email every three days and informed everybody about Rosario's health. Marcela Zubieta, founder at *Fundación Nuestros Hijos*, read the notebooks and suggested we publish them. That's how they became *La Pequeña Trapecista.* My mother dreamt Rosario was in a circus and had to fly in a trapeze as we were all on alert, sustaining the net in case she fell. That's where the book's title comes from."

"Rosario was always surrounded by **toys and books.** The first temptation was turning on the TV, but we tried to *avoid it.*"

3.

FACE THE DISEASE AS A FAMILY MILESTONE: "Some days after Rosario was diagnosed, while I was crying on my way home, I imagined a conversation between my oldest daughter, Magdalena, in her 20's, with some psychiatrist. She said: *I was abandoned by my parents.* So my wife and I shared the work: One was in charge of Rosario and the other one of her sisters. The one in charge of the sisters would be fully available for them: Check how they were doing, provide support and make them participants of what Rosario was living."

Gonzalo Muñoz

4.

EXPLAIN TO THE CHILDREN: "We always told her sisters everything, but were very aware of how they were taking things, and if there was any change in their behavior we immediately addressed it. . We coordinated with school, in order for both of them not to receive too much attention, and turn into weird kids."

"We started **recording** everything in two *giant* notebooks."

5.

GIVE MEANING TO THE EXPERIENCE: "Rosario's cancer made us aware of other children not having the access and opportunities we had, which is why we got involved with Foundation *Nuestros Hijos*. This marked a milestone in our lives, because we became aware of the fragility of life and of the importance of putting yourself at the service of good causes. My company, *Triciclos* was born out of that very experience of community recycling."

6.

TURN DRAMA INTO A GAME: "We created rituals to turn this drama into a big game. Rosario was always surrounded by toys and books. The first temptation was turning the TV on, but we tried to avoid it. In the end, she gave a meaning even to the floor tiles: She said the ships are over there, fishes are over there, this is the sea and that is an island. The infusion rod was a robot friend called *Rueditas*. We prepared two cups, one filled with marbles and the other one was empty. Each day, she took one marble and placed it in the empty cup to calculate how much time had to go by for her to get out of the clinic. It was a way of visualizing time."

7.

ALTERNATIVE THERAPIES: "We were willing to try any alternative therapy as long as it didn't expose Rosario to germs. We also tried massage, Bach flowers, music therapy.... We had people praying for her from around the world, a friend placed a pyramid underneath her bed... We believe there is an energy beyond faith: there were so may people to try healing Rosario, that for sure it helped her."

"This **marked** a **milestone** in our lives, because we became aware of the fragility **of life** and of the importance of putting yourself at the service of ***good causes."***

8.

FAMILY RE-EDUCATION: "Food needed to be very balanced. All food was sanitized, egg by egg, package by package. I taught my oldest daughters that in order for their hands to be totally clean, they had to count up to 20 when they washed them. And they counted! If any of my daughters felt they had a cold, they'd run to put on a mask."

9.

WHITE EUPHEMISM: *"We avoided using the word cancer with the girls because my grandfather had just passed away of that disease and they associated it to death. We talked about leukemia and explained them the disease using drawings."* ■

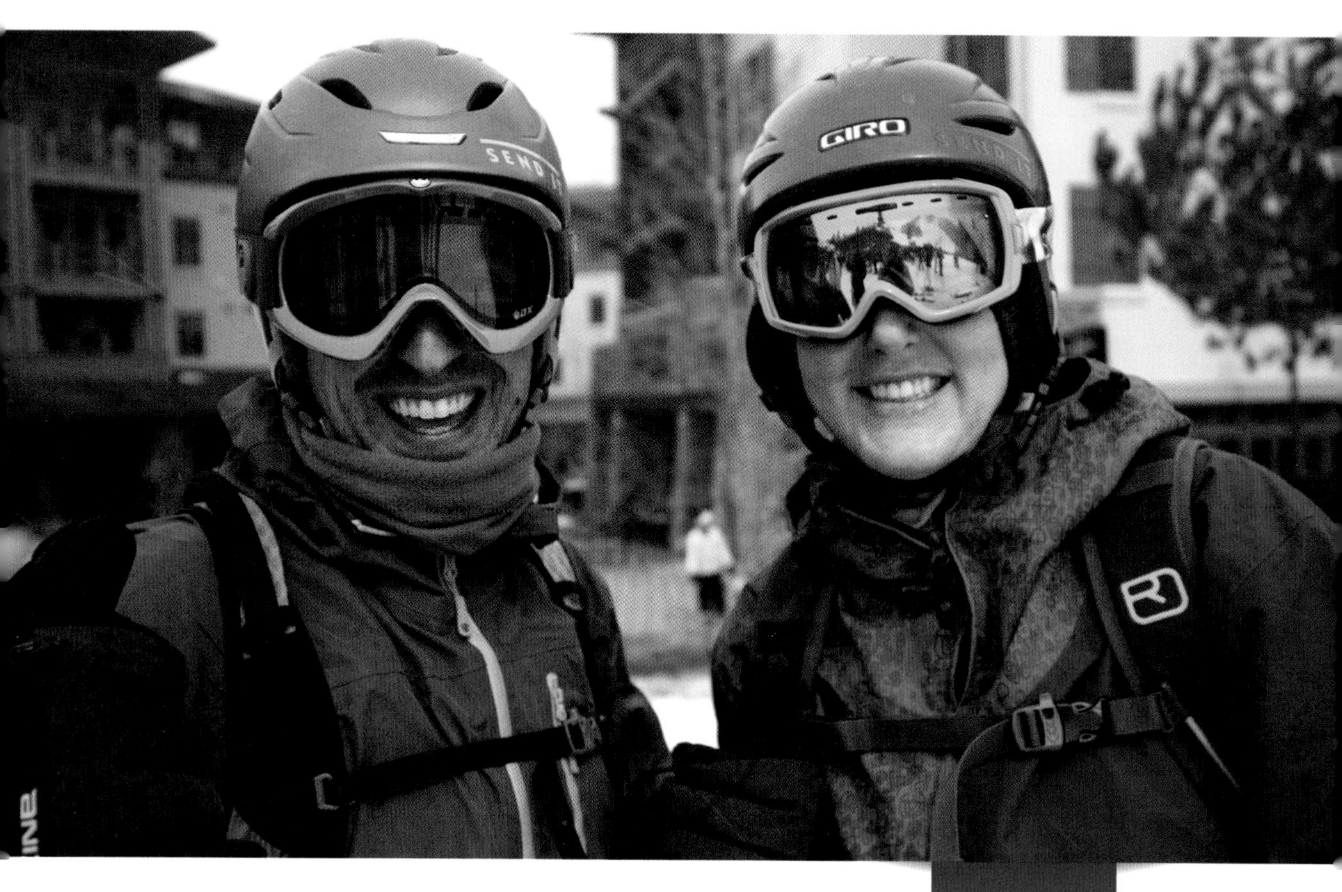

Dave Carbonell

leukemia

PATIENT

AGE: *34*

OCCUPATION: *Emergency Department Physician*

DIAGNOSIS: *T-cell acute lymphoblastic leukemia*

WHEN: *2012*

CONTEXT: *Four months before finishing my education as a doctor, I was diagnosed with my leukemia. I was so focused on finishing my apprenticeship that I ignored signs and symptoms that should have caused more concern. I entered an experimental trial, in which I underwent the same leukemia treatment that children undergo. After almost three and a half years of IV, spinal, and oral chemotherapy, as well as whole brain radiation, I have continued to be in remission and live my life to the fullest. I finished my education and practice as an ER doctor in California.*

1.

DIAGNOSIS AND TREATMENT IS OVERWHELMING. "There is lots of information presented to you in a short period of time. Have a friend or family member join you for discussions with your doctors, as well as at your treatments. Write down important things as you hear them, keep track of what medications you receive and how often you are supposed to take them. Don't try to remember it all.

2.

DON'T BE AFRAID TO ASK QUESTIONS!: "Your doctors and nurses want to help you. If you don't understand what you're going through, why you need a medication, how a treatment is supposed to help, bring it up! Your team might not always have answers or fixes for you, but the only way for them to help is if they know what you're curious about."

"**Write** down important things as you hear them. Don't try to *remember* it all."

3.

LONELINESS: "There are long stretches of time during treatment where you will be alone, and might feel lonely. Everyone has different ways to cope, and you might need to use different coping mechanisms at different times. Taking a mental summary of the different ways you can help yourself will help you through these isolating periods. It can be exercise, reading, meditation, stretching/yoga, nutrition, walks, movies/TV, time with family and friends."

4.

HUMANS THRIVE ON RHYTHMS AND PATTERNS: "Cancer tosses a wrench into those routines. Whatever you did before you got sick, try to keep it up through treatment, even if it's just a little bit. These connections to your old self will help keep you feeling like a human being, and not a guinea pig in a giant medical experiment."

5.

DON'T FORGET TO TAKE CARE OF YOUR MIND AND YOUR HEART: "Surround yourself with people that care about you. If you're exhausted and need time to yourself, take that time. You are in the fight of your life; you need all of the healthy support that you can get. Do not be afraid to let go of relationships or situations that are unhealthy for you." ■

6.

TAKE CARE OF YOUR BODY: "This means eating nutritiously, resting as needed, and also staying active."

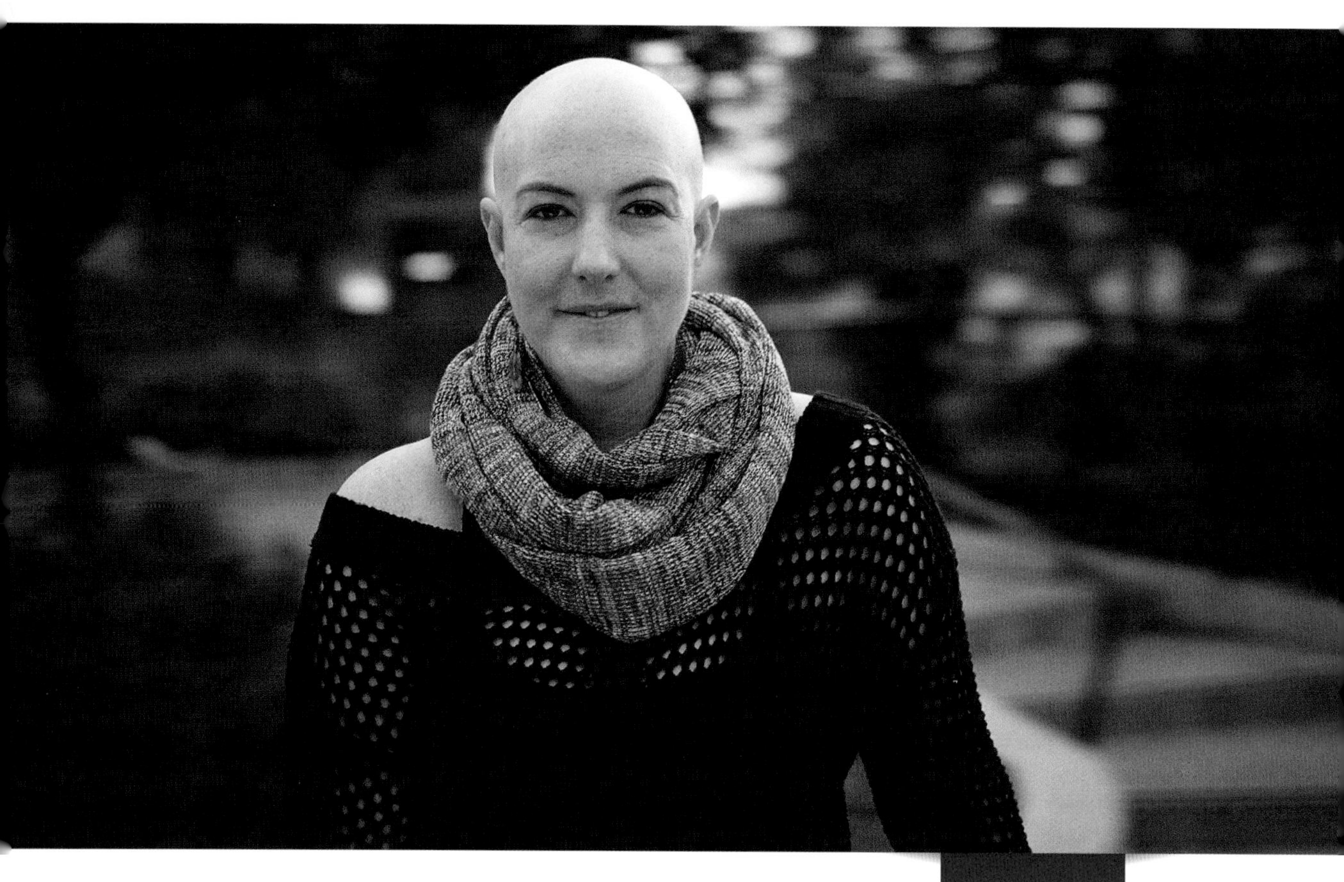

Abbie Alterman

leukemia

PATIENT

AGE: *33*

OCCUPATION: *Wildlife Biologist*

DIAGNOSIS: *Acute Lymphoblastic Leukemia*

WHEN: *2015*

CONTEXT: *At the time of my diagnosis I had been married for 6 months, living in Reno, Nevada with my husband and our dog. We were undergoing a remodel on our basement and back yard. I was working as a wildlife biologist, primarily doing avian and desert tortoise field survey work for large scale construction projects.*

1.

NAVIGATING THE MEDICAL SYSTEM:

"Someone early on in my cancer journey told me, "There is no one in the medical system that cares more about the outcome of your treatment than you (the patient)". That phrase stuck with me, and prompted me to stay as engaged and informed as possible. I researched every drug they gave me and I kept track of my own treatment schedule. I caught some mistakes and could correct them."

2.

FOR FAMILY AND FRIENDS: "Set up a calendar for people to prepare and deliver meals. Care packages are a great way to lift spirits. One friend gifted me movies on a thumb drive, another a magazine subscription. Humorous books, audio books and podcasts are all nice options for when a cancer warrior's eyes are tired. Helping with daily chores like laundry, dishes, housekeeping can be a tremendous favor to someone who is immune compromised."

3.

A SENSE OF SELF: "Know that maybe you will lose 'yourself' for a bit, but also know that it's possible to find a new return that could be even greater than your previous self. I tried to surround myself with familiar items and gifts from loved ones. I appreciated when family members would send me video chats from across the country to help feel more connected. "

"*Walk* as much as you can. Make daily **goals.**"

4.

HEALTHY LIFESTYLE/DIET: "Maybe that only looks like taking a shower, maybe it's walking around the block. Some medical facilities have access to cancer specific exercise resources, take advantage of them it will be a blessing to be around professionals who understand you may be experiencing side effects. Smoothies can be a helpful way to get in nutritious calories and can be easily customizable at home."

5.

EMOTIONS: "I think it is important to recognize that whatever emotion you are feeling, whether its anger, fear, sadness, resentment to be able to honor that feeling with acceptance. Speak to your medical team or social worker about mental health resources that may be available to you. Find articles or activities that soothes or comforts you, perhaps that's sitting in hot water, wrapping up in a soft blanket, listening to music, or petting your dog." ■

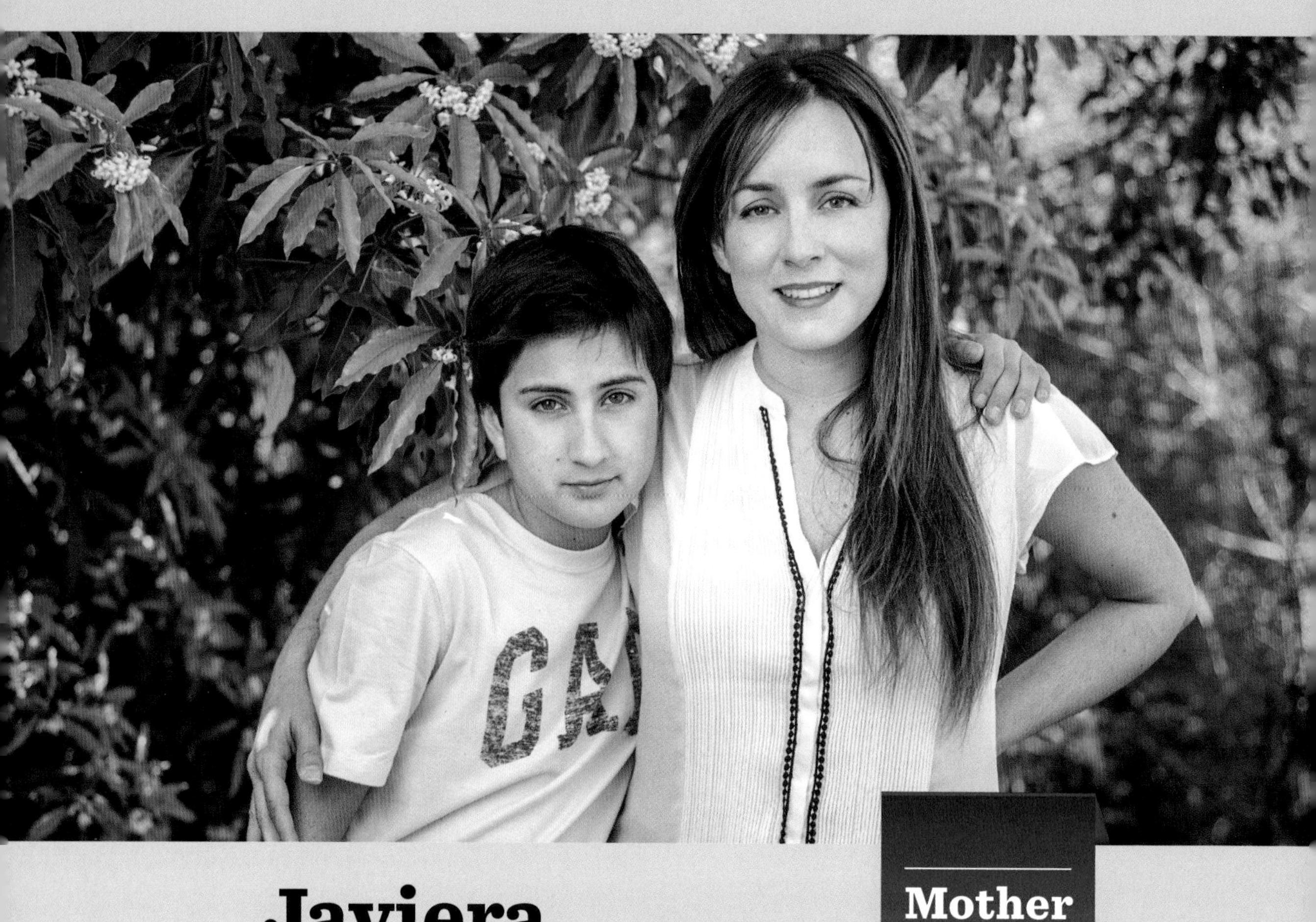

Javiera Chinchón

Mother *of* **leukemia patient**

AGE: *42*

OCCUPATION: *BA in business administration, human resources consultant*

RELATIONSHIP: *Mother of a leukemia patient*

WHEN: *2012*

CONTEXT: *Affected by a very rare type of pediatric cancer, chronic myeloid leukemia; Ignacio had a transplant on February 7, 2012. It was a very hard time for Javiera and her husband, filled with intense emotions, but of an almost unique closeness with the second of their three children. These are some of the tips Javiera wrote down during the long year and a half Ignacio's odyssey lasted; he is now close to turning 13 years old.*

1.

TRUTH WITH DRAWINGS: "One needs to explain everything to a child, because they want to know everything. I could never lie or hide information from Ignacio as he was interested in knowing about his state, we told him the truth. You need to use pedagogy, drawings when necessary, for explanations to be didactic and in his language. When some important change was imminent, we prepared him without him noticing: after hair loss, for example, we spoke about an older cousin who had shaved and everybody told him *how cool that you shaved.*"

2.

REALITY ADJUSTMENTS: "We realized that, as parents, we needed to build the 'glasses' through which Ignacio perceived the reality he was living. Although it was hard, it was necessary to have a positive attitude, always smile, see the good side of things, cry to laugh later and think with hope and faith that everything would come to an end."

"You need to use pedagogy, **drawings** when necessary, for explanations to be *didactic* and in their language."

3.

THE FRIENDS' WALL: "For Ignacio to be entertained, after the transplant we invented different activities and scheduled surprises for the end of the day. Each time Ignacio had visits, before the person left he had to draw a face on a wall we started building in his room."

4.

EVERY CLOUD HAS A SILVER LINING: "Sometimes, Ignacio tells me he misses the time when he was just transplanted, because he had a great time. It was a time in which we, as parents, were really close to him, and he tells me it would be nice to be like that again. Obviously, the leukemia was dreadful, but at the same time it was nice spending all that time together.

5.

FAMILY ASSISTANCE: "Both our families were very present. They took my children to and from school, did our grocery shopping and worried that my children got to birthday parties with presents. Sometimes, my mother-in-law or my mom went to the clinic to replace me so that I could escape for a while to be with my other children." ■

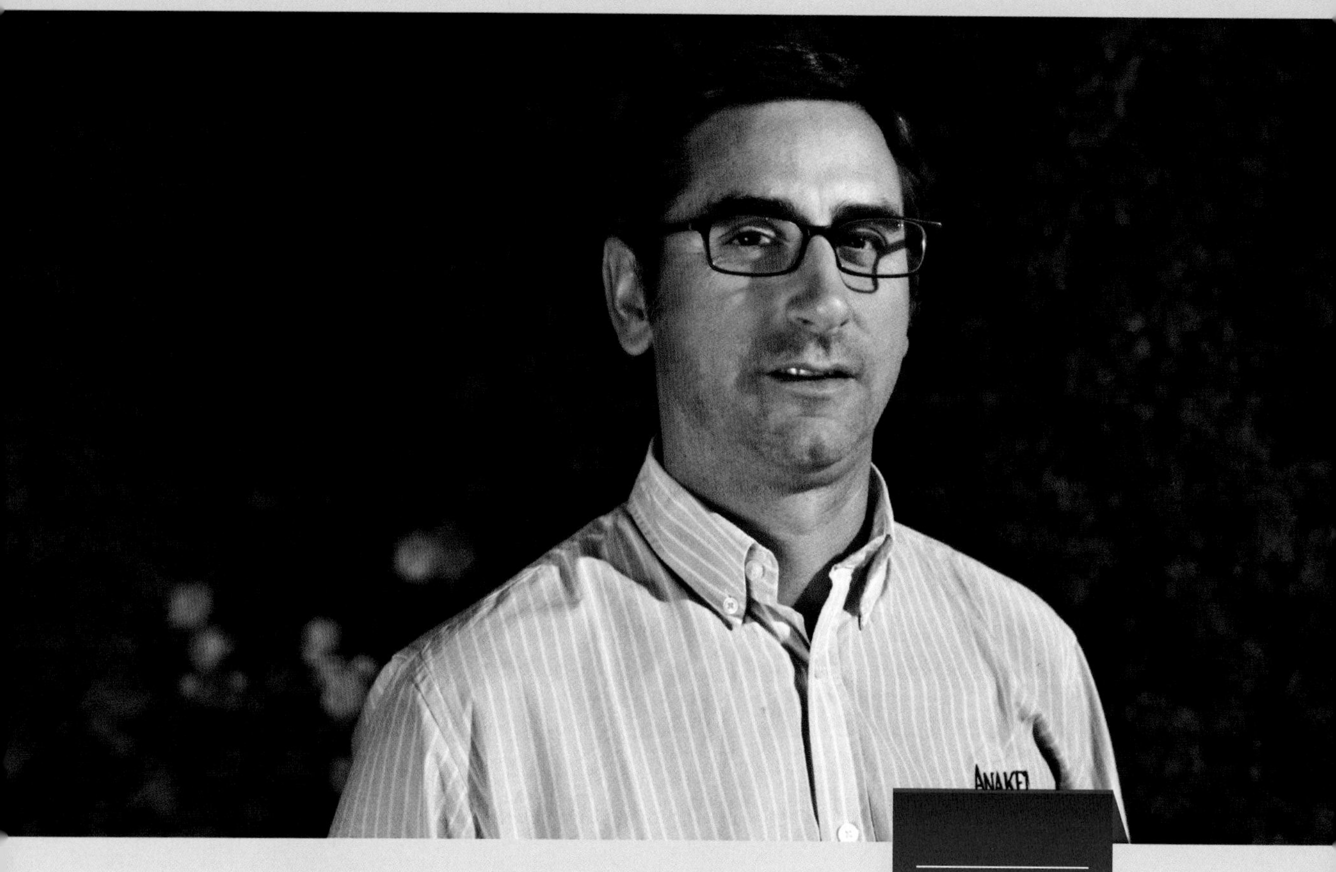

Juan Andrés Lira

Brother *of* **leukemia patient**

AGE: *43*

OCCUPATION: *Agricultural engineer*

RELATIONSHIP: *Brother of a leukemia patient*

WHEN: *1982*

CONTEXT: *Juan Andrés was 12 years old when he had to experience at first hand his 14-year-old brother's leukemia, José Manuel, who was called Jose. He was part of the incredibly hard journey his family went on which lasted until his brother died three years after being diagnosed. Currently, Juan Andrés keeps the memory of his brother alive by collaborating in the organization for children with cancer* Casa de la Sagrada Familia.

1.

KEEP THE MEMORY ALIVE: "We keep my brother's memory alive; we have dates that we all get together in his memory. Twenty years ago my mother decided that Christmas would always be celebrated on the December 23rd –my brother's birthday– with a mass and a big family reunion."

2.

SUBSEQUENT QUESTIONS: "In the years after his death I've had so many questions. From whether he should have been transplanted instead of being treated with drugs –I was the only compatible family member for organ donation–, or whether I'd have treated him any differently as an older brother if I'd known the truth about his condition. I think I probably would have. I treated him as someone completely normal, and perhaps this is why I never questioned my parent's hiding some of the information about his state from the rest of us."

"The patient is sometimes overprotected from things which they **can** actually **do** or tolerate *without* any problem."

3.

THE IMPORTANCE OF COMMEMORATING: "At those events they remember the jokes and fun times they had. Stories get repeated from one year to the next... It's a kind of therapy."

4.

HOW TO LIVE IT AMONG SIBLINGS: "I think a patient needs to feel that their siblings (and I'm emphasizing the sibling relationship as the relationship with parents is so different) are treating them as an equal and as somebody normal. Often people tend to overprotect them and try to stop them from doing things that actually they're quite capable of doing and would like to do, thereby altering their lives even more." ■

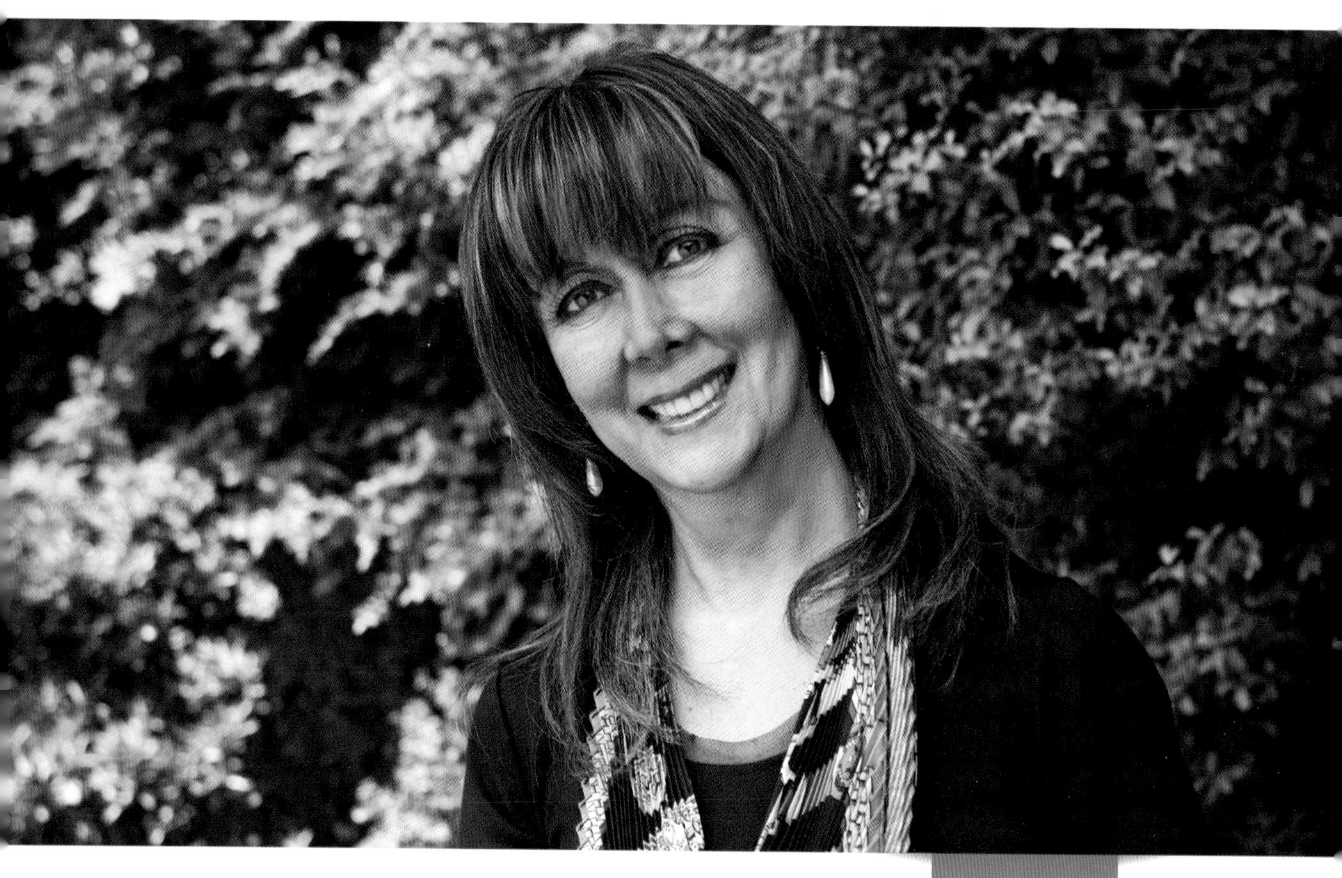

Leonor Gacitúa

ovarian cancer

PATIENT

AGE: *53*

OCCUPATION: *Trader*

DIAGNOSIS: *Ovarian cancer*

WHEN: *2007*

CONTEXT: *She was diagnosed with ovarian cancer in the final stage which had spread to the intestine, abdomen, uterus and the entire abdominal area. With strength and will to live, together with the help of Padre Pío –a Capuchin and Italian saint canonized in 2002–, she turned the prognosis around and smashed down the barriers the cancer had put up. She now lives free of the disease, living and fighting as she has always done.*

Tips

1.

NATURAL POTION: "Before each meal, I take two spoons of Aloe Vera, whisky and honey. It's not a magic potion, but whisky dilates pores and helps Aloe Vera penetrate into tissues; this calms inflammation, improves the digestion and helps the body respond to the chemotherapy. To prepare it, I cut a big leaf of Aloe Vera (without spines) into pieces, put it in the juicer and grind it. To avoid it being too dense, I strain half of it through a sieve and then mix this liquid with the other half. I add a tequila shot filled of whisky and half a cup of honey, and let it rest in the fridge inside of a glass for a day."

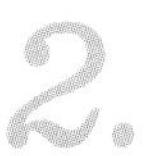

HEAL INJURIES: "I also take sodium bicarbonate that helps eliminating cancer according to Italian doctor Tullio Simoncini. I dilute a teaspoon in a glass of water and add the juice of a lemon. This was the only thing that healed the injuries that appeared in the mouth due to chemotherapy."

3.

RESCUING POISON: "Scorpion poison has helped in a great way to overcome chemotherapy. As far as I know, it's anti-inflammatory and has anticancer properties, and it stops cells from reproducing. It is sold by the Cuban laboratory *Labiofam*; I order it from people who travel there."

4.

DIET: "I use alkaline and acid foods as a guideline, like Roberto Ibáñez. I eat lots of fruits and vegetables, and eliminated refined salt and sugar, flour and white rice from my diet. Sometimes, when I am under chemotherapy, I take two sips of coffee to relax. As chemotherapy is so strong, I feel somehow protected, but in general I try not eating things that make me feel bad."

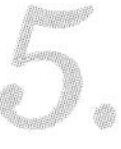

THE DOCTOR IS NOT GOD: "I learned doctors are not gods; they just studied some area of medicine. You need to worry about your disease, assume responsibility for it and be very alert. Don't trust doctors blindly. Even the best specialist may make mistakes." ■

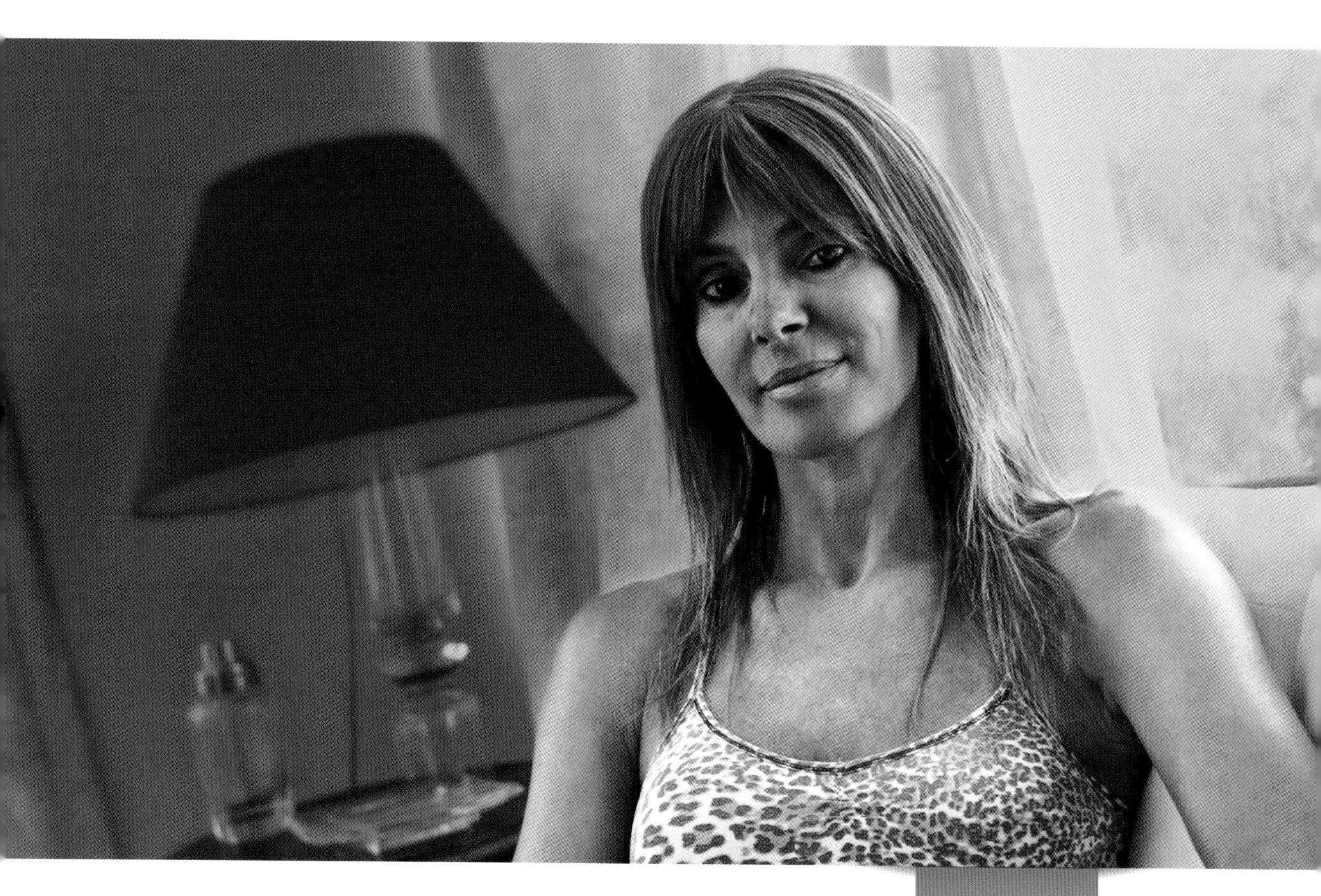

Isabel Mahou

ovarian cancer

PATIENT

AGE: *52*

OCCUPATION: *Nurse*

DIAGNOSIS: *Ovarian cancer*

WHEN: *2004*

CONTEXT: *During Christmas in 2004, Isabel told her family she had ovarian cancer: On December 31 she would undergo surgery to get the malignant tumor removed. She left the disease aside for almost a decade, but the aggressive nature of the cancer made it highly probable that she'd have a relapse and, in March 2012, tests showed she had metastases from the peritoneum to the lung pleural cavity. She started a new treatment.*

1.

THE BEST HELP: The will to live.

2.

DIGEST THE NEWS WITH THE FAMILY:

"Only those who have suffered from cancer know the terror and fear you feel when you're given your diagnosis."

3.

BE WELL INFORMED: "I'm a nurse who tends to be very scientific and pragmatic, but I realized it was not good for me to investigate everything in Google. It's good to do some investigation, but within limits, so that you lead as normal a life as possible."

4.

LOOK FOR POSITIVE STATISTICS:

"It's impossible not being frightened at first, but later your state of mind starts to become a very important factor. Statistics show that people who wait for death to come have a greater possibility of of relapse. I made an effort to maintain enthusiasm."

5.

LOOK TO YOUR SIDE: "A way of comparing the treatment you are receiving in Chile is reviewing protocols followed in the United States. You can find everything in the American Cancer Society website (cancer.org) and it's not hard to understand."

6.

WIG FROM THE BEGINNING: *"Personally, I couldn't stand the idea of seeing how I lost my hair little by little; so, I shaved my head before this happened and bought a wig. Being groomed helps your mood a lot."* ■

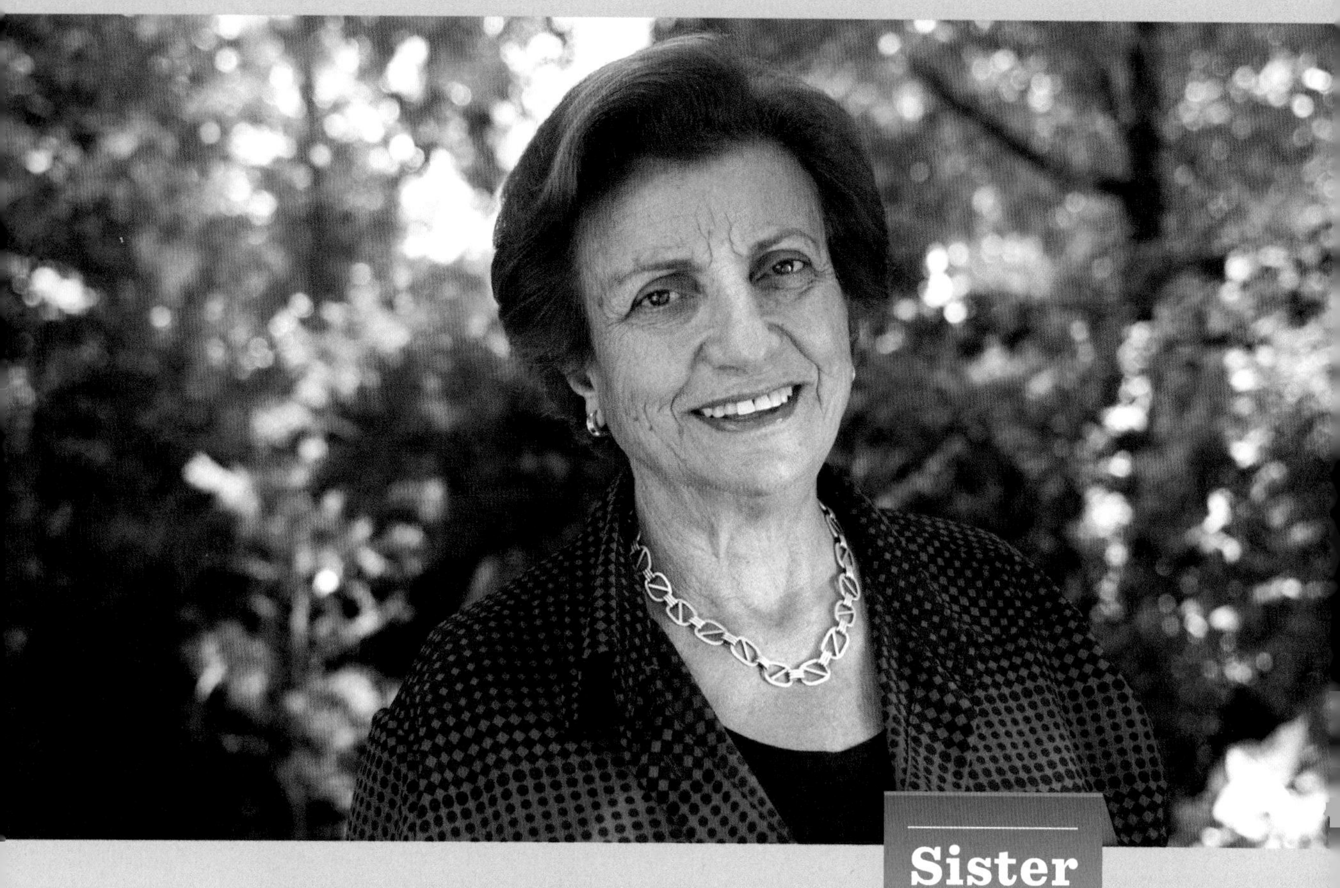

Jaennett Cattan Cattan

Sister *of* **ovarian cancer patient**

AGE: *70*

OCCUPATION: *Businesswoman*

RELATIONSHIP: *Sister of an ovarian, uterus and omentum cancer with metastasis in diaphragm*

WHEN: *1986*

CONTEXT: *When Jaennett learned her sister's condition was serious and that she needed to undergo emergency surgery, she remembered that her mother-in-law kept a newspaper clipping from 1980 about a person with cancer in whom doctors couldn't find any more tumor cells after the patient started taking the medication Lysate. She immediately started looking for the medication.*

1.

THE STORY OF LYSATE, A NATURAL DRUG: "Federico Díaz, the Uruguayan pharmacist says in the book *La batalla silenciosa* ("The Silent Battle") that he discovered Lysate by chance. He was given a dog that, in a short time, weakened and lost its hair. A friend suggested he should feed it with a cow's heart and keep it in a space with soil. He did and the dog changed its hair and recovered. Díaz wondered what had happened and his friend answered the dog was selfish, because he buried the heart, and when nobody saw it, it dug it out and ate it. Díaz decided to research on his own and discovered that at the depth at which his dog dug the piece of heart, proteins changed into amino acids. From that moment on, he started a scientific research and in 1960 he had synthesized Lysate."

2.

HE WHO SEEKS FINDS: "I was told that Lysate was not sold in Chile, but apparently a lady who lived in downtown Santiago, in *Echaurren* Street, sometimes had it. I asked for God's help and went house by house along *Echaurren* Street, business by business, until I collected some clues which took me to *Unión Latino Americana* Street. When I arrived, a woman dressed in light-blue told me that when God wanted to heal people, he sent them there. I bought the jar of Lysate capsules."

3.

THE EFFECTS: "Lysate had a wonderful effect since it allowed my sister to begin chemotherapy sessions with good creatinine, with her kidneys in a good state, and that allowed her to bear the treatment."

4.

LYSATE IN CHILE: "It's not sold here, you need to get to it through a contact or order it from Uruguay, where it can be bought at drugstores. After my sister's experience, I have been promoting its use for 26 years. Lysate boosts defenses in the organism to increase their state of alert and then the body is able to reject any invasion."

5.

ALL IN ALL, WHAT IS IT?: "Lysate is a natural product authorized in Uruguay. It helps keep the organism in good condition. It doesn't resuscitate people, but it has helped many people reduce their suffering in relation to a serious disease." ■

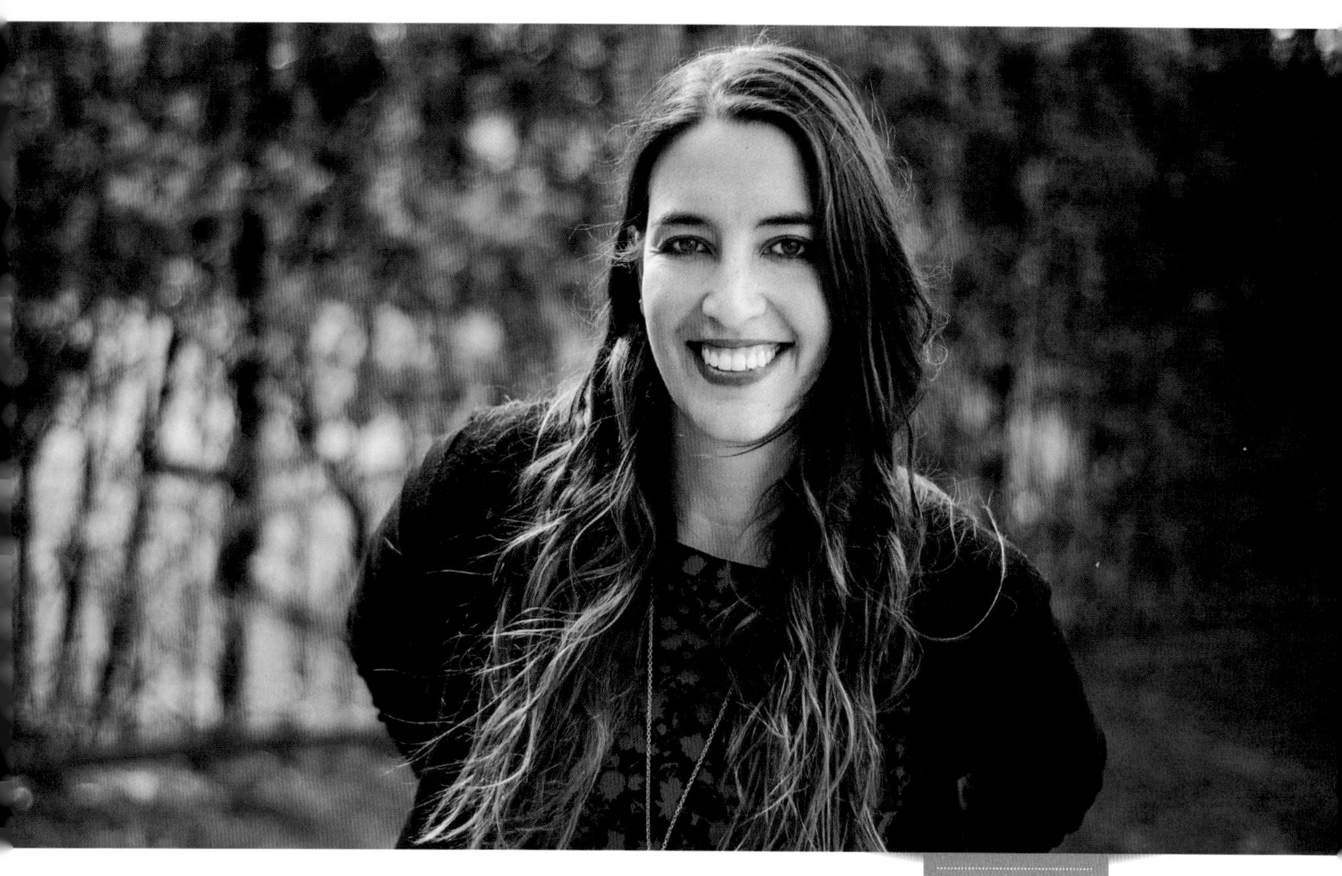

Daniela Rozental

papillary thyroid cancer

PATIENT

AGE: *28*

OCCUPATION: *Actress*

DIAGNOSIS: *Papillary thyroid cancer*

WHEN: *2010*

CONTEXT: *During a routine general check-up before travelling to New York to study, Daniela was diagnosed with a papillary carcinoma (thyroid cancer) with metastases in the lymph nodes in her neck. Her plans changed dramatically. On June 10 2010, the day she was meant to be leaving Chile, she was operated on. She had her thyroid and 70 nodes removed. She is now fully recovered, but looking back she is amazed at how quickly it all happened.*

1.

SEARCH THE REASONS WITHIN YOU: "I did it and understood I needed to stop swallowing my feelings. Although it's easier to blame life and the random factor exists, the body manifests and I believe that I got partly sick because I used to keep my feelings to myself. It's something I still need to work on one day at a time."

2.

BE REASONABLE AND EXHAUST ALTERNATIVES: "If you're told you need to take a test, do it; if you have to take a drug, take it, even if you want to look for other types of therapies."

3.

TALK ABOUT WHAT YOU'RE GOING THROUGH AND CHOOSE THE PERSON YOU WANT TO TALK TO: "I went to see a therapist with whom I felt really comfortable, because those who are closest to you speak from their own sorrow, from their own fears, while a therapist or psychologist helps you see everything from a different perspective."

4.

STAY CALM: "First, you need to think what having cancer means, what the possible treatments are, and who can provide you with more information. If you're not facing a rapid progress cancer, I would suggest taking some time before making any decision. I didn't have that alternative."

5.

ADVICE FOR THOSE WHO DON'T HAVE CANCER: "It sounds cliché, but never think it will never happen to you. Therefore, do what you want when you want to do it." ■

"I used to **bottle** my feelings up and I think that's one of the *reasons* I got sick."

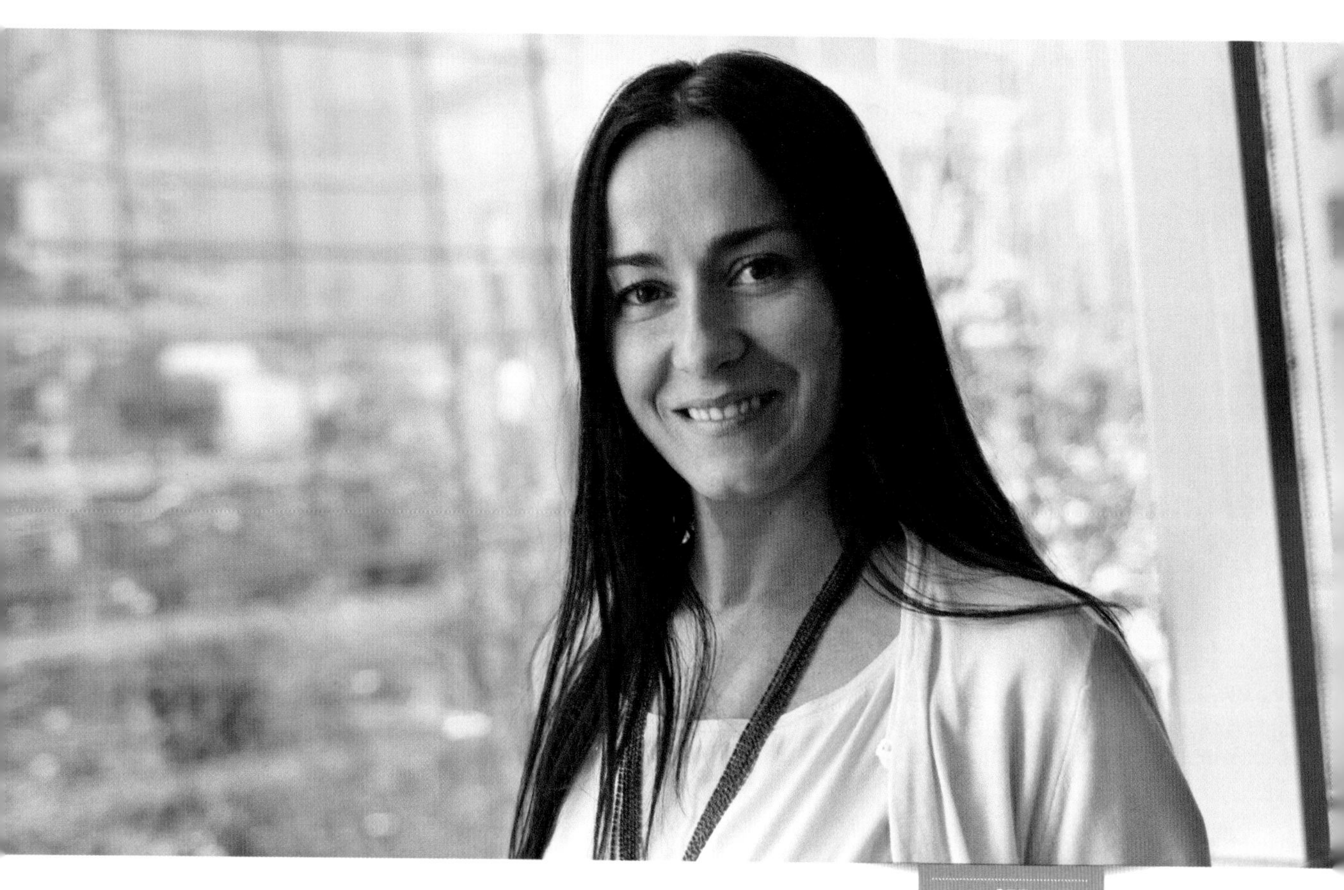

Loreto Wahr

papillary thyroid cancer
PATIENT

AGE: *40*

OCCUPATION: *Architect*

DIAGNOSIS: *Papillary thyroid cancer*

WHEN: *2009*

CONTEXT: *Thyroid cancer, although having one of the best prognoses, found Loreto Wahr in a very complicated time of her life: separated twice and with two small children. The hardest part to take on was the risk that her death would stop Blanca and Pedro, children from two different fathers, growing up together and sharing the memories that a mother builds up with her children. Nowadays the cancer is under control and she has twice-yearly check-ups. So her main focus is to put together enduring memories for her children.*

1.

PSYCHOLOGICAL THERAPY FOR SUPPORT: "Thanks to that therapy I managed to release the sorrow of my children potentially growing up separately. My mother has always helped me, but thinking about the effects my disease could have on my children made me sick. I was very independent and determined, but have little connection with my emotions: I lived without knowing if something was really what I wanted. Therapy helped me connect with my emotions and learn to say no."

"My two children and I became very *close*. We invented things such as the **'hug of three"**.

2.

LIVE INTENSELY: "You need to live intensely the process of the disease, but without any drama. In my case, it meant making a connection on the deepest level with people and building memories with my loved ones for when I was no longer alive. My two children and I became very close. We invented things such as the 'hug of three'. It was all to create memories, strengthen the bond, concretize projects, make their lives special for the day I would no longer be with them, so that they'd always have the memories to bring them together." ■

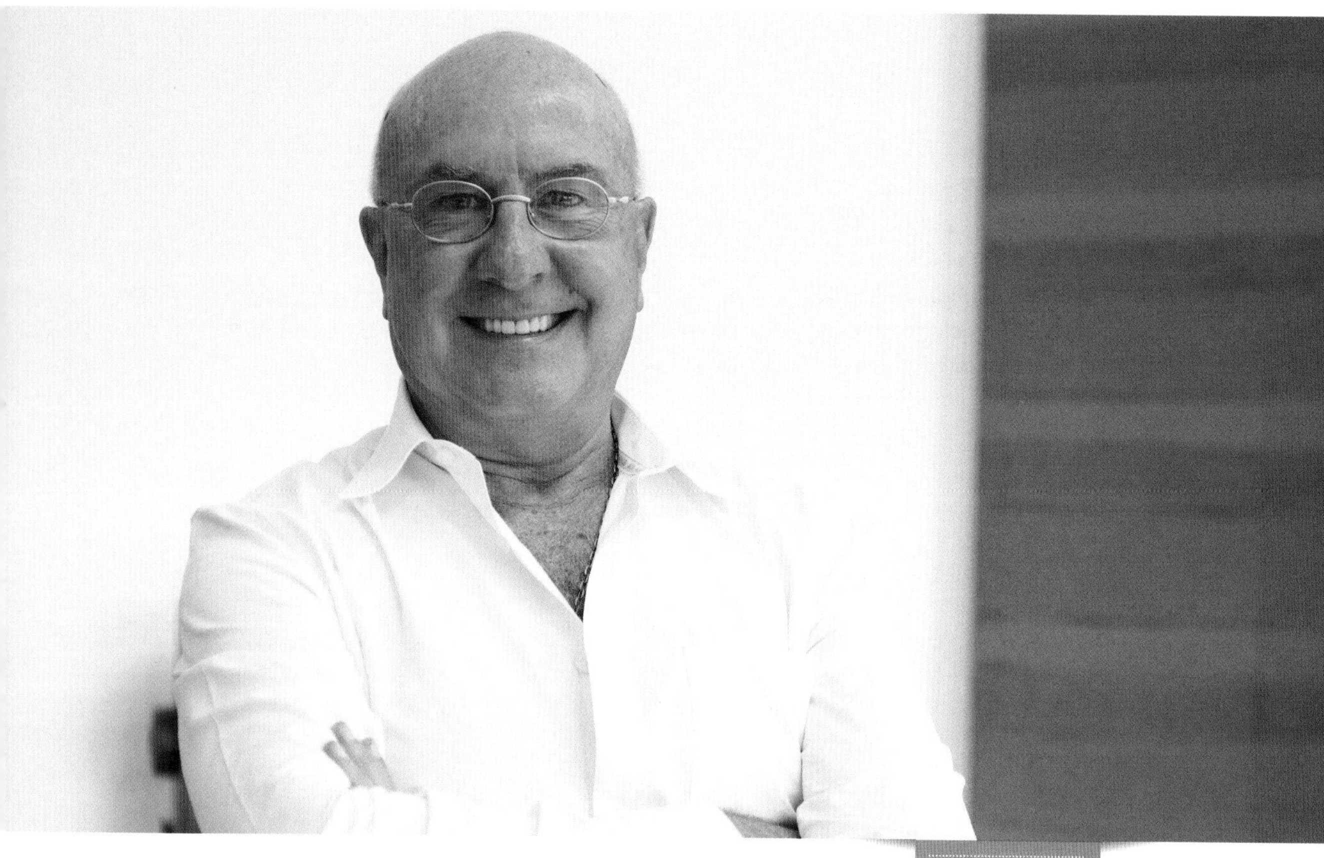

Adolfo Dammert

papillary thyroid cancer

PATIENT

AGE: *67*

OCCUPATION: *Publicist and Chairman of the Peruvian League against Cancer*

DIAGNOSIS: *Thyroid Cancer*

WHEN: *1981*

CONTEXT: *One morning, as I was tying my tie to go to work, I noticed a bulge on my neck. I thought it would go away alone, but it didn't. It had come to stay. Doctors, exams, and a surgery on Thursday, March 4, 1981. The following Tuesday, the surgeon called to say that it was thyroid cancer, and that some cells had escaped and were looking for fertile land for metastases. So, I had surgery again; this time to remove the entire area where the tumor had been. Then a third surgery; one that left me without my voice.*

1.

ACCEPT THE FEAR: "I was very afraid. My father had died of cancer a few months before, and I was paralyzed to think the same could happen to me. Fear paralyzes more than death, and that was clear to me. My children, very young at the time, only 4 and 2 years old, gave me the necessary strength. Thinking about them made me set fear aside."

2.

LOOK FOR ALL OPTIONS: "I looked at all the possible options to overcome my disease, and then I made all the important decisions regarding what was going to be performed on me. With good medical advice, of course."

"Every day, I wake up early and feel **thankful**".

3.

DON'T KEEP QUIET: "Back then, speaking about cancer meant speaking of sure death. Nowadays, that is not the case. I kept silent, of course. It was 1981. Today... talk; tell others how you feel and how you are doing. Your family and friends will be your support. The one I did not have, because I did not know how to speak up."

4.

WHATEVER HAPPENS, DON'T GIVE UP: "I was 32 years old, and – allegedly – had my whole life ahead of me. I had no voice, but the most important thing I kept: Life. It took me a year to be able to speak again, but I did it!"

5.

FEEL: "Feel life at its best. Watch that sunset. Enjoy that sunrise. Enjoy family and friends. You never know when you will have to face something hard. Don't be the one to regret things later on. If, right now, you don't say that loving word to, or make that kind gesture for, someone deserving it, afterwards it may be too late."

6.

BE THANKFUL. EVERY DAY: "Every day, I wake up early and feel thankful for cancer having been only an experience (I never call myself a 'survivor'). Thankful because I have seen my daughters grow and get married, and for having been able to see my grandchildren. I cried when I saw my daughters expecting, realizing that I was going to be able to meet them."

7.

HELP OUT: "Help. Help in everything you can. Giving is healing. It heals the soul, and it can cure cancer." ■

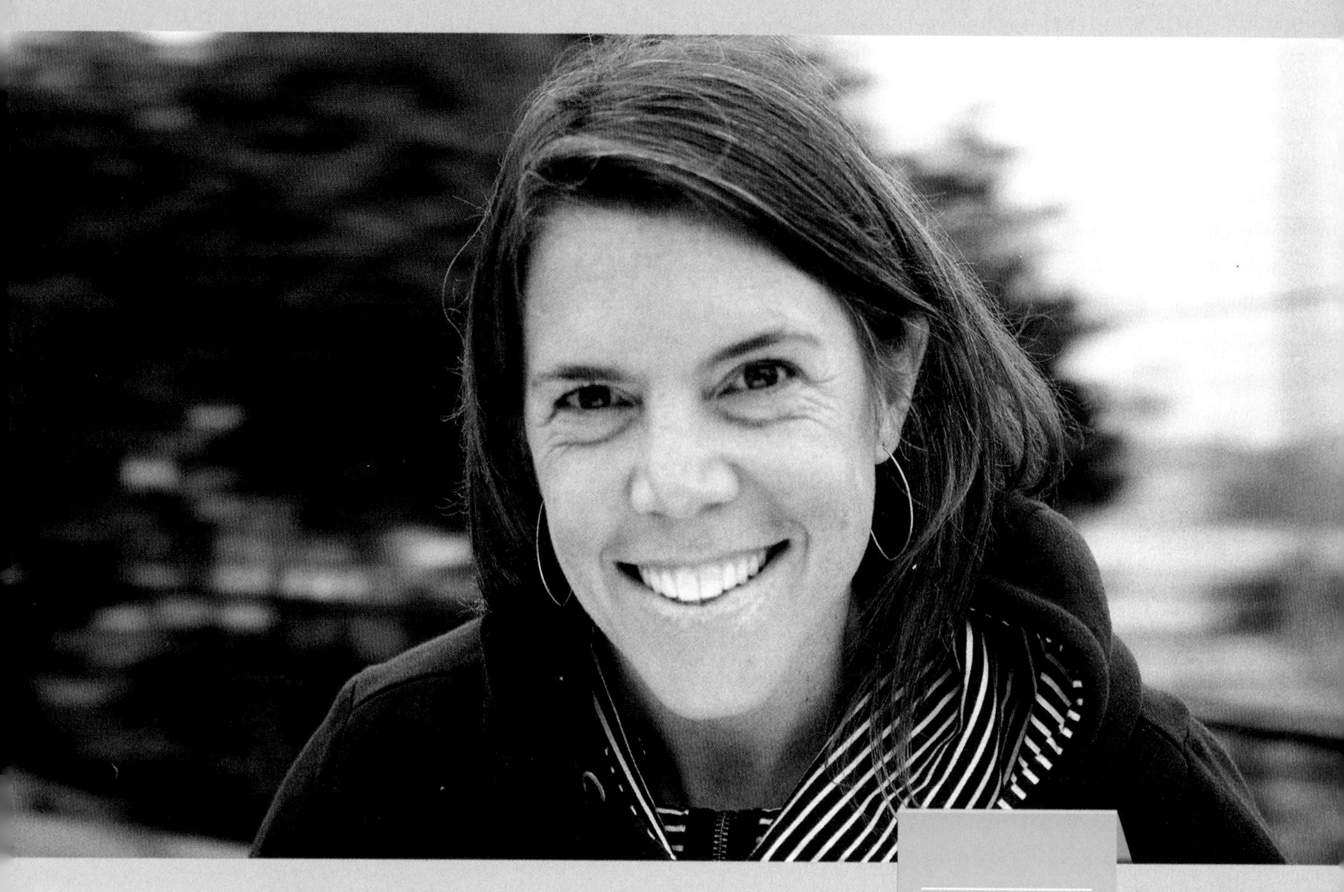

Katie Schou

Family *of* sarcoma patient

AGE: *36*

OCCUPATION: *Executive Director, Send It Foundation*

RELATIONSHIP: *Sister of a sarcoma patient*

WHEN: *2012*

CONTEXT: *Katie's older brother, Jamie, was diagnosed with a rare cancer at the age of 33. An avid skier and lover of all outdoor activity, Jamie found strength and courage in pursuing his passions outdoors. His vision was to bring the experiences that brought him so much life and joy, to others in the cancer fight. In the last year of his life, he founded the Send It Foundation to do just that. Today, Katie and her two sisters forge on with Send It, bringing Jamie's vision and legacy to life through meaningful adventures and a resource for peer support and community for young cancer fighters and survivors.*

1.

BELIEVE: "Jamie wrote in his journal, "Believe that you will succeed. Develop a deep conviction that you will win. The journey may get harder before it gets easier. Believe that anything is possible!" Hold onto this belief – as a patient, family member, or care-giver, we all must hold tight onto this conviction."

2.

PRACTICE GRATITUDE: "Practice gratitude - and, it's just that, a practice. Count your blessings every day. Be grateful for what you have and who you have. Take time to notice and reflect upon the things you're grateful for. The practice of gratitude helps you feel more present, and brings positivity, compassion, and kindness into your life. By simply writing down the moments we're grateful for, we can significantly increase well-being and life satisfaction."

3.

SET GOALS: "Big goals and little goals, every day, find something to aspire to. It may be as simple as taking a shower or going for a walk. Setting goals helps you keep moving forward. "What am I going to accomplish today?" Just answering that question opens the door to possibility, optimism, and positivity."

4.

COMMUNICATE: "Nobody should go through cancer alone - it takes a team. Don't be afraid to ask for help, and talk about what you're feeling and what you need. The people in your life want to help and they want to be there for you. Often, they simply don't know how or what to do. Help them be there for you - let them cook, drive you to appointments, deal with insurance companies, do your laundry, and handle life logistics. Your biggest job is your well-being and your health. Let your friends and family take care of the other stuff, so you can focus on you. And use these times to connect and spend time with your loved ones. It's healing and helpful for everyone."

5.

LAUGH: "Jamie wrote, "Keep a sense of humor and stay calm. Humor is a vital organ for survival, and helps keep a sense of sanity through the most challenging situations." There is humor everywhere - pay attention to it and keep laughing. AND, it's ok to cry! Cancer is scary and sad, you need to cry. And you need to laugh. Humor brings levity and lightheartedness when it's needed most. Laugh!"

6.

KEEP MOVING: "Movement is life. Keep moving, keep learning, keep growing." It's important to find something to engage your body and your mind, and keep moving forward. Exercise between treatments if it's possible for you, or strum a ukulele when you're lying low. Treatment is draining, and your regular life activities might seem out of reach. But as much as you can, keep moving!"

7.

SELF CARE: "Cancer is emotionally and physically exhausting for patients, and for family members and care-givers. As a care-giver, it's equally important to take care of yourself so you can be there for your loved ones. Practice self-care - rest, get outside, exercise, see friends, and live your life. And just as with patients, communicate what you need from your loved ones. Make sure to take a break and rejuvenate." ■

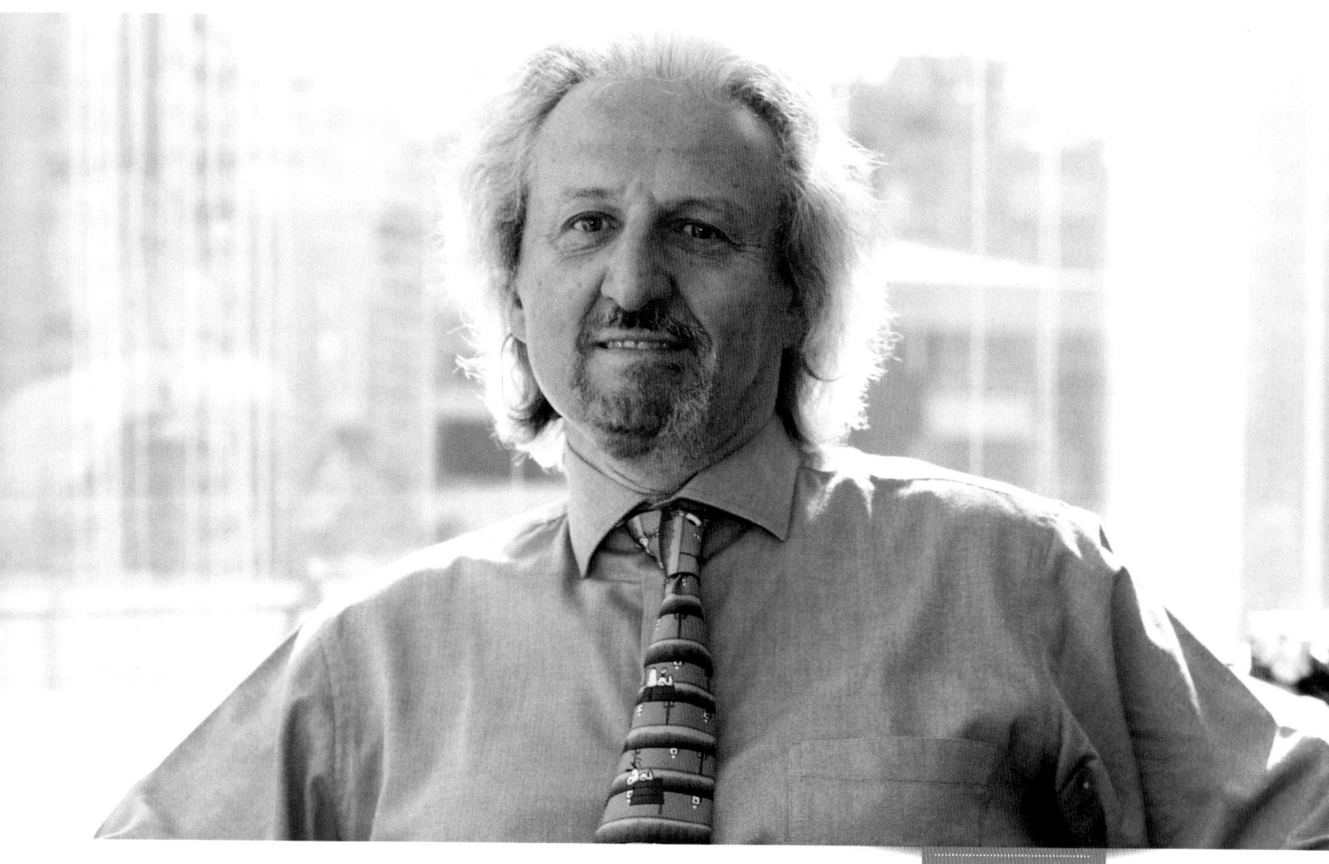

Francisco Javier Ibáñez

parotid gland cancer

PATIENT

AGE: *59*

OCCUPATION: *Lawyer*

DIAGNOSIS: *Parotid gland cancer*

WHEN: *2014*

CONTEXT: *A little bulge on the side of his jaw led Francisco Javier Ibáñez to a dental consultation, and one day of May 2014 he received a violent sentence: Parotid gland cancer, also known as tumor of the salivary ducts. After diagnosis and lung metastasis, he is now completely healthy.*

1.

DON'T RULE OUT ANY ALTERNATIVE TREATMENT THAT DOES NOT HURT YOU: "I took phytoplankton as dust, brought to me from abroad. It acts like a powerful antioxidant. It helps feed and detox cells, and it benefits the immune system, among other properties. I also had *reiki* done on me during the entire process, and it was an enormous relief, since the pain issue is complex, and you have to take everything that is palliative."

2.

A HEALTHY DIET IS ESSENTIAL: "I recommend a diet that is high in antioxidants, although at some point during my process I didn't have the strength, nor the will, to eat. Both my esophagus and mouth were full of ulcers and wounds, so I just had soups and juices made from food like berries and broccoli."

"Cancer is not *contagious,* but you have to understand why it **happened."**

3.

THREE KEY POINTS: "In my opinion, there are 3 keys matters to heal and move on. The first one is to believe in chemistry, in what you are taking in terms of medication, in your treatment, and in your medical team. Second, the will to get out of it. You have to have enormous enthusiasm, you have to be brave, and you must fight. Third, feel the love from your family, your partner, your friends. Realize how important you are for certain people. I had two grandsons on the way, and I felt I had to be healthy for them."

4.

UNDERSTAND WHY THIS HAPPENED TO YOU: "Cancer is not contagious, but you have to understand why it happened. The human body is like a colony: There is an army that stops bad guys from going through, and lets only the good guys in. When you are stressed out and worried about a lot of things, you become careless, your defenses barely stand the adrenaline and there comes a point in which the army gets weak, and so the bad guys get in. I had been so worried about other stuff that I had stopped taking care of myself."

5.

BE WILLING TO HELP THOSE IN NEED: "I tell my story to everyone who contacts me. I ask them what they fear, and I tell them "this is going to happen", or "this is going to hurt", etc. I'll listen to anybody who needs it about their doubts concerning medical procedures. I am always available to help in this way." ■

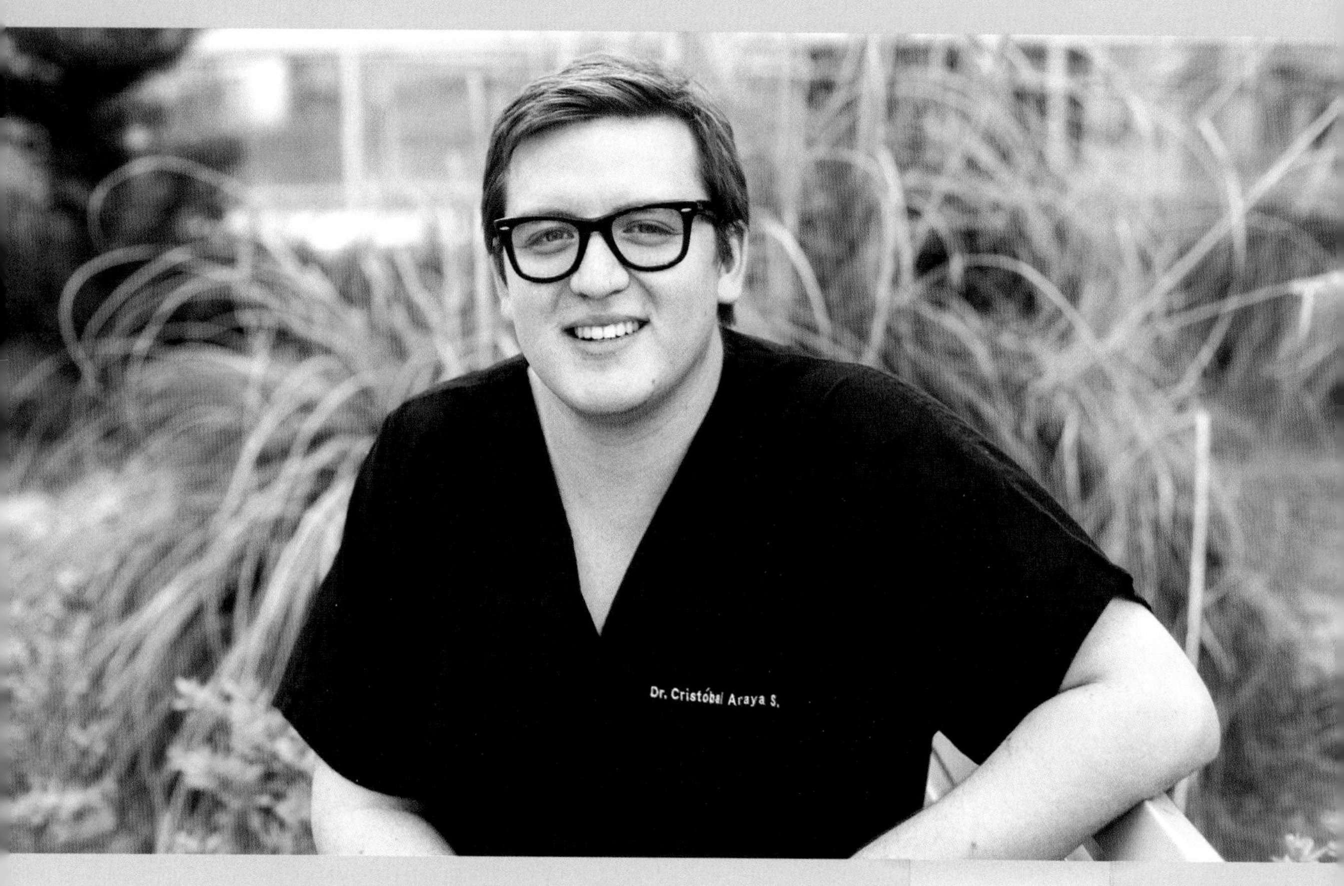

Cristóbal Araya

Dental surgeon

AGE: *27*

OCCUPATION: *Oral and Maxillofacial Pathologist*

CONTEXT: *Cristóbal Araya has focused on oral pathology since he began college, and now specializes in it. He has been long committed to his patients' health in his country's Public Health system. What follows are his tips and tools to prevent mouth cancer, also known as buccal or oral cancer.*

1.

MOUTH CANCER IS NO MYTH: "Ninety percent (90%) of mouth cancers correspond to the *squamous cell carcinoma*. Within the affected organs, we may find the tongue (most frequently its rim and lower section), lips, oral mucosae found on the inner face of cheeks, lips, and the hard and soft palate. Although it may be prevented, the biggest problem is that, up until now, cases of oral and maxillofacial cancer are only detectable at their advanced stages (stage III and IV). The greatest challenge faced by health professionals and specialists in the oral and maxillofacial field is, definitely, early detection."

"Oral sex with people carrying the disease may ***influence,*** along with other **factors,** the appearance of this type of cancer in young adults."

2.

HOW TO PREVENT IT: "There are certain habits and factors that have an influence in the appearance of oral cancer. Tobacco, for instance, is the main initiator and cause of this type of cancer. Also, an excessive consumption of alcohol, lack of hygiene, and continuous exposure to the sun with unprotected lips have an influence. Although the association of human papilloma virus with mouth cancer has not been proven, oral sex with people carrying the disease may influence, along with other factors, the appearance of this type of cancer in young adults."

3.

DETECTION AT AN EARLY STAGE: "There are some wounds that are deemed precursors of mouth cancer. Recognizing the latter as they appear may prevent the progress of oral cancer: white spots (*leukoplakia*), red spots (*erythroplakias*), or both simultaneously. Wounds and/or ulcers that do not heal in 2 weeks ought to be consulted for right away. Patients may also perform a self-examination in front of a mirror, so as to check the neck, internal surfaces of the cheeks, tongue (the rim and under part), gums, and palate. We, as specialists, also have the responsibility of thoroughly assessing our patients and of systematically performing an oral exam on them."

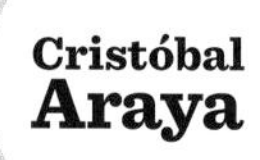

4.

MOUTH CANCER IS TREATABLE: *"Many people are scared of facing the disease, because they don't know how they will look after surgery, nor the impact it may have on the way they see themselves and on social reinsertion. Nowadays, in Chile, technology has really made huge progress, and people that undergo surgery and then supplementary radiotherapy and/or chemotherapy may get rid of the disease, meeting oncological, functional, and esthetical parameters, without any big negative impact."*

5.

5-STEP SELF-EXAMINATION IN FRONT OF THE MIRROR:

1. Touch your neck, looking for abnormal bulges.
2. Touch and observe your lips inside and out: look for changes in color, form, or consistency.
3. Observe and touch your gums, palate, and mucosae thoroughly. Look for the same changes described in step 2 above.
4. Stick out your tongue and thoroughly examine it. Move it from one side to the other, and pay attention to the rims, in search of any kind of alteration that stands out.
5. Raise your tongue and touch your palate with it. That way you will be able to have a look underneath your tongue and at the bottom part of your mouth. Run your finger from the back forward, and look for everything described in steps 1 to 4 above."

6.

GOOD EATING HABITS: "I recommend the consumption of flavonoids, which are abundantly found in food like black tea, onions, apples, black pepper, blueberries, plumbs, oranges, strawberries, and spinach. Flavonoids have several benefits as they have excellent antioxidant properties, and they contribute Vitamin C to the body. Plus, there are theories of their preventive role against cardiovascular diseases, arteriosclerosis, and some types of cancer."

"We, as ***specialists,*** also have the responsibility of thoroughly assessing our patients and of systematically performing an oral **exam** on them."

7.

POSITIVE AND PROACTIVE ATTITUDE: "It's the best tool the patient has to face the disease. The same applies to the specialist, who can make everything easier with a good attitude and disposition towards his/her patient. It is also advisable to include the family in the process, for them to actively (and also positively) participate in the treatment; you all fight together for a good cause. Beating cancer, that is." ■

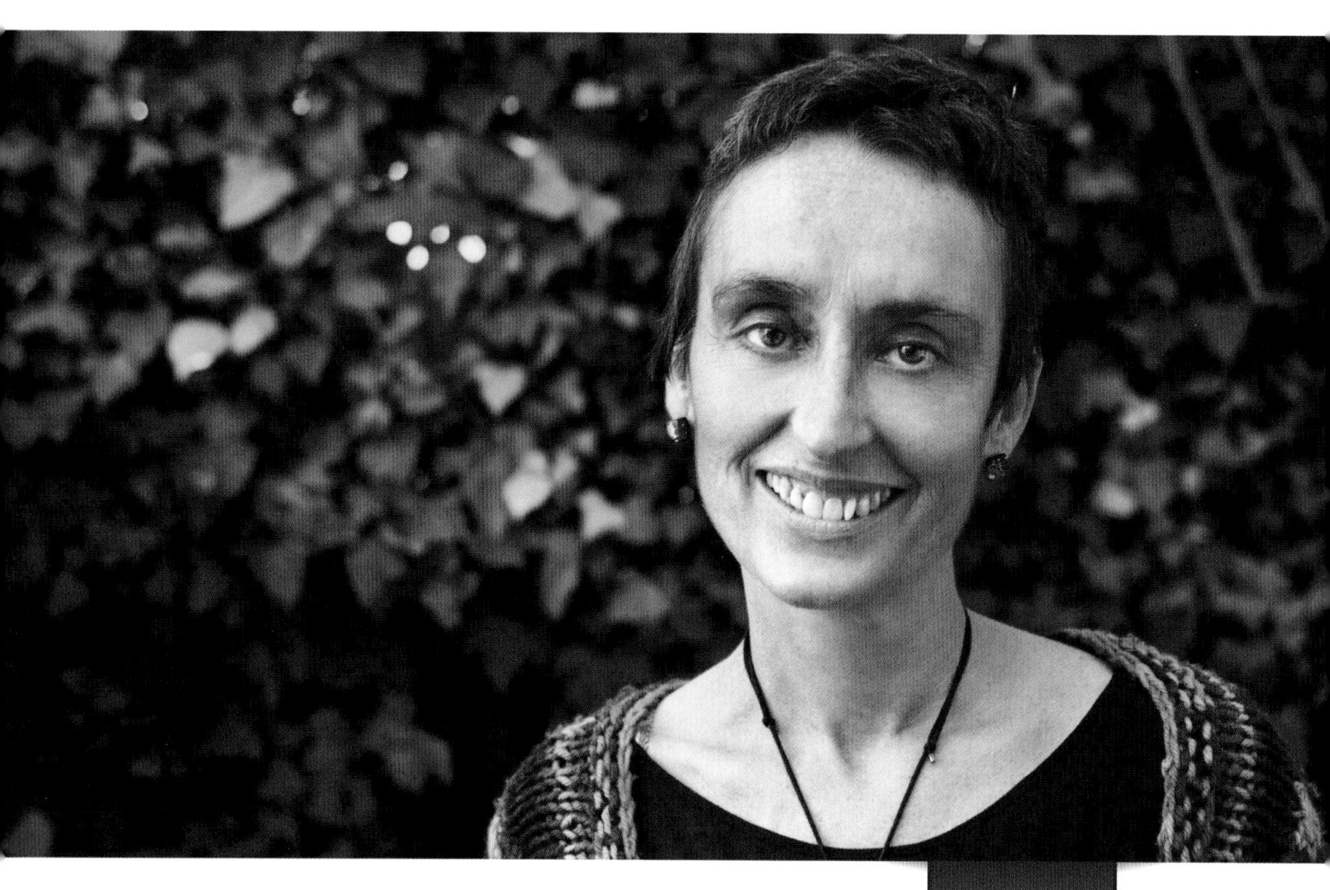

Carla Vidal

pancreatic cancer

PATIENT

AGE: *49*

OCCUPATION: *Psychologist*

DIAGNOSIS: *Pancreatic cancer*

WHEN: *2007*

CONTEXT: *From the moment she was diagnosed with a complex pancreatic cancer, Carla underwent a five-year treatment with more than 80 chemotherapy sessions. However, the disease had the last word and Carla died in November 2012. She undertook significant changes in her life to face the disease and was able to share some for this book.*

1.

OPEN UP TO THE WORLD AND TALK TO IT: "Writing my story opened a world to me. There's something emotional about belonging to the 'club' of cancer patients; and being open about it is like coming out of the closet. My testimonial was uploaded to different websites and ended up being public; I didn't control who had access to it. Thanks to that I met more sick people and we ended up creating a group who gets together once a month to share our processes, advice, diets and practical issues."

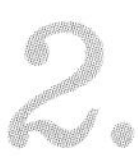

PAY FOR AN ONCOLOGICAL INSURANCE: "I took an insurance policy from the *Clínica Alemana* in 2002; a person close to me was selling it and I took it to help them. My husband and I thought about a possible accident or hospitalization, but never considered cancer. It ended up being that, in the event of cancer, the insurance didn't even have a deductible and we didn't pay a dime. Without that said insurance we could have paid one or two years, but in no way five. The difference, economically speaking, –but mainly in relation to emotional calmness– is huge."

"The hair was my *control* shelter and letting it go implied pure **lightness.**"

3.

WRITE DOWN YOUR DAY TO DAY: "When I started my testimonial I had been sick for five years and had gone through many things. I don't know if you can start writing from the beginning of the disease because your thoughts vary a lot. What I did was keep a kind of journal where I wrote about my everyday life, not just what I recalled. And I strongly suggest making this record because what you forget first is your everyday life."

4.

SMALL CHILDREN, BIG CHILDREN: "When I got sick, of my three children, the oldest was coming to the end of her schooling while the youngest was 10 years old. I always told them everything, but especially made sure to tell the youngest that I was sick, that I'd be undergoing treatment, that I might be very tired and would lose my hair. I focused on what the treatment would mean. It's important to be open with children, to lift the taboo, and to avoid them hearing things from other people."

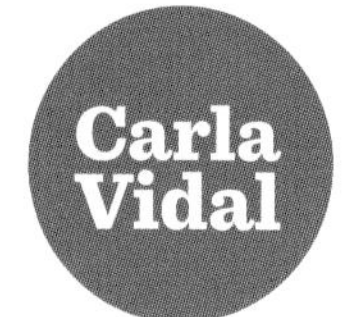

5.

ASSISTED FAMILY REORGANIZATION: "A colleague offered family therapy during the first year of the disease. It was a very positive experience, as it helped us adjust some family practices: As a mother, I used to work very much and, therefore, I was too controlling of domestic things. Therapy helped my children understand that in the future the house would have to work differently and they would have to do their part."

6.

THE HAIR RITUAL: "The hair loss process is terrible. You need to sweep the bathroom floor every day and it hurts because it opens your pores. When my time to shave arrived, I wanted to turn that moment into a meaningful activity and decided to make a family ritual instead of going to the hairdresser. We turned some music on and my husband shaved my head in front of my children. It was a really emotional moment. I asked for us to bury the hair and, while doing it, I was going to think what else I would like to bury with that hair, what stuff I would like to let go. We did it on a December 24th and it was so nice that, far from causing anguish or depressing me, it left me a feeling of lightness, because there was nothing else I needed to be holding."

8.

THE WIG: "I only wore the wig one day, and I couldn't bear it. In the end I put it away and wore scarves. That was liberating because my hair was the only thing I could control."

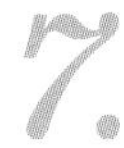

CREATE YOUR OWN SCENARIO: "Creating an environment is key. In all the chemotherapy session that I needed to be hospitalized (some were as an outpatient) I took chocolate candles to stop the room smelling like a hospital. I also took things to get distracted when I felt better, such as the computer; I had books, but reading is harder because you start feeling sick relatively quickly. Once I was back at home after chemotherapy, it was important to do fun activities. I watched movies, lots of movies."

9.

ASSERTIVENESS FIRST: "You have to be very clear about what does you good and what does not, and avoid doing things purely to meet other people's expectations. If people come to see you and you are not in the mood, they have to go, I'm sorry. It is not being ungrateful, but it's vital to maintain assertiveness. It was not easy for me, because the first year of my disease people would come like on a pilgrimage to my house, I was emotionally drained and I could see how absurd it was to subject myself to this on top of everything else you have to cope with. Chemotherapy can be like being in Hiroshima; that is why it is not always possible to meet social obligations normally."

10.

WHY DID THIS HAPPEN TO ME?: "The question is unavoidable and problematic. It has a bright side, because you start making useful adjustments in your new life. However, it also has a guilty side, which is macabre and whose other side is the fantasy that if you correct one thing you will heal, an expectation that can be exhausting. Getting out of that mortal trap is key and Buddhist psychology enabled me to do it, based on the idea that disease and death are natural situations, not personal failures."

11.

DON'T STRUGGLE, LIVE: "It's hard to understand, because one relates to being defeated, to losing the battle. And this is about leaving the fighting logic aside. It's not losing a battle, it's not winning, it's not losing. It's about escaping dichotomy and living."

13.

ANTHROPOSOPHIC MEDICINE: "I used it from the beginning as supplementary treatment, through injections in the stomach from a plant named *viscum* strengthening the immune system."

12.

THE VITALIZING ENZYME: "When people are about to die, they are full of energy the day before. An oncologist was obsessed with why that happened and discovered an enzyme that the body produces one day before it dies in order to vitalize you, which makes a goodbye possible. I undergo a treatment that lasts six months with this enzyme. It is a sublingual liquid, applied three times a day during the first week, the second week every 12 hours, and the third week only once a day. Then you control yourself once a month to ensure a good impregnation. The enzyme, together with other supplementary therapies like yoga, a no-sugar diet and meditation, have truly done wonders for me, because the level of energy I had this last year has been amazing. The first years at 9 p.m. I was already sleeping, and now I can go to bed at 12 without any problem."

"Diseases and death are natural situations, not a ***personal*** failure."

14.

SIMPLE THINGS: "I walk as much as I can and don't drive a car. I move from one place to another on foot and treasure those moments; even when I'm going somewhere specific I walk looking around. Those are very gratifying moments." ■

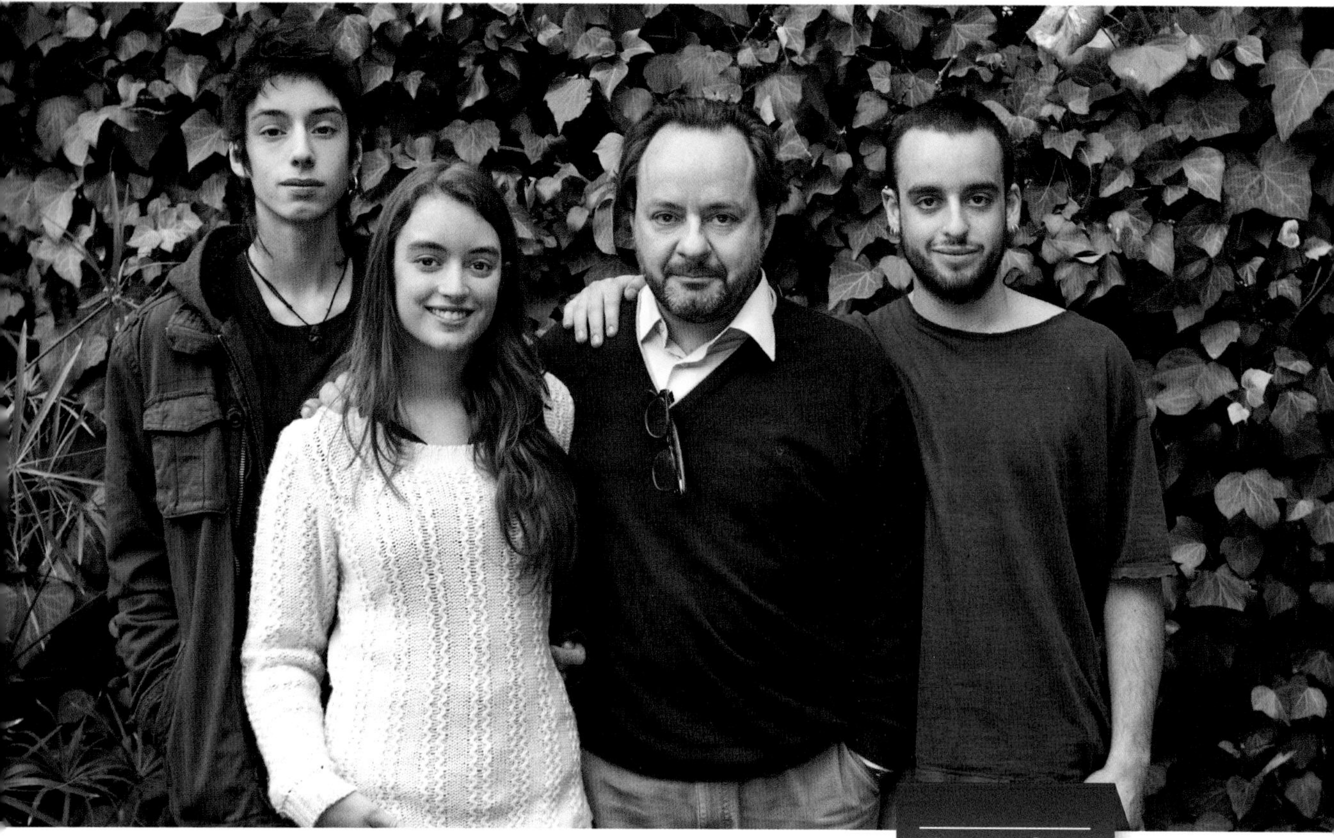

Familia Aguiló Vidal

Family of pancreatic cancer patient

Osvaldo Aguiló	Amparo	Bruno	Vicente
AGE: *56*	**AGE:** *26*	**AGE:** *23*	**AGE:** *18*
OCCUPATION: *Designer*	**OCCUPATION:** *Psychologist*	**OCCUPATION:** *Engineering student*	**OCCUPATION:** *Astronomy student*

CONTEXT: *Carla Vidal died in November 2012, some weeks before turning 50. When she was diagnosed with pancreatic cancer, the prognosis was she would live for a few more months, but more than five years had gone by when she died. Her husband, Osvaldo Aguiló, and their children Amparo, Bruno and Vicente, remember her as a woman who had a good life until the end. She asked for a white coffin for her family and friends to color it before taking her to the crematorium.*

1. RITES

AMPARO: "Rites are helpful, they help the issue not being so hard and the grief is shared collectively. On my mother's birthday, we threw her ashes and flower petals to the sea in *Algarrobo* [beach on the Chilean central coast]. People who joined us from the coast sang the mantras she liked; it made me feel at peace. It was a controlled, comforted grief. When I meditate, I invite her to chat with me. I have a small Buddhist altar in my room with her picture."

BRUNO: "My mother's funeral and burial left a big mark on me. I am very grateful to the priest who performed the liturgy. At one point we all painted the coffin, which was all white. Some took the brushes, others the paints. Some of my dad's friends played live music. When we left with the colorful coffin everybody clapped. I want to keep her alive in my mind, but, at the same time, I need to let her go a little, stop thinking about her death, about her not being here anymore, rebuild my life. I find this impossible, because my life is not the same since my mother died."

OSVALDO: "We practiced some rituals in the clinic and also after her death: a barbecue with the priest, a family ritual in *Isla Negra* (town in the central coast of Chile), celebrated New Year's Eve by the sea and planted a tree at her parents' house. This was the other side of what we lived just before: while Carla was in the clinic 50 or 80 people went to see her each day for three weeks; their company comforted us very much. But we also needed to demystify her a little bit: it is hard to deal with the image of a wife and mother who is up on a huge pedestal."

"Rites are *helpful,* they help the issue not being so hard and the grief is shared **collectively**"

2. EVERY ONE LIVES GRIEF THEIR OWN WAY

OSVALDO: "Each one of us is in his therapy, each one has lived this according to himself. We have tried to be careful and supportive towards each other, according to our own rhythms, according to the timings and character of each one of us."

AMPARO: "The process of learning to respect the different stages of grief that we all have was something we worked on. One expects that the others are living the same, but it is impossible. At one point, Bruno was very active with domestic chores and he demanded the same energy from us, but we were in different synchronies. For me, in another moment, I missed the collective rituals and wanted to be close to everybody, but Bruno told me: "Please respect me, I'm crying inside, I'm not interested in rituals at the moment." We can't demand that others are in the same place as we are."

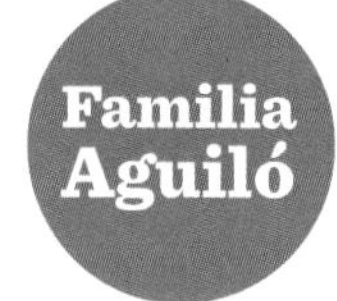

3.

WRITE

BRUNO: "Many people went to the clinic, but they couldn't all see my mother, so we handed around some notebooks and people wrote in them, and in the evening my father would read their notes. At least two notebooks were filled."

OSVALDO: "Like Carla said, for her it was important to write down everything that was happening. In fact, her notes were later published by Ediciones Catalonia as a book *Sin paréntesis* ("Without parenthesis", Catalonia publishing house)."

"When ***she*** died I thought **each one** would be locked in their bedrooms, it was a *relief* to discover that it was just a matter of time, since the four of us we like to sit and *talk*."

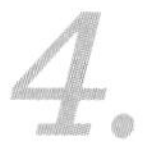

USE YOUR ROLE IN THE FAMILY

OSVALDO: "After Carla's death I was quite isolated in having to deal with the family's needs. Women seem to have a knack for remembering things to do with their children's medication, school dates, what they like and don't like... Talking to the children's godparents, with my sister-in-law and with Carla's friends really helped me try and take on that role."

AMPARO: "She was the one who kept everything in order in the family and without her things sort of fell apart, to the extent that we'd even forget to eat. I felt the pressure to try and bring everyone together, but I just didn't feel I could. She was the one who'd held us together, and when she died I really thought we'd all just disappear into our bedrooms on our own, but in fact it was a huge relief to discover that very quickly we all gravitated towards each other, just sitting and talking for ages."

BRUNO: "When my mother died I started doing the things that nobody seemed to be doing, like making lunch or taking the garbage out. One day I was about to have lunch with my brother and his girlfriend, and out of habit I said "Okay kids! Lunch time!". I was so tired around that time that for several months I didn't even have time to tidy my room."

VICENTE: "Mom was like a walking diary - she'd always remind us of things we had to do. Afterwards we became more proactive ourselves - I went to the dentist and realized I hadn't been in ages."

5.

THE DEATH TOPIC

OSVALDO: "There's no way to be specially prepared. During those five years Carla had cancer, we became somehow indecent in relation to the topic of death. We talked about it many times in the family, it was an open topic, it was never a private issue; in fact, we even joked about it; black humor. At many times the contact was more emotional, but the topic was always talked about in an open way. We started liking the way it was treated at the end."

6.

INTERFAMILIAL COMMUNICATION

BRUNO: *"We got used to receiving attention from everybody at the clinic, and for the family to be the center of attention, but we then realized that in our daily lives we only had each other. Luckily as a family we're good at talking about stuff. If we like something we can express that. This helps keep everything in perspective about one's own things and other people's."* ■

"We have tried to be *careful* and *supportive* to each other, according to our own rhythms, according to the ***timings*** and ***character*** of each **of us."**

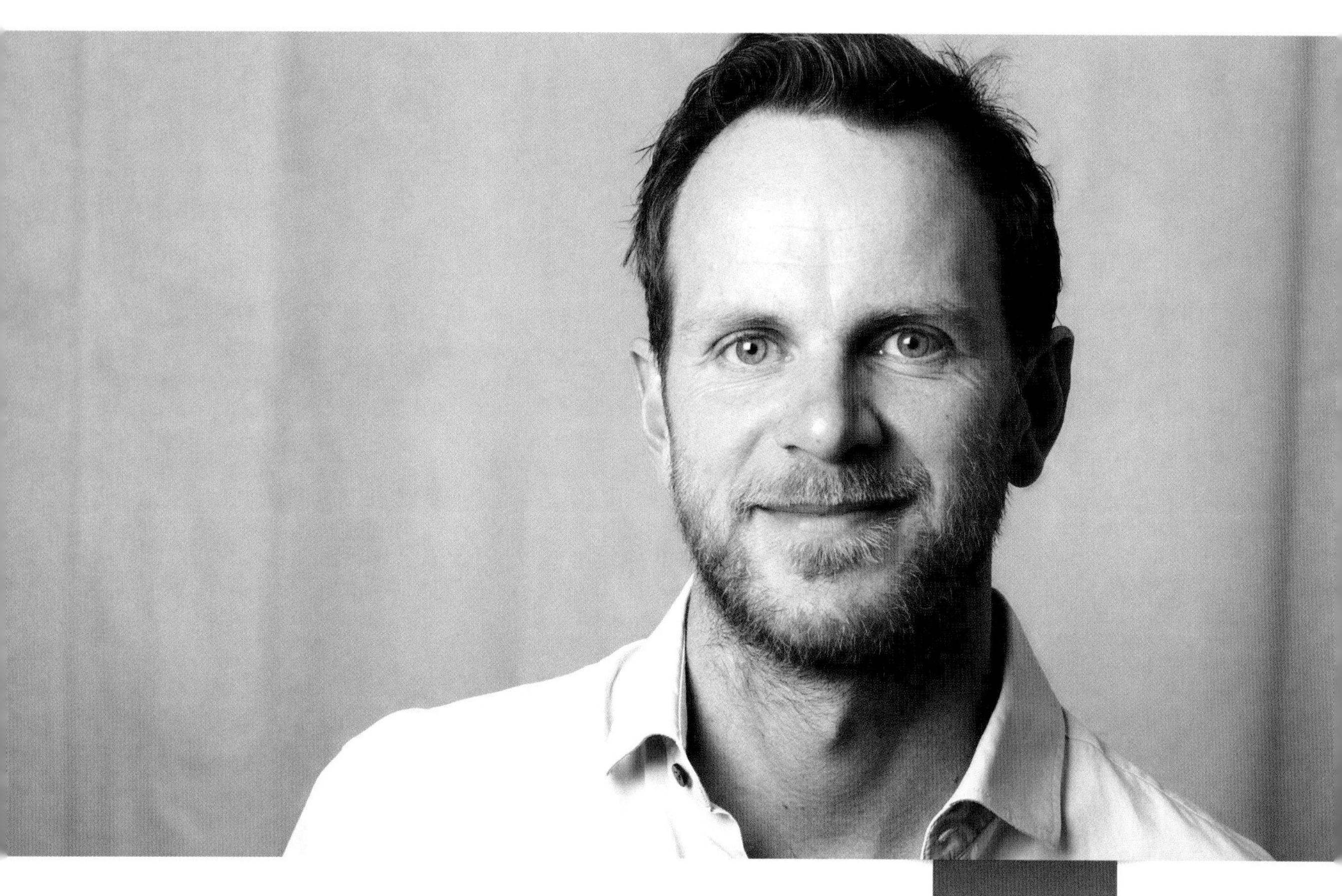

Martin Inderbitzin ✚

pancreatic cancer

PATIENT

AGE: *36*

OCCUPATION: *Neuroscientist, filmmaker and speaker*

DIAGNOSIS: *Pancreatic cancer*

WHEN: *2012*

CONTEXT: *Swiss citizen Martin Inderbitzin was diagnosed with an aggressive pancreatic cancer and, according to statistics, he only had 3 years left. Halfway through his treatment he decided to participate in a triathlon, despite never having practiced any high performance sports. Three months after ending his treatment, he crossed the finishing line of his first race. Martin documented this experience in order to inspire other cancer survivors around the world. That is how his website,* **MYSURVIVALSTORY.ORG**, *was born.*

1.

TO CRY IS HUMAN: "It is normal to feel devastated... sad... when you receive the diagnosis. It's OK to let these emotions flow. To cry and to be afraid is only human. Anything different would be odd."

2.

BREATHE: "After the initial shock, it was important for me sit down and breathe. To be quiet and realize that being diagnosed with cancer is not a death sentence. True, many people die from cancer, but many have survived, too; it is paramount not to forget that."

3.

YOU AND YOUR BODY ARE NOT A NUMBER: "As a neuroscientist, I know biology is not math. Nature is much more complex, and so is your body. Nobody knows how treatment or the disease is going to react in you. There are many examples out there, as well as in books, with evidence of you not being a number."

4.

FIND YOUR THING: "Each person reacts differently to cancer. Some need calm moments, others need to write a book. I myself had to run a triathlon, and others have changed their diets. Just ask yourself, what do I need? What is good for you?

"To *cry* and to be frightened is only human. Anything different would be **odd.**"

5.

DON'T JUDGE THOSE AROUND YOU: "Cancer doesn't only affect you. It also affects your family and friends. Different people deal with cancer in very different ways; some are really open about the subject while others just don't want to talk about it. Don't take it personally, it has nothing to do with you. They love you, but everyone has his/her own way of coping."

6.

SETTING GOALS: "One way of keeping your mind healthy is to set goals. The goal you choose does not really matter, just find one that suits YOU, and then divide it into stages. When I started my training for the triathlon, half way through chemo, I could not ride a bike for more than 10 minutes, but those 10 minutes made me feel happy. That was worth it."

7.

OPTIMISTS DIE HAPPIER: "I firmly believe in the power of a positive attitude. Clearly, that does not guarantee you will live more, but you will live happier for sure." ■

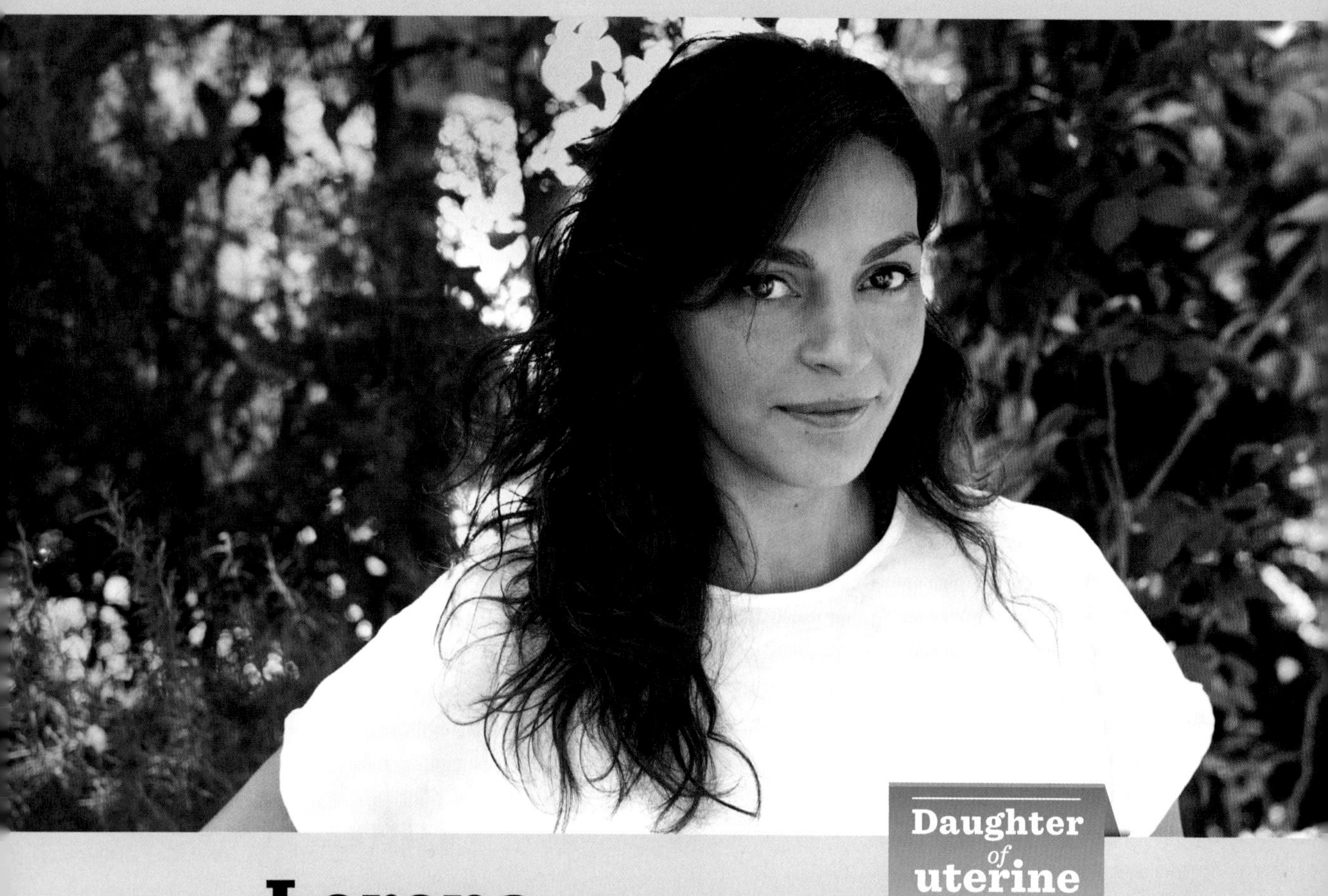

Daughter *of* uterine *and* cervical cancer patient

Lorena Penjean

AGE: *37*

OCCUPATION: *Journalist*

RELATIONSHIP: *Daughter of a Uterine and Cervical Cancer Patient*

WHEN: *2003*

CONTEXT: *When her mother, Nancy Cardenas, was diagnosed with uterine and cervical cancer, Lorena knew that she would be the one to keep her company through what was to come. She understood that the prognoses for her mother were not good, but she had no idea of how deeply the experience of keeping her mother company through the ordeal would affect her.*

1.

RESPECTING THE PATIENT'S DECISIONS: "When my mother had an infection, she was told *the only option we have to extend your life is to remove your uterus, ovaries and intestines and to leave you with a little bag for your needs.* She refused. She preferred to live what she had left of life well. I had no choice but to respect her decision. What was I going to do? I suffered from seeing her like that and could imagine how somebody must feel knowing that they are dying and that it is happening in the worst possible way."

2.

"ENSLAVEMENT TO PAIN": "Cancer is an illness that shows no mercy to people. Somehow, my mother's death freed me, and I was calmer when I stopped worrying about the hospital, the morphine, the doctors and the lab tests. But the enslavement to the pain remains. It is a pain with no sense at all."

3.

THE BIG DILEMMA: "The doctors were telling me that they could still dialyze, operate on her and a thousand of other things. I asked them what they would do in my place and one of them told me: *If it were my mom, I would leave her alone*. I spoke with my sister and obviously we did not want her to die, but we asked ourselves whether it was worth living like that. We made the decision on our own and decided to do nothing. It was terrible asking if she could stay in a hospice, where the terminally ill come to die in piece. Brutal."

4.

REINVENTING CHRISTMAS: "I began a charity campaign when my mother was still alive. Now I go to the hospital with my children; we gather gifts and I ask my friends for contributions, then I buy flowers for all the women in the hospital. It has already been six Christmases and I feel good doing it; it makes me happy and brings me peace. I am no Saint Teresa, but I channel positive energy and put it to good use in a place where people suffer."

5.

MOURNING TIME: "When my mother died, my entire childhood disappeared: when I learned to speak, when I learned to write, the homework. It is the womb. I still keep three items that are important to me: her phone, her hair band and her Bible. And a couple of boxes that I do not dare open, because I don't want to know what she was thinking when she was going to die. I still feel a lot of pain. A pain that stays. I feel it in my chest."

6.

HOPE FOR THE BEST AND PREPARE FOR THE WORST: "This saying is common among mountain climbers and it is my preferred attitude to face this process. I do not have an exact recipe, but you should keep the person company, be empathetic, and be as loving as you can; you should treasure memories and be a good person, because when people are gone, those are the only things that matter. You stay behind and you have to learn to live with that. I don't know what else. It is not much." ■

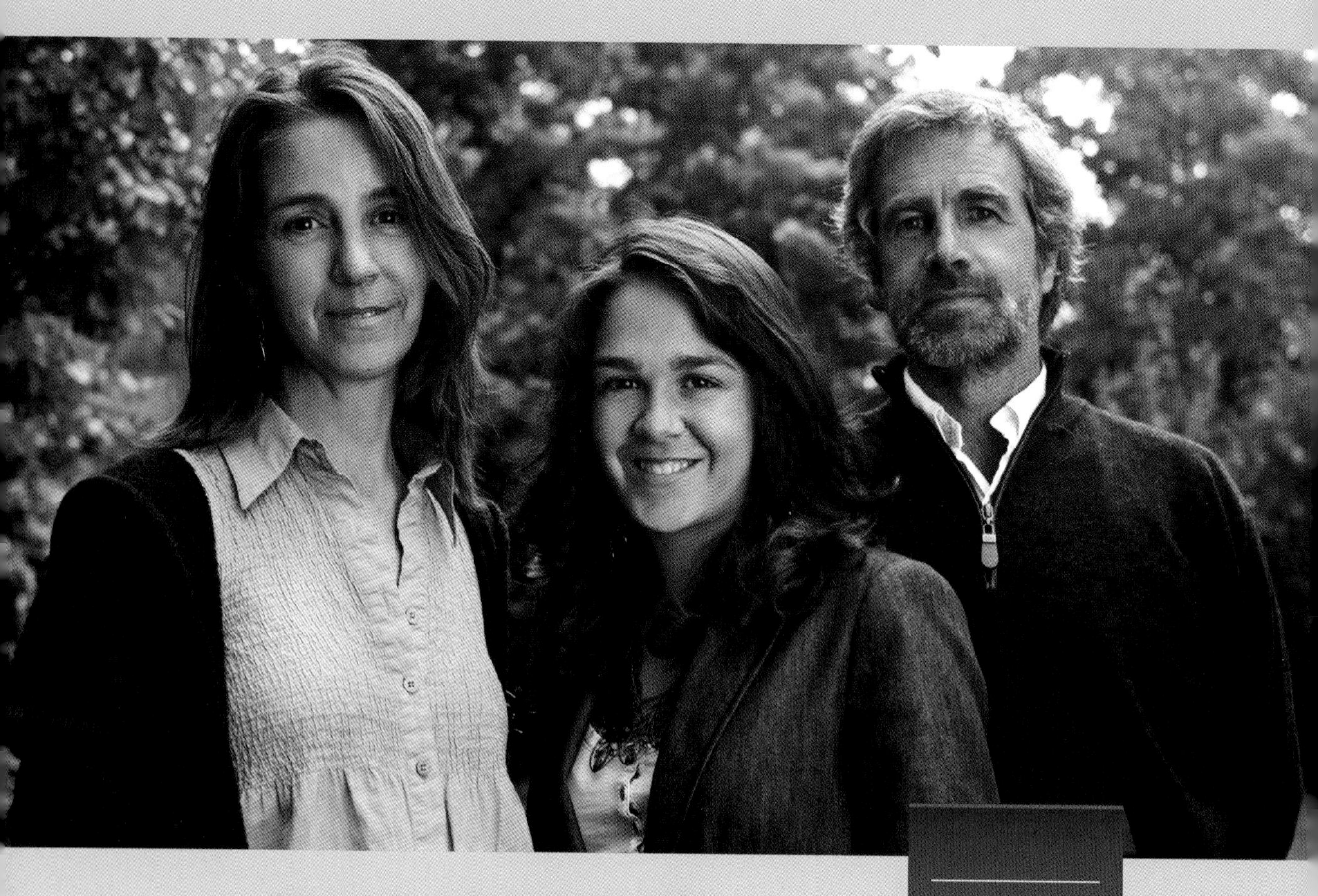

Juan Purcell & Isabel Salas

ELISA'S PARENTS

Parents *of* **osteosarcoma patient**

AGE: *48 & 47 respectively*

OCCUPATION: *Architect and teacher*

RELATIONSHIP: *Parents of osteosarcoma patient*

WHEN: *2010*

CONTEXT: *For the parents of Elisa Purcell the biggest challenge of their life came when she was 14 years old and was found to have a tumor in her knee, whose name and prognosis are ruthless: osteosarcoma. After a difficult period of therapy to contain the tumor, her doctors decided to give her a cutting edge prosthesis. Elisa's diagnosis and treatment generated a network of support, and great care from her parents; her siblings Pablo, Francisca and Pedro; her relatives; and many of her friends. Today everybody celebrates her triumph over this pitiless disease. This is her parents' testimony.*

1.

EVERYBODY IS A PATIENT: "Elisa was very patient when she received her treatment, and those of us who accompanied her had to be as well as we had to adjust to her needs: special meals, schedules, trips to places where she found happiness, visits that she wanted in spite of her low defenses, requests to change nurses and cleaning personnel, changes of bandages, etc. We tried to have everything so that she could get better."

2.

GIVE BACK: "Elisa had something change within herself, she acquired the marvelous capacity to keep others company. When she knows that somebody is suffering, she cannot be indifferent, she always makes loving gestures. She has been a great companion to people who have had it very rough. If she had not lived through what she lived through, perhaps that gift would have stayed dormant. Keeping others company is also very healing."

3.

ASK AND TAKE NOTE: "We tried to understand everything that was explained to us in order to make good decisions. We asked the doctors about everything and we wrote down what was happening. We found out about their experience with similar cases and we approached the doctors and medical centers with the most experience."

4.

FEMININE NOTES: "Taking care of Elisa's feminine charm, with scarves to cover her head, perfumes and nail polishes, lifted all of our spirits. Along with the doctors, we decided to suppress her period for some months with hormone injections. That way we spared her that physical exertion which was already uncomfortable and intensified by her low levels of platelets."

5.

AN ANGEL AT THE MINISTRY OF EDUCATION: "During Elisa's school tests, we received help from a professional at the Ministry of Education. We arrived at a tiny office and inside there was an angel. She was an expert in the area, and Elisa did not lose the two years even though she did not attend school regularly. One must pay attention to the appropriate people."

6.

PREVENT: "The extraction of ovarian tissue kept us calm knowing that Elisa could have children if she decides to. It is a technique brought to Chile from Belgium by the Catholic University. Only nine extractions had been done in Chile, but we did it because it ensured that Elisa could become a mother, considering that the chemos are strong. Her eggs are frozen and are viable." ■

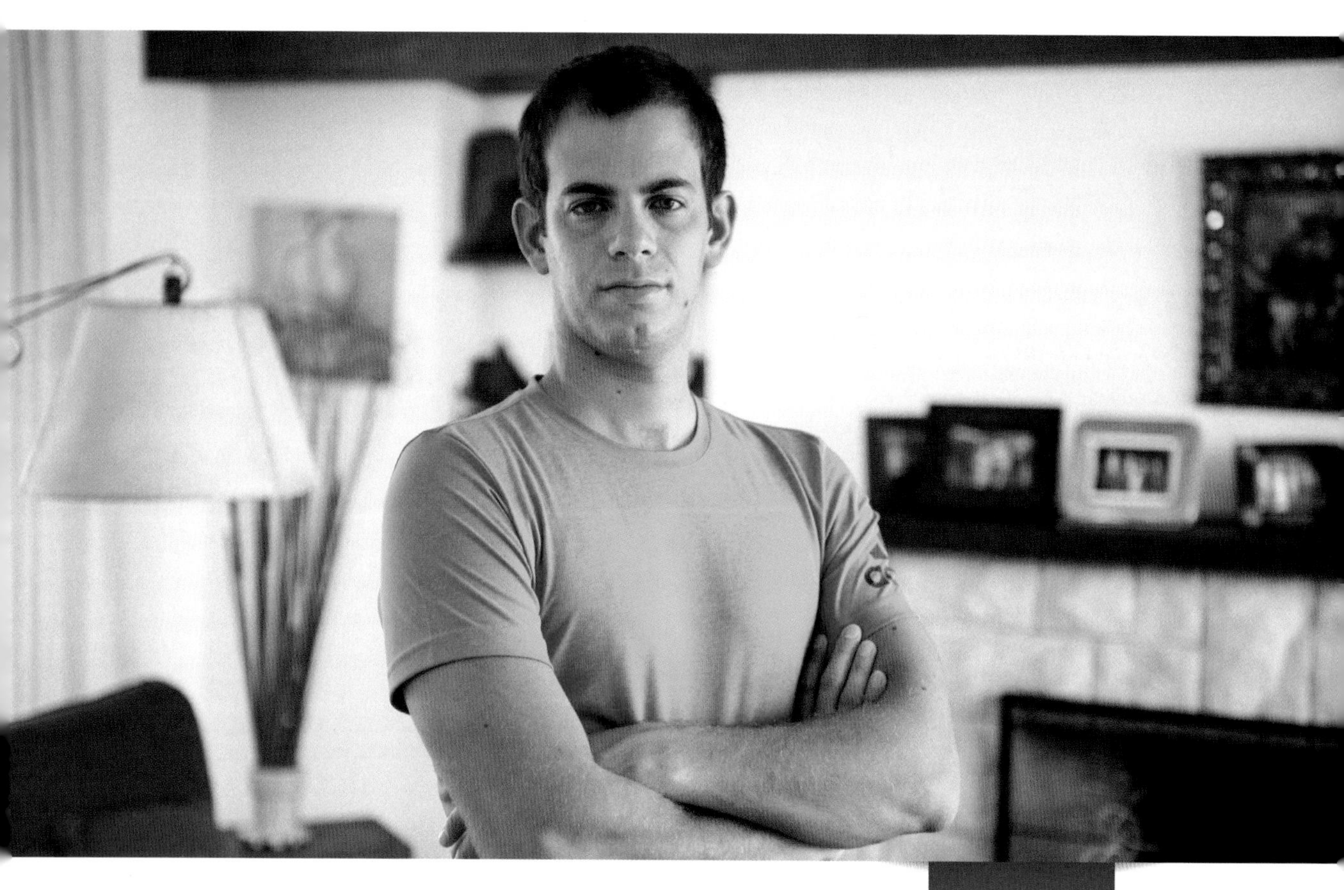

Pedro Pablo de Vinaeta

osteo sarcoma

PATIENT

AGE: *28*

OCCUPATION: *Athlete*

DIAGNOSIS: *Osteosarcoma*

WHEN: *2002*

CONTEXT: *Pedro Pablo de Vinaeta's life changed abruptly at the beginning of his teenage years, when he was diagnosed with bone sarcoma. He was 14 years old and loved sports. Thanks to his parents' enquiries, Pedro Pablo moved to Florence, Italy, where he underwent surgery that amputated his right leg. After several chemotherapy cycles and months in rehab, Pedro Pablo again embraced his passion for sports, and is today a courageous player of para-badminton.*

1.

OPTIMISM AND CERTAINTY: "I asked my doctor if my illness had a cure, and he said yes. With that, I assumed, and took for granted, that I would overcome cancer. Maybe I was naive, or even irrational, but I was certain I would get well. And that helped me a lot. I was always very optimistic. I was convinced that everything would turn out fine. And, despite the pain, I never gave up. I never said *no more chemo, please!* Nor did I ask *why me?* For me, that positive attitude from the very beginning was key to my recovery."

"You have to *make sure* that the patient feels as **happy** as possible, so that their anxiety level decrease."

2.

FOR A HAPPY PATIENT: "During those months in which I lived in a *pensione* in Italy, I was very happy despite the chemotherapy cycles, which were quite harsh. The reason was that I had my mom right there beside me, to hug her. Plus, the nurses were really nice to me, and they made me laugh a lot. My family would write to me from Peru, and whenever someone flew over to visit, that person would bring 50 stacks of cards and greetings from everyone. Thanks to the love I received from everywhere, my daily routine always had more minutes of happiness than sadness. So, you have to make sure that the patient feels as happy as possible, so that their anxiety level decrease."

3.

FAITH IS POWERFUL: "I am a practicing Catholic, and when all of that happened, my faith sort of shot up. Just as I was absolutely sure that I'd get better, I was also convinced that God listened each and every time I spoke to Him. Call it fate, but, my bedroom in that hostel was right across the street from a chapel. Even if I thought about something else, I had that constant reminder, and it was a great coincidence."

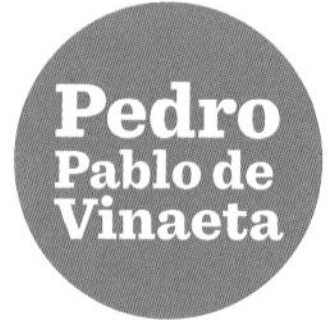

4.

LOOK FOR A SECOND OPINION: *"The first doctor I saw in Peru said that bone cancer treatment was just one and the same all over the world. That going elsewhere was pointless. He couldn't have been more wrong. He was sincere, very kind and nice, but he had made a mistake in trying to dissuade us from finding other treatments. When a patient is adult the responsibility falls on them, and they need to be fully informed and not rely totally on the doctors."*

5.

ENVISAGE THE FUTURE: "I had 2 things clearly in mind. First, the image of my grandparents on my mom's side. They had been married for almost 50 years, had 5 kids, and 14 grandchildren. Christmas and birthdays were a feast for the family. And so I thought, *if things don't work out here, I will never be able to experience that,* and I really believe it is one of the loveliest stages one can reach. I also used to envision things I'd do. Transcendental things. Stuff that would transform my country, that would change people's lives. And if my candle went out, so to speak, none of that would come true. The motivation I sought was a survival rope that kept pulling me forwards, that made me carry on walking."

6.

INTERNALIZE THAT NEW REALITY: "Losing my leg was harsh. The first few years I would not even wear shorts, and I used to feel very embarrassed if my prosthetic leg showed while walking. As much as I love the sea, I stopped going to the beach for 2 or 3 summers. The road to overcome that began with something my dad said to me: 'Look, Pedro Pablo, whether it's hard on you or not, whether you dare do it or not, at some point, you will overcome this. If you choose to send everything to hell, to dare do it and not feel ashamed, you will overcome it faster. If not, you'll be slow in overcoming it. But at some point you will.' That was the first push. The momentum I got to leave the trauma behind."

"The motivation I sought was truly a survival **rope** that kept pulling me *forwards*".

7.

POWER IS WITHIN YOU: "After psychotherapy in Peru and in Italy, I am convinced that change came about when I made the decision of daring to do it. When I said *to hell with what people say. To hell with their glances!* And all of that, you know. That's when I realized those were not piteous glances, but rather accepting glances. With that switch in my state of mind, I now understand that people do not need to look at me with pity, unless I am all nervous and scared, that is. It was a total flip-over of a situation." ■

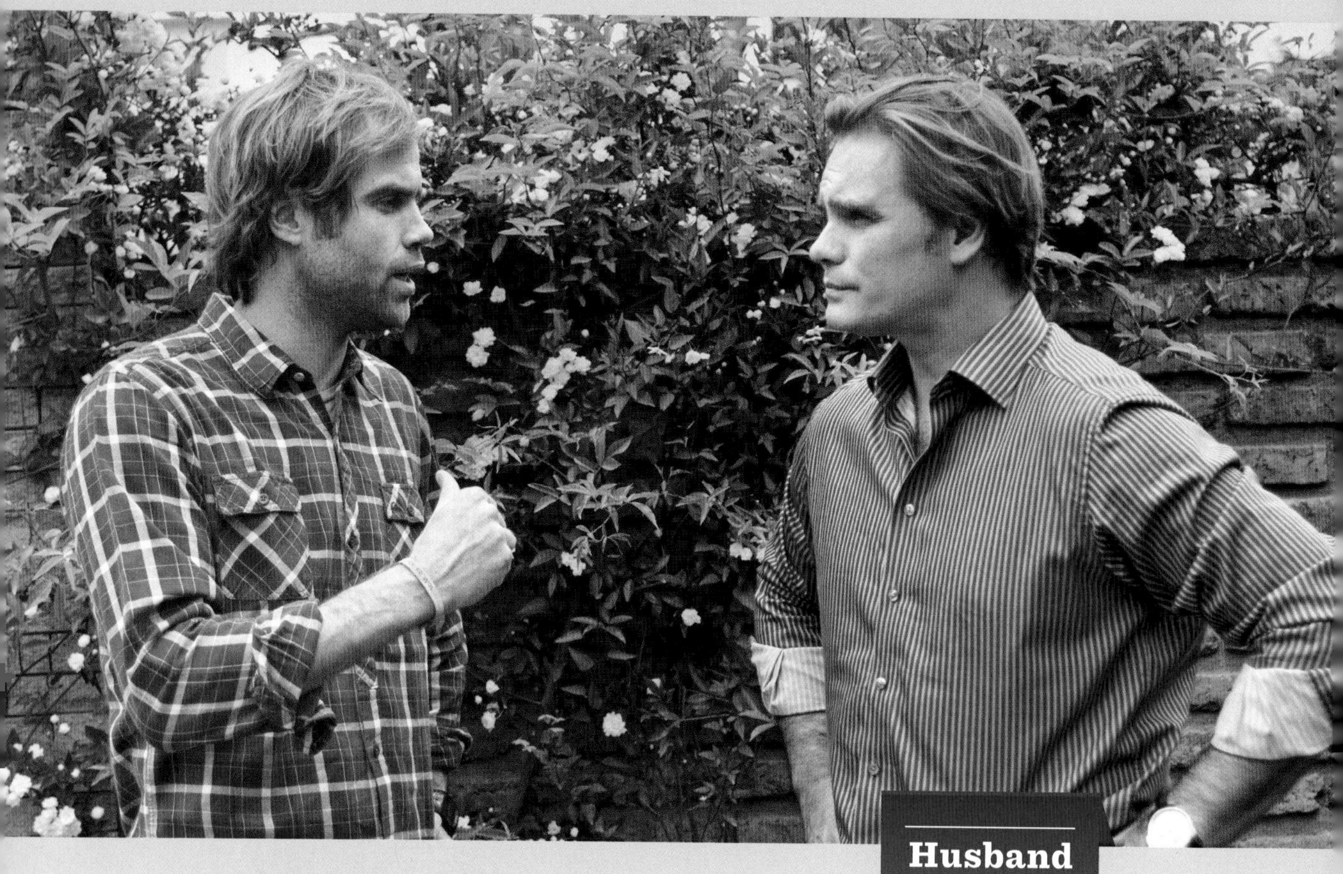

Husband *of* colon cancer patient

Amaro Gómez-Pablos

AGE: *47*

OCCUPATION: *Journalist*

RELATIONSHIP: *Husband of colon cancer patient*

WHEN: *1998*

CONTEXT: *The journalist and TV newscaster lost his first wife, Pilar Ruiz, after keeping her company through a rough five year battle against colon cancer. While already used to tough situations, the process left him with a hard lesson, where great sadness and lots of small happy moments intertwine. Pilar died in 2003 at the age of 30.*

1.

ALTERNATIVE THERAPIES: A MATTER OF FAITH: "It is true, there might be disappointments, but at the end of the day those therapies are an act of blind faith. What must be done is to clear the road and see what the best path is because there are therapies out there that have to be ruled out straight away. This part of the patient's process has to be respected."

2.

NO TO BLIND TRUST: I am personally interested in the exchange of opinions between professionals, and not in the blind trust placed in the latest fashionable treatment. I am interested in having a panoramic perspective in terms of how to tackle the disease. Therefore it is key to ask all the questions, even the ones related to looking for a second opinion. I want to be treated as an active patient. It is also crucial to ask the medical team not to scrimp on information but rather to present the big picture, without euphemisms.

3.

HUMANIZING THE PATIENT-DOCTOR RELATIONSHIP: "It is essential that the attending physician knows the name and last name of whoever they are treating. I also worry professionally about knowing the name and last name of whoever tells me a story, for example in a dramatic situation, and that is considering I am not intervening in their body."

"As a **husband,** you also have ***cancer.*** You do not suffer from it, but you understand its *psychology.*"

4.

HOW TO DEAL WITH SURVIVAL PROGNOSES: "While Pilar was anesthetized, an oncologist delicately told me her prognosis: "A year". We got married and lived together for 5 years. Generally, prognoses seem to me to be very respectable, yet I cannot give any specific advice as to how to deal with them. Sometimes they are not right, but other times they are useful because they give you an approximate idea of what is going to happen. The main problem is confusing it with a death sentence and to begin dying on the inside before it's time."

Amaro Gómez Pablos

5.

HOW TO UNDERSTAND THE PARTNER'S ROLE: "At one end, one must defy the sentence, because it is a fight, however, without dissociating from the word cancer, so that you are able to say it in front of your partner. As a husband, you also have cancer. You do not suffer from it, but you understand its psychology and realize that life is immanent."

6.

THE PATIENT CALLS THE SHOTS: "The patient controls all the emotions around their cancer, because the path forward depends on their attitude and they know, intuitively, that they trigger people's behaviors and attitudes about their disease. This includes doctors and the way in which information about their malady is delivered."

7.

LIVE HERE AND NOW: "To live here and now might only be an existential stance, but when a person whom you love has cancer, that ideal becomes a daily habit. It is very beautiful because then it becomes true."

8.

ONLY ONE ADVANTAGE: "The only advantage about cancer is that it is not traumatic, nor accidental. Therefore in one way or another you can get ready."

9.

"WHAT FOR" INSTEAD OF "WHY": "If you ask yourself why, you will enter a vicious circle out of which there is no escape: *why me, what happened?* Nevertheless, if you abandon that question and begin asking, *what am I going to live for*, that's a great existential question. A disease has taken over your body, but there is also a big question: *why am I here, where am I going, why do I want to keep living, what for?* Then you can establish a goal.

10.

DO NOT BURY MEMORIES: "Remembering and doing so with integrity. To remember is a very beautiful word, it comes from Latin. It is important not to bury any phases of your life, not even the cancer, rather you should look at it, contemplate it and fight it. Then, when it is not defeated, remember it."

11.

ANGELS ON THE ROAD: *"Cancer also brings about very beautiful things such as angels crossing your path. These angels are real people, tremendously generous, who in one way or another come to tell you that this disease can also be a beneficial stage in life."*

"It is *crucial* to ask the medical team ***not to scrimp*** on information and rather to present the **big picture,** without euphemisms."

12.

ON MATERNITY: "In the case of young couples, such as we were, the issue of maternity was unavoidable. And we talked about it, but we understood that it was like playing Russian roulette. In a woman's case, the growth of cancer spirals exponentially with pregnancy, unfortunately. That is also considering that your body is the host of toxic chemicals that can also affect the child. It was not easy to accept."

13.

TO GIVE UP OR NOT: "Another very important issue within the context of cancer is how to reconcile your role as a supporter to their willingness to live and their fighting spirit, while understanding their right to give up. Because sometimes this is so tiring, and suddenly you can get to the point where you recognize the limits of your own resistance. *We did not win, but we won a lot of time. Perhaps we did not win all of life, but we won time.* This can sometimes be transmitted by the patient themselves, but other times you have to have the intuition to recognize and accept it." ■

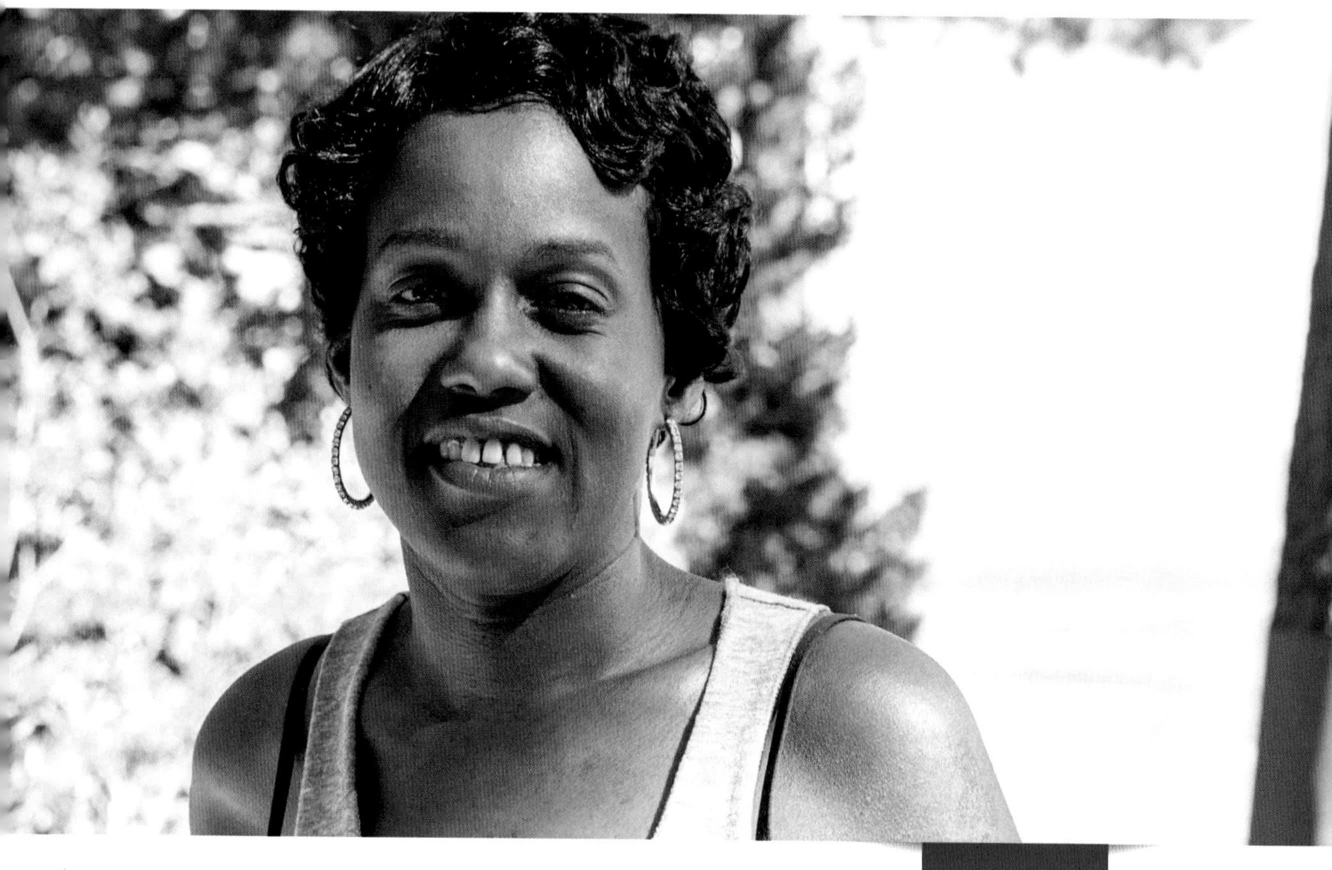

Yasmeem Watson

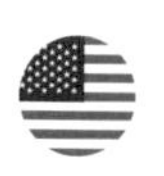

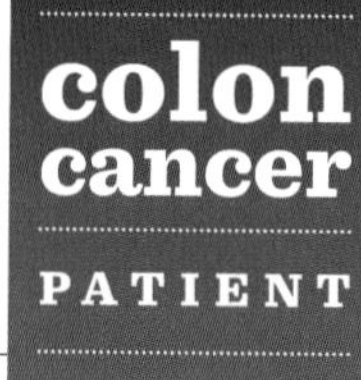

AGE: *39*

OCCUPATION: *Research Advocate and Contact Representative*

DIAGNOSIS: *Colon cancer*

WHEN: *2013*

CONTEXT: *Yasmeem complained about her symptoms for over a year to her doctor but was just told that she had IBS and to monitor her diet. This went on for over a year until Yasmeem began to advocate for herself and demand further testing. She was then diagnosed with stage III colon cancer. She had to have surgery and endure 8 months of chemotherapy. Colon cancer is preventable 90% of the time but the current screening guidelines leave the younger demographic to fend for themselves.*

1.

THANK GOD EVERY DAY FOR NEW MERCIES: "Thank God every day that your feet touch the floor, your life still has purpose, find it."

3.

TELL PEOPLE THE PEOPLE THAT MATTER THAT YOU LOVE THEM: "Tomorrow is not promised; seize every opportunity to spread LOVE."

5.

DON'T LET ANY GRASS GROW UNDER YOUR FEET: "Keep propelling forward never become stagnated."

6.

WRITE A BUCKET LIST THEN A F*CK IT LIST: "They are both equally important. If you love it, do it. If you don't, screw it."

8.

LOVE YOURSELF JUST AS YOU ARE: "You're not the same person you were prior to diagnosis, So What. Even a Caterpillar becomes a butterfly."

2.

TAKE THE PICTURE: "Even if your hair isn't combed, you can never replace memories."

"**Keep** propelling *forward* ***never*** become stagnated."

4.

WHO CARES IF THE GLASS IS EMPTY OR FULL: "Be happy that you have a glass, Go refill it."

7.

TAKE THE TRIP, ALONE: "Get to know yourself and bask in the transformation."

9.

BE THANKFUL, ALWAYS: "For everything." ■

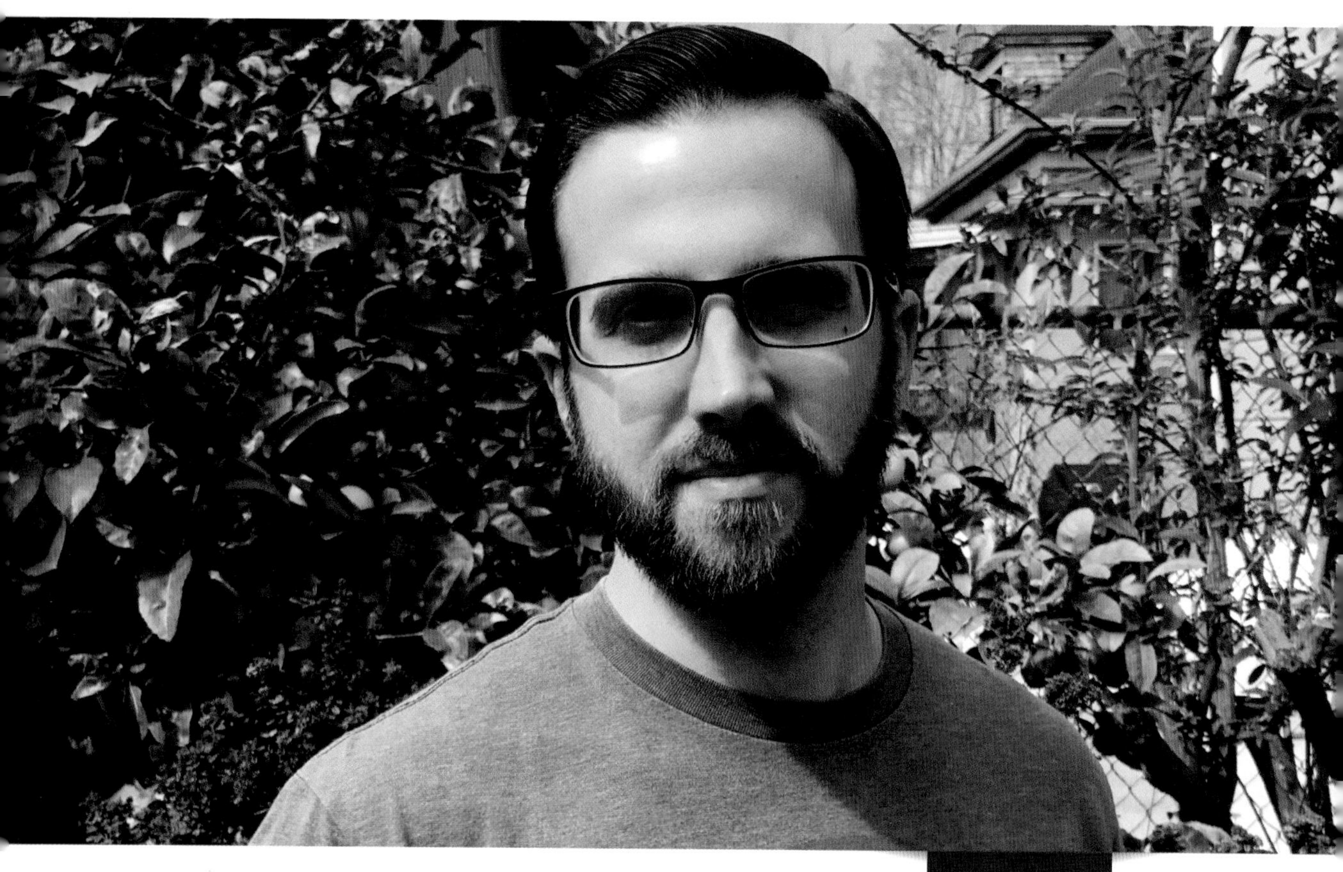

Erik Hale

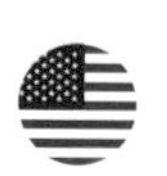

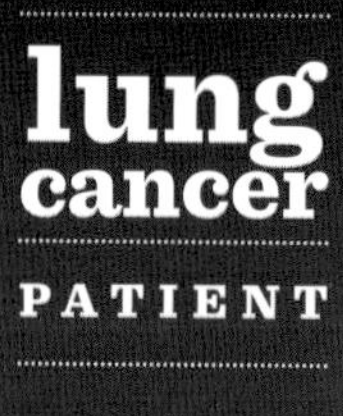

AGE: *34*

OCCUPATION: *Customer Relations*

DIAGNOSIS: *Stage 3A Adenocarcinoma (Lung Cancer in lower left lobe that spread to lymph nodes)*

WHEN: *2013*

CONTEXT: *I was diagnosed with lung cancer at the age of 30. I'm a non-smoker and was a preschool teacher at the time I was diagnosed. I was misdiagnosed for months and was told I had pneumonia and a fungal infection until finally a biopsy was performed and determined that I had a tumor in my lower left lobe. When I told my girlfriend my diagnosis, her response to me was simply, "We're getting married." Today we have been married for 2 years and live happily in the Bay Area.*

1.

BE YOUR YOUR OWN ADVOCATE: "If you aren't able to do it yourself have a strong network of friends and family to advocate for you. I thought all the doctors I spoke with just knew what was best. I didn't know I had to ask questions and push for results. You can and should take an active role in your treatment so don't be afraid to speak up."

2.

STAY BUSY: "I had to keep occupied through the long days at home while going through chemo. Find the activities that work for you because it can become overwhelming to just sit and ruminate on your own existence ad nauseum. If you have the energy for it try to go for walks as well. It seems like a lot when you're exhausted but being out in nature and sunshine helps keeps you in a positive frame of mind."

3.

KNOW YOUR LIMITS: "Give yourself time to talk with friends and family but know your limit. It's ok to tell a loved one you just can't talk right now. I realized this one day when I had 6 long conversations in a row essentially discussing my diagnosis. By the end of it I was mentally and emotionally drained. Your people will be there for you but know when you need to take care of you first."

"Stay **present,** enjoy the *small* stuff."

4.

ASK FOR HELP: "I can't stress this enough. I am a thoroughly independent person and don't ever want to feel like a bother. I did find that even though I'm stubborn and want to do everything myself it was so much nicer when I had a friend come to chemo with me or just sit and spend the afternoon with me. It's far too lonely to face this alone even if you've convinced yourself you're tough as nails and independent. Swallow some ego and pride and lean on those that want to help you."

5.

CULTIVATE YOUR TRIBE: "Have a toxic relationship in your life? No time like right now to dump it. It may seem selfish at first but you need to take care of you right now and we all have people in our lives who are, how can I put this gently, emotional vampires. Cultivate your tribe of strong, loving people."

6.

YOU WILL GET THROUGH THIS: "I know, it seems like too much. In the darkest times it's hard to see the future. Stay strong and know that you'll get your quality of life back. Don't lose the perspective you gain from this experience. I found that after my long recovery I did have a greater appreciation for my daily life. Stay present, enjoy the small stuff." ■

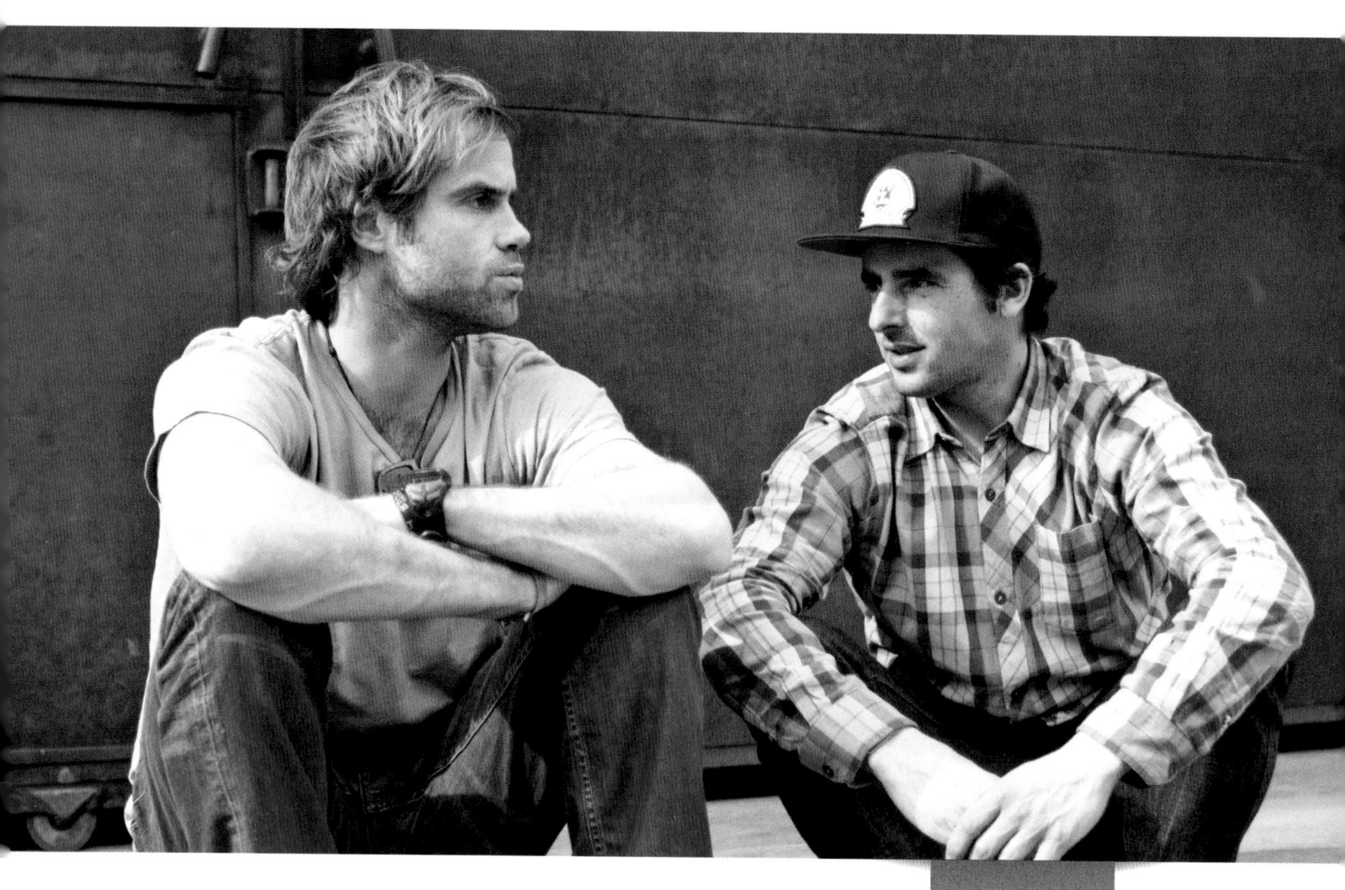

Carlos Ferrer

testicular cancer

PATIENT

AGE: *38*

OCCUPATION: *Aquatic sports photographer and commercial director of a production company*

DIAGNOSIS: *Testicular cancer*

WHEN: *1999*

CONTEXT: *When he was 20 years old, he received his diagnosis which seemed to rule out any possibility of fathering children. Thanks to good decision-making during the development of the disease, in spite of having had both his testicles removed, today he is the father, together with Javiera -his girlfriend of the time- of twins Angel and Amelia.*

1.

FREEZE YOUR SPERM!: "I decided to freeze my sperm, because with only one testicle you produce less sperm and the chemotherapy could damage the entire reproductive system."

2.

THE PROCESS IS PERSONAL, THE EXPERIENCE IS COLLECTIVE: "I definitely changed as a person, I became much more sensitive to certain things that I did not pay attention to before, I changed my attitude and I went from being a spoiled brat, who would fight with others, to being a guy who values life much more than money. The cancer not only affected my family and I, but also my group of friends. I feel like we all changed and I learned to recognize who my true friends were."

3.

NO PLACE FOR SHAME: "I always told my partners that I had had a testicular tumor, I was never ashamed. It was fun to talk about the plastic. I no longer produce sperm, because I don't have testicles. Instead I have prostheses. I want to highlight this, because many men are afraid of getting a prosthesis and it is important to do so, especially at the age when I went through that. It is as if you had silicone implanted, but in the form of a testicle. It is slightly harder than the natural one, but it's fine."

4.

FAMILY SUPPORT, ESSENTIAL: "When I was undergoing chemo at the private hospital I requested a special room at the end of the hall so that my friends could visit me at night and not bother the other patients while we were drinking beer and having a good time. There was a great atmosphere, they visited me every day."

"If I make a ***balance*** of all that I went through, the result is *good,* even with all the pain, suffering and uncertainty."

5.

THERE IS SPACE TO LAUGH (AND ENJOY): "When I had to give the sperm samples at the hospital, I went with Javiera, who was my girlfriend, and she dressed up as a nurse. We did not even need the porn movies that were available in the room. On top of that, every two seconds somebody was yelling: *"Are you ready with the sample?"* It was very funny. Having said that, my parents had no idea that I went with Javiera..." ■

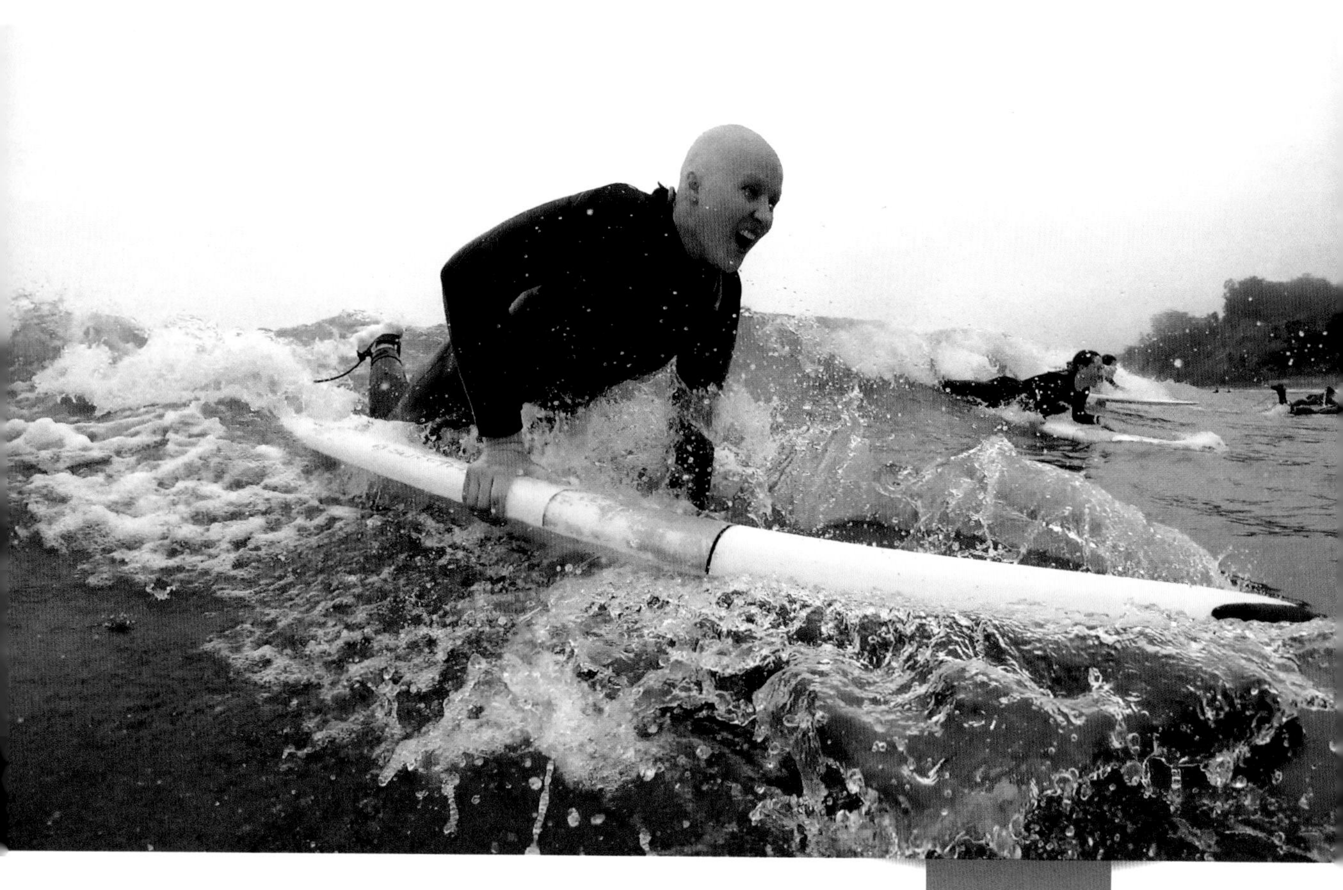

Geena Heaton

Ewing sarcoma
PATIENT

AGE: *25*
OCCUPATION: *Post Graduate*
DIAGNOSIS: *Ewing Sarcoma/Primitive neuroectodermal tumor*
WHEN: *2015*
CONTEXT: *I was diagnosed at 24 years old just entering the "real" world. I had just graduated college and was on my way to becoming a California Highway Patrol officer, when my life slammed on the brakes. I was diagnosed with a primitive neuroectodermal tumor, Ewings Sarcoma. An 8lb tumor on my rib cage. During my follow up appointment, I was told that I would be starting an aggressive chemotherapy plan. I spent the next year in the hospital, being blasted with chemotherapy. I am now cancer free and see cancer as a gift. It's allowed me to see life in a way that people dream of!*

1.

TREAT THE HOSPITAL AS A BUSINESS: "Your doctors are your managers, your nurses are your management team. You are the boss, you don't know everything but use your employees to benefit you. Your employees will help you. You are your best advocate. You need to speak up."

2.

TREAT YOUR BODY AS YOUR TEMPLE: "Feed yourself healthy fuel. But, who am I kidding I had ice cream every night!"

3.

MIND OVER Matter

4.

DO THE THINGS YOU ALWAYS DREAMED OF!: *"The time is now."*

"Treat your body as your **temple,** feed yourself healthy fuel."

5.

TIPS FOR A FRIEND: "This comes naturally! Cancer weeds out the people who aren't necessary in your life. The true friends will know how to support you naturally, or sometimes awkwardly."

6.

DO SOMETHING DAILY that gives you that feel good feeling. ■

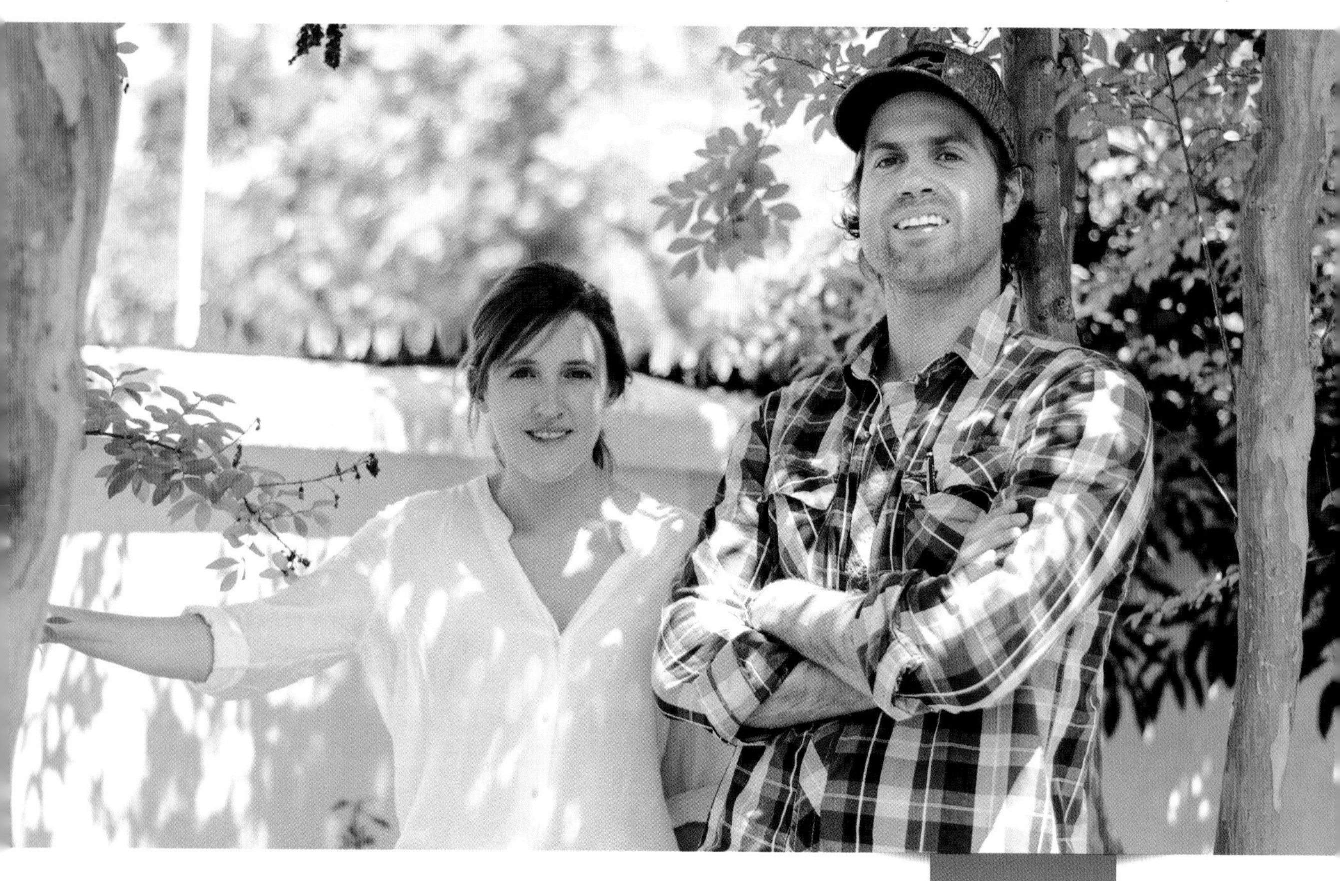

Carmen Hodgson

Ewing sarcoma

PATIENT

AGE: *29*

OCCUPATION: *Publicist*

DIAGNOSIS: *Ewing sarcoma*

WHEN: *2001*

CONTEXT: *When her cancer was discovered, Carmen was a freshman in high school. Today she works as a publicist and speaks with ease about the rough experience that she had as a teenager.*

1.

IT IS DIFFERENT TO GET TREATMENT IN CHILE: "My doctor consulted with other doctors and used the same treatments as a hospital in Houston, USA, and recommended I have the treatment in Chile. That was very important, because if I had left the country, I would have been on my own. Or perhaps with my mother, but without my siblings. I have no idea what would have happened, but having your family nearby is much better for recovery. When I had surgery, my entire school was outside the building, as well as my cousins, grandparents... I have never in my life felt so supported."

2.

THE IMPORTANCE OF FEELING LOVED: "Sometimes it was not good when people visited unannounced, because I was tired, but I only had those thoughts when the person first arrived. During the first two minutes of the conversation, they took me out of the world that I was living in. Everybody understood that before I did, which is why my family was with me every day and my school friends took turns so that I would never be alone. It was good to welcome them all."

3.

BEATING THE PAIN IS BEATING DEATH: "My doctor was incredibly good to me. I could ask him anything and he would answer: *"You are the one who's ill, I am going to tell you everything."* I never asked if I was going to die, because I knew that that would not happen. Perhaps I was too young to fully understand everything, but at the beginning I was certain that I was not going to die. I had plans for when I got out of the hospital. Afterwards, when I began feeling the terrible effects of the drugs, when I vomited up everything, then I thought I was going to die. Then I understood that I had two options: you give into death or you beat the pain and think that you only have two days left of chemo and after that you are going to feel better."

4.

THE FUTURE'S PROMISE: "The treatment consumes your life, and it excludes you from everyday life. Since I could not attend school, two teachers would give me homework, but I was not in the mood, nor did I have the strength to really study. Then, when you do not have the strength in that moment, you need to cling to the future and that's what I did: I clung to the future's promise, to what would happen when all of this was over."

5.

NO FORMAL PSYCHOLOGIST: "I never had a psychologist, my family was my psychologist. They took me to one once, because all the doctors recommended it for support, but, as a task, he asked me to write out my entire life and I said no."

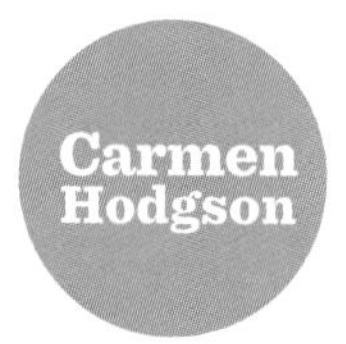

6.

GOD AND ANGER MANAGEMENT: "Never in my life had I been so close to God. It was the only thought that gave me peace, in spite of the occasional rage that I felt when I asked myself *why me, when I am not a bad person*. But then I thought about the fact that it could have been one of my siblings or my parents, and I preferred a million times that it was me."

7.

SEEING GOOD IN THE BAD: "There are people that have cancer and fall into despair. Looking back, I think that if I had fallen into despair I would have turned into a bitter person and I wouldn't have experienced everything I experienced , nor would I have learned everything that I learned, and my family would have not become so united. Why make worse what is already bad? Why not just enjoy the good moments in a bad situation? Just because you are at the hospital doesn't mean you are going to have a bad time if a cousin or a friend comes to visit you. Why would you not enjoy at least that?"

8.

THE BIG LESSON: "You begin to appreciate life, to think twice and to act with more conscientiousness. You see another side of things. You no longer live worrying about petty things that are not worth it, you understand that it is up to you how your life turns out. One way or another, cancer makes you a better person.

9.

IN RETROSPECT: "It was worth going through cancer. I do not regret it, nor would I change my story, because it opened my eyes. To me it is not traumatic to talk about my disease. It allowed me to meet people that I would have otherwise not met, it gave me wisdom and it showed me the people who are truly close to me. It is the ultimate test."

"Then I understood that I had two options: you give into death or you beat the pain and ***think*** that after that you are going **to feel better."**

10.

WHAT CANCER LEAVES BEHIND: *"In time the pain is forgotten, but the experience remains. I don't know what to say when I am asked what I felt, I only remember vomiting and not eating much. I know I was injected a lot and I know it hurt, but I don't know how much. I cannot relive that pain, I no longer feel it."*

11.

WORDS TO ANOTHER TEENAGER: "I would say to a 15-year-old girl who has cancer that it is difficult, but it is possible. Why tell them the bad things, when they are going to go through it anyway? I would also give them this to think about: the mistake is thinking exclusively about the disease. It is just like when people, who only think about work, are fired and then have nothing, this is the same: the important thing is to have something else. I would tell them not to forget that."

"You no longer live worrying about ***petty things*** that are not worth it, you understand that it is up to you how your life turns out."

12.

TOMATOES WITH ONIONS!: "Something happened to me with tomato with onions, and I am not sure why, but every time that I was released from the hospital, I would ask my mother to have ready tomato with onions. I cannot explain it, but the simple things begin to have new value."■

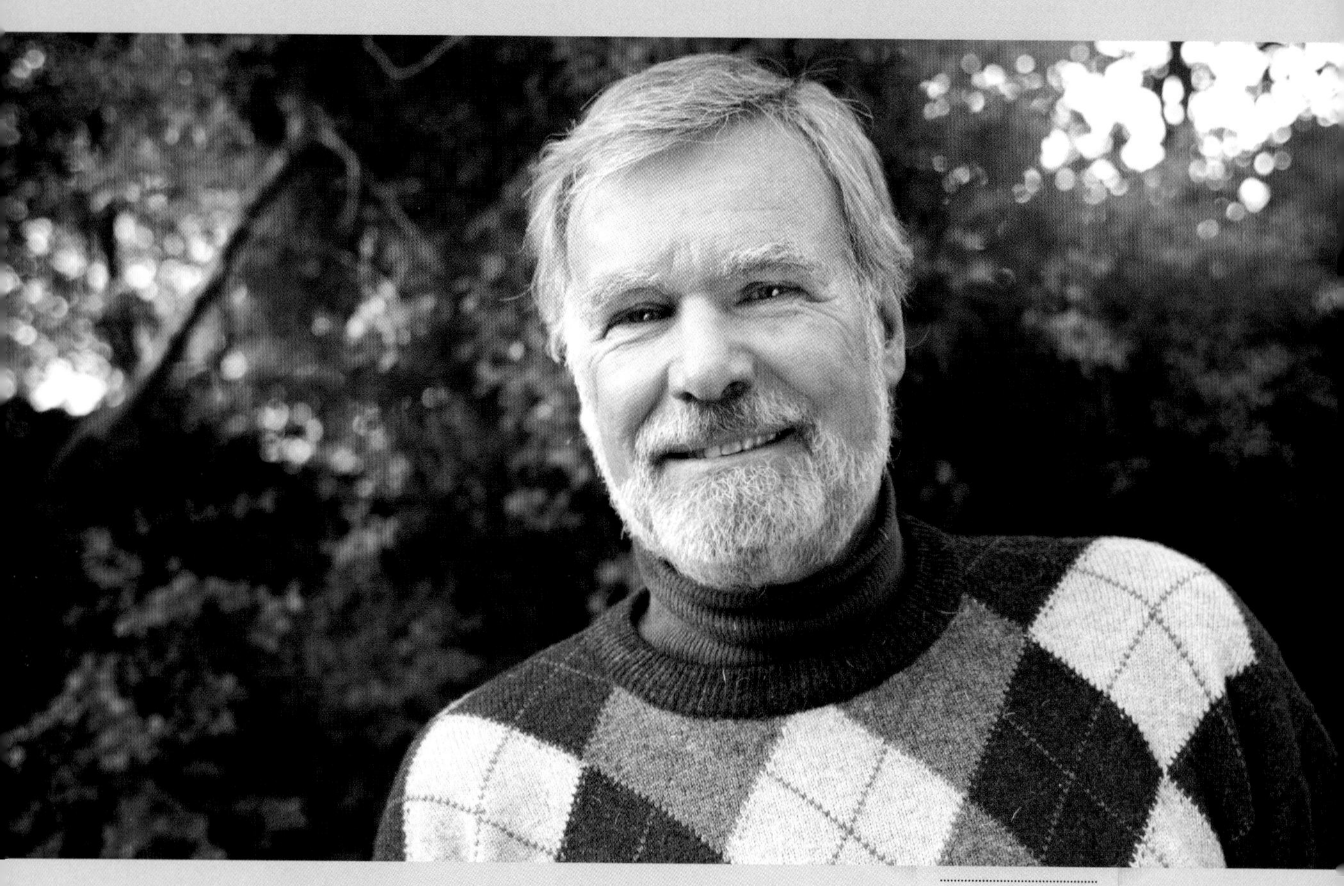

Rainer Schaale

prostatic cancer

PATIENT

THERAPIST

AGE: *65*

OCCUPATION: *Gynecologist and holistic therapist*

DIAGNOSIS: *Stomach & prostate cancer*

WHEN: *2004*

CONTEXT: *Almost 10 years ago he was, almost simultaneously, diagnosed with gastric cancer and prostate cancer. An unlikely coincidence given their different origins and lack of relationship, except for their hereditary factors: his father and sister had already been diagnosed with the disease. After that he spent his time trying to discover the roots of his cancer, he recovered and today he is a holistic therapist. In his practice he helps patients with an early cancer diagnosis recover and improves the quality of life of patients with advanced cancers through homeopathy and acupuncture without needles.*

1.

EXPLORE ROOT CAUSES: "Today it is known that over 70 or 80 percent of diseases have psychosomatic origins, psychic origins that favor or produce diseases."

3.

WHAT SCIENCE CANNOT PROVE: "If one of our parents had cancer at an early age, as happened in my case, it can unconsciously make the children develop a fear of getting cancer."

4.

HOLISTIC THERAPY: "Roger Callahan designed his therapy based on psychosomatics, but the teacher who trained me added genetic information, other people's life experiences and the treatment of non-psychic causes (toxins, deficiencies, neurobiological). He called it Thought Field Therapy, because it deals with everything. I use this therapy to help my patients today."

2.

COMPLEMENTING THERAPY AND SURGERY: "My prostate cancer improved for 10 years using the Thought Field Holistic Therapy. Then the antigens rose again, and a new biopsy revealed that the cancer was still there, but reduced. The urologist told me that I had gained those 10 years using that therapy. In any case, I decided to have surgery to be on the safe side, and the result was very positive."

"Rage, guilt, shame, fear and rejection are ***emotions*** that favor the cancer."

5.

HOLISTIC THERAPY AND ITS EFFECTIVNESS: "Undoubtedly the therapy extends and improves quality of life by removing negative energy generated by the cancer. It creates greater physical wellness and it prolongs survival.

6.

UNEXPRESSED EMOTIONS: "Rage, guilt, shame, fear and rejection are emotions that favor the cancer. Holistic therapy removes the roots of these emotions." ■

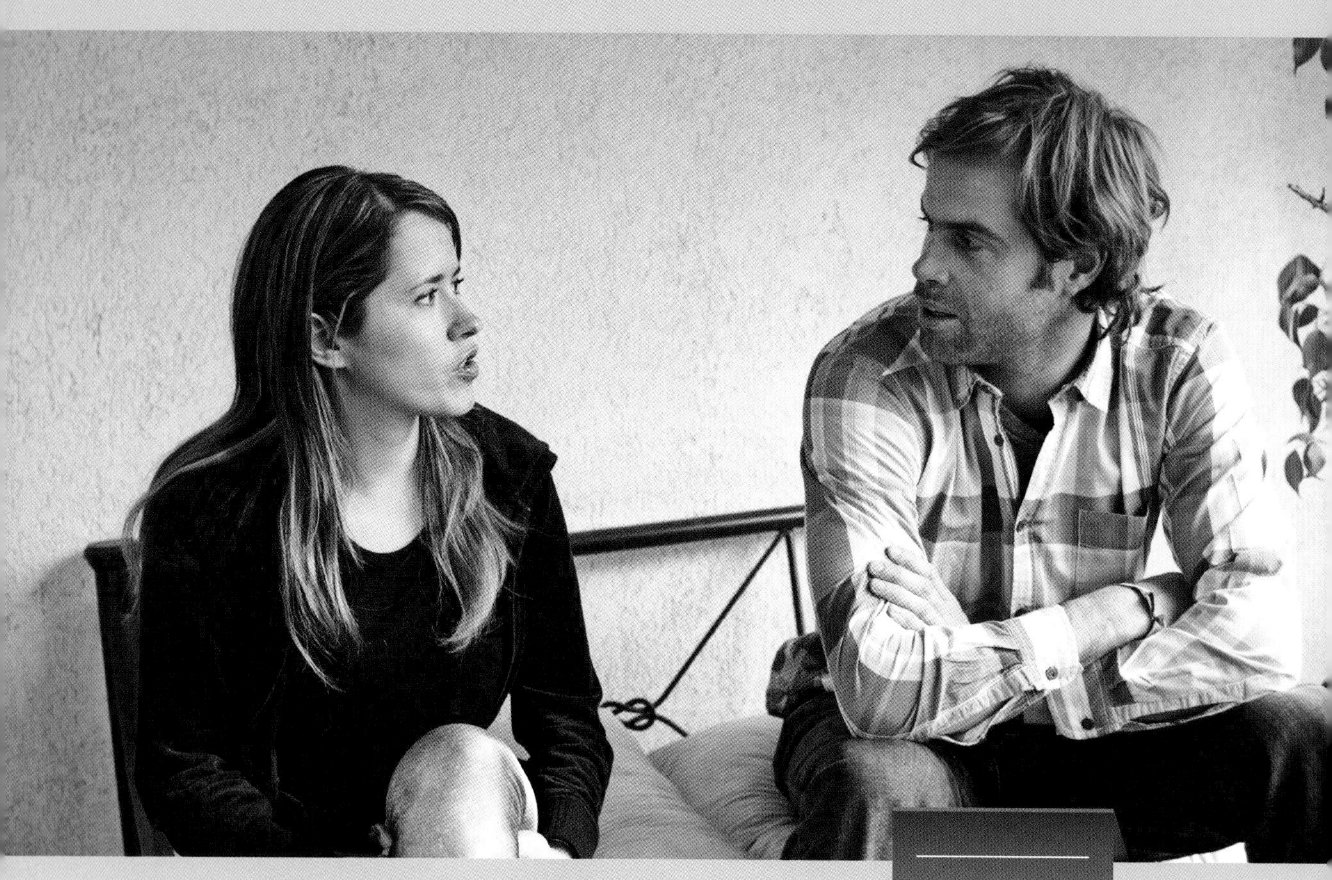

Constanza Larraín

Daughter of prostatic cancer patient

AGE: *31*

OCCUPATION: *Actress and singer*

RELATIONSHIP: *Daughter of patient with prostate cancer*

WHEN: *2011*

CONTEXT: *Fernando, the renowned Mago Larrain, famous on TV, is the father of seven children, Constanza being the youngest. Life circumstances made her decide to keep close company with her father in the last years of his prostate cancer.*

1.

THE WORDS THAT CAME: "The Larrain family shows love in very unconventional ways, mostly in the form of jokes. For example, I had never said to my father 'I love you' until the week when he was at the hospital, when I said it to him for the first time. Ever since I have said it to him every day, because we are not the family to say that every day."

2.

SHAMAN AND THE APRICOT STONE: "In the beginning, my father was very skeptical about non-clinical medicine, but later on he began trusting alternative therapies such as imams, reiki, iridology, the scorpion's venom ordered from Cuba, however, his attending physician was not very open to these ideas. He also tried apricot stones, which have vitamin B17 and are said to be very helpful. I remember writing on Facebook: *'I need apricot stones'* and I received tons of bags full of them."

"His disease made me **think** that he had a lot that went *unexpressed...*"

3.

PERSONAL OPINION: "The invasive interventions that he underwent –radiotherapy, strong drugs, morphine– began to wear my dad out. There were drugs that would make him wake up very drowsy all of a sudden, he said he saw aliens... When he lost his mobility –he could no longer walk on his own– he declined. I kept him company as much as I could and distracted him by showing him the funny side of everything. My father managed to keep his sense of humor until the very end."

Constanza Larraín

4.

DIFFERED TRUTH: "We always told him the truth, but if one morning he found out from some newspaper that an acquaintance had died, and in the afternoon we received news about his antigens going up we would choose to tell him about it later."

5.

THE REQUESTED FUNERAL: "On the day of the funeral it rained, so the church was overflowing with people and umbrellas. There were many people. But at the cemetery, things were more intimate. I hired a group that played balkan music, like from the Emir Kusturica movie, but it was a mess because of the rain. We had to rent the tent from some florist, so that the instruments would not get wet and the musicians were walking as people carried the tent over their heads. It was just like he requested: nothing depressing. I could not cry, because I was excited and truly felt like he was resting, certainly more than the rest of us were."

6.

THE EMOTIONAL THEORY: "I had never seen my father cry, and in the end, all of a sudden, he would become very sad. His disease made me think that he had a lot that went unexpressed... He was always very quiet about some things and I think he was aware of that. He joked about it, but not transcending his mother's or father's way of doing things was a heavy load for him to carry, they were cold and were never loving. They never told him 'We love you'. I actually think that that increased the chances of his life ending because of cancer."

"I distracted him showing the *fun* side of things. My father maintained his sense of **humor** until the end."

7.

POSTHUMOUS TALKS: "The last time I went to the cemetery, I think was on the one- month anniversary of his death. I like the cemetery in a very morbid way, I don't know why, but it has a very special energy. But now I prefer to speak with my dad "internally". I don't need to go there to do it, but of course there are people who enjoy that and it's alright."

8.

LAST WISHES: "He not only left me *El gran Libro de la Magia del Mago Larraín,* but he also asked me to practice everything that he had taught me over the years. Because, since I was a little girl, my dad would come to me to ask if the trick would work or not. He would teach me the tricks and made me promise that I wouldn't tell anybody how they were done, but I would not practice. Now I have begun to, because it was one of his last wishes."

9.

PROMISES ARE TO BE KEPT: "I knew that the first Christmas after his death was going to be hard. My dad and I went to the Calvo Mackenna Hospital, because he had been asked to perform for the children with cancer. I went with him and my dad was super excited to be surrounded by little children, with no hair, who were connected to tanks. He was so amazed by the energy springing from the children's happiness that he requested that I do the same thing every year. I said yes right away, feeling a tightness in my throat, because he also had cancer. Next year we could not go, because he was not doing very well. Then he died, but for the first Christmas without him, I decided to fulfill our promise on my own." ■

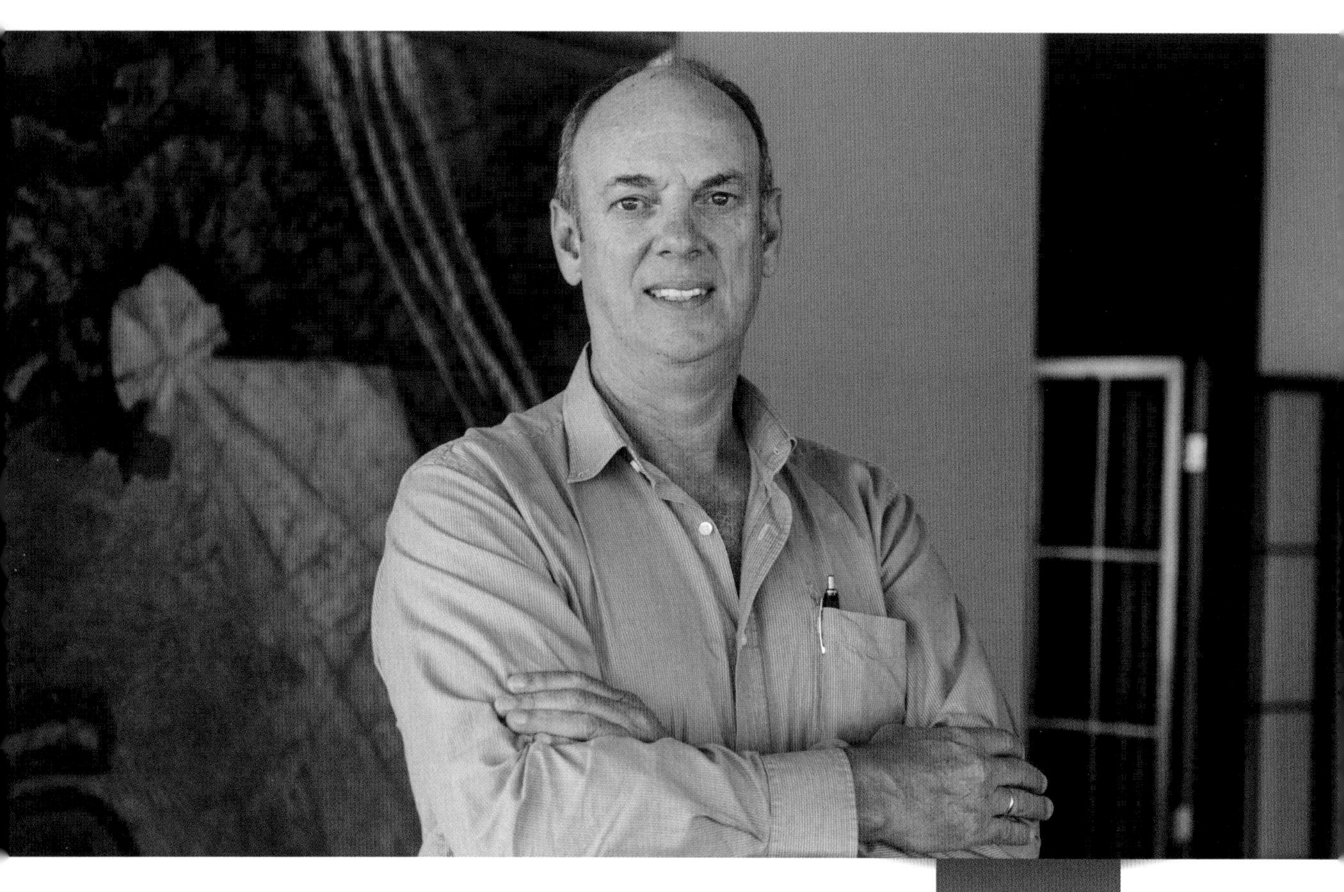

Juan Antonio Dibos

prostate cancer

PATIENT

AGE: *55*

OCCUPATION: *Race car driver and sports manager*

DIAGNOSIS: *Prostate cancer*

WHEN: *2011*

CONTEXT: *Once a year, Peruvian race car driver Juan Antonio Dibos subjects himself to routine medical tests as a requirement to obtain his sports license for competitive car racing. In June of 2011, a sign for a urological test 'magically' caught his eye, and at the last minute, he decided to ask for a check-up. The result? He was diagnosed with prostate cancer that required immediate surgery. Juan Antonio scheduled his surgery for right after his 51st birthday, which he celebrated among family and friends. It was a sort of farewell from him without them learning about the seriousness of the case. Luckily, his cancer is nowadays under control.*

1.

FACE CANCER FEARLESSLY: "You only have one life; you'll die anyway, maybe earlier, maybe later; due to an accident or old age or a disease. So, why fear it? My sister Solange taught me that it is YOU who lives life, not the disease. She was a year younger than I was, and died of cancer 14 years ago, after an intense fight that lasted 18 months. Do not fear the disease, 'cause maybe it'll teach you the meaning of a joyful life."

2.

TRUST YOUR DOC: 'You don't get a good vibe from him/her? Change docs if necessary, until you feel at ease. It is paramount that you understand whatever he/she explains to you, and for you to act on that. You don't have to disregard your own research. The Web has tons of information. What's important is to look for reliable and documented sources and sites. And remember that trust is a 2-way street: the doctor you end up trusting will know how to best lead your treatment in terms of your mood and in terms of its course."

"Do not **fear** the disease, 'cause maybe it'll teach you the meaning of a *joyful life.*"

3.

DO NOT GIVE UP ON YOUR PROJECTS BECAUSE OF YOUR ILLNESS: 'I didn't know if I'd get rid of the cancer. But why make it a victor from the very beginning? My cancer was diagnosed in June of 2011, and in May I had signed up for the Dakar, which was being organized in Peru for the first time. After my surgery in August, I continued to visit potential sponsors... And I got financial sponsorship from my oncological insurer! A month later I gradually resumed physical exercise to face the challenge that the Dakar Rally is."

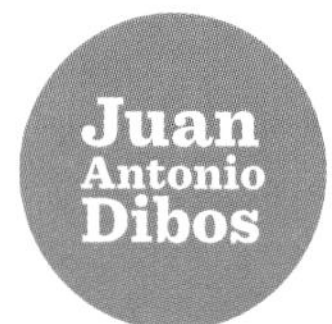

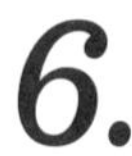

MAKE YOUR FAMILY FEEL CONFIDENT: I never showed an ounce of fear in front of my 3 daughters, my wife, my mother, and my 10 siblings. On the contrary, I comforted them saying everything would be fine. Maybe I did worry about abandoning them early, so to speak, but not fear. Not even when I had a relapse 14 months after the surgery. If they see you well, they will in turn convey to you a higher degree of confidence, of certainty, and everything else you need to overcome this. It's not about denial in the face of the disease, it's just a way of looking at it with faith."

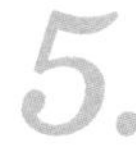

LAUGHTER IS THE BEST MEDICINE: 'Appointments with the doctor had their serious moments, but also their funny ones, even amid the tensest of situations. Before my treatment, the doc explained to me I'd be given radiotherapy, and that they'd give me oncological and hormonal pills. Four months later, my nipples felt hot and itchy. I'd also gained weight, so I didn't realize I'd grown breasts! Hahahah! I couldn't believe it! But, at the same time, I couldn't help but joke about it with everyone around. I even booked an appointment with my wife's and daughters' OBGYN. 'Doc', I asked, 'this will flatten out once I go off the pills, right?' The answer, amid laughter, was 'no...so start looking for a plastic surgeon.' I still have them, 'cause I'm definitely not going through a NipTuck! Hahhahahah!'

6.

THE RELEVANCE OF AN ONCOLOGICAL INSURANCE: 'I used to have a medical insurance with full coverage. The kind that cost an eye and a leg. One day things weren't going well, from a financial standpoint, so I drastically cut down my expenses, including that insurance. We only had the school/university insurance for my daughters, plus another one from a local private hospital, for emergency matters. One day I told myself: 'I have to save up on something else, because I cannot leave my family without an oncological insurance.' I took out that insurance towards the end of 2010. And I was diagnosed with cancer by mid- 2011. Was I lucky? Yes, very much so. So go out there and get oncological insurance right now!'

7.

CONVEY TO OTHERS WHAT YOU LEARN: 'You'll learn more and more about your cancer with every day. I learned several things about prostate cancer. The main thing: go get your physicals when you should. Don't you dare talk to me about the rectal exam not being for manly men. I get furious just thinking that there were men that left this world leaving their family behind, unprotected, just because they were scared of having a doctor placing a finger up their butt! To find out what's going on with your prostate, the doctor needs that rectal exam, the ultrasound, and the PSA (prostatic specific antigen, which you get from a blood test). Only through those 3 elements can you be forwarded to the biopsy that determines the progress status of the cancer and the treatment to be followed."

8.

THE JOB AND DAILY LIFE AFTER CANCER: *'I now don't only think about a job that gets me enough money. I also think about my life/job. I look for jobs associated to my passion, car racing, and although in Peru that's not something from which to make a comfortable living, well... here I am, opening up new roads so that making a living off it can be just like anywhere else in the world. I don't compete anymore (though I don't lose hope of that changing at some point), and I'm now more involved in the managing part of the business. What do my wife and children think? I have their 100% support, even if I sometimes don't see then for 20 days in a row. For the moment, all I ask is for God to give me enough life to walk my girls down the aisle.'* ■

"I didn't ***know*** if I'd get rid of the cancer. But why *make* it a victor from the very **beginning?"**

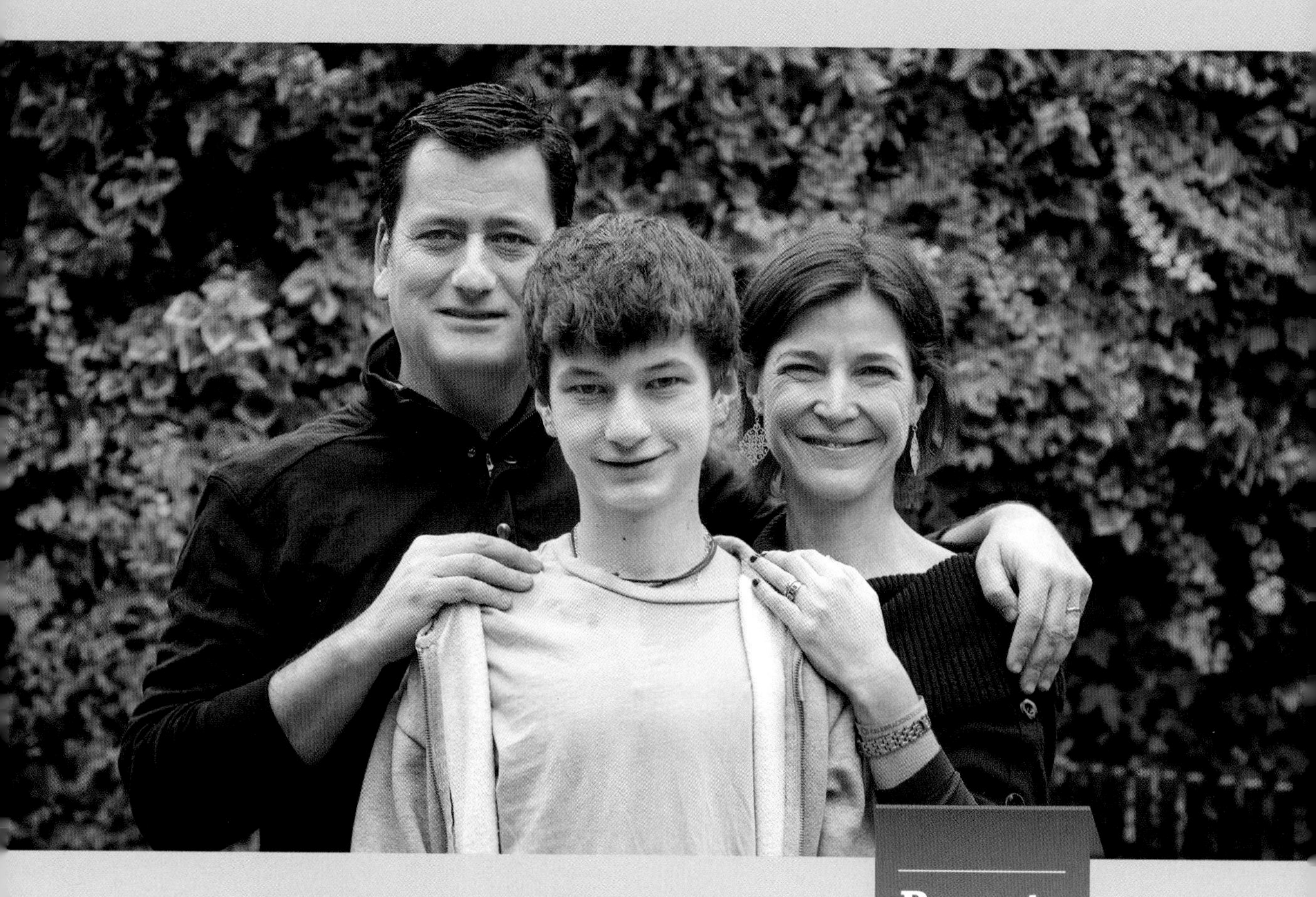

Pablo Allard
& Alejandra Méndez

PABLO'S PARENTS

Parents *of* **clear-cell sarcoma patient**

AGE: *44 & 46, respectively*

OCCUPATION: *Architect and teacher*

RELATIONSHIP: *Parents of clear-cell sarcoma patient*

WHEN: *2002*

CONTEXT: *When he was two and his family lived in the United States, Pablo Allard's oldest son was diagnosed with clear-cell sarcoma, a rare and aggressive tumor that formed in his kidneys and medulla. In 2004, the tumor metastasized to his brain and in 2006 it reached his thyroid gland, both were treated with chemo, radiation, a bone marrow transplant and surgeries. Today, after a childhood marked by oncologic treatments, Pablo Allard Mendez is 16 years old, has two younger siblings, plays soccer, organizes activities at school and lives a teenager's normal life.*

1.

GETTING BACK TO NORMAL: "We decided to go back to having a normal life and not become that family that overcame cancer and is going around telling everybody what they lived though. We won and that means that we left the realm of cancer. That is why Pablo has a normal life today and we have learned to go on trips without the children, as well as to not be apprehensive and let him go out with his friends. Today he parties, dates, eats anything, and climbs mountains. He is a teenager like everybody else, and we push for everybody to see it that way as well."

2.

TAKE ADVANTAGE OF THE VOLUNTEERS: *"The Ronald McDonald House Charities have a shelter in Boston for families that come from afar, and they gave us a room for Pablo. One day we were in the playroom with him and a woman approached us and asked if we wanted to go out for lunch while she took care of him. That is how the volunteers were. Every thursday afternoon they went to play with the children, so that the parents could rest, be together, even cry. It was a tremendously good surprise. Pablo's grandmother, his mother and I work today as volunteers at Foundation* Nuestros Hijos *(Our Children) in Chile."*

3.

GOING THE EXTRA MILE: "In a certain way our motto was working and not thinking. We focused on saving our son and to do that we had to work and fight every day. Looking back, that strength and conviction were crucial, because at no point did we say let's leave it in God's hands. We were not going to give in to death for a second, nor were we going to let it take away the pleasure of being together and enjoying life. In 18 years of being married, we have never been happier as a couple and family than when we were fighting together."

4.

ENJOYING DAILY LIFE: "For example, seeing our son with his girlfriend are things that we value much more now."

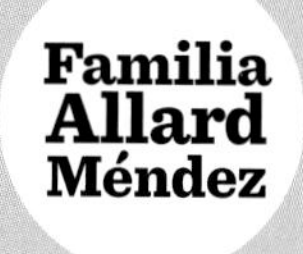

5.

CLOSING A CHAPTER: "Cancer has to be beaten not only by removing it from the body, but also from the head. You could write a book about your experience, publish it, launch it and then close the chapter. One should not stay stuck in the issue, because if it is in your mind, perhaps it is because you haven't beat it yet."

6.

CONTROLLING EMOTIONS: "You should never lie to the person who is ill. Whenever possible we tried to create the most positive environment. Nor did we allow ourselves to break down, express anger or anguish in front of Pablo. We always tried to protect him from resentfulness, because that energy is transmitted and has consequences."

"We were not going to **give** in to death, but it was not going to take away the happiness of being together and *enjoy.*"

7.

INFORMED INTUITION: "Decisions must be made all the time. For example, deciding what type of chemotherapy Pablo should take on and weighing up the associated risks. We had never made such hard choices as the ones then, and we learned how to choose based on some sort of informed intuition. We read a lot, searched the internet, asked the doctors, but finally we would make the decisions on our own."

8.

DO NOT UNDERESTIMATE SMALL GESTURES: "Oh, are they important! We learned that when somebody close goes through a difficult situation and is having a rough time, receiving a message or getting a cup of coffee can be very valuable gestures that make a huge difference.

9.

GET AWAY: "Each cancer is different, in its roots and processes. In our son's case, our latest therapy was getting away from it. Statistically, there is always the chance that the cancer could come back, but we decided to not get stuck on that, and instead decided that everybody should live a normal life. I remember a very concrete moment: Pablo had finished his treatment not too many months ago, we were back in Chile, and I was stuck in traffic, annoyed and complaining about the heat. All of a sudden I realized that I was living the same moment as any other woman in Santiago. Then, I got away, it's over. Back to my life. I stopped pitying myself and I felt like part of the crowd again.

10.

AWAY FROM PESSIMISM: "It is hard to explain, but had we been in Chile, it would have been more complicated to focus without avoiding pessimism. Living far away saved us from constant visitors, the sad and pitying expressions. That social pressure of being around people all the time overwhelms and tires you, and it is contagious."

"Each cancer is *different,* in its reasons and processes. In the case of my son, our therapy was to get **out of there."**

11.

THE AMERICAN DOCTOR: "American doctors are, in my opinion, more reserved than the ones in Chile, who assume you are more ignorant and can make decisions on your behalf. When we were there, sometimes we would ask our doctor what he would do in our shoes, but he refused to give us that answer. They are all like that, because that way they also avoid insurance or lawsuit risks. So they do not compromise for one second. They are very strict and rigorous."

12.

THE POWER OF TESTIMONY: "One day when we were at the foundation, a couple arrived with their son who was then 15 years old. When he was six, he fell ill from cancer and nobody believed that he would recover. From that moment onwards, they came back every year to share their experience of hope with other families in a similar situation. That brief encounter pushed us forward, because even though we were focused, we did not give ourselves the right to imagine Pablo in the future. Hearing that testimony and imagining ourselves coming back one day to the hospital to tell other families that it is indeed possible to move forward was of great help; it gave us hope. On the 10th anniversary of his treatment, we went back with Pablo to Boston Children's Hospital not only to thank the nurses and doctors, but also to give back. We met with other parents who were also fighting, and it was very intense. Giving them a hug was very meaningful." ■

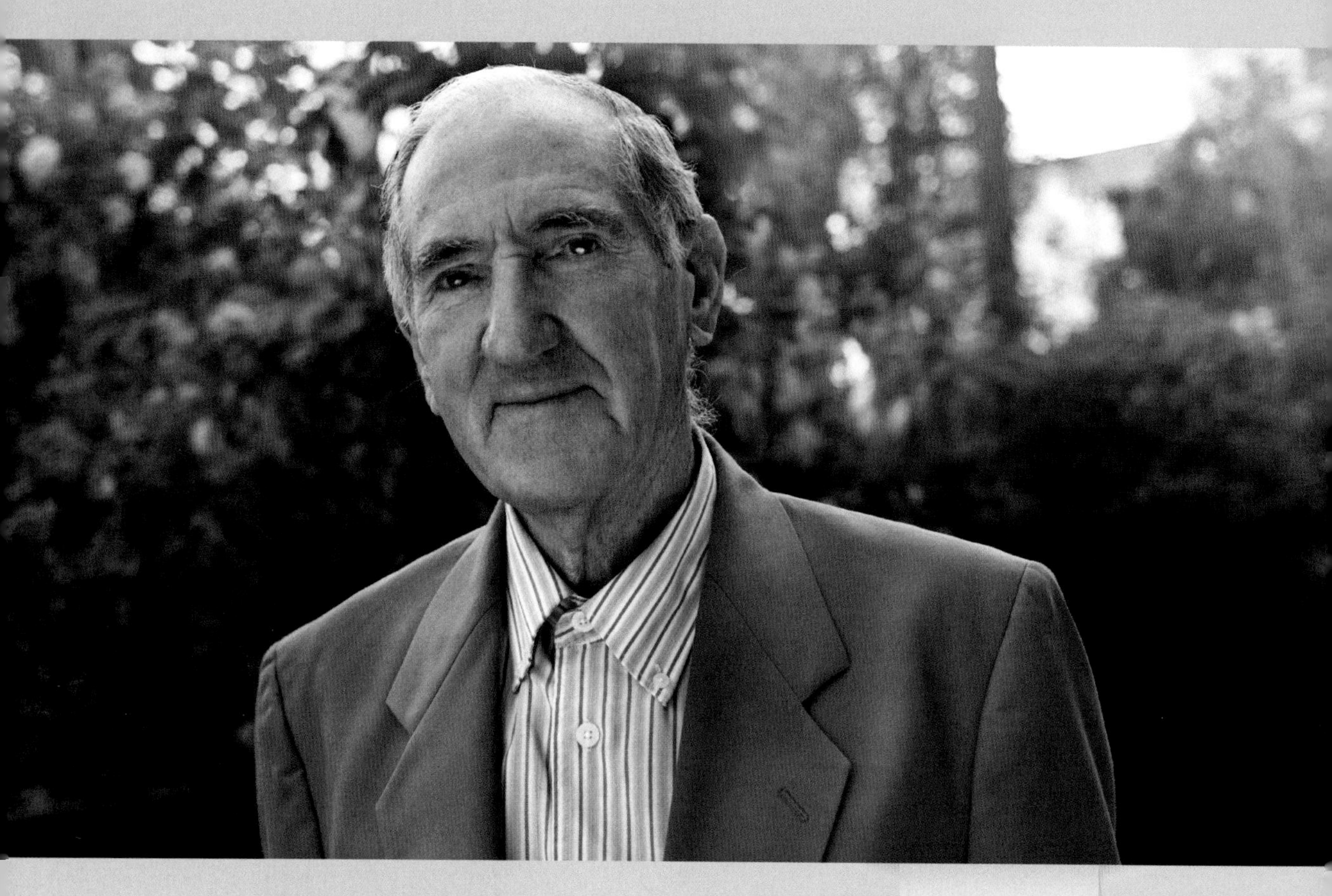

Roberto Williams

Therapist

AGE: *79*

OCCUPATION: *Engineer and herbalist*

CONTEXT: *His father died at 98 and his mother at 92. To Roberto Williams, plants condense all of mankind's knowledge of himself throughout the history of his own evolution. He asserts that the basis for its effects on the organism lies in the sublingual consumption.*

1.

TWO APPLES A DAY: "Natural medicine immensely improves an organism's functioning. Two apples leave the brain very active, because it is the organ that consumes the most sugar. You eat one in the morning and one in the afternoon, thus introducing the biggest amount of pulp in your mouth. It is very healthy."

2.

HOW ALOE VERA ACTS: "This plant has been used for a long time, but it was never known why it healed. In 1988, a wise Japanese man discovered that it contains an active ingredient, vegetal germanium. Specifically, after the aloe has purified your blood, the germanium forces the cancerous cell to breathe the purified oxygen from your blood, which is why this cell tends to recover its benignity."

"**Goosegrass** helps the organism encapsulate tumors. This is why when I am on the street and I see this plant, I caress it, because I know what *it does.*"

3.

ALOE VERA, HONEY AND A GOOD DISTILLED DRINK: "There are around 470 types of Aloe Vera and they are all medicinal. It should be mixed with honey and a good distilled drink, because honey is a food that has the capacity to move through the entire body, except very small tissue, such as cartilages, lungs and testicles. The distilled drink helps dilate and widen the capillary vessels."

4.

LIKE WILD WEEDS FOR TUMORS: "Goosegrass is the popular name given to *Galium aparine*, a plant which is used to increase milk production among first-time mothers, but a German woman wrote a book about how she cured cancer patients with it. This weed helps the organism to encapsulate tumors, which means that no blood vessel continues to supply it with blood, and if it is encapsulated it begins to shrink. It can be ingested as drops or as homeopathic globules. This is why when I am on the street and I see this plant, I caress it, because I know well what it does." ■

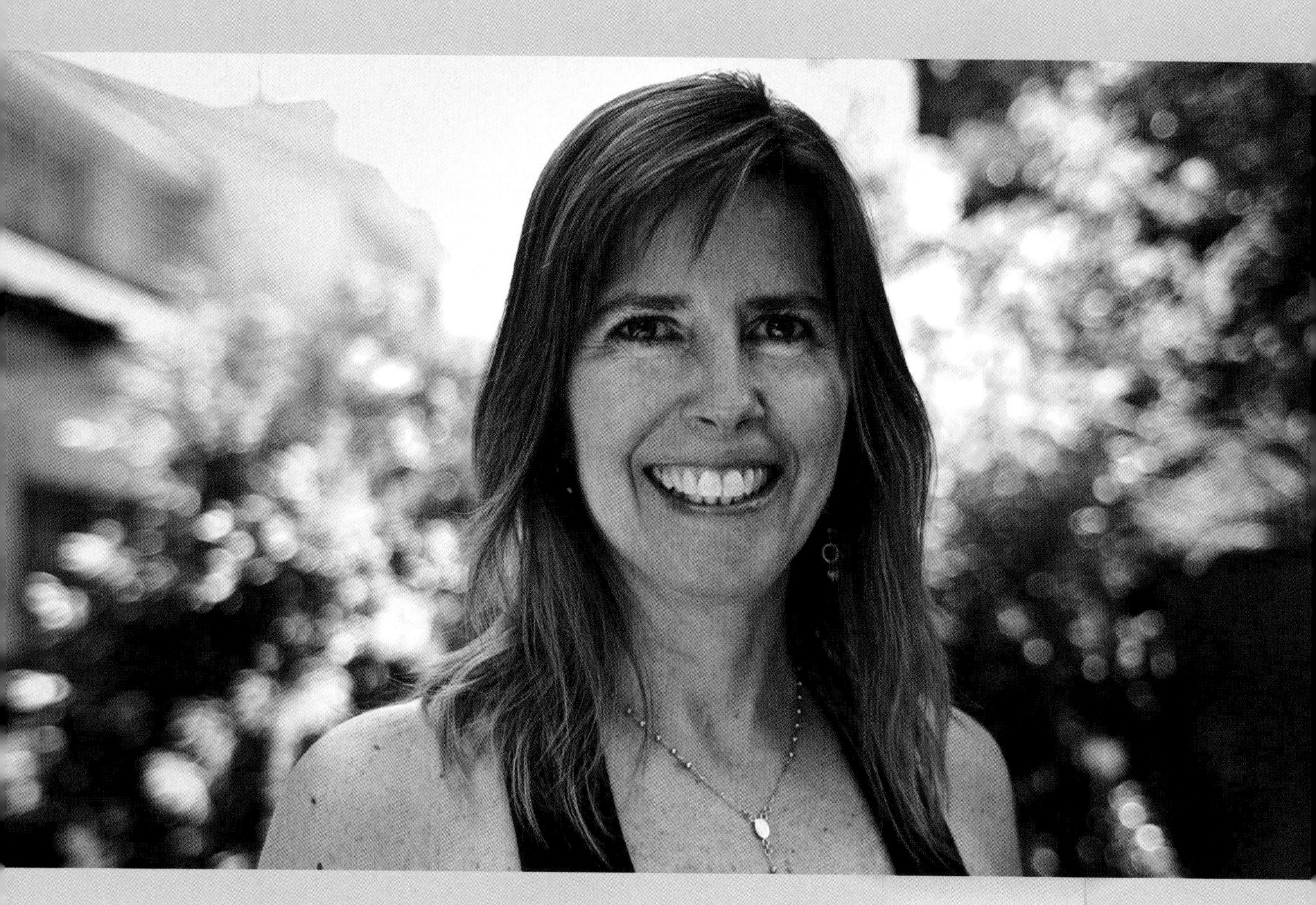

Patricia Eing

Therapist

AGE: *50*

OCCUPATION: *Pilates instructor and technical director of the Laurus center*

CONTEXT: *Her decades of work are based on a movement that helps harmonize the body. When this harmony is cultivated, we balance the organism and can recover from anything from the common cold to an autoimmune disease. To Patricia, disease appears when we forget our body.*

1.

MENTAL, PHYSICAL AND ENERGETIC BODY: "The three are inseparable. My knowledge consists of adapting the body's movement according to what is needed, depending on the pains or aches, activating different chakras and regulating energy. Healing processes are unique and individual, where therapy through movement is a complement that helps the person feel better and put their systems in order."

2.

HOW THE THERAPY WORKS: "When you conduct a physical analysis, you see which muscular imbalances are there; what the joint limitations are; and what the pains and inflammations are. These are normally attached to blockages of energy flow. These blockages prevent the organisms' autoregulation process and we can improve it using the appropriate movement. There are also studies that explain the relationship between posture, breathing patterns and unexpressed emotions. For example, if you are dealing with restricted breathing, you are seeing a person who is going through emotional hardships which cause this patterns. Sometimes simply improving these patterns is enough for a meaningful liberation."

3.

WE ARE WHAT WE EAT: "Diets are directly related to the body's well-being. We often miss this factor. When you carry out an analysis of a person's diet, you can improve the performance of the organs. The liver, for example, has a very important role in the process of detoxification, especially for cancer."

4.

WORKING FROM THE BODY: "Sometimes working from the emotions, like psychologists do, can be painful for the patient. This is why I am not interested in being a psychologist, nor a healer, rather a facilitator for personal processes from my own experience with movement. There are certain organs in the body that are connected with different emotional blocks and I work from that perspective, without interfering with that person's deep feelings. Improving breathing patterns with physical exercises can lead to unblocking deep emotions. Not mentally, because sometimes the mind is our worst enemy."

5.

HOW THE THERAPY PROCEEDS: "You begin with a preliminary evaluation. If it is somebody with a disease, you begin with a conversation to understand what their process and history have been, and that guides me to design the most appropriate exercise guidelines."

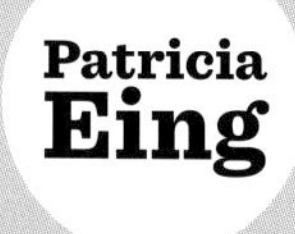

6.

THE BODY WARNS US: "Our body is a mirror of ourselves. Learning to listen to it is the best self-knowledge and disease-preventing tool. People speak of diseases as unexpected, however, many times they occur because one has not been capable of seeing what the body is showing us."

7.

ILLNESS AS A GROWTH OPPORTUNITY: "Very frequently the recovery process from a disease or an accident is very tough, but the learning curve is so steep that you end up being grateful for the experience."

8.

THE AUTOIMMUNE DISEASES BOOM: "Medicine has made many advancements. Diseases from yesterday are very much under control, but the challenge lies in today's autoimmune diseases, which have to do directly with today's stress levels and the world's competitiveness. On top of that, add the sedentary crisis, which does not allow the body to get rid of that load. Our body was made to move around, not sit around. If you help it move again, in a healthy environment, you can find that balance. I say healthy environment, because there are people that *say if he was an athlete, why did he get sick?* Well, perhaps the chosen sport was not appropriate for him. It is important to evaluate what the physical activity's suitable intensity for the person is. This is done according to age, sex and physical traits, among other factors."

9.

LOSING THE FEAR TO FACE ONESELF: *"Finding spaces in silence, leaving the mundane noise aside to connect with oneself and that way lose the fear and to realize that the disease could be self-produced. Diseases are not external. You have to lose the fear to face yourself. I know it is hard, and it is easier said than done."*

"Our body was made to **move** around, not *sit around.*"

10.

MOVEMENT AND CANCER: "For people who are suffering or recovering from cancer the techniques of movement therapy offer the possibility to experience a world of self-knowledge. To do that, the process has to be tackled not from fear, but rather from a desire to learn and understand why the body is ill and what the soul needs. Our body creates what we need, nobody injected us with the disease." ■

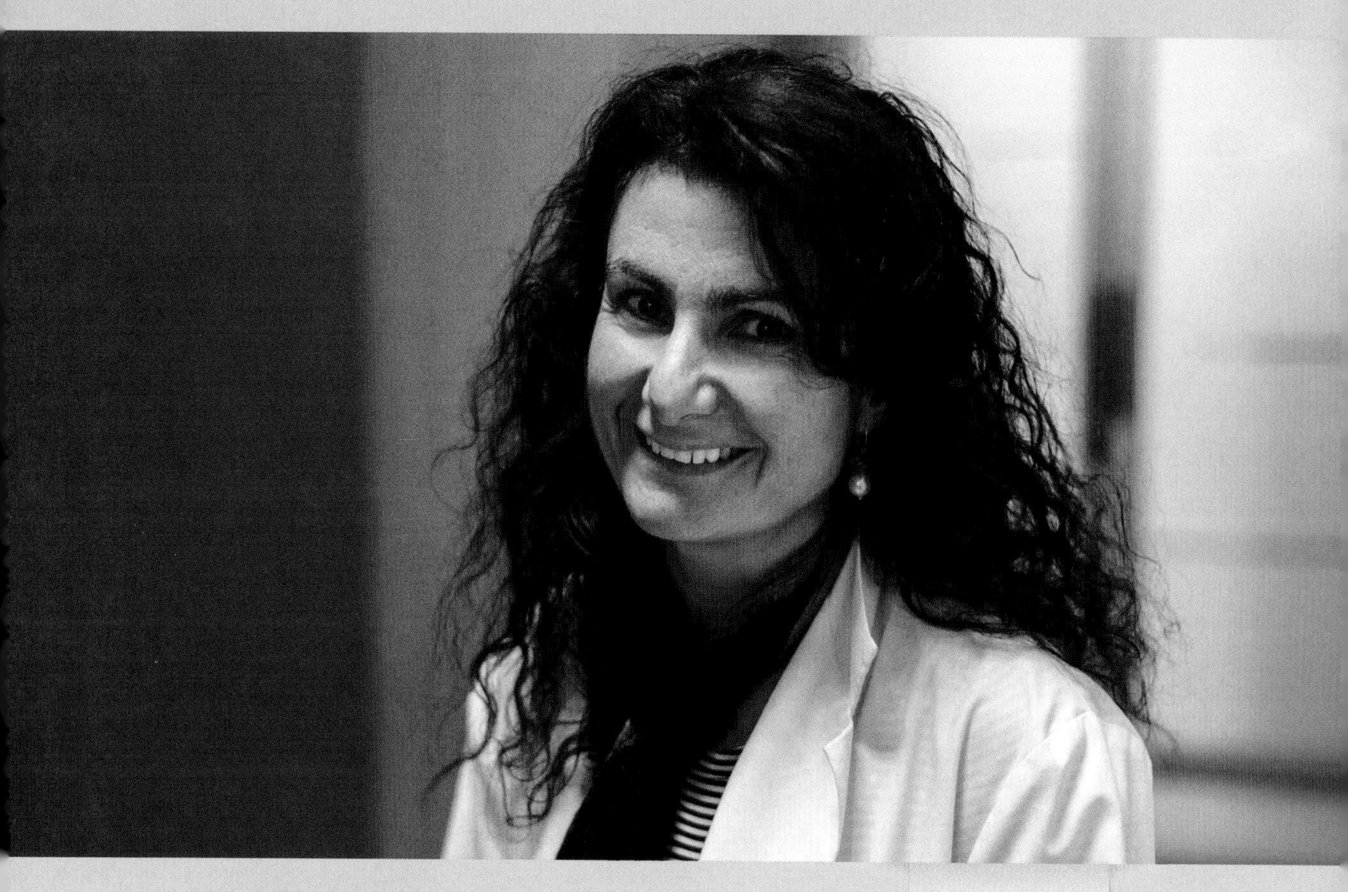

Pamela Salman

Doctor

AGE: *45*

OCCUPATION: *Oncologist*

CONTEXT: *Even though she sees her occupation as tough and consuming, this oncologist from the* Arturo López Pérez *Foundation has also been able to see the gratifying side of her job. Even when there is no cure, it is possible to help the patients and their families have a better quality of life and prepare for death.*

1.

THE DIFFERENCE OF A SPECIALIZED HOSPITAL: "I work at a specialized oncologic hospital which is focused exclusively on treating all types of known cancers. All the specialties are covered, there is hospitalization available for surgeries and we have the most innovative treatments and equipment. The advantage of this type of hospital as opposed to big hospitals is that they are less impersonal and all of the resources and efforts are focused on oncology."

2.

FREE TREATMENTS?: *"The treatments that we offer are free for the people eligible for certain research trials. They are expensive treatments, but these studies allow for some people to obtain them free of charge."*

"In the *Arturo López Pérez* foundation we have *all* the latest drugs that ***exist*** on the market."

3.

***ARTURO LÓPEZ PÉREZ* FOUNDATION:** "Here we have all the latest drugs that exist on the market. At this center we conduct clinical studies, which are research protocols with new drugs that come from abroad. These are different for people with certain types of pathologies."

4.

CUTTING-EDGE TECHNOLOGY: "We were the first institution to offer the PET scan, which is the most effective cancer-detecting method, and we are the only center in Chile that offers intraoperative radiation therapy for mammary tumors. The radiation therapy, instead of being performed for a long time after the surgery, is performed during the surgery. Soon we will have the cutting-edge radiation therapy equipment and we will be the only center in Latin American with it. This has always been the institution's spirit: being a center of high complexity for cancer treatment and clearly this goal has been reached over the years." ■

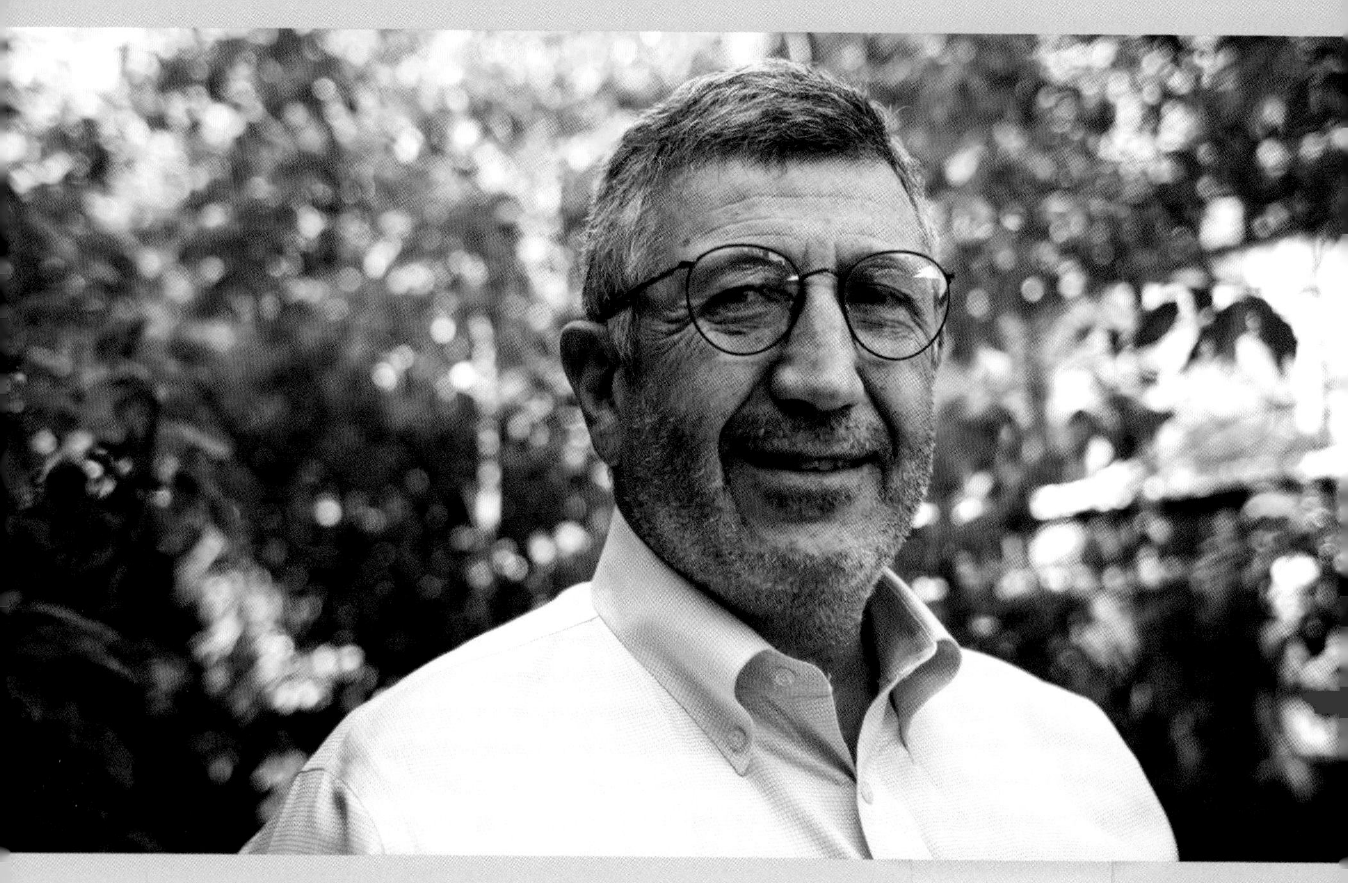

Benjamín Paz

Doctor

AGE: *56*

OCCUPATION: *Oncologist*

CONTEXT: *Roberto Ibáñez had one of the most illuminating conversations with Benjamin Paz about cancer. The doctor, based in LA, USA, spoke with inspiring and wise words. He took the time to listen and support. He was not the attending physician, but his contribution to the recovery process was enormous. Roberto wrote down the most eloquent phrases of the conversation that they had, and here they are.*

1\.

"All life experiences are good life experiences. Good always comes out. From that point of view, there are **no wrong decisions."**

2\.

"Probabilities are in your favor and, only because of probability, they are against the tumor."

3\.

"There are some experiences that make the window you are looking out of shift. Cancer is one of them. **Remember that nobody looks at the world from the same window.** There are as many points of view as there are people in the world."

4\.

"You are going to have cancer days and cancer moments. Take the time you need to think. Also tell your loved ones how you feel, and that will help them to get in tune with you, to understand you and to understand how they have to react in these moments."

"All experiences in **life** are good experiences."

5\.

"Just like Bill Gates' father wrote: **you need to show up for life,** *you cannot just watch."*

6\.

"When a person says *I do not feel well,* the immune system is working on something. It does not matter whether it is psychological or physical, it is working nonetheless. Therefore, **protect your immune system.** This is one of the most important things for me."

7\.

"You must worry about living a good life, live well. You need to be happy in life. I am going to repeat this: **Just live well."**

8\.

"Sleep at least eight hours a day. The body and the immune system regenerates best when you are asleep. Less than eight hours a day is almost as if you had not slept at all."

9\.

"At this very moment you are 100% healthy. You cannot give the tumor any chances. **You have to live a healthy life."**

10\.

"Have a good breakfast and a healthy lunch. These are the most important meals of the day. Remember to stop whatever you are doing and sit at a table. Do not do two things at the same time. As you grow older, you will understand what I am telling you." ■

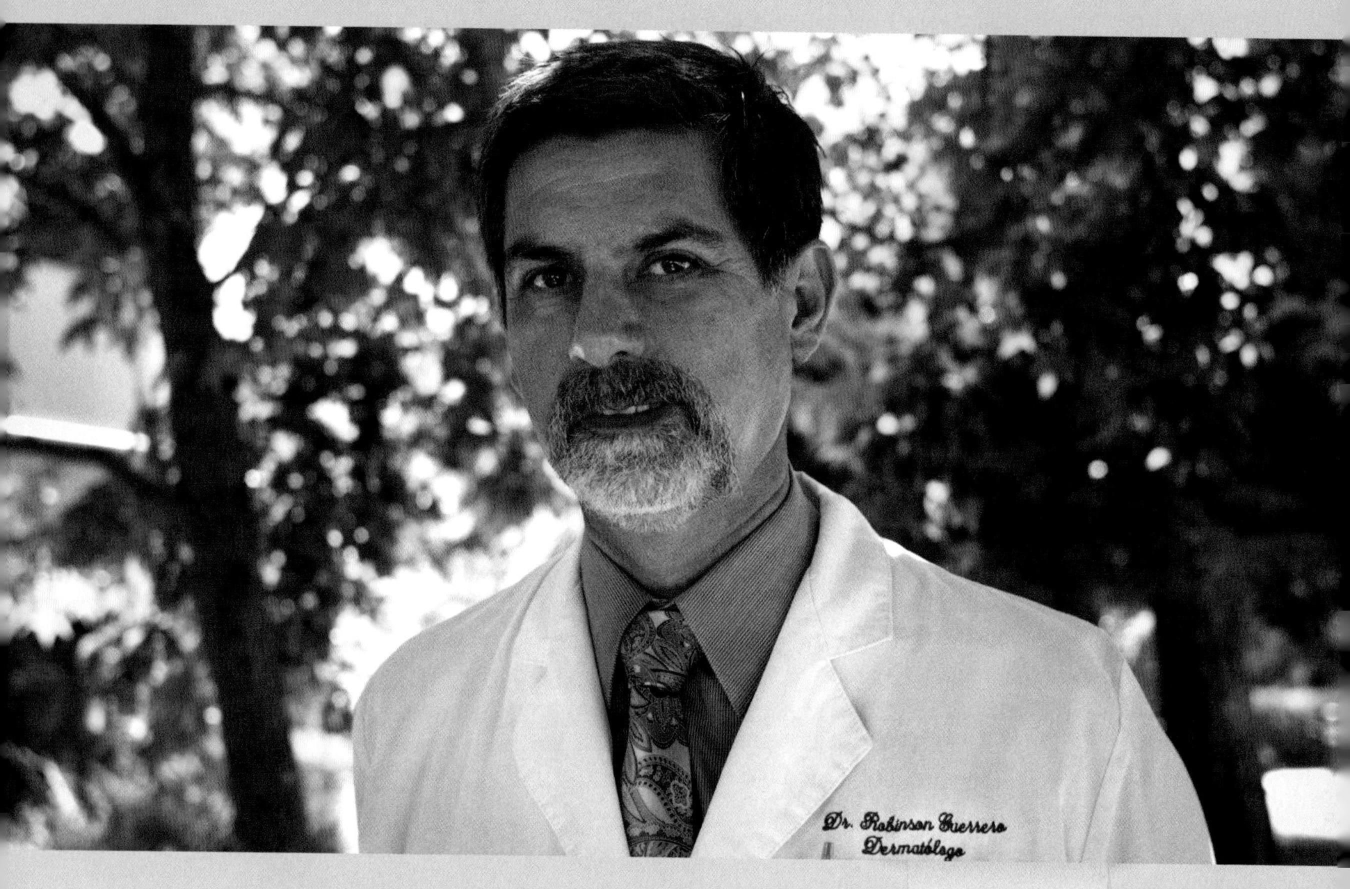

Robinson Guerrero

Doctor

AGE: *59*

OCCUPATION: *Dermatologist*

CONTEXT: *With over 30 years of experience detecting and diagnosing moles, the uninterrupted practice of his profession has allowed him to become a first-class witness to the substantial increase in skin cancer and melanoma. Dr. Guerrero diagnosed the woman who inspired this book, Loreto Agurto's, first melanoma.*

1.

DISTINGUISHING BETWEEN SKIN CANCER AND MELANOMA: "People speak about 'melanoma skin cancer' and 'non-melanoma skin cancer'. The latter originates from skin cells and evolves into relatively benign cases, without metastasis, called basal cell carcinoma, or into more aggressive cases, with metastasis, called squamous cell carcinoma.
The melanoma originates from the pigmented skin cells and it can form from a mole or in situ. It is malignant unless it is detected in an intraepidermal stage. When a mole produces cancer, it is a melanoma. If it is a wound that looks like a wart or a wound that does not scar, it is important to discard skin cancer."

2.

NOT CONVENIENT TO PREVENT HAIR LOSS: "The hair always grows back after a chemotherapy. Yet, there are techniques such as compressing an area during the application of the chemo to prevent it from affecting the scalp and thus limiting the hair loss. But what happens if a cancerous cell is somewhere around the scalp? I prefer to have the chemo effects reach the entire body.

3.

CAREFUL, CASES ARE INCREASING: "I have been a dermatologist for over thirty years, and when I began practicing, I saw a melanoma every five years. Now I see around five melanomas a year. There are people who say that the diagnosis has improved, but between the ozone layer and our survival rates increasing, I hold that, in some way, the genetics have changed."

4.

THE IMPORTANCE OF ATTITUDE TOWARD LIFE:
"You die when you want to die, when you give up your defenses. This is not to be written in a science book, because it has not been proven yet, but I have seen it in many patients: when beating cancer, the attitude towards life and the emotional side are very important".

5.

PREVENTING SKIN CANCER AND MELANOMA:
"Self-examination is crucial: look on your own body for moles. Moles follow the ABCDE model: Asymmetry, Border, Color, Diameter, and Evolution. If it is more than 5mm in diameter, you need to pay close attention to it. Same thing, if the color changes or the borders are irregular. If it has grown within a year, it is better to remove it. New moles, small and black, should also be removed.

6.

NEW PHOTOPROTECTION OPTIONS: "To prevent skin cancer there exist photoprotection capsules, which are self-tanning. At pharmacies you can ask for them to be prepared with components such as Biotin, which stimulates cellular regeneration and nourishes the skin, nails and hair; Silymarin, which protects the liver, is a photo-protector and helps against rosacea; Vitis vinifera, is an antioxidant extract from grape seeds, and green tea that you take once a day for a month, during the greatest periods of solar radiation." ■

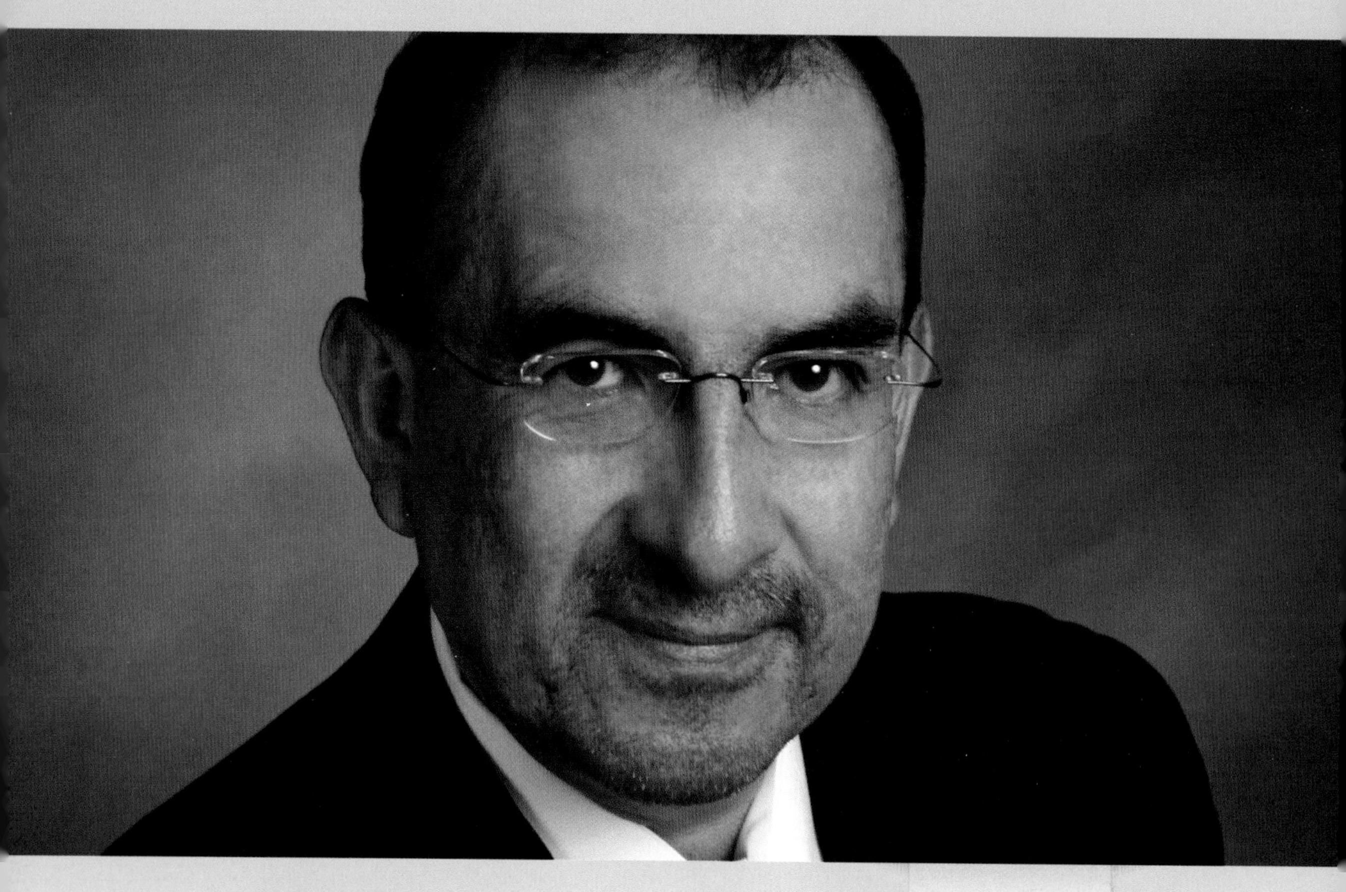

Elmer Huerta

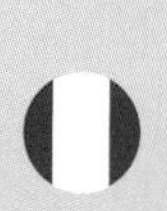

Doctor

AGE: *63*

OCCUPATION: *Oncologist*

CONTEXT: *Doctor Elmer Huerta is the founder and current Director of the Cancer Preventorium, a division of the Washington Cancer Institute at MedStar Washington Hospital Center, in the U.S., a hub concerned exclusively with the prevention of diseases in healthy patients. With an expertise of more than 20 years in the field, Dr. Huerta is considered a world leader in the fight against cancer.*

1.

DON'T BE SCARED: "Cancer can be controlled, and even cured. Back in 1960, only 30% of those developing cancer lived beyond the 5 years following their being diagnosed. Currently, approximately 80% of people suffering from cancer surpass those first 5 years with an excellent quality of life."

2.

LOOK FOR A SECOND OPINION: *"It is very important that when a patient receives a cancer diagnosis, he/she seeks a second opinion regarding treatment, and also to confirm the diagnose."*

Currently, approximately ***80%*** of people suffering from cancer surpass those first 5 years with an excellent quality of *life*."

3.

CHOOSE A CANCER SPECIALIST:

"To begin treatment, look for an oncologist, an oncological surgeon, or an oncological radiotherapist. Let that specialist see you, diagnose you, and properly take care of you."

4.

GET PROPERLY INFORMED: "You have to be very careful with what you read on the Internet, because it's equivalent to the old snake oil seller tale; it can be anything. Ask your doctor, so as to make sure that the information you find is the most suitable one. Here in the US, I recommend sites ending in *gov*; government material, that is. There are other reliable sources with tons of information in Spanish, such as the American Cancer Society (**CANCER.ORG**), the National Cancer Institute (**CANCER.GOV**), and the American Society of Clinical Oncology (**ASCO.ORG**)."

Elmer Huerta

5.

DON'T BELIEVE EVERYTHING THEY SAY: *"People speak because they have a mouth. When cancer is detected, there is always the friend, aunt, cousin, that says "look, milk causes cancer", or "you can't eat meat, anymore", or even that "Cuban blue Scorpion cures cancer". Plus, there are all those other "look at this" and "look at that". Consult only your doctor."*

6.

CARRY A JOURNAL: "If you are a patient, use a journal to take notes on a daily basis about the medication you take, how you feel, what effects those drugs have on you, etc. This is paramount. Because then, when you go to the doctor and are asked "have you used this drug before?", you can check the journal and say: "yes I have, I have it here in my journal."

7.

TAKE CARE OF YOUR MENTAL HEALTH: "Cancer diagnosis may cause post-traumatic stress syndrome; it may cause a huge emotional impact. Just as a person takes care of his/her body and physical health, he/she must take care of his/her mental health. That's why you should consult a psycho-oncologist. This specialist can help patients find what relaxes them. And so then, the patient can choose a sport, or yoga, or a hobby. Because there are thousands of ways to channel the emotional internal energy."

8.

LEAD A HEALTHY LIFESTYLE: "A healthy diet. Daily physical activity. Not smoking cigarettes, of course. Sleeping properly. And dealing with stress. A patient's lifestyle must be taken care of during cancer."

9.

BE PATIENT: "Take things as they come, day by day. I always recommend my patients to cross that bridge when they come to it. Many people with cancer tend to think about the future in a very "untidy" manner. For example, the doctor prescribes some medication, and before they take it, they say: "I have heard this drug has such and such side effects; what happens if this or that occurs? That type of questions only helps increase anguish and anxiety. Some people are simply not reactive to medication, and yet, they worry too much about what *could* happen to them."

"If you are a patient, use a journal to take notes on a **daily** basis about the medication you take, how you *feel,* what effects those drugs have on you."

10.

PRESERVE YOUR REPRODUCTION CHANCES: *"Chemotherapy and radiotherapy treatments may reduce fertility. That's why I recommend, especially young people, to consult their doctors on freezing their sperm or eggs for the future before undergoing such therapies."* ■

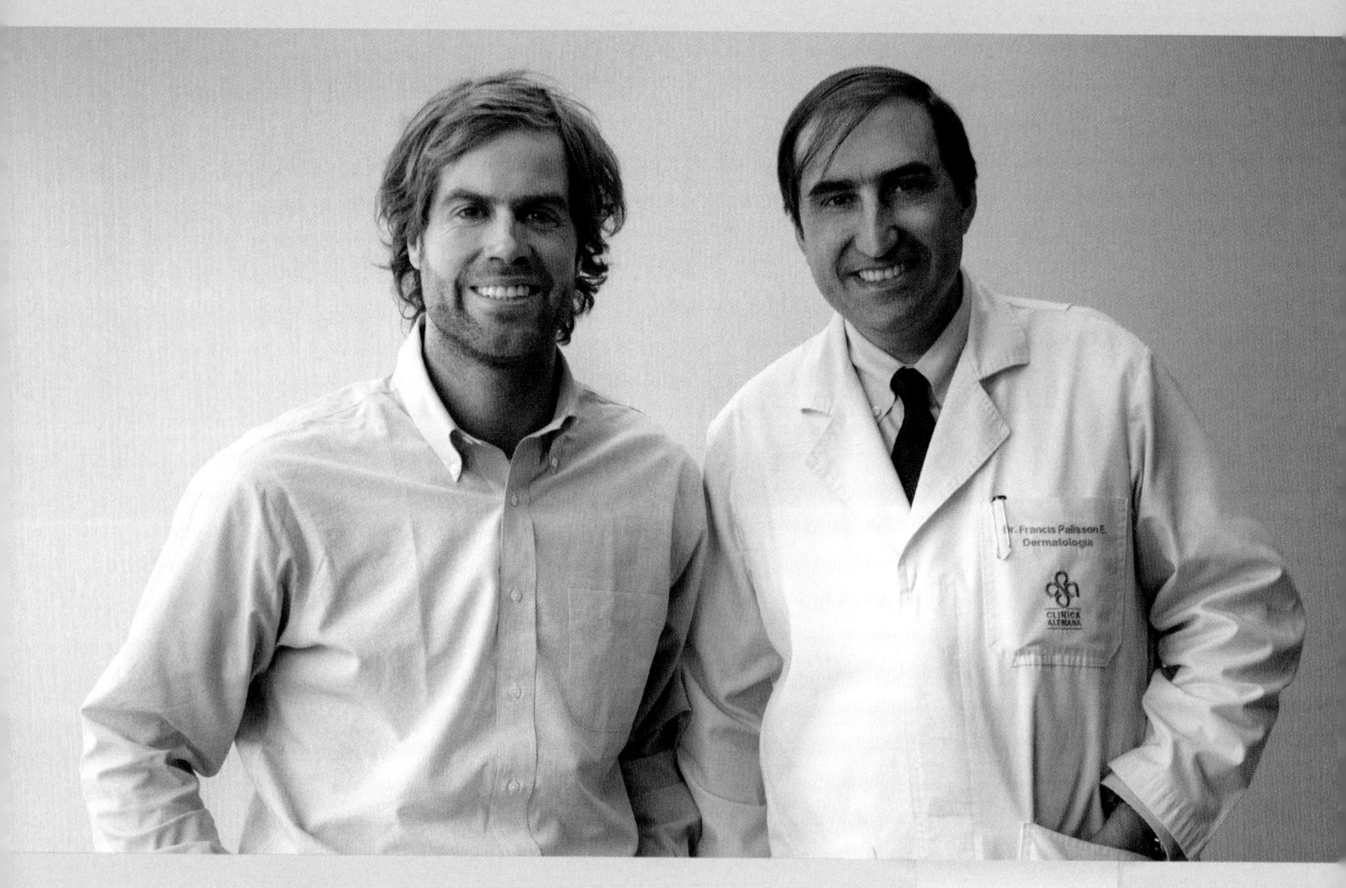

Francis Palisson

Friend and dermatologist

AGE: *47*

OCCUPATION: *Dermatologist*

CONTEXT: *The vocation of Francis Palisson was strongly influenced by a melanoma that his father had on his left hand. This fact was key to his professional life and it led him to have a special sensitivity about this disease. At this point, after the mandatory biannual tests and the long conversations that took place, Dr. Palisson has become a friend of Roberto Ibáñez and has been a guide in his recovery process.*

1.

MELANOMA FACTORS: "There is a genetic basis, which includes factors expressed in the DNA received from parents, and other environmental factors, within which ultraviolet radiation is amongst the most important. This is so clear that there are family melanomas, which only affect certain types of skin and people that have a first-degree relative with melanoma history."

2.

EARLY DETECTION: "If you have an early diagnosis, when the depth is less than a millimeter, the patient has a 90% probability of recovery. One millimeter is the depth at which melanoma is still considered thin. The risk of metastasis overall can begin when the depth goes beyond 0.75 millimeters."

3.

PROLIFERATION: "The growth speed of a melanoma on the skin is relative. It depends on the immunological system, the mutation that defined the melanoma growth, the nutritional condition of the patient, as well as the exposure to ultraviolet light. Personally, I am a fan of the whole nutritional and healthy lifestyles issues, even though there are not enough studies to prove it in detail. The use of sun protectors is a key factor in preventing melanoma and there is sufficient medical literature to support this."

4.

PROGRAMMED EVOLUTION: "When a mole disappears, it does not mean that everything went with it. The immune system can detect a bad mole and destroy it on the surface. It is like wounding a shark's fin and leaving a wound under the skin that has the capacity to spread to other organs."

5.

PERIODICAL CHECK-UPS: "Early melanoma diagnosis allows for a survival rate of over 9%, therefore it is key to undergo periodical checkups with a specialist at least once a year, or more, depending on the patient's medical history. The skin test must cover the entire skin surface." ■

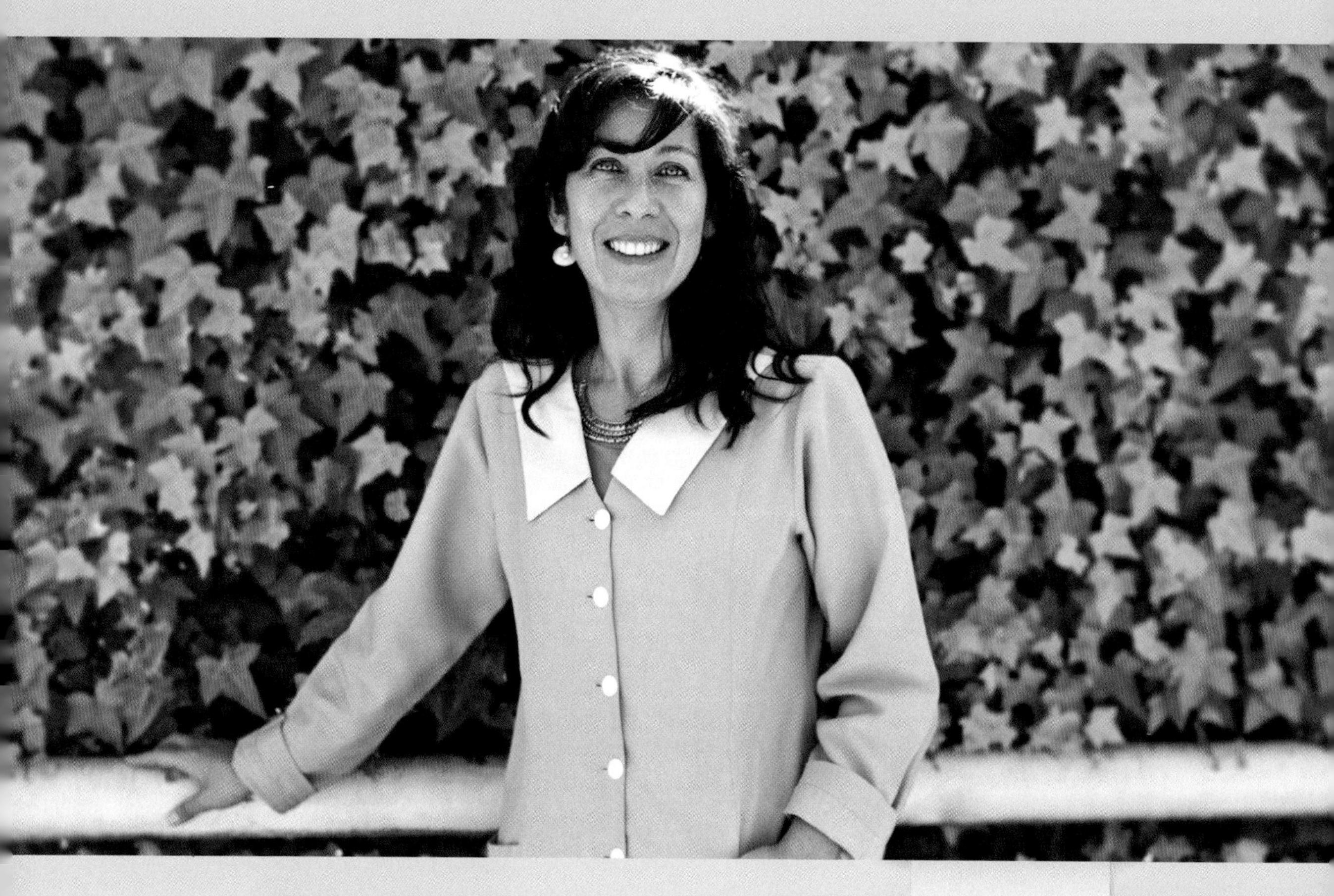

Isabel González

Social worker

AGE: *45*

OCCUPATION: *Social assistant for Oncology and Palliative Care,* Sótero del Río *Hospital*

CONTEXT: *Isabel has been working for 22 years in the public health system and in the last 12 in the Program of Oncology and Palliative Care (adults) of Hospital* Sótero del Río. *Her mission is to support, guide, inform and articulate the social networks in connection to financing of treatments not covered by the health system.* "I see the patient, manage their anguish and rage, which tends to be a lot, I interview and orient them about the possibilities that exist in our society to obtain resources," *she explains.*

1.

REAL EXPECTATIONS: "The first recommendation for a patient with cancer, whose treatment funding is not guaranteed by the public health or AUGE systems, is to have real expectations and to realize that the social network is complementary with the work of the family network. If a patient assumes beforehand that the government must cover all the treatments indicated, it is very hard to move forward. Great governmental efforts have been made in this regard, and we are waiting for the *Ricarte Soto* Act to come into effect, but the expectations must be real: public resources are finite and the oncological needs are endless. The social worker cannot solve the root of the problem, but when working together (institutional networks, family networks and even lab contributions, considering donations), you are able to finance the high-cost treatments in the public sector."

2.

DO NOT WAIT FOR GOVERNMENT HELP TO BEGIN THE TREATMENT: "If a patient waits for the funds from the municipality or the state government to be approved, they are going to waste valuable time. It is more convenient to consider these contributions as a life saver to finance the middle or end cycles, never to begin the treatment. It is much better to begin immediately with the available resources."

3.

CHARITY EVENTS: "The situation of some oncological patients sensitizes their surroundings. In these cases, one can mobilize acquaintances, neighbors, work colleagues and the community to organize events with charitable purposes. In the more vulnerable areas, lots of charity events take places, such as raffles, bingos and shows where artists and famous people also participate."

4.

EVALUATING COST-BENEFIT: "I recommend speaking with the oncologist and asking what the prognosis of the patient is and what the goal of the treatment is: whether the treatment is curative or palliative. Many people in despair sell their possessions, incur expenses and even debt, and that is perhaps only for a treatment that will improve the patient's life, which is very important, but perhaps it is not to cure the disease. One must be very well informed to make those decisions and plan expenses."

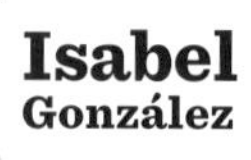

5.

DO NOT BUY THE ENTIRE TREATMENT: "Experience shows me that although the patient has the possibility to finance the entire oncological treatment, it is advisable to purchase it cycle by cycle. After each cycle, the oncologist requests tests from the patient to assess the results. Sometimes the patients do not respond how they were expected to and the specialist could change the drugs or modify the procedure. In most cases, there is no reimbursement for purchased chemotherapies."

6.

TRUST THE PUBLIC HEALTH SYSTEM: "People tend to believe that treatments in public hospitals are of lower quality and many express publicly their frustration to be in that system. The truth is that we do not have the accomodation or the appropriate infrastructure, but our specialists are the same ones that work in the private system, and the quantity of cases that are seen in the public sector exceeds the private sector, so the public officer's eye is much more developed and trained, so there must be trust in the treatment offered here."

"It is much better to begin ***immediately*** with the available resources, rather than losing valuable time waiting for help to arrive."

7.

ATTEND YOUR THERAPY: "Cancer is a very powerful disease which affects all of the patient's surroundings, which is why emotional and psychological support is needed. Some public hospitals have psychologists in their oncology departments, but this resource is never sufficient. Ideally, people would get in touch with support groups from the institutions that specialize in their type of cancer to look for opportunities of psychological support, or alternative and complementary therapies. Since 2005 at the *Sotero del Rio* Hospital, we have an agreement with the *Yo Mujer* Corporation, which offers workshops for patients with breast cancer, as well as providing information about oncological treatments and psychotherapy."

8.

RATIONAL DECISIONS: *"When an adult patient proposes the possibility of taking out a loan to get treatment –and incur debt–, the first thing I tell them is to speak with the doctor and ask them what can be achieved with the chemotherapy and what would their survival rate be if they undergo the treatment. Then they should evaluate. For example, if they tell me that my chemotherapy is not curative, but palliative, then I have a good prognosis of the situation, and I think it is worth it. But if even with the chemo the estimation is short, and it is limited to months, it seems to me that it should be thought through with more care, especially if within the family group there are children in a development stage. Life, after the patient passes away, continues."*

"Although the patient has the possibility to finance the entire oncological treatment, it is ***advisable*** to purchase it cycle by cycle."

9.

HAVE A COMPANION: "If a patient is not fit to go through the processes alone, they should have a companion. Hopefully the companion would always be the same, so that when the patient cannot attend something, they feel ill, the companion could replace them and get the information about the treatment and developments that the patient is going through. If the patient keeps changing companions, the process is much slower, and the transfer of information is less fluid which can hamper the treatment."

10.

PALLIATIVE CARE AND PAIN RELIEF: "If the cancer progresses, in spite of the treatment, the patient is not unprotected. The public health system has palliative care and pain relief units for advanced cancer patients which are covered by the AUGE. This includes analgesic therapy for pain control, care by a multidisciplinary team (doctor, nurse, psychologists and social workers), home visits when the patient is too weak, workshops for the caretakers and mourning support for the main caretaker after the patient passes away. No patient, even when their cancer is past medical help, deserves to die in pain or suffering." ■

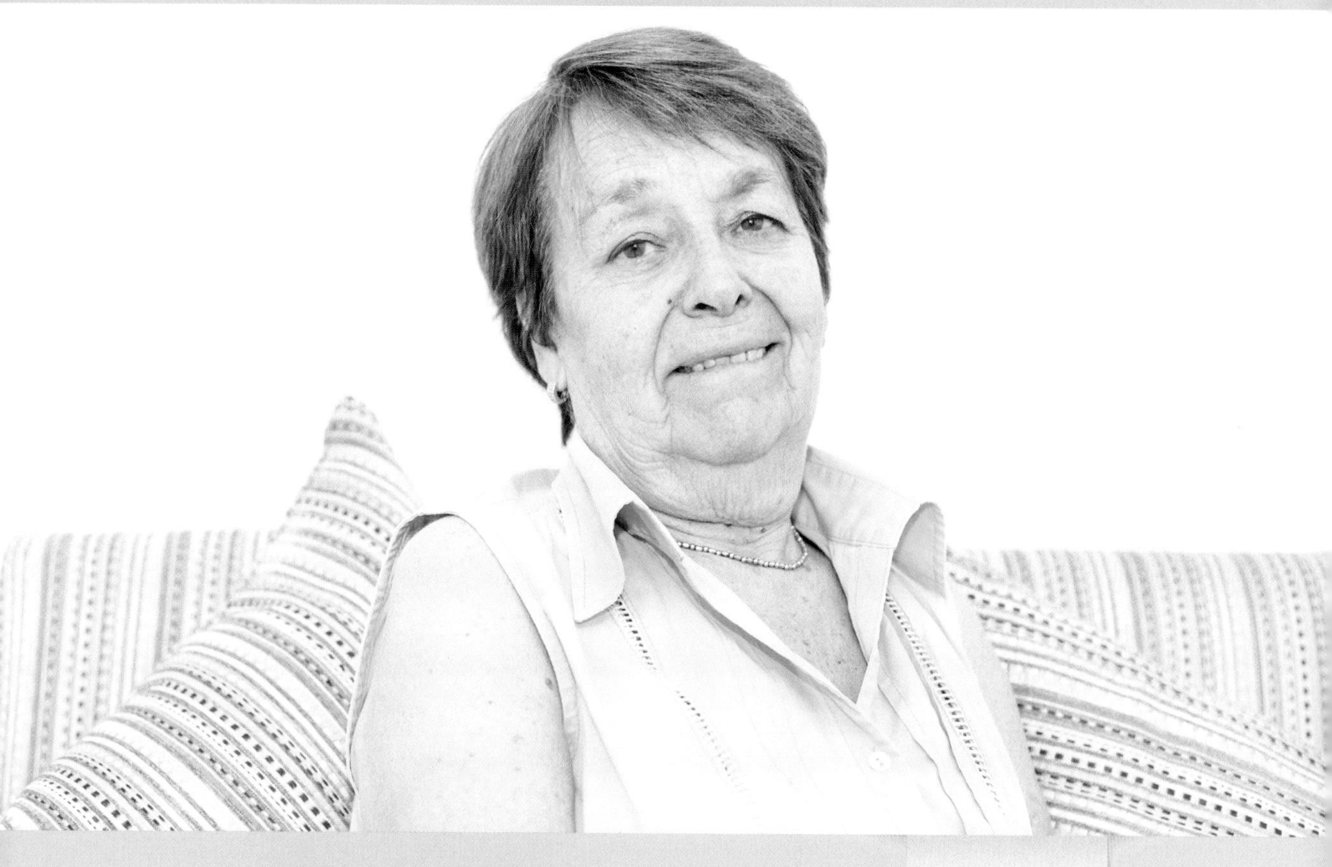

Jennifer Middleton

Psychologist

AGE: *67*

OCCUPATION: *Clinical psychologist specialized in psycho oncology*

CONTEXT: *A psycho-oncology pioneer in Chile, she has worked with cancer patients since 1979 and authored* Yo (no) quiero tener cáncer *("I Don't Want to Have Cancer"), where she deals with how the lifestyle and the decisions of a person can have an effect on their body, one of the principles of proactive psycho-oncology. This specialty –which gravitates between medicine and psychology– analyses the link between the patient's behavior and their disease, the prevention and a treatment that addresses healthy habits and changes in their form of life.*

1.

THE DIFFERENCE BETWEEN GUILT AND RESPONSIBILITY: "Proactive psycho-oncology, such as the one I practice, supports the theory that the disease is the result of a person's self-abuse. Sometimes that is confused with guilt and what a cancer patient needs the least is to feel guilty. But they do have to assume responsibility. If you smoked two packs of cigarettes a day and now you have lung cancer, let's assume smoking is the cause and let's see what can be done. Perhaps you can begin to understand why you smoked those two packs and how you can begin leading a healthy lifestyle and perhaps reverse the disease. It is your responsibility to figure out how you modify that."

2.

CHANGING VITAL PRIORITIES: "If a person wants to recover, they need to reconnect with themselves on a very deep level to change their vital priorities. When the most important thing in somebody's life is to have economic success (with its high stress levels), to be liked by everybody or to have prestige, working with themselves they will realize that that is not fundamental. What is important is to feel realized as a person."

3.

THREE INSPIRING BOOKS: "Ian Gawler is an Australian author and he wrote *You Can Conquer Cancer.* Doctors told him he had two or three weeks left, but he knew that meditating strengthened the immune system. Then, he said: well, I am going to meditate five hours a day. Over twenty years have passed since then, he completely recovered and today he owns a recovery center in Sidney for those who have cancer. Greg Anderson wrote *Cancer: 50 Essential Things To Do.* He had lung cancer. He was in a wheelchair and had already lost one lung, but he said I am going to get better. And he got better. Then he surveyed 13,000 people who, in spite of a terminal diagnosis, had been saved and identified the common denominators that helped them recover. They are all in his book. Another very good book is *Making Sense of Illness* by Jean Shinoda. She writes about what it means and the meaning behind becoming ill, how you can enrich your life and that of others in the process, instead of wasting it. She proposes that if you are already sick, use it to grow, to relate better with other people and to love life again."

Jennifer Middleton

4.

CANCER IS NOT ANY BATTLE: "You must work full time to get better. If you say *"I am going to meditate"* but then you cannot find the time, that is not an acceptable excuse when you have a serious cancer. You are fighting against death, so you should work hard to get better. Many people deny the gravity of the disease and do not work in-depth to make those changes. Nobody can cure other people, you have to heal yourself."

"*Proactive* psycho-oncology, as the one I exercise, sustains the theory that the disease may be the result of a self-abuse of the person ***himself.***"

5.

FAMILY'S ROLE: The family has to understand the process the patient is going through, and they must be willing to tolerate some changes, which are not always going to be pleasant. For example, most women with breast cancer are extremely generous and when they begin their process, they become, so to say, selfish. And you have to accept that."

6.

SPEAKING ABOUT DEATH IN THE FAMILY: "Having a patient in the family is not only critical for the patient, but also for the entire family. Roles are switched, and there are economical, social and work repercussions. It is important that the family members express their feelings and manifest their rage and doubts. Above all, I recommend allowing the patient to speak about death. This doesn't mean that they want to die, but that they have anxieties that they need to share."

7.

BIOLOGY AND INTELLIGENCE: "When we submit biology to intelligence, every time our stomach hurts because we are tense, then we rationalize: *Sure, it hurts, but I shouldn't be tense, so I can keep going.* It is a different thing to say okay, what is happening to me? Why am I tense? What is scaring me about the future? What can I do to tackle this threat in a different way? That, instead, is submitting intelligence to my emotions, and therefore, my biology."

"If the **patient** at a certain moment wants to speak about death, it does not mean he wants to die."

8.

INTEGRATIVE APPROACH: "It is not only the psychological dimension that acts upon us, many things converge: how you relate with people, what you eat, how you manage your time. To some it is more important to emphasize one thing over another, but integrating everything, I believe, makes cancer reversible. However, you have to work and work hard on a full-time schedule to get better. You're fighting against death, so you must work really hard."

9.

FROM FEAR TO ACTION: *"Some people experience denial in regard to the seriousness of the disease so they do not work deeply enough to make the necessary changes. Other people, who are very scared, are willing to do whatever it takes. I believe that fear, and seeing death from up close, can be very mobilizing."*

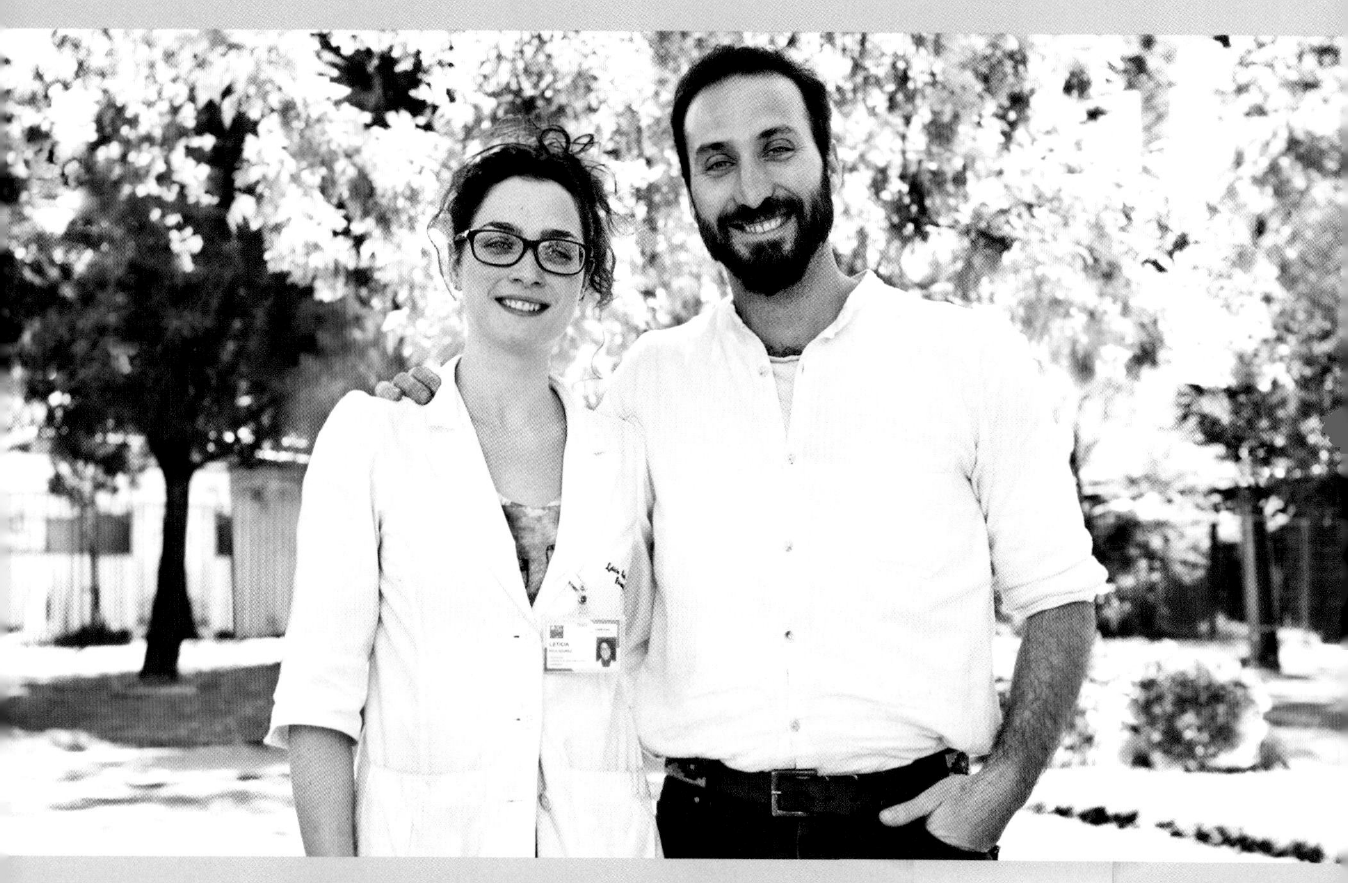

Christopher Scott & Leticia Rojo

Psychologists

AGE: *32 and 28, respectively*

OCCUPATION: *Psychologists from the mental health team at the Palliative Care Unit from* Sotero del Rio *Hospital*

CONTEXT: *Leticia and Christopher receive patients with advanced cancer and help them channel their mental pain, so that they can be better off during the final chapter of their lives. Everybody has the right to do psychotherapy, although it might be hard at the beginning due to the patients' prejudices. Many of them say that they go to the 'crazy doctor', but at the end the vast majority wind up valuing the psychologists, they say. Nowadays they see patients as well as their families. On top of treating them in their practices, they organize home visits, and they also incorporated group therapy.*

1.

MENTAL PEACE: "The purpose of psychological therapy is to help the patients find mental peace in this difficult moment. They know that they are going to die, but it could be years, and that uncertainty generates anxiety, anguish, and depression."

2.

CONNECTION WITH THE PATIENT: "What's important is to continue to connect with the patient. Most times they don't show signs of connection with the outside world, sometimes because of the drugs or because of some type of defense. Keeping the connection between the patient and the people that surround them is the beginning of actively reconnecting with reality: talking to them, taking care of them, cleaning them, reading books, telling them what you've done during the day, telling them what you want, always respecting each other's ways. If you do not speak very much, but know how to hug, then it is important to double or triple the hugs."

"At the end of ***life,*** existential crises are generally unleashed, and the patient has the **necessity** to fulfill certain *wishes.*"

3.

BEING HUMAN: "Family members feel the pressure to be noble and to stay strong in the face of the disease, but there are emotions and human qualities that sometimes we forget that we can feel. For example, ambivalent feelings: I love my wife, but what is happening to her makes me angry. The husband has to tell his wife that he loves her and keeps his anger inside, but hopefully he should feel the freedom to express what is happening to him and show his pain during the process. It is paramount that he learns how to validate his feelings and not feel guilty."

Scott & Rojo

4.

FAMILY UNITY: "It is key that the family remains a solid clan. To do this, it is recommended to create opportunities to express emotions. The invitation is to break that ice, sit down with the family and talk about things. Even if everybody ends up crying, they are going to feel each other's support."

5.

PSYCHOLOGY'S ROLE: "We are here to contain, to help in the search for mental resources available to the person so that they can find their own ways. So we try to stabilize them, to improve their life conditions."

"It is **key** that the ***family*** remains a *solid* clan."

6.

CREATE SUPPORT NETWORKS: "It is recommended that the patient and his family get in touch with people who are undergoing a similar process. This way there is contention: they are not the only ones and they are not alone in this process."

7.

EVERYBODY HAS THEIR TIPS: "This is a very personal process, so every patient has their own tips. Our support consists in helping them finding their own."

8.

CLOSING THE CYCLE: *"At the end of life, existential crises are generally unleashed, and the patient has the necessity to fulfill certain wishes. It is important to identify what the most urgent wishes before dying are and to try to fulfill them. Closing this cycle is very unique: it could be speaking with the child that was never noticed, eating toasted flour with sugar, writing the will or seeing the stars. But, in general, the patient lives more in the moment, has the need to feel closer to the people that they love and to make the most of the time they have left."*

"Mourning *actively* starts with **maintaining** a link between the patient and the people surrounding him."

9.

BE GENEROUS: "Sadness hurts, and it is hard to express, that is why people tend to remain silent and live the pain individually. But it is best to do the opposite, because shared misfortunes are better lived." ■

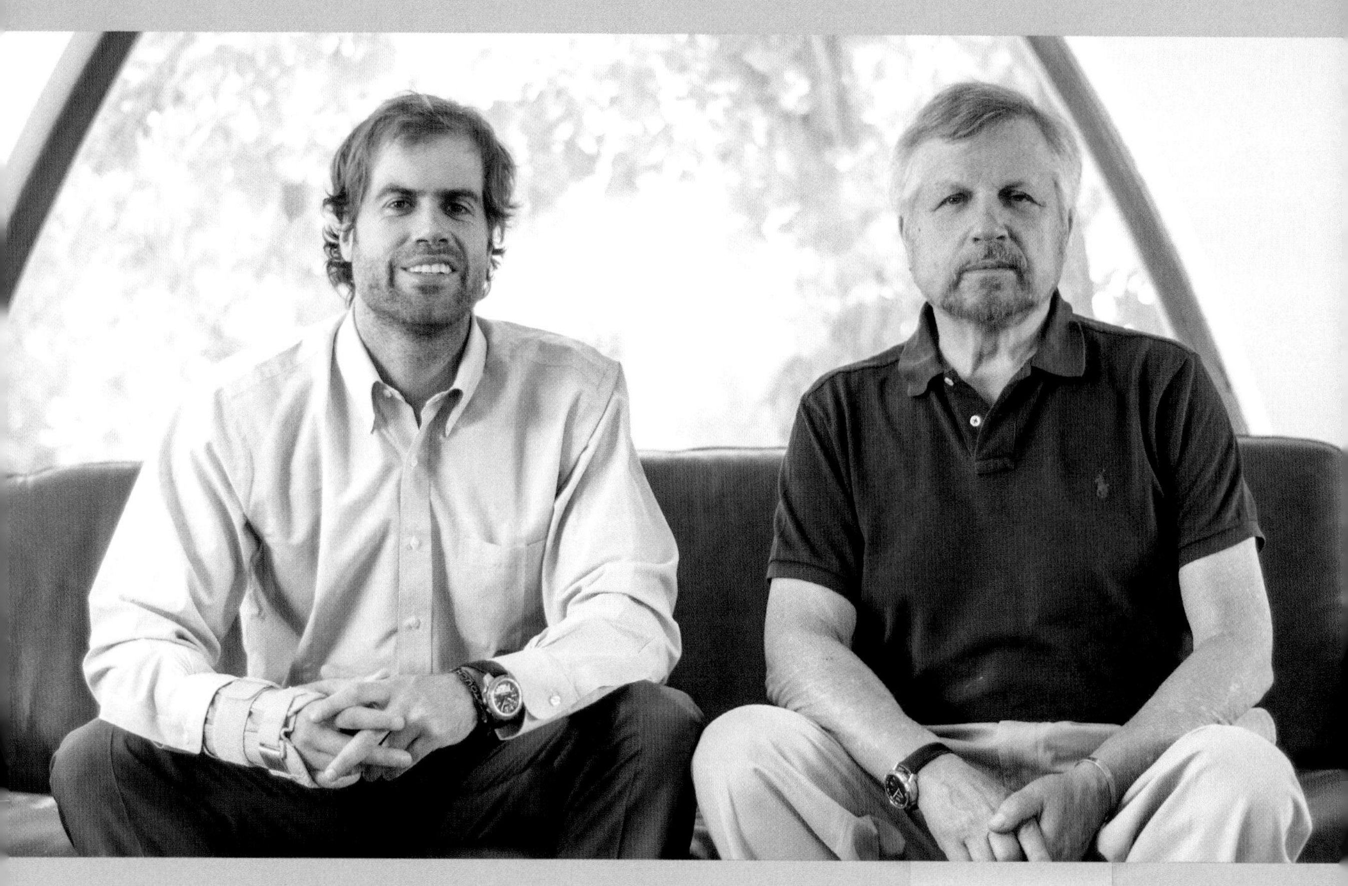

Iván Mimica

Friend and businessman

AGE: *73*

OCCUPATION: *Scientist and businessman*

CONTEXT: *For Roberto Ibáñez, his friend Ivan Mimica is one of Santiago's best kept secrets. Thanks to him, he managed to get to Mark Mincolla's practice in the US, the natural therapist who designed a special diet for Roberto according to his own needs. Together with Ivan, Roberto has scrutinized the issue of diet from every point of view. He has reviewed books and has tried supplements such as* Delphinol, *a peanut concentrate developed by Ivan. According to Roberto, Ivan's advice –he's an encyclopedia of alternative medicine and natural diets– have been essential to his recovery.*

1.

THERE'S NO RULE FOR EVERYBODY:
"Every person has a different story that must be unraveled to understand the disease. Its metabolism and constitution have to be studied."

2.

SUGAR CAN PRODUCE INFLAMMATORY PROCESSES:
"You have to pay special attention to this issue, because we eat 'disguised' sugar all the time: pasta, white rice, white flour. When it comes to sugar, it is important to include the foods composed mostly of carbohydrates and especially those rich in starch. Natural fructose in some foods can also be harmful for the body, although not every organism responds in the same way to sugar ingestion. There are people who simply have better metabolisms."

3.

A MOSTLY ALKALINE DIET: *"This is the diet that every human being should have. Acidity can lead to death and a body low in alkaline will try to obtain the resources needed to alkalize from the bones, where you can find calcium, potassium and magnesium. A mostly alkaline diet (70% alkaline and 30% acidic) must have foods low in the glycemic index, so mostly fruits and vegetables, and it should be complemented with fish, almonds, nuts, beans, lentils and chickpeas. Potatoes, rice, pasta, meat, milk and all proteins are acidic."*

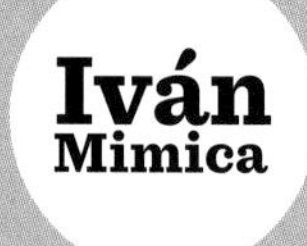

4.

MILK, IN GENERAL, IS DAMAGING FOR HEALTH: "Just like its derivatives, milk can produce many allergies and inflammation in the human body. These weaken the immune system, thus opening the door to a wide range of inflammations. According to the Japanese doctor Hiromi Shinya, milk is like a dead food. It has been warmed up to high temperatures to kill bacteria. However, this process also kills the enzyme required to digest the milk properly. Breast milk? It is healthy and fundamental in a specific life stage, but adults do not need to consume milk products, even for the calcium, because the calcium in milk is lost due to phosphorus contained by processed milk. It is much better to obtain calcium from vegetables, like broccoli."

5.

MANAGING STRESS, EMOTIONS AND THOUGHTS: "When a person gets stressed or has negative thoughts, their organism responds by producing a damaging amount of cortisol, which produces inflammation. According to Mark Mincolla, one of cortisol's many functions is to regulate inflammation in the organism by giving the immune system the instructions to either decrease or increase production. In a period of stress, cortisol levels rise with the purpose of making more 'emergency' energy available. But chronic stress reduces the tissues' sensitivity to cortisol, due to the continued exposure, which has an effect on the body's capacity to respond to infections; for example, when an inflammation is supposed to bring white blood cells to the affected area to enhance immunological defenses."

6.

BE AWARE OF CONSUMED TOXICITY: "Many foods contain large amounts of parasites and heavy metals. Therefore, it is better to consume fruits and vegetables of a known origin, from your garden, or organic."

7.

THE IMPORTANCE OF CONSUMING FATTY OILS IN A BALANCED WAY: "There are three types of fatty oils: Omega 3, Omega 6 and Omega 9. The amounts required to consume them in a balanced manner depend on the health condition of a person. The healthiest are Omega 3, because they can be found in bluefish such as tuna, horse mackerel, sardines, harvestfish, sole, anchovies, cod, herring and salmon. All of them contain more than 5 grams of fat for every 100 grams of edible meat (5%), which is different from white fish, which has a lower index. Omega 3 can also be found in lobster, shrimp, crab, calamari and octopus, egg yolk, rabbit meat, chia seeds, sprouts, pineapples, nuts, almonds, chickpeas, spinach, strawberries, lettuce, cucumber, parsley, cauliflower, soy, purslane and pumpkin. Ideally, you would consume these fats in a balanced manner: three portions of Omega 3 per one of Omega 6. Nowadays, it is normal to consume 12 portions of Omega 6 per one of Omega 3, which causes inflammation in the body."

"Each person has a **different** story that has to be ***unraveled*** to understand the disease."

8.

ATTENTION TO THE WHAT AND THE WHEN: *"Raw foods have more active enzymes than cooked food. Enzymes as well as other nutrients that are found in fresh and raw foods are very sensitive to heat, and are destroyed at temperatures over 30°C. This is why frying food is one of the worst methods of cooking. Nevertheless, it is important to give the body space to digest. The biggest recommendation is to respect meal times, and that the last meal of the day takes place three or four hours before going to sleep."* ■

MY TIPS

Many of these tips and recommendations are located throughout this book, but I wanted to gathered them in one chapter, in order for them to be available and easy to find.

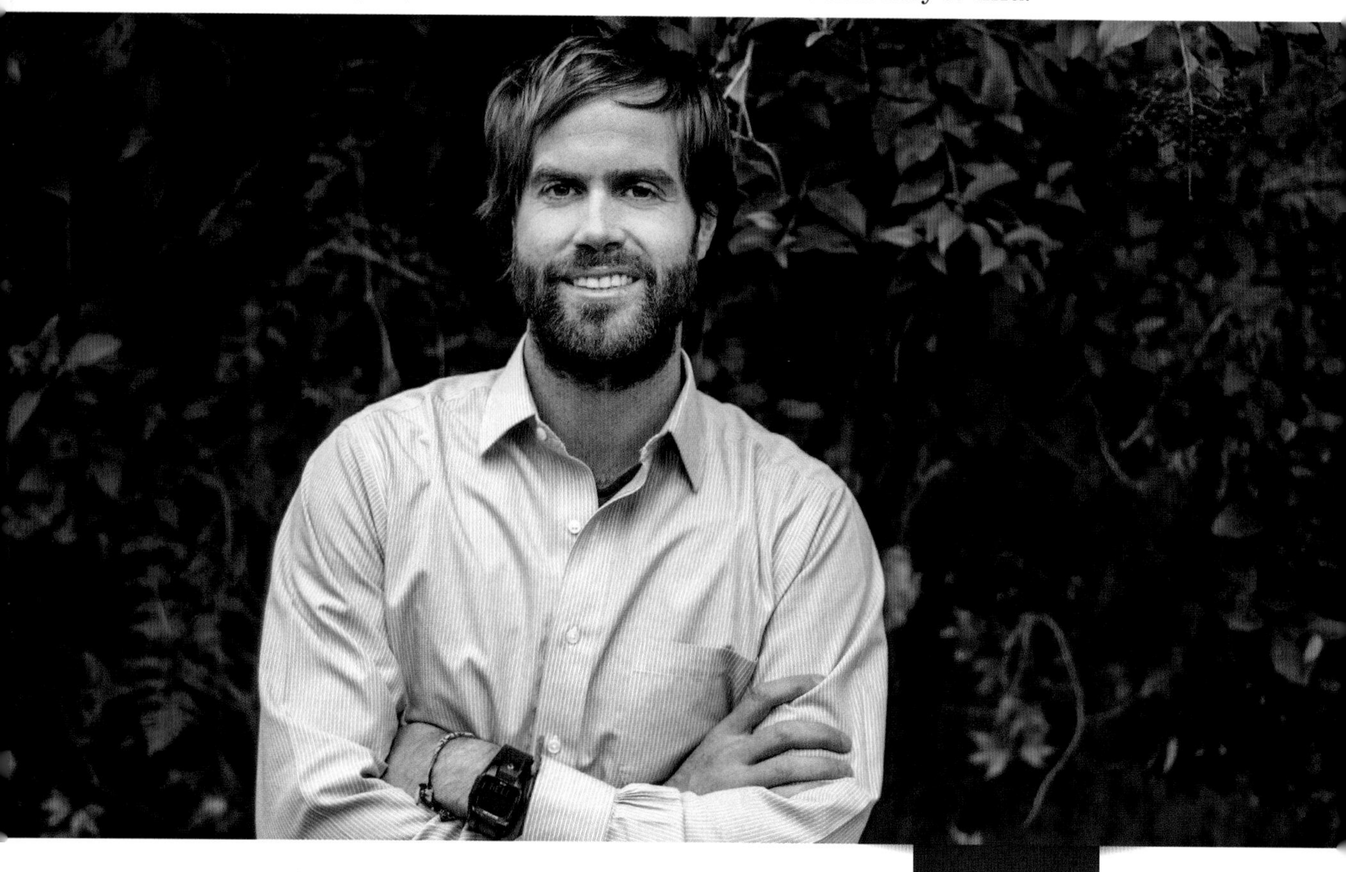

Roberto Ibáñez

melanoma
PATIENT

AGE: *32*

OCCUPATION: *Businessman*

DIAGNOSIS: *Melanoma*

WHEN: *2011*

CONTEXT: *My life changed forever after receiving the diagnosis of melanoma. With the support of my family, friends and work colleagues, and after seeing the most suitable specialists in as quickly as possible, I moved forward while making the commitment to myself that I would share my knowledge and the experience brought to me, unexpectedly, by cancer.*

1.

ENCOURAGE FAMILY SPACES: "It could be once a month or once a week, but it is necessary to get together and speak about everything freely. It is important to speak with your family and tell each other everything about the disease. If the news is hard, or very hard to bear, we support each other. I think that's the lesson that we, the Ibañez-Atkinson family, learned through all this.

2.

THINK POSITIVELY AND FOCUS ON THE GOOD PROGNOSES: "I decided to focus on the 80% chance of living, leaving the other dark 20% probability of metastasis under the rug, forgotten. This wasn't my automatic reaction, it took me a while to assimilate the news and change my outlook to a positive one, in the understanding that optimism can work wonders."

3.

PROVIDE A GUESTBOOK: "I wish I'd thought earlier of getting a guestbook for visitors at the hospital. I didn't think of it at the time but it's a great idea."

4.

CANCER MODE 'ON': "This is like a certificate that excuses you from responsibilities and gives you space to live those cancer moments when you just can't face everyday tasks. I think it is a very useful tool, and that cancer patients should use it when they are sick of everything and don't want (or do want to) do something. Having cancer gives you the freedom to have the cancer mode 'ON'. What's important is to use it appropriately and responsibly."

5.

CANCER DOESN'T HAVE TO BE A LONELY ROAD: "In spite of the fact that you can have a lot of company, you internally live a process that is very personal. It is difficult to let others in, especially when you feel capable of controlling all the variables. The trust is that you have to learn to accept that certain things are simply not within your reach and that it is impossible to know their outcome. Therefore, it is better to take decisions with someone at your side."

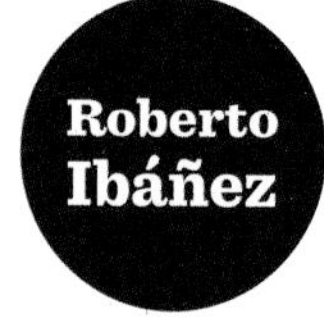

6.

SHARE AND LEARN TO RECEIVE: "What's yours or of the other person. Emotions, thoughts, material and immaterial things, are better enjoyed in the company of someone else. Love yourself and let yourself be loved."

7.

BEING AFRAID IS LEGITIMATE: "Everybody is afraid, and what you have to do is understand it and accept it. Fear is not bad, because it is a driver that leads you to act and make decisions. It is complicated not to understand it. What I am most scared of is uncertainty. I hate losing control of things. But when I am in nature and I am afraid of the unknown, an engine switches on and it does not stop until I find a way to solve it."

8.

HOW TO HANDLE UNCERTAINTY: *"You have to learn to accept that certain things are just not within our reach."*

9.

THE 8 SACRED HOURS: "You have to have a minimum of 8-hours sleep in order for the body and mind to rest and recover correctly. A minimum of 8 hours sleep a night has been by far the best remedy prescribed by allopath and naturopath doctors."

10.

WRITE: "Is a tremendous tool to express, develop or understand emotions. Writing was one of my greatest allies during the hardest moments of the cancer journey."

11.

DON'T WAIT FOR SOMETHING BAD TO HAPPEN BEFORE YOU MAKE CHANGES: "It sounds so obvious, but it's actually hard to change your outlook on life until something bad happens to force that change. 'Bad' in quotation marks, because that something negative can of course become the motor for positive change. So try to make the change without the need for the 'bad' thing to catalyze it."

12.

THE WAY DOES NOT DEFINE THE ESSENCE: "It is hard to find the correct way to say things, to communicate to a loved one good or bad news. What people say often comes out wrong but that doesn't mean that it wasn't intended kindly. It's important to understand the essence of what someone is saying before judging them. Especially people who are close to you."

13.

NOT ONLY THE PATIENT HAS CANCER: "Every family member goes through the process in a different way during the disease and during the recovery. I get a deep vibe of understanding, love and unconditional support from my family, who have always been there, but today it is even stronger."

14.

GET CLOSE TO NATURE AND SPORT:

"They are the best doctors. They develop your body and soul, and they never fail."

"Telling someone that *I don't want* to do something because I have cancer, is a very **valid** excuse."

15.

EVERYONE HAS THEIR OWN STORY:

"Respect the decisions taken by those close to you. In the end it's their life, not yours."

16.

LIVE FOR TODAY, NOT YESTERDAY NOR TOMORROW: "Just like the word says, the present is a gift. We can't change the past, only learn from it and try not to let it define us. Live in the present, enjoy it and look forward to the future without expecting anything from it."

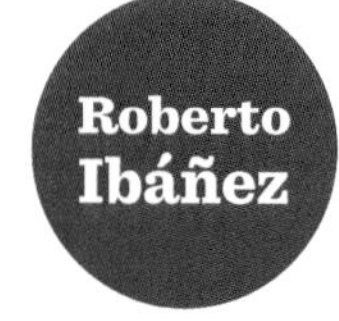

17.

LEARN TO SAY NO: "Don't get involved in things you don't like doing. Sounds stupid, but many people do it every day. Learn to say no, it's a tremendous help to finding your path and marking out your own space."

18.

LIVE FOR THE *WHAT FOR* AND NOT FOR *THE WHY*: "Cancer underlines what is worth living, and spending time and energy on. The 'what for'. The 'why' will just paralyze you, but 'what for' is a steam train of energy."

19.

LEAVE YOUR LEGACY WHILE YOU ARE ALIVE: *"A lot of people worry about what they'll leave when they're gone, but the truth is that you're a lot more use alive than dead. So if you have a dream or a goal that you think might help others, then live that dream and fulfil that goal!"*

20.

GOOD BYE EGOS: "Reconciliation and compromise is almost always a better tool than protecting the ego, bottling things up or fighting. Understanding others helps reduce anxiety, gives you peace and makes you happier."

21.

WE ARE WHAT WE EAT: "After my experience, I concluded that the mind is an indissoluble part of your body. If you are happy or sad, it has a repercussion on your health. And of course diet is key. We are what we eat and if we don't take care of our body we damage it. And then, our body reacts intoxicating itself, reducing immunity or with the unexpected appearance of cancer or any other serious disease."

"I will not get tired of insisting that ***family*** is key in this process. The first thing you **have** to do, is *thank* them."

22.

THERE ARE ALTERNATIVE ROADS: "After examining the options I decided to follow a treatment that combined natural methods and traditional medicine. My surgeries were performed by an oncologist, but afterwards my healing method was through natural drugs, a change in the way I ate, and in my lifestyle."

23.

LISTEN TO YOUR BODY: "My immune system was screwed up for at least three years, and I did not pay attention to the signs that it was sending me. If for some reason you find yourself saying "I don't feel good" (physically or mentally), it's because something is happening that you have to resolve."

"Cancer has been an enormous pain, but also a ***gift:*** it has been a time of **reassuming** bonds, *healing* wounds from the past and **changing** attitudes."

24.

PREVENTING MELANOMA REAPREANCE: "The main tips I receive from doctors to take care from a reappearance was to use 50 SFP solar protector, take Vitamin D every day (since I cannot be exposed to the sun, and Vitamin D comes from the sun), have an annual eye check-up (since melanoma can reappear in the eye), individually check my own skin once a month, and get checked out by a dermatologist every three months."

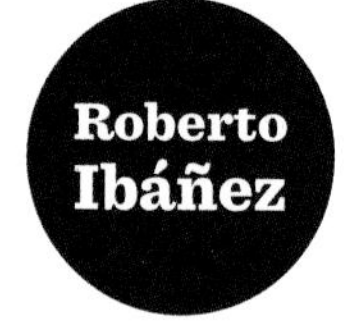

25.

PROTECT YOURSELF AGAINST UV RAYS!: "This is the most efficient way of decreasing melanoma risk. You have to avoid excessive sun exposure to avoid sunburns. You should cover yourself with hats, parasols or anti-UV clothes, if possible. I always use sunscreen before doing sport, when I take a walk or before heading to the office. During winter and summer my skin is always protected, whatever the weather."

26.

CHECK YOUR GENETIC HISTORY: "The risk of getting a melanoma is higher if one or more direct relatives (mother, father, sibling, and children) have had it. In my family there was no history, but two of my siblings, motivated by my cancer, have had suspicious malignant moles removed. Someone with many moles has a greater propensity to generate the illness. Specialists also say that people with freckles and red-haired people present more melanomas than others."

27.

THE FIRST ONE TO UNDERSTAND THE DISEASE MUST BE THE PATIENT: "In the beginning, I had trouble connecting with my disease, and that was why it was hard to participate in the decision-taking process. Fluidness in the doctor-patient relationship eventually comes, but for this to happen you have to accept your disease, empower yourself as a patient, ask everything you need to ask and resolve your doubts."

28.

IT IS YOUR RIGHT TO GET EXPLANATIONS: "They have to answer your questions and explain to you everything that you do not understand. They have to show you all the possible roads that you can take, with their positive and negative effects. Everybody must understand that if you are a patient you need to be as active and empowered as possible."

29.

THE INTERNET WILL NOT ANSWER EVERYTHING: "The information source chosen by the patient to answer their questions is very important. A piece of advice offered to me by Dr. Gustavo Vidal was not to look for answers on the internet, because it could make me assume the worst. Or even confuse me. I looked for all the medical opinions available; I asked and I compared differences. Yet, if it is going to relieve you to look for information on your own, it is convenient to at least ask your doctor what the most legitimate websites are."

30.

ORGANIZE AND FILE ALL THE INFORMATION: "My family created a file with everything that we gathered on a daily basis. This helped us maintain order, and since it was so much information, it allowed us to find something when we wanted to counteract opinions or we didn't remember something. Everything was there: hundreds of research pages, doctors' opinions in Chile, tips about doctors in the USA, cancer research centers in Europe, different treatments, and pros and cons of each, telephone numbers and contact emails, etc."

32.

THE POWER OF ALKALINE FOOD AND IONIZED WATER: "We know that cancer in order to occur needs an acid environment, this is a low pH, which means that chemistry favors the proliferation of the disease. We have to maintain a relation of four alkaline foods per one acid food (see chapter, You are What you Eat, page 170). Another excellent way of maintaining the body alkaline, is consuming water ionized in a high pH. I take more than 3 liters of this water per day. I recommend the book *The Miraculous Properties of Ionized Water: The Definitive Guide to the World's Healthiest Substance*, by Bob McCauley. Reading it I realized the incredible benefits of ionized water, because it counteracts the effects of acid food in the body, among other things. I have an ionizing machine to alkalyze water. From there I take my daily consumption to take and cook. The machine can be purchased through **SHITIVEGOTCANCER.COM**"

31.

LEARN MEDICAL NOMENCLATURE:

"It is very useful so that you can understand everything that the doctors tell you. Helps you better understand the information you research and speeds up the conversations with specialists."

"Everything is *enjoyed* best when you are in the company of someone you love. Love yourself and let yourself **be loved."**

33.

THANK, THANK AND THANK MORE: "I am not going to get tired of insisting that the family has been essential in this process. The patient's experience of cancer is 100% influenced by how their family reacts and supports them. Sometimes you don't see this. Grab every opportunity to thank them for what they're doing for you. A simple hug or a "thank you", always are welcome, consolidate bonds and only build positively towards the future." ■

Final *words*

Overcoming a disease like cancer has a life-lesson for everyone, especially the patient. Despite the difficulties, it also leaves good things in its wake. In Roberto Ibáñez's case, it brought close support from his family, as well as from many friends. I saw that directly.

In a way cancer also allows you to take a fresh look at life and see what is worth it. This is why patients usually improve their relationship with their family and they grow personally and spiritually. From this perspective, I value the intention of *Shit, I've got Cancer, what do I do?*, of cooperating in order for patients to better face their disease and handle it in a suitable way, with minimum collateral conflicts.

Gustavo Vial, Oncological Surgeon.

For most of my life I've had the privilege of being surrounded and inspired by thousands of people with cancer. At this point, more of my close friends have had cancer than haven't. Through countless conversations, usually after a day of adventure, I've learned a lot about life, love, laughter and the fight against cancer. Through them all a few consistent themes have resurfaced time and time again, and all of them point to this book being a valuable tool for anyone fighting cancer, and the ones who love them.

By consolidating mountains of knowledge, personal experience, resources, research, tips and inspiration, this book serves as the guidebook to navigate the uncertain and overwhelming path of life post diagnosis.

And while cancer may immediately threaten to break spirits, shatter lives, cast doubt, isolate, alienate and depress, there is another, brighter path presented to all who choose to walk it. A path filled with awakening, new adventures, and meaningful relationships. By reading this book, you're taking the first step down that brighter path and joining a huge tribe of others doing the same.

BRAD LUDDEN, FOUNDER OF FIRST DESCENTS.

Final *words*

I never could have imagined how drastically my life would change with my brother's diagnosis, and that I would someday be doing meaningful work with young adults in the cancer fight. I wish every day that I could talk to my brother, share life with him, and have him back. Simultaneously, I am filled with a deep sense of gratitude and appreciation for the life I live, and the people in it, more than I ever would have been able to otherwise. Somehow, that is the gift that he has left. Cancer is devastating and cancer has a way of bringing to light life's most profound beauty.

Nobody should go through the experience of cancer alone. If you are reading this book, your life has likely also been turned upside down, and you're seeking the stories, insights, and human experiences of others to help guide your journey.

This book showcases the courage, perseverance, strength, and love that rises out of our souls through the most adverse circumstances. With pain and fear and sadness, there is love and connection and beauty. Let these stories hold you and support you and alleviate some of the fear. With or without cancer, our time is precious and today is a gift.

KATIE SCHOU- EXECUTIVE DIRECTOR OF THE SEND IT FOUNDATION.

When we faced the word cancer for the first time, the feeling was one of fear, profound worry and confusion.

Shit I've got cancer! What do I do? To whom do I get close? How do I face this nightmare?

However, there are tons of reasons to remain calm, be optimistic, and to keep looking at life joyously. Because we live in privileged times, marked by the greatest scientific developments in human kind. What was unknown and deadly only a few years ago, is nowadays researched, prevented, or cured. The research in clinics, labs, and universities is unstoppable, and progress is made every day. A lot can be done to achieve a cure in many cancer cases.

Just as I was told by a very good friend who was forced to look cancer in the eye, it is necessary to remain calm, seek good advice, and "occupy, rather than preoccupy, yourself with it." That got to us, and it was from that springboard, so to speak, that we organized ourselves to methodically and in an organized way tackle the *tsunami* affecting Roberto. The important thing was to assess the situation correctly, so as to hopefully make timely and right decisions.

We admire our son Roberto for the way in which he has faced the challenge of his disease, and we applaud him for his generosity in sharing his experience, along with the experience of many others in this precious book, filled with life experiences, anecdotes, reflections, information, and suggestions that also turn it into a consultation and prevention text.

We believe life is a gift from God, and that it should be looked at positively. The sole fact of "being" is something so wonderful and mysterious that has to be treasured, no matter what the condition of our existence in this earth is. Roberto, thank you for letting us live together through this process. We have been enriched as individuals and as parents, and we have perceived, clearer and clearer as time goes by, your outstanding personal characteristics.

DAD AND MUM.

Table of contents *by key word*

Diet

Acid food 72, 174, 180, 185, 190, 469
Alkaline food 72, 174, 180, 185, 190, 469
Antioxidant 175, 176, 177, 178, 185, 221, 439
Delphinol 177, 185, 458
Glutathione 175, 176, 177, 178, 221
Gluten 171, 185
Holistic therapist 203, 408, 458
Inflammatory food 173, 174, 178, 186, 191, 459
Ionized water 185, 469
Milk 72, 73, 91, 171, 172, 179, 180, 184, 185, 187, 190, 191, 342, 407, 459, 460
Omega 3 174, 175, 188, 297, 461
pH 72, 173, 174, 175, 180, 181, 185, 190, 467
Sugar 72, 73,171, 172, 173, 174, 175, 177, 178, 179, 180, 182, 183, 185, 186, 190, 191, 317, 363, 375, 429, 457, 459
Toxicity 171, 183, 184, 188, 190, 200, 213, 214, 217, 460
Water 64, 77, 158, 169, 172, 174, 181, 185, 186, 285, 287, 307, 363, 469
Vitamin 73, 78, 79, 99, 176, 177, 178, 183, 190, 221, 237, 417, 465

Financing

AUGE 218, 223, 321, 334, 447, 449
Financing 321, 446, 447
GES 218, 223, 225
Health/oncologic Insurance 117, 219, 224, 383, 427
Municipal funds 225, 293, 321
Public system 198, 199, 218, 223, 320, 321, 333, 334, 447, 448

Prevention

Check-up 73, 74, 104, 155, 162, 236, 303, 368, 445
Family background 157, 159, 162, 169, 176, 184, 282, 445, 466
Genetic 86, 155, 158, 169, 181, 190, 208, 222, 296, 415, 439, 445, 466
Mammogram 11, 12, 278, 282, 287
Prevention 162, 166, 177, 210, 221, 225, 226, 251, 269, 335, 432, 439, 445, 450, 465, 466, 473

Rest 118, 126, 284, 406, 425
Self-care 226, 227, 257, 299, 324
Self-examination 439
Sport 24, 32, 42, 46, 73, 75, 110, 131, 158, 159, 169, 176, 178, 184, 263, 295, 321, 432, 468
Stress 40, 64, 70, 74, 77, 79, 80, 119, 134, 136, 142, 143, 160, 171, 174, 176, 178, 179, 184, 187, 189, 190, 191, 201, 218, 222, 263, 270, 299, 307, 312, 321, 432, 451, 460
Sun / solar rays 15, 33, 73, 111, 155, 156, 157, 158, 159, 166, 167, 169, 190, 251, 466
Sunscreen / solar protector 15, 73, 78, 157, 158, 166, 167, 251, 445, 465, 466

Melanoma

Autoimmune vaccine 82, 83, 85, 86, 88, 89, 90, 91, 99, 164, 165, 197, 237, 297
Clinical trial 62, 64, 79, 82, 117, 164, 198, 221
Dermatologist 7, 52, 73, 74, 75, 78, 82, 97, 155, 156, 159, 162, 236, 237, 251, 438, 439, 444, 465
Immunotherapy 78, 163, 164, 217
Interferon 66, 70, 71, 75, 76, 77, 78, 79, 80, 82, 164, 179, 217
Ipilimumab 64, 79, 164, 198
Nodes / Sentinel node 11, 38, 40, 41, 42, 43, 44, 45, 46, 52, 54, 56, 65, 67, 78, 79, 80, 97, 106, 122, 123, 124, 128, 130, 155, 161, 162, 163, 209, 210, 272, 292, 320, 345, 368
Oncobiomed 86, 87, 99, 164, 237
Pathologist 34, 65, 67
Tacos 65

Treatments, procedures

Biopsy 19, 34, 36, 39, 65, 74, 97, 103, 157, 162, 163, 196, 209, 210, 215, 240, 256, 300, 310, 341, 368, 415
Catheter 90, 108, 267, 343, 356
Chemotherapy 54, 98, 103, 104, 108, 120, 125, 136, 138, 155, 163, 176, 182, 190, 203, 210, 212, 213, 214, 216, 224, 270, 273, 274, 280, 283, 284, 287, 288, 291, 309, 317, 321, 323, 324, 327, 329, 337, 342, 351, 357, 363, 367, 382, 384, 395, 409, 411, 426, 439, 448, 449
Magnetic resonance 209, 210, 291
Mastectomy 276, 277, 300, 301
Palliative care 163, 203, 211, 212, 219, 220, 223, 393, 446, 449, 454
PET 66, 67, 75, 76, 78, 80, 82, 134, 136, 175, 209, 210, 435
Prosthetics 110, 293, 394, 409
Radiotherapy 54, 108, 155, 163, 203, 212, 214, 215, 216, 219, 278, 283, 284, 287, 288, 302, 305, 326, 330, 337, 417, 435
Surgery 11, 46, 65, 78, 124, 127, 212, 214, 215, 222, 250, 338, 415, 424, 435
Transplant 106, 117, 215, 216, 217, 266, 267, 359, 424

Cancer

Benign, malign tumor 65, 78, 81, 87, 90, 103, 104, 107, 108, 139, 155, 156, 157, 159, 160, 161, 162, 163, 164, 168, 169, 175, 178, 191, 195, 207, 208, 209, 210, 212, 214, 215, 217, 220, 221, 223, 287, 333, 409, 429, 435, 437

Breast cancer 11, 12, 125, 129, 209, 210, 217, 219, 223, 226, 272, 276, 278, 282, 283, 286, 290, 292, 296, 298, 300, 301, 302, 304, 318, 435, 448, 452

Colon cancer 58, 161, 197, 209, 210, 223, 286, 400, 404

Diagnostic 24, 37, 38, 43, 70, 86, 95, 106, 113, 160, 161, 163, 166, 184, 196, 198, 199, 202, 203, 204, 210, 211, 214, 215, 218, 219, 220, 224, 249, 257, 279, 303, 309, 335, 349, 365, 405, 435, 439, 445, 451

Gastric cancer 223, 414

Incidence 158, 165, 209, 220, 221, 223

Immune system 66, 79, 80, 81, 87, 110, 119, 160, 161, 162, 163, 164, 166, 171, 174, 175, 178, 181, 185, 187, 207, 208, 209, 214, 216, 217, 221, 258, 324, 342, 385, 437, 445, 451, 460, 466

Leukemia 59, 105, 106, 109, 113, 209, 210, 216, 217, 223, 291, 327, 335, 343, 344, 345, 348, 350, 353, 354, 356, 358, 359, 360

Lymphoma 125, 182, 197, 209, 216, 217, 223, 306, 310, 314, 316, 320, 322, 326, 328, 330

Lung cancer 125, 134, 157, 207, 209, 210, 222, 223, 246, 320, 406, 407, 451

Malign cells 38, 155, 164, 207, 212

Metastasis 11,35, 36, 38, 40, 43, 44, 45, 46, 48, 52, 54, 55, 65, 66, 75, 76, 78, 79, 87, 97, 107, 110, 122, 128, 155, 156, 157, 160, 161, 162, 163, 165, 166, 168, 207, 208, 209, 210, 212, 215, 236, 272, 278, 292, 320, 364, 366, 368, 424, 439, 445, 464

Mourning 50, 202, 387, 449, 455, 456, 457

Neuroblastoma 340, 341

Osteosarcoma 382

Ovarian cancer 108, 172, 210, 223, 278, 362, 364, 366, 393

Pancreatic cancer 210, 281, 382, 386, 406

Pediatric cancer 209, 332, 333, 334, 335, 336, 340, 344, 350, 354, 356, 358, 424

Prostate cancer 90, 164, 172, 203, 209, 210, 217, 223, 414, 415, 416

Recovery 43, 46, 52, 57, 64, 134, 182, 184, 193, 213, 220, 222, 224, 240, 268, 286, 301, 307, 311, 436, 444, 451, 458

Relapse 107, 109, 117, 122, 134, 140, 284, 302, 306, 310, 364, 365

Sarcoma 103, 161, 194, 209, 394, 410, 424
Skin cancer 19, 35, 36, 37, 92, 151, 155, 156, 158, 159, 166, 167, 209, 246, 250, 251, 256, 266, 438, 439
Survival rate 40, 65, 80, 139, 161, 163, 164, 165, 194, 211, 212, 217, 218, 265, 334, 337, 401, 415, 445, 449
Symptoms 66, 99, 114, 135, 172, 183, 189, 208, 211, 212, 213, 215, 218, 220, 221, 306, 321, 336, 405
Terminal cancer 163, 199, 211, 362, 392, 393, 451
Testicular cancer 110, 210, 408, 409
Therapist 150, 203, 204, 215, 219, 369, 414, 428, 430, 458
Therapy (hormonal, antioxidant, physical, sports, etc.) 79, 90, 164, 175, 176, 177, 179, 190, 197, 204, 210, 211, 212, 217, 219, 220, 221, 225, 263, 265, 280, 297, 319, 323, 342, 353, 357, 361, 369, 384, 385, 401, 415, 417, 427, 431, 433, 447, 448, 449
Thyroid cancer 107, 210, 217, 368, 369, 370, 424
Uterine and cervical cancer 210, 223, 392

Patient

Couple/marriage 13, 41, 53, 58, 114, 118, 126, 140, 144, 239, 289, 338, 339, 402, 403, 409, 425, 427, 471
Drugs 64, 177, 183, 189, 191, 203, 212, 217, 224, 225, 319, 334, 455
Faith 92, 288, 321, 349, 353
Family/family members 40, 43, 44, 46, 53, 55, 58, 59, 60, 61, 91, 96, 97, 98, 106, 110, 112, 118, 126, 129, 138, 139, 179, 193, 195, 201, 211, 218, 222, 227, 239, 242, 243, 263, 288, 301, 305, 315, 325, 327, 331, 341, 351, 359, 361, 365, 384, 388, 389, 405, 409, 411, 447, 452, 455, 456, 464, 465
Friends 48, 50, 52, 54, 60, 84, 110, 113, 119, 201, 202, 227, 242, 253, 275, 269, 301, 311, 319, 325, 338, 359, 409, 411, 465
Internet 54, 103, 131, 199, 281, 321, 426, 463
Psychological support 219, 222, 226, 279, 295, 297, 305, 319, 342, 343, 357, 369, 371, 448
Second opinion 97, 198, 205, 218, 219, 401
Support network 54, 113, 242, 311, 334

Secondary Effects

Burns 158, 167, 178, 283, 288, 466
Fertility 214, 217
Hair loss/wig 90, 104, 118, 120, 131, 201, 213, 273, 289, 291, 303, 329, 343, 359, 365, 383, 384, 419, 439
Nausea 104, 211, 212, 213, 285, 287
Scars/healing effect 47, 59, 67, 71, 98, 122, 131, 139, 143, 156, 162, 163, 201, 202, 277, 285, 288, 301, 315, 439
Secondary Effects 64, 75, 77, 79, 78, 90, 164, 165, 179, 183, 197, 198, 203, 204, 212, 213, 214, 217, 219, 220
Ulcer/wounds 111, 258, 277, 363, 467

Alternative medicine, other therapies

Allopathic medicine 64, 183, 184
Aloe vera 279, 281, 288, 317, 363, 407, 429
Alternative medicine 183, 203, 249, 458
Aromatherapy 342
Bach Flowers 280, 353
Heart lysate 270, 366, 367
Homeopathy 183, 357, 414
Holistic therapy 415
Magnets 203, 280, 417
Massages 98, 265, 353
Meditation/relaxation 226, 247, 280, 303, 306, 307, 309, 317, 319, 324, 385, 451, 452
Music Therapy 265, 342, 353
Natural drugs 229, 287, 467
Reflexology 324
Reiki 203, 280, 312, 319, 324, 357, 417
Scorpion poison 321, 363, 417
Yoga 222, 247, 280, 295, 317, 385